AF412689

ALCOHOLIC LIVER DISEASE

Pathology and Pathogenesis

For my children
Elisa and Ross

ALCOHOLIC LIVER DISEASE

SECOND EDITION

Pathology and Pathogenesis

EDITED BY

Pauline Hall

MB, BS, FRCPA

Senior Consultant in Pathology
Department of Histopathology, Flinders Medical Centre
Adelaide, South Australia
Associate Professor of Pathology
The Flinders University of South Australia

FOREWORD BY

Peter J. Scheuer

MD, DSc (Med), FRCPath

Edward Arnold
A member of the Hodder Headline Group
LONDON BOSTON MELBOURNE AUCKLAND

First published in Great Britain 1995 by
Edward Arnold, a division of Hodder Headline PLC,
338 Euston Road, London NW1 3BH

Distributed in the Americas by
Little, Brown and Company
34 Beacon Street, Boston, MA 02108

Whilst the advice and information in this book is believed to be true and
accurate at the date of going to press, neither the author nor the publisher
can accept any legal responsibility or liability for any errors or omissions
that may be made. In particular (but without limiting the generality of the
preceding disclaimer) every effort has been made to check drug dosages;
however it is still possible that errors have been missed. Furthermore,
dosage schedules are constantly being revised and new side effects
recognized. For these reasons the reader is strongly urged to consult the
drug companies' printed instructions before administering any of the drugs
recommended in this book.

British Library Cataloguing in Publication Data
A catalogue record for this book is available from the British Library

ISBN 0 340 57194 2

1   2   3   4   5   95   96   97   98   99

Typeset in 10 on 11pt Plantin by
Paston Press Ltd, Loddon, Norfolk
Printed and bound in Great Britain by
The Bath Press, Lower Bristol Road, Bath BA2 3BL

Foreword

A decade has passed since the publication of the first edition of this book. In spite of intensive research into many aspects of alcohol-related liver disease during this time, there remains an almost endless list of important and challenging questions which need to be answered if the deleterious effects of alcohol are to be reduced or eliminated altogether. The problems span many disciplines, including pathology, epidemiology, biochemistry, immunology, virology and clinical medicine; all are represented in the second edition, in sections written by an international panel of distinguished workers in the field.

Three problems seem to me, as a histopathologist, to be of particular interest. The most intriguing of these three is the apparent latent period, supported by examination of serial liver biopsies, between the onset of heavy drinking and the development of steatohepatitis. In some subjects this latent period may be as long as ten years or more. What happens during this period, and why is the onset of the lesion delayed? In the answer may lie the key to susceptibility and pathogenesis. Better knowledge of both would go a long way towards providing an effective strategy for prevention.

New knowledge of the role of Ito cells (lipocytes or fat-storing cells) has somewhat shifted the emphasis of thinking on the pathogenesis of alcohol-related liver disease from the hepatocyte to the cell population of the sinusoid and perisinusoidal space. Is the fibrosis for which the Ito cells appear to be largely responsible the key event in the pathogenesis of steatohepatitis and, by extension, cirrhosis? Is it possible for instance, that new collagen and other matrix components isolate hepatocytes so effectively from their neighbours that cell damage is initiated or accelerated? It would be interesting in this respect to supplement the many helpful recent and current biochemical studies of cytokines and collagen synthesis with purely morphological research on the three-dimensional structure of the newly-formed fibrous network.

Third, why is alcohol-related steatohepatitis, or alcoholic hepatitis, so very similar morphologically to non-alcoholic steatohepatitis? The two are often indistinguishable under the microscope, suggesting a common pathogenetic pathway the nature of which remains a mystery.

Clearly there remains much to be done. Pauline Hall and her panel of authors have fully addressed the many relevant questions in the second edition, which she has wisely made into a new book rather than a simple update of the first edition. Like the late and much missed Hans Popper, who wrote the foreword to the first edition, Pauline Hall's interest and understanding go well beyond her main discipline of pathology. This has ensured the scope and value of the second edition, and its potential appeal to a wide readership.

Hans Popper commented that many contributors to the first edition, including himself, believed that moderate drinking could add to the enjoyment of their lives. I share this view, and express the hope that with continuing and strenuous efforts, perhaps supported by the alcohol industry itself, the serious and worldwide problems of alcohol-related liver disease may be significantly reduced.

Peter J. Scheuer
London, 1994

Preface

Work on the first edition of *Alcoholic Liver Disease* was completed ten years ago and the book was published in 1985. The long delay between the two editions is difficult to explain in view of the considerable advances in knowledge and the changing attitudes to alcoholic liver disease. The focus of the second edition has been changed primarily to reflect the growth in knowledge of pathogenic mechanisms involved in alcohol-associated liver injury. Nevertheless, it was with considerable reluctance that I decided not to include and expand the epidemiology and clinical sections of the first edition. I hope my colleagues who contributed to the many excellent chapters to these sections in the first edition will forgive me for not including them in the second. The epidemiological chapters provided a wealth of factual information about drinking patterns around the world; however, when I was planning the first edition Hans Popper warned me that my focus on epidemiology was unlikely to generate any new information about risk factors or pathogenic mechanisms for alcoholic liver disease. My decision not to include a clinical section in the second edition was based on my knowledge that a number of clinical books on liver disease were currently in preparation. In order to maintain the emphasis on pathogenic mechanisms, I decided that it would be interesting to have a chapter on therapeutic agents written from the viewpoint of the insights that the use of drugs such as propylthiouracil have provided into mechanisms of liver injury. Nevertheless, Professor Willis Maddrey, after reading all the other contributions, kindly decided to remedy what on balance seemed to be a deficiency in the book, by including a section on clinical aspects and management of alcoholic liver disease, in particular the role of liver transplantation, in his introductory chapter as well as providing an excellent overview highlighting many of the important aspects of the following chapters.

One of the major advances in knowledge of alcoholic liver disease that has occurred in the ten years relates to the role of the Ito cell (lipocyte) in hepatic fibrosis. Consequently, the majority of contributors included a detailed discussion of Ito cells in their chapters. Although I have attempted to allow each chapter to exist as an entity, I have also been firm in my editorial approach and have removed considerable amounts of text. I would therefore like to apologize to any contributor who feels disappointed by my exclusion of some of their material, but this was always done to reduce duplication of information.

On the other hand, I have exercised editorial restraint about matter such as literary style and usage of terms such as Ito cell or lipocyte, acetaminophen or paracetamol, to reflect the country of origin of the contributor. Since all of the contributors are widely published and have highly characteristic styles of presenting their work, I decided not to impose a uniform, bland editorial style. I hope the reader will enjoy contributions such as Professor Maddrey's graphic description of the hostile microenvironment induced in the liver by alcohol and the resultant chaos inside the hepacoyte.

All the chapters have been written by leading authorities on the various aspects of pathology and pathogenesis of alcoholic liver disease and many of the contributors have generously included unpublished results of recent studies as well as references to papers in press in 1994. Many of the contributors have also outlined new areas for future study. Another edition of this book may well appear in only a few years, reflecting the use of molecular biology techniques in advancing our knowledge of pathogenic mechanisms for hepatocyte injury and hepatic fibrosis, and of factors stimulating hepatocyte regeneration. A third edition of this book would certainly include a section on liver transplantation and the recurrence of alcoholic liver disease in the transplanted liver. The apparent acceleration of progression of alcohol-related liver injury in the transplanted liver should lead to studies that may provide valuable insights into pathogenic mechanisms of liver injury.

This book is directed at all researchers who are studying alcohol-associated liver injury; hepatologists, gastroenterologists, and general physicians caring for patients with alcoholic liver disease, and pathologists with an interest in liver disease. In addition, I hope the book will become a definitive reference for both undergraduate and postgraduate students who are studying alcoholic liver disease; I hope the book will be made available in medical libraries throughout the world.

I am greatly honoured to have the foreword for the book written by Professer Peter Scheuer. Professor Scheuer provided me with invaluable support and guidance through all the stages of production of this second edition. I hope the finished product and the critical response to the book will justify his support.

P. de la M. Hall
Adelaide, 1994

Acknowledgments

The production of this book would not have been possible without the personal support and encouragement of Professor Douglas Henderson, the head of the Histopathology Department, Flinders Medical Centre. In particular, I am most appreciative of the use of office and photographic facilities.

Professor Willis Maddrey was one of the reviewers who gave the publisher Edward Arnold advice about my outline for the second edition. Not only have I incorporated all of his valuable suggestions into the content of the book, but I have been able to include an outstanding introductory chapter by Professor Maddrey for which I am most grateful. I would also like to thank the other anonymous reviewers who also advised the publishers. A number of excellent suggestions about content have been included in the book.

Colleagues who kindly assisted me were Associate Professors Tony Seymour and Malcolm Mackinnon, who gave critical but highly constructive advice about my chapters, and Dr John Plummer, who provided invaluable proof-reading assistance with a number of chapters. Mrs Cathy Fox, assisted by Mrs Joanna Fenton and Ms Marlene Newland, provided me with excellent secretarial assistance. The high quality of the final text is due to the meticulous work by Mrs Fox who played a major role in the editing process.

Particular thanks are due to Mr Peter Eime who spent many hours in the dark room to produce the high-quality black-and-white photographs for my chapters. Of equal quality are the electron micrographs kindly provided by Mr Peter Leppard.

I am indebted to pathologists and clinicians, particularly those working in Flinders Medical Centre, but also those in other teaching hospitals and in private practice both in Adelaide and many parts of Australia, who over the years have contributed liver biopsy material for my opinion.

I would also like to thank my children Elisa and Ross, and my friends Dr Christine Lunam, Mrs Beverley Dimond, Mrs Nathalie Leader and Dr Rodney Hall for their support and encouragement, and for tolerating my neglect during the past year.

Finally I am indebted to all the contributors without whom the book would not have eventuated, and the many people at Edward Arnold who have helped with the various stages of planning, editing and promotion of the book.

P. de la M. Hall
Adelaide, 1994

Contributors

Amela M. Arria, School of Hygiene and Public Health, Johns Hopkins University, Maryland, USA

Michael K. Bay, Department of Medicine, Division of Gastroenterology and Nutrition, University of Texas Health Science Center at San Antonio, 7703 Floyd Curl Drive, San Antonio, Texas 78284–7878, USA

George L.A. Bird, Senior Registrar and Honorary Clinical Lecturer, Department of Medicine, Gartnavel General Hospital, Glasgow G21 0YN, Scotland

Laurence M. Blendis, Department of Medicine, Toronto General Hospital, 9th Floor, Room 9–220 Eaton Wing, Toronto, Ontario M5G 2C4, Canada

F.J. Lou Carmichael, Anaesthetology Department, Toronto Western Hospital, 399 Bathurst Street, Toronto, Ontario M5G 2C4, Canada

Valeer J. Desmet, Pathologische Ontleedkunde II, U.Z. Sint-Rafael, Katholieke Universiteit Leuven, Minderbroedestraat 12, B-3000 Leuven, Belgium

Rita De Vos, Pathologische Ontleedkunde II, U.Z. Sint-Rafael, Katholieke Universiteit Leuven, Minderbroederstraat 12, B-3000 Leuven, Belgium

Bruce R. Dobbs, Scientific Officer, Department of Surgery, Canterbury Area Health Board, Christchurch, New Zealand

Lawrence Feinman, Associate Professor of Medicine, Chief GI Section, 111D, Veterans Affairs Medical Center, 130 West Kingsbridge Road, Bronx NY 10468, USA

Linda M. Fletcher, Liver Unit, Queensland Institute of Medical Research and University of Queensland, Bancroft Centre, Brisbane, Queensland 4029, Australia

Robin Fraser, Associate Professor, Department of Pathology, Christchurch School of Medicine, PO Box 4345, Christchurch, New Zealand

Samuel W. French, Professor of Pathology, Department of Pathology, UCLA School of Medicine, Harbor-UCLA Medical Center, 100 West Carson Street, Torrance, CA 90509, USA

Scott L. Friedman, Associate Professor of Medicine, Liver Center Laboratory, San Francisco General Hospital, Building 40, Room 4102, 1001 Potrero Avenue, San Francisco, CA 94110, USA

Judith S. Gavaler, Chief, Women's Health Research Program, Oklahoma Medical Research Foundation, and Chief, Women's Research, Oklahoma Transplantation Institute, Baptist Medical Center of Oklahoma, 3300 NW Expressway, Oklahoma City, Oklahoma 73112, USA

Pauline de la M. Hall, Senior Consultant in Pathology, Department of Histopathology, Flinders Medical Centre, Bedford Park, South Australia 5042; Associate Professor of Pathology, Flinders University of South Australia, Adelaide, South Australia; Honorary Consultant, Queen Elizabeth Hospital, Woodville, South Australia, Australia

June W. Halliday, Liver Unit, Queensland Institute of Medical Research and University of Queensland, Bancroft Centre, Brisbane, Queensland, 4029, Australia

Richard Hift, Senior Lecturer and Senior Specialist, Liver Research Centre of the Medical Research Council (MRC) and University of Cape Town, Cape Town, South Africa

Kamal G. Ishak, Chairman, Department of Hepatic Pathology, Armed Forces Institute of Pathology, Washington, DC; Clinical Professor of Pathology, Uniformed Services University for the Health Sciences and Medical Care Consultant, National Institutes of Health, Bethesda, Maryland; Consultant, Department of Pathology, College of Physicians and Surgeons, Columbia University; Professorial Lecturer, Mount Sinai School of Medicine, New York, USA

Ralph E. Kirsch, Professor of Medicine, Co-Director Medical Research Council/Liver Research Group, Department of Medicine, Medical School, Observatory 7925, Cape Town, South Africa

Charles S. Lieber, Professor of Medicine and Pathology, Mount Sinai School of Medicine; Director, Section of Liver Disease and Nutrition, Alcohol Research and Treatment Center and GI-Liver Program, Veterans Administration Medical Center, 130 West Kingsbridge Road, Bronx, NY 10468, USA

Roderick N. M. MacSween, Professor and Honorary Consultant Pathologist, University Department of Pathology, Western Infirmary, Glasgow G11 6NT, Scotland

Robert S. McCuskey, Head and Professor, Departments of Anatomy and Physiology, College of Medicine, University of Arizona, Tucson, Arizona AZ 85724, USA

Willis C. Maddrey, Professor of Internal Medicine, Executive Vice-President for Clinical Affairs, University of Texas, Southwestern Medical Center, Dallas, Texas, USA

Jacquelyn J. Maher, Assistant Professor of Medicine, Liver Center Laboratory, San Francisco General Hospital, Building 40, Room 4102, 1001 Potrero Avenue, San Francisco, CA 94110, USA

Michio Morimoto, Department of Pathology, UCLA School of Medicine, Harbor-UCLA Medical Center, 100 West Carson Street, Torrance, CA 90509, USA

Kunihiko Ohnishi, Associate Professor of Medicine, The First Department of Medicine, School of Medicine, Chiba University, 1–8–1 Inohana, Chiba City (280), Japan

Kunio Okuda, Emeritus Professor of Medicine, Director, The First Department of Medicine, School of Medicine, Chiba University, 1–8–1 Inohana, Chiba City (280), Japan

Hector Orrego, Addiction Research Foundation, 33 Russell Street, Toronto, Ontario M5S 2S1, Canada

Lawrie W. Powell, Director, Queensland Institute of Medical Research, Bancroft Centre, 300 Herston Road, Brisbane, Queensland 4029, Australia

George W.T. Rogers, Research Fellow, Department of Histopathology, Canterbury Area Health Board, Christchurch, New Zealand

Steven Schenker, Department of Medicine Division of Gastroenterology and Nutrition, University of Texas Health Sciences Center at San Antonio, 7703 Floyd Curl Drive, San Antonio, TX 78284, USA

Peter J. Scheuer, Emeritus Professor of Histopathology, Royal Free Hospital School of Medicine, University of London, UK

Michael F. Sorrell, Director, Alcohol Research Center, Department of Veterans Affairs Medical Center, 4101 Woolworth Avenue, Omaha, NE 68105, USA

Hidekazu Tsukamoto, Department of Medicine, Case Western Research University, MetroHealth Medical Center, Cleveland, OH, USA

Dean J. Tuma, Scientific Director, Alcohol Research Center, Department of Veterans Affairs Medical Center, 4101 Woolworth Avenue, Omaha, NE 68105, USA

Peter Van Eyken, Pathologische Ontleedkunde II, U.Z. Sint-Rafael, Katholieke Universiteit Leuven, Minderbroederstraat 12, B-3000 Leuven, Belgium

Hyman J. Zimmerman, Professor of Medicine, Emeritus, George Washington University; Distinguished Scientist, Emeritus, Armed Forces Institute of Pathology, 2825 16th Street NW, Building 54, Washington, DC 20306–6000, USA

Contents

Part I
Introduction

1 Alcohol and the liver: An overview

Willis C. Maddrey

Introduction

The cascade of events initiated by the excessive ingestion of alcohol and culminating in acute and chronic liver diseases has fascinated generations of clinicians and clinical investigators. Alcohol use and its effects – both favourable and unfavourable – has affected human health greatly, and the pivotal role of alcohol in causing liver disease has been increasingly defined. Excessive use of alcohol remains the most important cause of cirrhosis in the Western world and a leading cause of death and mortality during mid-life.

As is amply demonstrated in this volume, there continues to be great interest in learning how alcohol and its metabolic products injure the hepatocyte and how such increased understanding of the mechanisms of injury might be used to fashion approaches that prevent or at least minimize injury (Maddrey 1988, 1990). Excessive use of alcohol clearly causes liver injury in a somewhat dose-related manner. However, the variability in expression and extent of injury is remarkable (Grant *et al.* 1988). There are individuals who seem to be especially susceptible to the injurious effects of alcohol and an even greater number who have tolerances that border on legendary. Clearly, it is not only how much alcohol is ingested but by whom.

Mechanisms of alcohol-induced liver injury

Cellular injury from alcohol develops predominantly as a consequence of the direct cellular toxicity of acetaldehyde, the major metabolite of alcohol (Lieber 1993; see Chapter 2). Recognition that acetaldehyde is the most important agent causing alcohol-induced injury led to studies of mechanisms of damage and fostered searches for ways to limit acetaldehyde production, speed its elimination, or minimize its effects.

Throughout this volume, there are extensive discussions of many cell-damaging consequences of acetaldehyde (see Chapter 5). Undoubtedly there are important contributions from the oft-associated nutritional deficiencies, which determine the type, rate of progression and extent of injury (Mezey 1991). For a detailed discussion, see Chapter 8.

Factors influencing susceptibility to alcohol-induced injury

Major efforts have been undertaken to determine the amount of alcohol that must be ingested to cause liver injury (Pequignot and Cyrulinik 1970; Lelbach 1975). These studies are all beset by daunting problems in obtaining an accurate history of how much alcohol has been ingested and for how long (Orrego *et al.* 1979b). There is no question that individual responses to alcohol vary across a remarkable range. The idea of an alcohol dose–response curve in relation to causing liver injury only gets us so far. There is compelling evidence that the tendency to alcoholism is inherited (Bosron *et al.* 1993). Of particular importance to hepatologists is the additional question of whether the likelihood of developing liver injury from alcohol is influenced by heredity. The observation that only 1 in 12 alcoholics develops evidence of severe liver injury, while interesting, can be turned round to stimulate consideration as to why the majority of heavy users *do not* develop tissue damage. Inherited differences in preference (even need) for alcohol, differences in the rate or response of metabolism by isoenzymes, and altered responses to acetaldehyde, all offer areas for study which are fully discussed in this text.

Clinicians from around the world are generally convinced that females are at greater risk of developing alcohol-induced liver disease than males, even when such factors as body weight and amount of alcohol ingested are considered (Schenker and Speeg 1990). However, why females are at increased risk is not known. The suggestion that females have relatively less gastric mucosal alcohol dehydrogenase than males, thereby allowing more of a given amount of alcohol to reach the liver, is interesting (Frezza *et al.* 1990; Lieber 1993; see Chapter 2). Whether this is of clinical importance remains to be established. Sex differences in the rates of metabolism of alcohol and the characteristics of the various enzymes involved in metabolism of alcohol have been vigorously pursued but definitive answers are not yet available (see Chapters 7 and 18 for detailed discussions of risk factors).

Factors promoting the appearance and progression of liver injury

There have been numerous efforts to identify coexistent factors which may affect the rapidity of onset or progression of alcohol-induced injury. Attention has been directed towards the effects of malnutrition on metabolism and on the immune system, as well as studies of factors that promote an increased susceptibility to infection. The well-established impairment of the ability of the liver to regenerate in the chronic alcoholic is of undoubted importance (Diehl *et al.* 1988; see also Chapter 8).

Surely, there is more than just long-term ingestion of large doses of alcohol that leads to liver injury. Changes in nutrition or the superimposition of some other disease process may tip the scales. There has been much interest in, and investigation of, the role of coexistent viral infections in initiating or worsening of underlying alcohol-induced liver injury. Patients who are chronic alcoholics and who also have chronic viral hepatitis seem more likely to progress to cirrhosis than individuals who have only one of these conditions. Some studies have reported that patients with alcoholic cirrhosis are much more likely to have concomitant chronic hepatitis C than is found in a control population of alcoholics who do not have hepatitis C (Pares *et al.* 1990). The additive nature of the liver injuries appears to promote progression to cirrhosis. Furthermore, there is evidence that chronic alcoholics who also have evidence of hepatitis B infection are more likely to develop progressive liver disease leading to cirrhosis and portal hypertension than their alcoholic counterparts who do not have chronic hepatitis B (Mills *et al.* 1979). Possibly the concurrent hepatitis B infection serves as an additive insult to the liver. The intriguing possibilities of alcohol–viral interactions warrant further exploration (see Chapter 9 for a detailed discussion).

Various cytokines may have roles in promoting liver disease in the chronic alcoholic patient (McClain *et al.* 1993). Exposure to endotoxin derived from Gram-negative bacteria is a known cause of liver damage (Nolan 1989). Endotoxin may affect hepatocytes directly or indirectly through release of additional mediators of injury, such as superoxide and tumour necrosis factor (TNF) from Kupffer cells. The identification and definition of the role of the many cytokines has been an active, productive and confusing field. Various cytokines, probably of great importance in alcohol-induced liver disease, include TNF, interleukin-1 (IL-1), interleukin-6 (IL-6), the transforming growth factors (TGFα and TGFβ), and platelet-derived growth factor (PDGF) (McClain *et al.* 1993). Cytokines may reinforce cellular injury, and several promote the transformation of lipocytes to fibroblasts leading to collagen production. Interleukin-8 appears to have an important role as a chemoattractant of polymorphonuclear cells (Sheron *et al.* 1993). Issues that need further investigation include to what degree an alcohol-induced liver injury is augmented by the effects of one or more cytokines. As more is learned, therapies directed towards ways of blocking the production of specific cytokines or inhibiting their effects at a cellular level may become relevant. The correlation of serum levels of specific cytokines (e.g. IL-6 and TNF) may prove to be useful predictors of prognosis in patients with alcohol-induced liver disease (Hill *et al.* 1992; Bird *et al.* 1990; see also Chapters 4 and 6).

The adverse hepatotoxic effects of selected therapeutic drugs may cause an acute liver injury in a chronic alcoholic (Seeff *et al.* 1986). The best studied of these potentially toxic drugs is acetaminophen (paracetamol). Chronic users of alcohol have induction of cytochrome P4502El (CYP2E1), which is also the P450 subtype involved in the metabolism of acetaminophen (Tsutsumi *et al.* 1989). Alcohol-related induction of CYP2E1 subtype may lead to an increased rate of conversion of acetaminophen to a toxic intermediate (NADQI). In these patients, toxic metabolites may accumulate in dangerous quantities even when the dose of acetaminophen ingested has been relatively modest and not taken with suicidal intent. In normal individuals, acetaminophen intermediates are bound by glutathione and excreted in urine as mercapturic acid. Glutathione, the major hepatoprotectant guarding against the effects of toxic intermediates of acetaminophen, is decreased in chronic alcoholics and impaired defences may contribute to the likelihood of injury (Jelell *et al.* 1986; for a detailed discussion, see Chapter 16).

Clinical manifestations

There is a broad spectrum of clinical manifestations of alcoholic liver disease ranging from few or minimal symptoms to life-threatening fulminant liver injury. There is often little correlation – occasionally even considerable dissociation – between the apparent severity of injury based on clinical findings and those found on liver biopsy (MacSween and Burt 1986).

The progression of alcohol-induced injury is not orderly. Alcoholic hepatitis is often found superimposed on already established cirrhosis, and the clinical manifestations result both from acute alcoholic hepatitis and from problems arising as complications of cirrhosis. Alcoholic hepatitis is considered at least partially reversible. Alcohol steatosis is considered largely reversible. Even at the stage of alcoholic hepatitis when there is early fibrosis, the possibility exists that some (if not most) of the injury may be reversible. Many patients have coexistence of fatty liver, alcoholic hepatitis and cirrhosis.

Percutaneous liver biopsy is useful in the evaluation of chronic alcoholic patients for determining the stage of the illness and providing at least a rough guide to prognosis. In addition, a liver biopsy may provide evidence of associated disorders which may be important.

Diagnosis of alcoholic liver disease

The diagnosis of alcoholic hepatitis – indeed of any alcohol-induced liver disease – requires consideration in any patient in whom there is a history of regular alcohol use. Confirmation of the diagnosis and assessment of the extent of injury is best established by performing a liver biopsy. The liver biopsy provides at least a rough guide to prognosis (see Chapter 3). There are no biochemical tests that have proven sufficiently helpful to enable the presence (or extent) of alcohol-induced injury to be established with confidence. A non-invasive test that would obviate the need for liver biopsy would be most useful. Unfortunately, no such test is yet available.

Even with a liver biopsy, we can only guess at the extent of reversible injury. However, there are several histologic clues worthy of mention and these are fully discussed throughout this volume (MacSween and Burt 1986). Undoubtedly, the extent and activity of active and established fibrosis is important. Alcohol and its metabolites transform hepatocytes from well-organized, functioning units to somewhat isolated cells with disrupted communications both internally and to the extracellular environment. Nutrients have trouble getting to and through the cell surface as the result of many factors, including the loss of fenestrae in the endothelial cells lining the sinusoids (defenestration), as well as the barrier presented by accumulation of collagen and other proteins in the space of Disse. At the surface of the hepatocyte the plasma membrane is disorganized, and within the cell, multiple hostile microenvironments are found. Variable oxygen availability, pH changes, toxic metabolic products, a decreased pool of mitochondrial glutathione, and damaged microfilaments needed to hold the organelles in place all contribute to the chaos. Which of these processes signals irreversible injury continues to be an area of active investigation. The cumulative effects of these injuries plus an impaired hepatocyte regeneration determines to a large extent the clinico-pathologic manifestations and the likelihood of a successful outcome, even if the patient stops using alcohol.

In most Western patients, alcoholic hepatitis is a necessary step in the development of alcohol-induced cirrhosis. However, studies from Japan in particular have indicated that in some patients alcohol may stimulate the production of fibrosis and cirrhosis without requiring alcoholic hepatitis as an intermediate lesion (Uchida *et al.* 1987). Furthermore, in the alcohol-fed baboon model, fibrosis and cirrhosis also developed in the absence of alcoholic hepatitis (Lieber 1993).

Histopathologic abnormalities

Several rather well-defined cellular and subcellular alterations in patients with alcoholic hepatitis have been recognized (MacSween and Burt 1986; French *et al.* 1993). The problem is in the evaluation of the prognostic value of any given subcellular alteration in order to determine if the alteration is itself predictive of a serious problem or is just another non-specific result of damage. Characteristically, alcohol-induced injury leads to cell necrosis. Inflammation may be scant or plentiful. If inflammation is present, polymorphonuclear leucocytes are usually the predominant infiltrating cells, although there may be a mixed cellular infiltrate which includes lymphocytes.

Mallory bodies, intracellular eosinophilic inclusions located predominantly around nuclei, are often found in patients with active alcohol-induced liver disease. Mallory bodies represent masses of intermediate filaments (French *et al.* 1993). The presence of Mallory bodies in a patient with alcoholic hepatitis suggests a more serious disease than is present in an alcoholic patient who does not have these alterations (Harinasuta and Zimmerman 1967). Cells containing Mallory bodies, often ringed with polymorphonuclear leucocytes, are marked for imminent death. Some studies suggest that immunologic reactions directed against the Mallory bodies may be important in the pathogenesis of alcohol-induced liver injury (Paronetto 1993; Zetterman *et al.* 1976; also see Chapters 3 and 6).

Much attention has been directed towards alcohol-induced changes in perisinusoidal cells and the effects these changes have on sinusoidal blood flow and the orderly exchange of constituents between the sinusoids and hepatocytes. Alterations in the space of Disse are important in determining if free exchanges of constituents from blood to hepatocytes are able to occur. The space of Disse may be filled with several types of collagen, non-collagenous proteins and immunoglubolin A (IgA) in patients with alcohol-induced liver injury. A basal lamina underlying the endothelial cells is often found, adding to the barrier to free exchange between blood in the sinusoid and the plasma membrane of the hepatocyte. The basal lamina is extracellular and contains various proteins including type IV collagen and fibronectin. The barriers to free exchange serve to isolate the hepatocytes from the portal blood. A further consequence of the development of barriers to access in the space of Disse includes increased pressure within the sinusoid (for a detailed discussion, see Chapters 14 and 15).

Hepatocytes are considerably and irregularly enlarged in patients with alcohol-induced liver injury. Enlargement results from an increase in intracellular lipids and also secretory proteins whose transport from the hepatocyte has been inhibited (Baraona *et al.* 1977). The irregularly enlarged hepatocytes may impinge on the sinusoidal lumen contributing to increased pressure (Vidins *et al.* 1985).

There are alcohol-related problems with the manufacture of proteins and movement of proteins to sites for discharge into the blood (Tuma and Sorrell 1988; Diehl 1992). Injury to the Golgi apparatus with disruption of the endoplasmic reticulum contributes to impairment of protein secretion.

Particular attention has been directed towards the increased collagen in the space of Disse (Orrego *et al.* 1979c; Friedman 1993; see Chapter 4). Much of the collagen is produced by Ito cells (also known as lipocytes), which are transformed by exposure to alcohol to become fibroblast-like cells (Weiner *et al.* 1990). In this transformation, the Ito cell loses its characteristic fat droplets and the amount of rough endoplasmic reticulum increases. Recognition of the importance of transformation of Ito cells to fibroblasts and the effects of the collagen produced by these cells has added greatly to our understanding of how alcoholic-induced injury leads to cirrhosis (Mak and Lieber 1988; Friedman 1993). Lipocytes have been established as the site of formation of proteoglycans (Arenson *et al.* 1988). The deposition of collagen in the space of Disse is especially prominent in zone 3 (Horn *et al.* 1985). A further finding in patients with alcoholic hepatitis is increased numbers of myofibroblasts in zone 3 of the hepatic acinus (Mak and Lieber 1986). These cells characteristically contain microfilaments and alpha-actin.

The site of excessive production and deposition of collagen has been suggested to be of importance in determining the likelihood of progression to cirrhosis (Van Waes and Lieber 1977). There is more rapid progression in individuals in whom there is evidence of excessive collagen deposition around the terminal hepatic venule (zone 3). Similarly, in a baboon model, those animals who had perivenular deposition of collagen early in the course of alcohol-induced injury were at much greater risk of progressing to cirrhosis (Lieber 1993).

Defenestration leads to loss of access of plasma within the sinusoid to the space of Disse (Horn *et al.* 1987). Electron microscopic studies in patients with alcoholic hepatitis have suggested that endothelial defenestration is a prominent feature especially likely to be found in zone 3 (for a detailed discussion, see Chapter 15).

Elevated serum IgA levels are characteristically found in patients with alcoholic hepatitis and cirrhosis (Van de Wiel *et al.* 1988). The deposition of IgA along the plasma membrane may serve to increase the barrier affecting transfer from blood to hepatocytes. One suggestion is that IgA triggers the release of TNF by monocytes in patients, with the cytokine then augmenting the damage (Deviere *et al.* 1991; see also Chapter 6).

There is clearly a zonal selectivity in alcohol-induced liver injury. Many of the histologic abnormalities found in patients with alcohol-induced liver injury are more fully expressed in the perivenular (zone 3) region of the hepatic acinus (Horn *et al.* 1986; see also Chapters 3 and 17). The perivenular region is furthest from the entry site for oxygen into the hepatic acinus and therefore has relatively less oxygen available. The relative hypoxia of zone 3 may be exacerbated by the oft-associated anaemia and by the increased demands of an alcohol-induced hypermetabolic state. Other characteristics of zone 3 which are undoubtedly important in determining the site of injury, include the heightened concentrations of cytochrome P450 enzymes and alcohol dehydrogenase relative to other parts of the acinus (Lieber 1993; see also Chapter 19).

Management of alcoholic hepatitis

One goal of understanding how alcohol damages the liver is to fashion a way to prevent or minimize injury. For some patients with alcoholic liver disease, there is little hope that any treatment will make a difference. There is a point beyond which it is just too late to achieve benefit from abstinence. However, even an extensively remodelled cirrhotic liver may hold on for a long time if the assaults cease. More specific ways of regulating fibrogenesis and of possibly blunting the role of short-lived immunologic responses to acetaldehyde adducts are needed.

Whether supplemental vitamins affect recovery from liver damage is also unknown. Clearly, ingestion of excessive vitamin A may promote additional injury (Lieber 1993). A role for supplemental polyunsaturated lecithin, which has been shown to decrease the rate of production of collagen by Ito cells exposed to alcohol and to prevent the progression of alcohol-induced injury in the baboon, is under investigation (Lieber *et al.* 1990; Li *et al.* 1992; see also Chapter 8).

Once a patient has developed clinical and histologic evidence of alcoholic hepatitis, there is no question that a potentially life-threatening liver disease is present. By this time in the illness, the moment is past during which it is likely that abstinence from alcohol will lead to complete restoration of a normal liver. In fact, many of the patients included within the broad spectrum of *alcoholic hepatitis* have already moved to a stage of active cirrhosis.

There are several issues to consider in the treatment of a patient with alcoholic liver disease. One is whether it is likely that the patient already has established cirrhosis and is undergoing another wave of alcohol-induced necrosis or if there are elements of reversible disease. Another is to determine if the patient is bereft of defences. If so, the major therapeutic thrusts may relate to the need for support or treatment of coexisting problems of gastrointestinal bleeding, infection, ascites or hepatic encephalopathy. Additionally, it is necessary to determine if there are coexisting disorders such as iron overload or chronic viral hepatitis that must be considered when planning treatment.

For the great majority of patients with alcoholic liver disease, there is as yet no definite therapy that will do more than can be achieved by abstinence and good diet administered by medical personnel aware of, and ready to respond to, associated complications (Maddrey 1990; Mezey 1993). However, efforts continue to find approaches that will benefit the patient. That little progress has been made is not the result of a lack of trying.

Important approaches to patient management build on supportive care, with the emphasis on abstinence from alcohol, correction of nutritional deficiencies and treatment of associated problems, especially infections. For patients with mild disease, abstinence and support may lead to gradual restitution of the liver towards normal. For extremely ill patients with hepatocellular decompensation, bleeding disorders and encephalopathy, the prognosis is unfavourable despite support. The patient with alcoholic hepatitis who does not have irreversible cirrhosis is at a pivotal stage. In these individuals, some forms of treatment may make a difference.

Several experimental therapies have been evaluated in attempts to stabilize patients during the acute phases of alcoholic hepatitis, thereby reducing short-term mortality and, possibly, preventing the development of cirrhosis (Maddrey 1990; Mezey 1993). These therapies include corticosteroids, evaluated because of the established anti-inflammatory and anti-fibrotic effects of these drugs; propylthiouracil, given in a effort to decrease the hypermetabolic state and reduce zone 3 (perivenular) hypoxic injury; insulin and glucagon, to stimulate hepatic regeneration; anabolic-androgenic steroids, in efforts to promote an anabolic state; and intravenous nutritional support, to reverse catabolism. Each of these approaches is worthy of consideration: on the one hand, because there may be some demonstrable beneficial effects; on the other, because of what has been learned in therapeutic trials regarding the natural history of alcohol-induced liver disease.

Corticosteroids

Corticosteroids have been extensively evaluated in alcoholic hepatitis randomized in several double-blind trials (Maddrey 1990; Imperiale and McCullough 1990). These agents are of proven value in the treatment of auto-immune hepatitis, and their known effects on the immune response, hepatic inflammation and the regulation of cytokines and collagen production has led to evaluations in patients with alcoholic liver disease.

Favourable corticosteroid effects include stimulation of the production of albumin and inhibition of the production of collagen types I and IV through effects on gene regulation (Jefferson *et al*. 1985; Weiner *et al*. 1987). Some studies of corticosteroid therapy in patients with severe alcoholic hepatitis have shown an apparent favourable outcome in short-term mortality, whereas others have shown no benefit (Maddrey 1990). There is now some agreement regarding what these results show and support

for the use of these drugs in patients with severe acute alcoholic hepatitis (Maddrey 1990; Imperiale and McCullough 1990; Ramond *et al*. 1992).

Factors associated with an adverse prognosis in patients with alcoholic hepatitis include hepatic encephalopathy, marked prolongation of the prothrombin time and considerable elevation of serum bilirubin (Maddrey *et al*. 1978). A discriminant function was derived by stepwise regression, which allows assessment of the severity of the alcoholic hepatitis based on the prothrombin time and serum bilirubin. The prognostic value of the discriminant function as a useful guide to prognosis has been confirmed in several additional trials (Carithers *et al*. 1989; Ramond *et al*. 1992). In severely ill patients, there have been significant improvements in survival for those who have received corticosteroid therapy.

The efficacy of corticosteroid therapy in the treatment of patients with severe alcoholic hepatitis, especially in those who have hepatic encephalopathy, has been further validated by metanalysis of the reported trials. In one metanalysis of 11 randomized trials, a protective efficacy of 37 percent (95 percent confidence interval 20–50 percent) was attributed to the use of corticosteroids (Imperiale and McCullough 1990).

Therefore, there may well be a subgroup of patients with alcoholic hepatitis in whom the disease is severe enough to cause early death during the acute illness and yet not so severe as to preclude any positive effect of therapy. These patients may benefit from short-term corticosteroid therapy. Whether corticosteroid therapy makes any difference in long-term survival in alcoholic hepatitis, and whether long-term treatment interferes with the subsequent development of cirrhosis, has not been adequately evaluated (see Chapter 19 for a detailed discussion).

Propylthiouracil

The evaluation of propylthiouracil as a treatment for alcoholic hepatitis was based in part on observations that the most severe alcohol-related injury is often in the perivenular (zone 3) region and often has many of the characteristics of an ischaemic injury (Orrego *et al*. 1987). Through a decrease in the hypermetabolism, propylthiouracil potentially provides a way to reduce oxygen consumption and protect the vulnerable zone 3 from the effects of hypoxia.

As is the case with corticosteroid therapy, some trials have supported the use of the drug and others have shown no benefit (Orrego *et al.* 1987; Halle *et al.* 1982). In one large trial, there was a statistically significant reduction in mortality at 2 years in patients who received propylthiouracil (Orrego *et al.* 1987). There were no complications from propylthiouracil, including no evidence of a treatment-induced hypothyroidism. However, these favourable results with propylthiouracil were not found in another double-blind controlled trial. The putative role for propylthiouracil therapy in patients with alcoholic liver disease warrant further study (see also Chapter 19).

Anabolic-androgenic steroids

Anabolic-androgenic steroids have been used in alcoholic hepatitis to reverse an often present catabolic state and promote hepatic regeneration. There has been intermittent interest for years in the use of these agents in the treatment of alcoholic liver disease (Maddrey 1986). Early studies suggested that anabolic-androgenic steroids hastened the resolution of alcoholic fatty liver (Leevy 1962). However, there was scant evidence of any favourable effects in patients with more severe forms of alcoholic liver disease and interest waned for two decades (Fenster 1966).

A role of anabolic-androgenic steroid therapy was reconsidered in a multicentre cooperative trial evaluating prednisolone, oxandrolone and placebo therapies in patients with alcoholic hepatitis (Mendenhall *et al.* 1984). There were no differences in survival for the three groups during the early months of the study. However, there was a suggestion that oxandrolone improved long-term survival. The statistical analysis (conditional survival) required that a patient survive the acute phase of the illness in order to be considered for analysis in longer follow-up. No ready explanation for these somewhat puzzling findings are available, and the results have not been subsequently confirmed (Mendenhall *et al.* 1993).

Insulin and glucagon therapy

Insulin and glucagon are established stimulants of hepatic regeneration (Leffert *et al.* 1979). The excessive use of alcohol impairs the ability of the liver to regenerate. A number of stimulants to regeneration have been identified, including insulin, glucagon, epidermal growth factor and glucocorticoids. Of these, infusions of insulin and glucagon have been most widely studied.

Controlled trials of insulin and glucagon infusions in patients with severe alcoholic hepatitis have been reported with conflicting results (Baker *et al.* 1981; Feher *et al.* 1987; Bird *et al.* 1991; Trinchet *et al.* 1992). All were of 3 weeks duration with daily 12 h infusions of insulin and glucagon. Enthusiasm for this approach has waned.

However, it stands to reason that stimulation of liver regeneration should help. It is doubtful whether insulin and glucagon infusions will prove to be the answer – hypoglycacmia is too easy to induce and is too dangerous. There are also issues as to whether these stimulants of regeneration can be taken up successfully and used by injured cells. The stimulant needs to get into a cell that is capable of responding in order to exert an effect (Dalke *et al.* 1990).

Nutritional therapy

Clinicians and investigators now readily recognize the multiple evidences of malnutrition often found in patients with alcoholic liver disease (Mezey 1991; Lieber 1993). Previously, a pivotal role for malnutrition in promoting the development of alcoholic liver disease was widely considered (and often accepted). Following recognition that much of alcohol-induced injury was the result of direct toxicity (most likely from acetaldehyde), interest in the role of nutrition in the pathogenesis of alcoholic liver injury waned. However, there have been several re-evaluations of the roles of protein–calorie malnutrition and vitamin deficiency as promoting factors in the development of alcoholic hepatitis and cirrhosis.

The results of many trials of amino acid infusions in the treatment of alcoholic hepatitis have not been consistent (Munoz 1991; Mezey 1991). Part of the problem may relate to the difficulties in identifying comparable treatment groups. However, convincing improvements in survival have not been established.

There is ample evidence that patients who have received several types of infusions have benefited, with a better nitrogen balance and increases in serum albumin, prealbumin, transferrin and retinol binding protein levels (Diehl *et al.* 1985; Mezey *et al.* 1991; Bonkovsky *et al.* 1991a, b). The issue is not whether nutritional support is helpful, but rather what type of support is most effective, to what extent and at what cost.

Liver transplantation in the treatment of alcoholic liver disease

No overview of alcoholic liver disease in the 1990s would be complete without consideration of the role of liver transplantation in treatment. The considerable mortality among patients with decompensating alcoholic cirrhosis and the increasingly favourable results with liver transplantation have led to evaluations and re-evaluations of the role of liver transplantation (Starzl *et al.* 1988; Schenker *et al.* 1990). The issues under active evaluation focus on whether patients with alcoholic liver disease should have equal access to transplantation (Lucey *et al.* 1992). These matters have been fraught with controversy and emotion (Cohen and Benjamin 1991; Moss and Siegler 1991). Early in the development of liver transplantation, few patients with alcoholic liver disease were transplanted and the mortality was high in those who had the operation. In many liver transplantation programmes, patients with alcoholic liver disease were not deemed to be suitable candidates for transplantation.

Several centres, however, pressed forward and in several series survival following liver transplantation in alcoholic patients was similar to that found in patients who did not have alcohol-induced injury (Starzl *et al.* 1988; Kumar *et al.* 1990). Major debates began. There are those who conclude that in light of the relatively small number of livers available for transplantation, it is not appropriate to use these scarce organs for individuals who have alcohol-induced disease, thereby denying patients with other types of diseases an opportunity to have a transplant. The alternative argument is that since it has been established that alcoholism is a disease, there is no justification for denying these patients access to what may be a life-saving procedure.

There are many issues to be considered even if it is decided that a history of alcohol abuse alone should not exclude a patient from consideration of transplantation. Patients with alcoholic liver disease often have additional major medical problems. These include cardiomyopathy, pancreatitis, neuropathy and cerebral atrophy. Any of these conditions or the sepsis often found in patients with alcoholic liver disease may reduce or obviate the candidacy.

Another issue is whether there should be a documented required interval of abstinence prior to acceptance of a patient as a candidate for liver transplantation. Even in this area, the requirements are changing. Some proceed to liver transplantation in individuals who have relatively acute disease with evidence of recent drinking. However, most centres do not consider liver transplantation an appropriate treatment unless commitment to abstinence is demonstrated.

Today, liver transplantation for patients with alcoholic liver disease has evolved to a position in which most centres evaluate and accept some alcoholics, especially those who have demonstrated the ability and commitment to remain abstinent and to participate appropriately in making life decisions which will help ensure graft survival.

References

Arenson, D.M., Friedman, S.L. and Bissell, D.M. (1988). Formation of extracellular matrix in normal rat liver: Lipocytes as a major source of proteoglycan. *Gastroenterology* **95**, 441–447.

Baker, A.L., Jaspan, J.B., Haines, N.W., Hatfield, G.E., Krager, P.S. and Schneider, J.F. (1981). A randomized clinical trial of insulin and glucagon infusion for treatment of alcoholic hepatitis: Progress report in 50 patients. *Gastroenterology* **80**, 1410–1414.

Baraona, E., Leo, M.A., Borowsky, S.A. and Lieber, C.S. (1977). Pathogenesis of alcohol-induced accumulation of protein in the liver. *Journal of Clinical Investigation* **60**, 546–554.

Bird, G.L.A., Sheron, N., Goka, A.K.J., Alexander, G.J. and Williams, R.S. (1990). Increased plasma tumor necrosis factor in severe alcoholic hepatitis. *Annals of Internal Medicine* **112**, 917–920.

Bird, G., Lau, J.Y.N., Koskinas, J., Wicks, C. and Williams, R. (1991). Insulin and glucagon infusion in acute hepatitis: A prospective randomized controlled trial. *Hepatology* **14**, 1097–1101.

Bonkovsky, H.L., Fiellin, D.A., Smith, G.S., Slaker, D.P., Simon, D. and Galambos, J.T. (1991a). A randomized, controlled trial of treatment of alcoholic hepatitis with parenteral nutrition and oxandrolone. I. Short-term effects on liver function. *American Journal of Gastroenterology* **86**, 1200–1208.

Bonkovsky, H.L., Singh, R.H., Jafri, I.H., Fiellin, D.A., Smith, G.S., Simon, D., Cotsonis, G.A. and Slaker, D.P (1991b). A randomized, controlled trial of treatment of alcoholic hepatitis with parenteral nutrition and oxandrolone. II. Short-term effects on nitrogen metabolism, metabolic balance and nutrition. *American Journal of Gastroenterology* **86**, 1209–1218.

Bosron, W.F., Ehrig, T. and Li, T.-K. (1993). Genetic factors in alcohol metabolism and alcoholism. *Seminars in Liver Disease* **13**, 126–135.

Carithers, R.L., Jr., Herlong, H.F., Diehl, A.M., Shaw, E.W., Combes, B., Fallon, H.J. and Maddrey, W.C.

(1989). Methylprednisolone therapy in patients with severe alcoholic hepatitis: A randomized multicenter trial. *Annals of Internal Medicine* **110**, 685–690.

Cohen, C. and Benjamin, M. (1991). Ethics, alcoholics, and liver transplantation. *Journal of the American Medical Association* **265**, 1299–1301.

Dalke, D.D., Sorrell, M.F., Casey, C.A. and Tuma, D.J. (1990). Chronic ethanol administration impairs receptor-mediated endocytosis of epidermal growth factor by rat hepatocytes. *Hepatology* **12**, 1085–1091.

Deviere, J., Vaerman, J.-P., Content, J., Denys, C., Schandene, L., Vandenbussche, P., Sibille, Y. and Dupont, E. (1991). IgA triggers tumor necrosis factor and secretion by monocytes: A study in normal subjects and patients with alcoholic cirrhosis. *Hepatology* **13**, 670–675.

Diehl, A.M. (1992). Alcohol-related trafficking accidents. *Hepatology* **15**, 964–966.

Diehl, A.M., Boitnott, J.K., Herlong, H.F., Potter, J.J., Van Duyn, M.A., Chandler, E. and Mezey, E. (1985). Effect of parenteral amino acid supplementation in alcoholic hepatitis. *Hepatology* **5**, 57–63.

Diehl, A.M., Chacon, M. and Wagner, P. (1988). The effect of chronic ethanol feeding on ornithine decarboxylase activity and liver regeneration. *Hepatology* **8**, 237–242.

Feher, J., Cornides, A., Romany, A., Karteszi, M., Szalay, L., Gogl, A. and Picazo, J. (1987). A prospective multicenter study of insulin and glucagon infusion therapy in acute alcoholic hepatitis. *Journal of Hepatology* **5**, 224–231.

Fenster, L.F. (1966). The nonefficacy of short-term anabolic steroid therapy in alcoholic liver disease. *Annals of Internal Medicine* **65**, 738–744.

French, S.W., Nash, J., Shitabata, P., Kachi, K., Hara, C., Chedid, A. and Mendenhall, C.L. (1993). Pathology of alcoholic liver disease. *Seminars in Liver Disease* **13**, 144–149.

Frezza, M., DiPadova, C., Pozzato, G., Terpin, M., Baraona, E. and Lieber, C.S. (1990). High blood alcohol levels in women. *New England Journal of Medicine* **322**, 95–99.

Friedman, S.L. (1993). The cellular basis of hepatic fibrosis. *New England Journal of Medicine* **328**, 1828–1835.

Grant, B.F., Dufour, M.C. and Harford, T.C. (1988). Epidemiology of alcoholic liver disease. *Seminars in Liver Disease* **8**, 12–25.

Halle, P., Pare, P., Kaptein, E., Kanel, G., Redeker, A.G. and Reynolds, T.B. (1982). Double-blind, controlled trial of propylthiouracil in severe acute alcoholic hepatitis. *Gastroenterology* **82**, 925–931.

Harinasuta, U. and Zimmerman, H.J. (1967). Alcoholic steatonecrosis: Relationship between severity of hepatic disease and presence of Mallory bodies in the liver. *Gastroenterology* **60**, 1036–1045.

Hill, D., Marsano, L., Cohen, D., Allen, J., Shedlofsky, S. and McClain, C.J. (1992). Increased plasma interleukin-6 activity in alcoholic hepatitis. *Journal of Laboratory Clinical Medicine* **119**, 547–552.

Horn, T., Junge J. and Christoffersen, P. (1985). Early alcoholic liver injury: Changes of the Disse space in acinar zone 3. *Liver* **5**, 301–310.

Horn, T., Junge, J. and Christoffersen, P. (1986). Early alcoholic liver injury: Activation of lipocytes in acinar zone 3 and correlation to degree of collagen formation in the Disse space. *Journal of Hepatology* **3**, 333–340.

Horn, T., Christofferson, P. and Henriksen, J.H. (1987). Alcoholic liver injury: Defenestration in non-cirrhotic livers. A scanning electron microscopic study. *Hepatology* **7**, 77–82.

Imperiale, T.F. and McCullough, A.J. (1990). Do corticosteroids reduce mortality from alcoholic hepatitis. *Annals of Internal Medicine* **113**, 299–307.

Jefferson, D.M., Reid, L.M., Giambrone, M.-A., Shafritz, D.A. and Zern, M.A. (1985). Effects of dexamethasone on albumin and collagen gene expression in primary cultures of adult rat hepatocytes. *Hepatology* **5**, 14–20.

Jelell, S.A., DiMonte, D., Gentile, A., Guglielmi, A., Altomare, E. and Albano, O. (1986). Decreased hepatic glutathione in chronic alcoholic patients. *Journal of Hepatology* **3**, 1–6.

Kumar, S., Stauber, R.E., Gavaler, J.S., Basista, M.H., Dindzans, V.J., Schade, R.R., Rabinovitz, M., Tarter, R.E., Gordon, R., Starzl, T.E. and Van Thiel, D.H. (1990). Orthotopic liver transplantation for alcoholic liver disease. *Hepatology* **11**, 159–164.

Leevy, C.M. (1962). Fatty liver: A study of 270 patients with biopsy proven fatty liver and a review of the literature. *Medicine* **41**, 249–278.

Leffert, H.L., Koch, K.S., Moran, T. and Rubalcava, B. (1979). Hormonal control of rat liver regeneration. *Gastroenterology* **76**, 1470–1482.

Lelbach, W.K. (1975). Quantitative aspects of drinking in alcoholic liver cirrhosis. In: *Alcoholic Liver Pathology* (Edited by Khanna J.M., Israel Y., and Kalant H.), pp. 1–18. Addiction Research Foundation of Ontario, Toronto.

Li, J., Kim, C., Leo, M.A., Mak, K.M., Rojkind, M. and Lieber, C.S. (1992). Polyunsaturated lecithin prevents acetaldehyde-mediated hepatic collagen accumulation by stimulating collagenase activity in cultured lipocytes. *Hepatology* **15**, 373–381.

Lieber, C.S. (1993). Biochemical factors in alcoholic liver disease. *Seminars in Liver Disease* **13**, 136–153.

Lieber, C.S., DeCarli, L.M., Mak, K.M., Kim, C.-I. and Leo, M.A. (1990). Attenuation of alcohol-induced hepatic fibrosis by polyunsaturated lecithin. *Hepatology* **12**, 1390–1398.

Lucey, M.R., Merion, R.M., Henley, K.S., Campbell, D.A., Turcotte, J.G., Nostrant, T.T., Blow, F.C. and Beresford, T.P. (1992). Selection for and outcome of liver transplantation in alcoholic liver disease. *Gastroenterology* **102**, 1736–1741.

MacSween, R.N.M. and Burt, A.D. (1986). Histologic

spectrum of alcoholic liver disease. *Seminars in Liver Disease* **6**, 221–229.

Maddrey, W.C. (1986). Is therapy with testosterone or anabolic-androgenic steroids useful in the treatment of alcoholic liver disease. *Hepatology* **6**, 1033–1035.

Maddrey, W.C. (1988). Alcoholic hepatitis: Clinicopathologic features and therapy. *Seminars in Liver Disease* **8**, 91–102.

Maddrey, W.C. (1990). Alcoholic hepatitis: Pathogenesis and approaches to treatment. *Scandinavian Journal of Gastroenterology* **25**, 118–130 (suppl 175).

Maddrey, W.C., Boitnott, J.K., Bedine, M.S., Weber, F.L., Jr., Mezey, E. and White, R.I., Jr. (1978). Corticosteroid therapy of alcoholic hepatitis. *Gastroenterology* **75**, 193–199.

Mak, K.M. and Lieber, C.S. (1986). Portal fibroblasts and myofibroblasts in baboon after long-term alcohol consumption. *Archives of Pathology and Laboratory Medicine* **110**, 513–516.

Mak, K.M. and Lieber, C.S. (1988). Lipocytes and transitional cells in alcoholic liver disease: A morphometric study. *Hepatology* **8**, 1027–1033.

McClain, C., Hill, D., Schmidt, J. and Diehl, A.M. (1993). Cytokines and alcoholic liver disease. *Seminars in Liver Disease* **13**, 170–182.

Mendenhall, C.L., Anderson, S., Garci-Pont, P., Goldberg, S., Kiernan, T., Seeff, L.B., Sorrell, M., Tamburro, C., Weesner, R., Zetterman, R., Chedid, A., Chen, T. and Rabin, L. (1984). Short-term and long-term survival in patients with alcoholic hepatitis treated with oxandrolone and prednisolone. *New England Journal of Medicine* **311**, 1461–1479.

Mendenhall, C.L., Moritz, T.E., Roselie, G.A., Morgan, T.R., Nemchausky, B.A., Tamburro, C.H., Schiff, E.R., McClain, C.J., Marsano, L.S., Allen, J.I., Samanta, A., Weesner, R.E., Henderson, W., Gartside, P., Chen, T.S., French, S.W. and Chedid, A. (1993). A study of oral nutritional support with oxandrolone in malnourished patients with alcoholic hepatitis: Results of a Department of Veterans Affairs cooperative study. *Hepatology* **17**, 564–576.

Mezey, E. (1991). Interaction between alcohol and nutrition in the pathogenesis of alcoholic liver disease. *Seminars in Liver Disease* **11**, 340–348.

Mezey, E. (1993). Treatment of alcoholic liver disease. *Seminars in Liver Disease* **13**, 210–216.

Mezey, E., Caballeria, J., Mitchell, M.C., Pares, A., Herlong, H.F. and Rodes, J. (1991). Effect of parenteral amino acid supplementation on short-term and long-term outcomes in severe alcoholic hepatitis: A randomized controlled trial. *Hepatology* **14**, 1090–1096.

Mills, P.R., Pennington, T.H., Kay, R., MacSween, M. and Watkinson, G. (1979). Hepatitis B antibody in alcoholic cirrhosis. *Journal of Clinical Pathology* **32**, 778–782.

Moss, A.H. and Siegler, M. (1991). Should alcoholics compete equally for liver transplantation? *Journal of the American Medical Association* **265**, 1295–1298.

Munoz, S. (1991). Nutritional therapies in liver disease. *Seminars in Liver Disease* **2**, 287–291.

Nolan, J.P. (1989). Intestinal endotoxins as mediators of hepatic injury – an idea whose time has come again. *Hepatology* **10**, 887–891.

Orrego, H., Kalant, H., Israel, Y., Blake, J., Medline, A., Rankin, J.G., Armstrong, A. and Kapur, B. (1979a). Effect of short-term therapy with propylthiouracil in patients with alcoholic liver disease. *Gastroenterology* **76**, 105–115.

Orrego, H., Blendis, L.M., Blake, J.E., Kaput, B.M. and Israel, Y. (1979b). Reliability of assessment of alcohol intake based on personal interviews in a liver clinic. *Lancet* **ii**, 1354–1356.

Orrego, H., Medline, A., Blendis, L.M., Rankin, J.G. and Kreaden, D.A. (1979c). Collagenisation of the Disse space in alcoholic liver disease. *Gut* **20**, 673–679.

Orrego, H., Blake, J.E., Blendis, L.M., Compton, K.V. and Israel, Y. (1987). Long-term treatment of alcoholic liver disease with propylthiouracil. *New England Journal of Medicine* **317**, 1421–1427.

Pares, A., Barrera, J.M., Ercilla, G., Bruguera, M., Caballeria, L., Castillo, R. and Rodes, J. (1990). Hepatitis C virus antibodies in chronic alcoholic patients: Association with severity of liver injury. *Hepatology* **12**, 1295–1299.

Paronetto, F. (1993). Immunologic reactions in alcoholic liver disease. *Seminars in Liver Disease* **13**, 183–195.

Pequignot, G. and Cyrulinik, F. (1970). Chronic disease due to overconsumption of alcoholic drinks (excepting neuropsychiatric pathology). *International Encyclopaedia of Pharmacology and Therapeutics* **2**, 375–412.

Ramond, M.J., Poynard, T., Rueff, B., Mathurin, P., Theodore, C., Chaput, J.-C. and Benhamou, J.-P. (1992). A randomized trial of prednisolone in patients with severe alcoholic hepatitis. *New England Journal of Medicine* **326**, 507–512.

Schenker, S. and Speeg, K.V. (1990). The risk of alcohol intake in men and women. *New England Journal of Medicine* **322**, 127–130.

Schenker, S., Perkins, H.S. and Sorrell, M.F. (1990). Should patients with end-stage alcoholic liver disease have a new liver? *Hepatology* **11**, 314–319.

Seeff, L.B., Cuccherini, B.A., Zimmerman, H.J., Adler, E. and Benjamin, S.B. (1986). Acetaminophen hepatotoxicity in alcoholics. *Annals of Internal Medicine* **104**, 399–404.

Sheron, N., Bird, G., Koskinas, J., Portmann, B., Ceska, M., Lindley, I. and Williams, R. (1993). Circulating and tissue levels of the neutrophil chemotaxin interleukin-8 are elevated in severe acute alcoholic hepatitis, and tissue levels correlate with neutrophil infiltration. *Hepatology* **18**, 41–46.

Starzl, T.E., Van Thiel, D., Tzakis, A.G., Iwatsuki, S., Todo, S., March, J.W., Koneru, B., Staschak, S., Stieber, A. and Gordon, R.D. (1988). Orthotopic liver transplantation for alcoholic cirrhosis. *Journal of the American Medical Association* **260**, 2542–2544.

Trinchet, J.-C., Balkau, B., Poupon, R.E., Heintzmann, F., Callard, P., Gotheil, C., Grange, J.-D., Vetter, D., Pauwels, A., Labadie, H., Chazouilleres, O., Mavier, P., Desmorat, H., Zarski, J.-P., Barbare, J.-C., Chambre, J.-F., Pariente, E.A., Roulot, D. and Beaugrand, M. (1992). Treatment of severe alcoholic hepatitis by infusion of insulin and glucagon: A multicenter sequential trial. *Hepatology* **15**, 76–81.

Tsutsumi, M., Lasker, J.M., Shimizu, M., Rosman, A.S. and Lieber, C.S. (1989). The intralobular distribution of ethanol-inducible P450IIE1 in rat and human liver. *Hepatology* **10**, 437–446.

Tuma, D.J. and Sorrell, M.F. (1988). Effects of ethanol on protein trafficking in the liver. *Seminars in Liver Disease* **8**, 69–80.

Uchida, T., Shikata, T., Govindarajan, S. and Kronborg, I. (1987). The characteristics of alcoholic liver disease in Japan: Clinicopathologic comparison with alcoholic liver disease in the United States. *Liver* **7**, 290–297.

Van de Wiel, A., Van Hattum, J., Schuurman, H-J. and Kater, L. (1988). Immunoglobulin A in the diagnosis of alcoholic liver disease. *Gastroenterology* **94**, 457–462.

Van Waes, L. and Lieber, C.S. (1977). Early perivenular sclerosis in alcoholic fatty liver: An index of progressive liver injury. *Gastroenterology* **73**, 646–650.

Vidins, E.L., Britton, R.D., Medline, A., Blendis, L.M., Israel, Y. and Orrego, H. (1985). Sinusoidal caliber in alcoholic and nonalcoholic liver disease: Diagnostic and pathogenic implications. *Hepatology* **5**, 408–414.

Weiner, F.R., Czaja, M.J., Giambrone, M.-A., Takahashi, S., Biempica, L. and Zern, M.A. (1987). Transcriptional and posttranscriptional effects of dexamethasone on albumin and procollagen messenger RNAs in murine schistosomiasis. *Biochemistry* **26**, 1557–1562.

Weiner, F.R., Giambrone, M.-A., Czaja, M.J., Shah, A., Annoni, G., Takahashi, S., Eghbali, M. and Zern, M.A. (1990). Ito-cell gene expression and collagen regulation. *Hepatology* **11**, 111–117.

Worner, T.M. and Lieber, C.S. (1985). Perivenular fibrosis as precursor lesion of cirrhosis. *Journal of the American Medical Association* **254**, 627–630.

Zetterman, R.K., Luisada-Opper, A. and Leevy, C.M., (1976). Alcoholic hepatitis: Cell-mediated immunological response to alcoholic hyaline. *Gastroenterology* **70**, 382–384.

2 Metabolism of alcohol: An update

Charles S. Lieber

Introduction

In nature, ethanol is produced mainly by fermentation of carbohydrates by yeast, but it can also be found in mammals in trace amounts. Bacterial fermentation in the gut is one way in which ethanol is produced in the body and the function of the enzyme alcohol dehydrogenase may be to rid the body of this alcohol. After ingestion ethanol is readily absorbed from the gastrointestinal tract. Only 2–10 percent is eliminated through the kidneys and lungs; the rest is oxidized in the body, principally in the liver. The rate of removal of ethanol from the blood is remarkably decreased by hepatectomy or procedures damaging the liver (Thompson 1956). The hepatocyte contains three main pathways for ethanol metabolism: the alcohol dehydrogenase (ADH) pathway in the cytosol, the microsomal ethanol oxidizing system located in the smooth endoplasmic reticulum, and catalase located in the peroxisomes (Fig. 2.1).

The alcohol dehydrogenase (ADH) pathway

A major pathway for ethanol metabolism involves ADH, an enzyme that catalyses the conversion of ethanol to acetaldehyde.

Multiple forms of ADH

Studies over the past 15 years on ADH molecular forms in human liver have revealed a degree of complexity in ADH isoenzymes that has no counterpart in lower animal species (Bosron *et al.* 1993). Human ADH is a dimeric zinc metalloenzyme for which several classes have been distinguished (Jornvall *et al.* 1987). Subunits hybridize within but not between classes. Human liver ADH exists in multiple molecular forms which arise from the association of different types of subunits into active dimeric molecules. A genetic model accounts for this multiplicity as products of seven gene loci, ADH1 through ADH7 (Bosron *et al.* 1993). Polymorphism occurs at two loci, ADH2 and ADH3, which encode the β and γ subunits. These homodimeric and heterodimeric isoenzymes have been isolated and purified to homogeneity. Class I isozymes migrate cathodically on starch gel electrophoresis. There are three types of subunit, α, β and γ in class I. The primary structures of all three forms have been established, as well as the overall properties and the effects of the amino acid substitutions between the various forms. Each subunit has 374 residues, of which 35 exhibit differences among the α, β and γ chains. Corresponding cDNA structures are also known, as are the genetic organization and details of the gene structures. Allelic variants occur at the β and γ loci. Corresponding amino acid substitutions have been characterized, and enzymatic differences between the allelic forms are

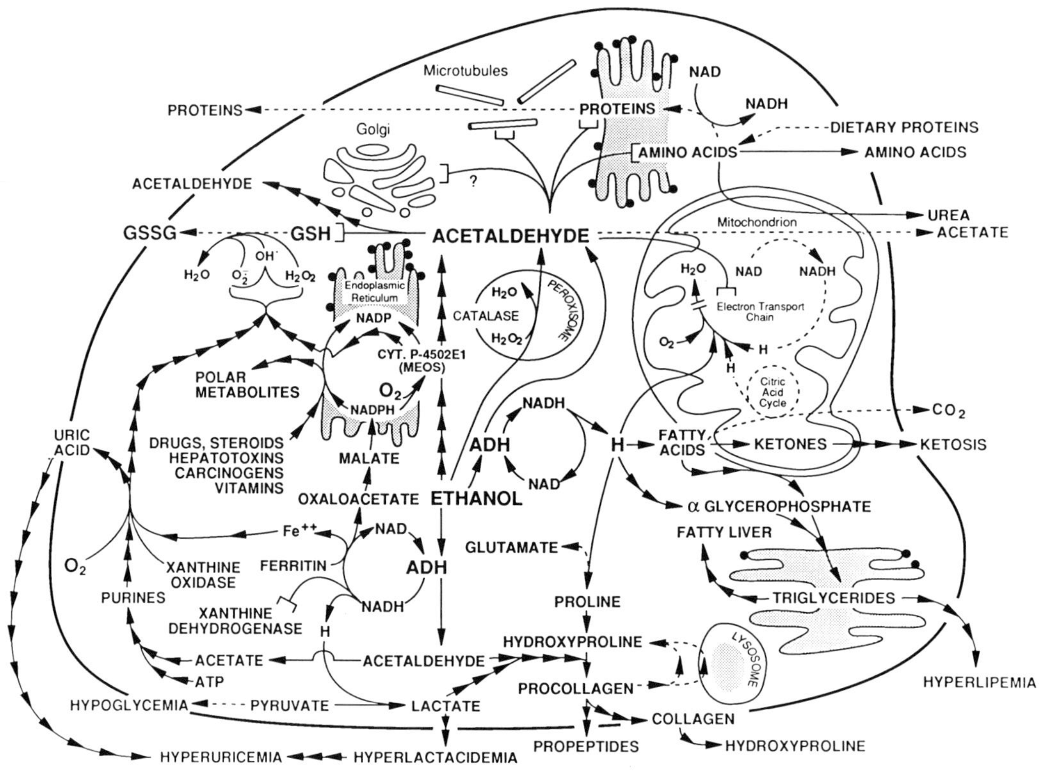

Fig. 2.1 Oxidation of ethanol in the hepatocyte. Many disturbances in intermediary metabolism and toxic effects can be linked to (1) alcohol dehydrogenase (ADH) mediated generation of NADH, (2) the induction of the activity of microsomal enzymes, especially CYP2E1, and (3) acetaldehyde, the product of ethanol oxidation. NAD, nicotinamide adenine dinucleotide; NADH, reduced NAD; GSH, reduced glutathione; GSSG, oxidized glutathione. The broken lines indicate pathways that are depressed by ethanol, whereas repeated arrows reflect stimulation or activation. The symbol -[denotes interference or binding. Reproduced with permission from Lieber (1994).

explained by defined residue exchanges. The subunits of class I are derived from at least three genetic loci (Smith *et al.* 1971; von Bahr-Lindstrom *et al.* 1986; Duester *et al.* 1986) and constitute the α subunit (the major form expressed in fetal liver), different β subunits, distributed non-identically in various populations (β_1 common in Caucasian populations, β_2 common in Oriental populations and β_3 found at least in some African populations) (von Wartburg *et al.* 1965; Jornvall *et al.* 1984; Bosron *et al.* 1983), and the two allelic types of γ subunit (γ_1 and γ_2, both of high frequency). Von Wartburg *et al.* (1965) first differentiated the normal ADH of human liver (pH optimum 10.5) from the so-called atypical type (pH optimum 8.8), which shows a several-fold higher activity. The main normal human ADH has only the β_1 subunit, whereas the atypical type also has the β_2 subunit. Both subunits are controlled by the ADH2 locus. The atypical

form of ADH occurs in frequencies between 5 and 20 percent in European populations: English 10 percent (Smith *et al.* 1971); Swiss 20 percent (von Wartburg and Schurch 1968); German 9 percent (Harada *et al.* 1978). In Mongoloid populations, the frequency is up to 90 percent (Stamatoyannopoulos *et al.* 1975). The K_i values for 4-methylpyrazole inhibition of the class I isozymes are in the μM range.

Other data also reveal the genetic organization and the gene structures (Duester *et al.* 1986), as well as the protein structures, of subunits of the class II type and subunits of the class III type. Class II isozymes migrate more anodically than class I isozymes and, unlike the latter, which generally have low K_m values for ethanol, class II (or π) ADH has a relatively high K_m (34 mM) and an insensitivity to 4-methylpyrazole inhibition with a K_i of 2 mM at pH 7.5 (Li and Magnes 1975; Bosron *et al.* 1979). Class III (χ ADH) does not participate in the oxidation of ethanol in the liver because of its very low affinity for that substrate; it is not inhibited by 12 mM 4-methylpyrazole (Pares and Vallee 1981). More recently, a new class (IV) of ADH has been identified in human stomach (Hernandez-Munoz *et al.* 1990), so-called σ- or μ-ADH (Yin *et al.* 1990; Moreno and Pares 1991), its full length cDNA established (Yokoyama *et al.* 1994), and a cDNA encoding yet another new class of ADH (V) in liver and stomach was reported (Yasunami *et al.* 1991).

Large differences in K_m for NAD^+ at pH 7.5 (7.4 μM for β_1 to 710 μM for β_3) and alcohol (0.049 mM for β_1 to about 35 mM for β_3) have been reported. The V_{max} for ethanol oxidation at pH 7.5 varies from 0.23 U/mg for β_1 to 8.6 U/mg for β_2 (Bosron *et al.* 1993). In the rat (Julia *et al.* 1987) and the baboon (Holmes and VandeBerg 1987), isoenzymes of ADH have been characterized that exhibit many analogies with human ADH classes.

Lobular (acinar) distribution of ADH

Early histochemical studies on rat liver showed either maximal ADH activity in the periportal regions (Greenberger *et al.* 1965) or a uniform distribution within all regions of the liver lobule (Berres *et al.* 1970). In contrast, microquantitative measurements by Morrison and Brock (1967) revealed maximal activity of ADH in the perivenular (zone 3) region in human liver, while in female rats the activity in zone 3 was about 1.7 times higher than in the periportal region (zone 1). Modern immunohistochemical techniques have shown that ADH is located mainly in the zone 3 hepatocytes (Buehler *et al.* 1982), even in cirrhotic livers (Sokal *et al.* 1993). More recently, microchemical assays were performed in microdissected tissue samples from the whole length of the sinusoid (Maly and Sasse 1991): the ADH activity in men < 50 years of age showed an increase in the gradient from zone 1 to zone 3; furthermore, ADH activity was significantly higher in women. After the age of 53 in men and 50 in women, the sex difference in the distribution profiles was no longer apparent. Immunoelectron microscopy has shown the enzyme within the cytoplasm of hepatocytes (Haseba *et al.* 1991). Separation of periportal and perivenular hepatocyte populations, employing ante-retrograde and retrograde collagenase perfusion in the male rat liver, led to the conclusion that there were no regional differences in ADH activity in the rat (Vaananen *et al.* 1984) and, in rat hepatocytes, the class I enzyme was expressed

equally in periportal and perivenular regions (Chen *et al.* 1992). However, microdissection techniques have shown an intermediary peak at the end of the second third of the sinusoidal length in male rats, and a gradual increase in activity, beginning periportally and increasing in the direction of the perivenular region (zone 3) in females (Maly and Sasse 1987). The high activity of liver ADH in adult females relative to adult males in some rodent strains does not constitute a general phenomenon, but depends on the species and strains of animals studied (Maly and Sasse 1985).

Redox change

In ADH-mediated oxidation of ethanol, hydrogen is transferred from the substrate to the cofactor nicotinamide adenine dinucleotide (NAD), converting it to its reduced form (NADH), and acetaldehyde is produced (Fig. 2.1). The dissociation of the NADH–enzyme complex has been shown to be a rate-limiting step in this reaction (Theorell and Chance 1951). As a net result, the first step in the oxidation of ethanol generates an excess of reducing equivalents in the cytosol, primarily as NADH. Thus, in normal rats given alcohol, there is a marked shift in the redox potential of the cytosol, as measured by changes in the lactate and pyruvate ratio (Domschke *et al.* 1974). The altered redox state, in turn, is responsible for a variety of metabolic abnormalities. Some of these, such as hyperlactacidaemia, are linked to the utilization of the excess NADH in the cytosol (Fig. 2.1). The reducing equivalents can also be transferred to NADPH, and the increased NADPH can be utilized for synthetic pathways in the cytosol and microsomal functions.

Some of the hydrogen equivalents formed in this reaction are transferred from the cytosol into the mitochondria. The mitochondrial membrane is impermeable to NADH and the reducing equivalents are thought to enter the mitochondria via shuttle mechanisms such as the malate cycle (quantitatively, probably the most important), the fatty acid elongation cycle and the α-glycerophosphate cycle. In these cycles, NADH reduces the oxidized partner of the shuttle pair (i.e. oxaloacetate) in the presence of the cytoplasmic enzyme (malate dehydrogenase), thereby regenerating NAD. The reduced component (i.e. malate) now traverses the mitochondrial membrane where it reacts with the mitochondrial enzyme and NAD (or FAD in the case of α-

glycerophosphate) to generate NADH or FADH plus the oxidized partner. FADH and NADH are then oxidized by the respiratory chain, and the oxidized partner enters the cytoplasm where it is available for another round of the shuttle cycle. Normally, fatty acids are oxidized via β-oxidation and the citric acid cycle of the mitochondria, which serves as "hydrogen donor" for the mitochondrial electron transport chain. When ethanol is oxidized the generated hydrogen equivalents – which are shuttled into the mitochondria – supplant the citric acid cycle as the source of hydrogen. Following the administration of ethanol, the mitochondria are shifted to a more reduced redox state as measured by changes in the ratio of β-hydroxybutyrate to acetoacetate (Domschke *et al.* 1974).

Gastric ADH and other sites of extrahepatic ethanol metabolism

Although the liver is the main site of ethanol metabolism, some extrahepatic metabolism occurs; oxidation of ethanol has been reported in the stomach of the rat (Lamboeuf *et al.* 1981, 1983) and has been related to the presence of ADH (Hempel and Pietruszko 1979; Pestalozzi *et al.* 1983). At least three different forms of ADH exist in the stomach (with the $\gamma\gamma$, $\sigma\sigma$ and $\chi\chi$ isoenzymes) with either high or low K_m's for ethanol (Hernandez-Munoz *et al.* 1990). Because of the extraordinary high gastric ethanol concentration after alcohol ingestion, even the gastric ADH with the high K_m for ethanol can become active, and significant gastric alcohol metabolism may ensue (Julkunen *et al.* 1985a, b). Ethnic variability is possibly involved, since 80 percent of Japanese were found to lack significant expression of one of the gastric isozymes (Baraona *et al.* 1991). The concentration of alcohol in the beverage affects the amount metabolized in the stomach and consequently in the rat – which has only the high K_m enzyme – relatively high concentrations of ethanol are required for significant first-pass metabolism to be observed (Roine *et al.* 1991). When only 2.5 percent ethanol was used, no first-pass metabolism was measurable (Smith *et al.* 1992). Also, when low concentrations are used, relatively large volumes are involved, which may accelerate gastric emptying, thereby also resulting in less gastric metabolism.

The first-pass metabolism decreases the bioavailability of ethanol and represents a "protective barrier" against systemic effects, at least when alcohol is consumed in small amounts as in "social drinking". This "gastric barrier" disappears after gastrectomy (Caballeria *et al.*, 1989a) and may in part be decreased in the alcoholic (Di Padova *et al.* 1987; Frezza *et al.* 1990), because of a decrease in gastric ADH activity. Some commonly used drugs inhibit gastric ADH activity *in vitro* for example aspirin (Roine *et al.* 1990) and H_2-blockers such as cimetidine and ranitidine (Caballeria *et al.* 1989b, 1991), and result in increased blood alcohol levels (Caballeria *et al.* 1989b; Di Padova *et al.* 1992); this interaction is particularly striking at low doses of alcohol, as described by Caballeria *et al.* (1989b) and Hernandez-Munoz *et al.* (1990). Whether the H_2-blockers' effect on blood alcohol can be demonstrated with higher doses of alcohol has been the subject of controversy (Roine *et al.* 1992), but a positive interaction has been reported by several groups (Seitz *et al.* 1984; Di Padova *et al.* 1992).

Women have a lower gastric ADH activity than men (Frezza *et al.* 1990), at least below the age of 50 (Seitz *et al.* 1990). As a consequence, for a given intake their blood alcohol levels are higher, an increase that is compounded by differences in body composition (more fat, less water in women) and, on average, a lower body weight. The higher blood alcohol level, in turn, may contribute to the greater susceptibility of women to alcohol (see also Chapter 7).

Lung slices and microsomes can convert ethanol to acetaldehyde (Pikkarainen *et al.* 1981), but pulmonary ADH is thought to make only a minor contribution to ethanol metabolism *in vivo* (Bernstein *et al.* 1990). The quantitative role of such extrahepatic oxidative pathways is unsettled and may vary from species to species.

Rate-limiting factors in ADH-mediated ethanol metabolism

According to classic concepts, the major rate-limiting factor in the metabolism of ethanol by the ADH pathway is the capacity of the liver to reoxidize the NADH produced from the reduction of NAD by the hydrogen from the ethanol. Studies in humans given low doses of ethanol have shown that as long as hepatic blood flow is not limiting, the rate of ADH-catalysed elimination of a small dose of ethanol *in vivo* is limited by the dissociation of NADH from the enzyme and by the rates of oxidation of acetaldehyde and reoxidation of NADH (Cronholm *et al.* 1988). These views are supported by recent observations that amino acid substitutions at position 47 of human $\beta_1\beta_1$ and $\beta_2\beta_2$ ADH affect hydride transfer and coenzyme dissociation rate constants, and that the different activities of $\beta_1\beta_1$ and $\beta_2\beta_2$ for alcohol oxidation and acetaldehyde reduction are caused primarily by different coenzyme dissociation rates (Stone *et al.* 1993), and by the observation in a group of 25 alcoholics with varying degrees of liver injury (from normal liver to cirrhosis) and in six non-alcoholic cirrhotics, that the alcohol metabolic rate was related to hepatic functions and was independent of the activity of hepatic ADH (Panes *et al.* 1993).

ADH is not necessarily present in excess and under a variety of circumstances it is the level of the enzyme itself that actually becomes one of the rate-limiting factors (Crow *et al.* 1977). The concept that rates of ethanol metabolism may be determined by the level of ADH activity has been the subject of controversy for many years. The "atypical" ADH isolated by von Wartburg *et al.* (1965) has, *in vitro*, a much higher activity at physiologic pH than the normal variety. Although those individuals with "atypical" ADH have enzyme activities several times higher than normal, *in vitro*, this is not accompanied by an acceleration of the metabolism of ethanol *in vivo* (Edwards and Price-Evans 1967). Similarly, marked modifications in ADH activity found in patients with alcoholic liver disease are not accompanied by parallel alterations in the kinetics of alcohol disappearance (Zorzano *et al.* 1989). Furthermore, human liver showed higher K_m ADH and lower K_m ADH activity than rat liver, whereas ethanol metabolism of rats was much faster than in human subjects. This discrepancy supports the view that in the process of alcohol oxidation, ADH itself may not be the major rate-limiting factor, provided at least a normal amount of ADH is present. Under these conditions, velocities may depend on the availability of the cofactor NAD and the capacity of the cell to dissociate the ADH–NADH complex and reoxidize NADH.

Although ADH activity above normal may not increase the rate of ethanol oxidation, diminution of ADH activity can reduce it; for example a low-protein diet has been shown to diminish hepatic ADH levels in rats (Horn and Manthei 1965; Bode *et al.* 1970; Wilson *et al.* 1986) and to slow the metabolism of ethanol considerably, both in rats (Bode *et al.* 1970; Pekkanen *et al.* 1978; Wilson *et al.* 1986) and humans (Bode *et al.* 1971). Bode and Thiele (1975) showed that prolonged fasting markedly slows the metabolism of ethanol. In liver cells isolated from fed rats, the rate of ethanol oxidation was about twice that in the fasting state. Since the concentrations of malate, aspartate and α-glycerophosphate in liver cells from fed rats were higher than in the cells from starved rats, it seems likely that the higher rate of ethanol oxidation in the liver cells from fed rats was caused by increased activities of the hydrogen-transport cycles. In contrast to starved rats, malate addition was rather ineffective in stimulating ethanol oxidation in the liver cells of fed rats, indicating that the hydrogen-transport cycles were not rate-limiting. Under these conditions, it might be expected that reoxidation of reducing equivalents would be rate-limiting in ethanol oxidation. Indeed, the addition of uncoupling agents caused a large stimulation of ethanol oxidation, suggesting that in livers of fed rats the mitochondrial reoxidation of NADH, whether transported from the cytosol or generated directly in the mitochondria by ADH, is a rate-limiting step. Similarly, treatment of rats with 3,3′,5-triiodo-L-thyronine (T3) for a period of 6 days led to a 45 percent decrease in total liver ADH, but the rate of ethanol elimination *in vivo* was the same as in control animals (Smith and Dawson 1985). These results do not support the notion that ethanol elimination *in vivo* is normally governed primarily by the level of ADH under these conditions.

A word of caution is needed concerning the possible variability in ethanol metabolism caused by species differences. For instance, in spontaneously hypertensive rats, rates of ethanol metabolism appear to be modulated by ADH activity, which in turn is strikingly affected by sex hormones, with inhibition by testosterone and stimulation by oestradiol (Rachmamin *et al.* 1980). In conventional rats as well, a number of studies, reviewed by Lieber (1984, 1987), have shown hormonal influences. The interaction between sex hormones and ethanol-metabolizing enzymes was tested in detail by Teschke *et al.* (1986). Oestradiol increased the hepatic activities of ADH and catalase in both ovariectomized and sham-operated female rats on the control diet, whereas this enhancing property was virtually lost in animals on the ethanol diet. According to Lumeng and Crabb (1984), changes in ethanol elimination rates produced by fasting and castration mainly reflected changes in the V_{max} of liver ADH. It has been shown that a decrease in the rate of degradation is the principal cause for the increase in liver ADH following castration (Mezey and Potter 1985). Similarly, stimulation of protein degradation (or possibly effects on translation) may explain why corticosterone induces rat liver ADH mRNA but not enzyme protein or activity (Qulali and Crabb 1992). In mice also, changes in the mRNA levels after ethanol feeding could not be directly related to the changes seen in enzyme activity (Bond and Singh 1990). In general, in most species tested, ethanol feeding causes an apparent reduction in hepatic ADH enzyme activity regardless of corresponding mRNA changes.

Another key factor in the rate of ethanol metabolism is the accumulation of acetaldehyde. In hepatocytes from fed rats, the "flux control coefficient" for ADH decreased with increasing acetaldehyde concentration, suggesting that, as acetaldehyde concentrations rise, control of the pathway shifts from ADH to other enzymes, particularly aldehyde dehydrogenase (Page *et al.* 1991). Thus, there does not appear to be a single rate-determining step for the ethanol metabolism pathway via ADH.

Metabolic changes associated with ethanol oxidation

In ADH-mediated oxidation of ethanol, acetaldehyde is produced and hydrogen is transferred from alcohol to the cofactor nicotinamide adenine dinucleotide (NAD), which is converted to its reduced form (NADH) (Fig. 2.1). The acetaldehyde produced again loses hydrogen and is converted to acetate, most of which is released into the bloodstream. As a net result, ethanol oxidation generates an excess of reducing equivalents in the liver, primarily as NADH. The large amounts of reducing equivalents produced overwhelm the ability of the hepatocyte to maintain redox homeostasis and a number of metabolic disorders ensue.

Hyperlactacidaemia, hyperuricaemia, ketonaemia, acidosis
The enhanced NADH/NAD ratio reflects itself in an increased lactate/pyruvate ratio that results in hyperlactacidaemia because of both decreased utilization (Greenway and Lautt 1990) and enhanced production of lactate by the liver. The hyperlactacidaemia contributes to the acidosis and also reduces the capacity of the kidney to excrete uric acid, leading to secondary hyperuricaemia (Lieber *et al.* 1962). Alcohol-induced ketosis (Lefevre *et al.* 1970) and enhanced purine breakdown (Faller and Fox 1982) may also promote the hyperuricaemia. Another possible consequence of enhanced purine degradation is increased production of activated oxygen species by xanthine oxidase, as suggested by

the protective effect of allopurinol against the alcohol-induced lipid peroxidation (Kato *et al.* 1990). Hyperuricaemia may be related to the common clinical observation that excessive consumption of alcoholic beverages commonly aggravates or precipitates gouty attacks.

Enhanced lipogenesis and depressed lipid oxidation
The increased NADH/NAD ratio also raises the concentration of α-glycerophosphate that favours hepatic triglyceride accumulation by trapping fatty acids. In addition, excess NADH may promote fatty acid synthesis (Lieber and Pignon 1989). The activity of the citric acid cycle is depressed, partly because of a slowing of the reactions of the cycle that require NAD, and because the mitochondria use the hydrogen equivalents originating from alcohol, rather than those derived from the oxidation of fatty acids that normally serve as the main energy source of the liver.

Theoretically, lipids that accumulate in the liver can originate from three main sources: (1) dietary lipids, which reach the bloodstream as chylomicrons, (2) adipose tissue lipids, which are transported to the liver as free fatty acids and (3) lipids synthesized in the liver itself (Lieber and Savolainen 1984). These fatty acids accumulate in the liver primarily because of (1) decreased lipid oxidation in the liver, (2) enhanced hepatic lipogenesis, (3) decreased hepatic release of lipoproteins, (4) increased mobilization of peripheral fat and (5) enhanced hepatic uptake of circulating lipids. Most commonly, decreased fatty acid oxidation results in the accumulation of dietary fat in the liver (Lieber and Spritz 1966; Lieber *et al.* 1966). In addition, chronic ethanol consumption results in changes in mitochondrial function, in particular a decreased capacity to oxidize fatty acids. The decreased fatty acid oxidation, whether as a function of the reduced citric acid cycle activity (secondary to the altered redox potential) or as a consequence of permanent changes in mitochondrial structure, offers the most likely explanation for the accumulation of fat in the liver, especially fat derived from the diet. In addition, with stressful amounts of ethanol and/or fasting conditions, some mobilization of fatty acids from adipose tissue may also contribute to the accumulation of lipids in the liver.

Ethanol and protein metabolism
Inhibition of protein synthesis has been observed after the addition of alcohol to various preparations

in vitro (Rothschild *et al.* 1971; Jeejeebhoy *et al.* 1975). *In vivo*, the acute effects of ethanol on protein synthesis have been less consistent. The perivenular region of the hepatic acinus, which is already somewhat hypoxic in the normal state, may represent an area of exaggerated toxicity (Jauhonen *et al.* 1982). Indeed, this zone shows a striking exaggeration of the ethanol-induced redox changes; the latter may be sufficient to impair protein synthesis.

Ethanol and glucose metabolism

Acute ethanol intoxication occasionally causes severe hypoglycaemia, which can result in sudden death. As reviewed elsewhere (see Lieber 1992), hypoglycemia is due in part to a block of hepatic gluconeogenesis by ethanol, again as a consequence of the increased NADH/NAD ratio in subjects whose glycogen stores are already depleted by starvation or who have pre-existing abnormalities in carbohydrate metabolism. Under other conditions, ethanol may accelerate rather than inhibit gluconeogenesis. Indeed, hyperglycaemia may occur in association with alcoholism.

Miscellaneous redox-associated effects

Other metabolic effects of ethanol attributed to the generation of NADH include interference with the metabolism of galactose, serotonin and other amines. The increased availability of NADH results additionally in alteration of hepatic steroid metabolism in favour of the reduced compounds.

Zonal distribution of the pathologic effects associated with ADH-mediated ethanol metabolism

A characteristic feature of early alcoholic liver disease is the presence of steatosis and other lesions in the perivenular (centrilobular) region, that is zone 3 of the hepatic acinus. The mechanism for this zonal selectivity of the toxic effects involves several distinct and not mutually exclusive mechanisms. One of these, namely the hypoxia hypothesis, originated from the observation that liver slices, from rats chronically fed alcohol, consume more oxygen than those of controls. It was then postulated that the enhanced consumption of oxygen would increase the gradient of oxygen tensions along the sinusoids to the extent of producing anoxic injury of perivenular hepatocytes (Israel *et al.* 1975). Indeed, both in alcoholics (Kessler *et al.* 1954) and in animals chronically fed ethanol (Jauhonen *et al.* 1982; Sato *et al.*

1983), decreases in either hepatic venous oxygen saturation (Kessler *et al.* 1954) or PO_2 (Jauhonen *et al.* 1982) and in tissue oxygen tensions (Sato *et al.* 1983) have been found during the withdrawal state. However, the changes in hepatic oxygenation found during the withdrawal state disappeared (Shaw *et al.* 1977; Jauhonen *et al.* 1982) or decreased (Sato *et al.* 1983) when alcohol was present in the blood. Acute ethanol administration in cats did not alter O_2 uptake (Greenway and Lautt 1990). In naive baboons, alcohol increased splanchnic oxygen consumption but the consequences of this effect on oxygenation in the perivenular region were offset by increased blood flow resulting in unchanged hepatic venous oxygen tension (Jauhonen *et al.* 1982). Ethanol in fact induces an increase in portal hepatic blood flow (see Chapter 14). In baboons chronically fed ethanol, defective O_2 utilization rather than the lack of a blood O_2 supply characterized liver injury produced by high concentrations of ethanol (Lieber *et al.* 1989). We postulated that the low oxygen tensions normally prevailing in perivenular regions could exaggerate the redox shift produced by ethanol (Jauhonen *et al.* 1982). To study the magnitude of such a shift in the baboon, the effects of ethanol on the lactate/pyruvate ratio in hepatic venous blood (an approximation of that in perivenular hepatocytes) were compared with the ratio in total liver. Ethanol increased the lactate/pyruvate ratio and decreased pyruvate more in hepatic venous blood than in total liver. In isolated rat hepatocytes, the ethanol-induced redox shift was markedly exaggerated by lowering the oxygen to a tension similar to that found in perivenular regions. The process was also assessed in the isolated perfused rat liver, by varying the oxygen supply, to reproduce the oxygen tensions prevailing *in vivo* along the sinusoid (Jauhonen *et al.* 1985). It is noteworthy that hypoxia increases NADH, which in turn inhibits the activity of NAD^+-dependent xanthine dehydrogenase, thereby favouring that of oxygen-dependent xanthine oxidase (Kato *et al.* 1990), see Fig. 2.1. It has been postulated that, due to the acetate derived from ethanol, purine metabolites accumulate and could be metabolized via xanthine oxidase. This process may lead to the production of oxygen radicals, which may mediate toxic effects towards liver cells, including peroxidation. Physiologic substrates for xanthine oxidase, hypoxanthine and xanthine, as well as AMP, significantly increased in the liver after ethanol, together with an enhanced urinary output of allantoin (a final product of xanthine metabolism). Allopurinol pre-treatment resulted in 90 percent inhibition of xanthine oxidase activity, and also significantly decreased ethanol-induced lipid peroxidation (Kato *et al.* 1990).

The zonal distribution of some enzymes can influence the selective perivenular toxicity. Proliferation of the smooth endoplasmic reticulum (SER) after chronic ethanol consumption is maximal in the perivenular region, with associated enzyme induction and related effects. Furthermore, human ADH has now been demonstrated mainly in hepatocytes around the terminal hepatic venule. Thus, a presumably higher level of ethanol metabolism in the perivenular region could contribute to the selective injury in this region, for instance by providing (together with the "induced" microsomal pathway) an increased amount of the toxic metabolite acetaldehyde (Lieber 1985). However, after chronic ethanol consumption, unlike the activity of MEOS which is induced, the activity of ADH may not change or even may decrease (Lieber and DeCarli 1970; Brighenti and Pancaldi 1970; Salaspuro *et al.* 1981); decreased hepatic ADH activity may occur even in the absence of liver damage (Ugarte *et al.* 1967). A modest decrease in ADH activity may not affect rates of ethanol metabolism (and hence of acetaldehyde production), but a severe decrease could offset, at least in part, the enhanced metabolism resulting from MEOS induction.

Microsomal ethanol oxidizing system

The first indication of an interaction of ethanol with the microsomal fraction of the hepatocyte was provided by the morphologic observation that in rats, ethanol feeding results in a proliferation of the SER (Iseri *et al.* 1964, 1966; Lane and Lieber 1966). This increase in SER resembles that seen after the administration of a wide variety of hepatotoxins (Meldolesi 1967), therapeutic agents (Conney 1967) and food additives (Lane and Lieber 1967). Since most of the substances that induce a proliferation of the SER are metabolized, at least in part, by the cytochrome P450 enzyme system that is located on the SER, the possibility that ethanol may also be metabolized by enzymes was raised. Such a system has been demonstrated in liver microsomes *in vitro* and found to be inducible by chronic ethanol feeding *in vivo* (Lieber and DeCarli 1968) and was named the microsomal ethanol oxidizing system (MEOS) (Lieber and DeCarli 1968, 1970). It was concluded that the

MEOS was distinct from both ADH and catalase, and was dependent on cytochrome P450 because of (1) isolation of a P450-containing fraction from liver microsomes, which although devoid of any ADH or catalase activity, could oxidize alcohol as well as higher aliphatic alcohols (e.g. butanol which is not a substrate for catalase) (Teschke *et al.* 1972, 1974) and (2) the reconstitution of ethanol-oxidizing activity using NADPH-cytochrome P450 reductase, phospholipid and either partially purified or highly purified microsomal P450 from untreated (Ohnishi and Lieber 1977) or phenobarbital-treated (Miwa *et al.* 1978) rats. Chronic ethanol consumption results in the induction of a unique P450, as shown by Ohnishi and Lieber (1977) using a liver microsomal P450 fraction isolated from ethanol-treated rats. An ethanol-inducible form of P450 (LM3a), purified from rabbit liver microsomes (Koop *et al.* 1982), catalysed alcohol oxidation at rates much higher than other P450 isozymes, and also had an enhanced capacity to oxidize 1-butanol, 1-pentanol and aniline (Morgan *et al.* 1982), acetaminophen (Morgan *et al.* 1983), carbon tetrachloride (CCl_4) (Morgan *et al.* 1983), acetone (Ingelman-Sundberg and Johansson 1984; Koop and Casazza 1985) and *N*-nitrosodimethylamine (Yang *et al.* 1985). Similar results have been obtained with cytochrome P450j, a major hepatic P450 isozyme purified from alcohol- or isoniazid-treated rats (Ryan *et al.* 1985, 1986). Others have also provided evidence for the existence of a P450j-like isozyme in humans (Song *et al.* 1986; Wrighton *et al.* 1986). Subsequently, a purified human protein (now called CYP2E1) was obtained in a catalytically active form, with a high turnover rate for ethanol and other specific substrates (Lasker *et al.* 1987). Using antibodies against this CYP2E1, and the Western blot technique, a 5- to 10-fold induction was found in biopsies of recently drinking subjects (Tsutsumi *et al.* 1989), see Fig. 2.2. Compounds other than ethanol (e.g. acetone) can also serve as CYP2E1 inducers, but it has been shown in rats that the activity of CYP2E1 can be induced by ethanol, even in the absence of acetonaemia or hepatic steatosis (Lieber *et al.* 1988). In monkey livers, a mRNA was isolated having 92–94 percent homology of the deduced amino acid sequence of human CYP2E1, if induced by either 3-methylcholanthrene or PCB (Komori *et al.* 1992). The mechanisms for the increase in CYP2E1 after chronic ethanol consumption are still the subject of debate, and include increased enzyme synthesis (Tsutsumi *et al.* 1993) and decreased enzyme degradation. Research with a

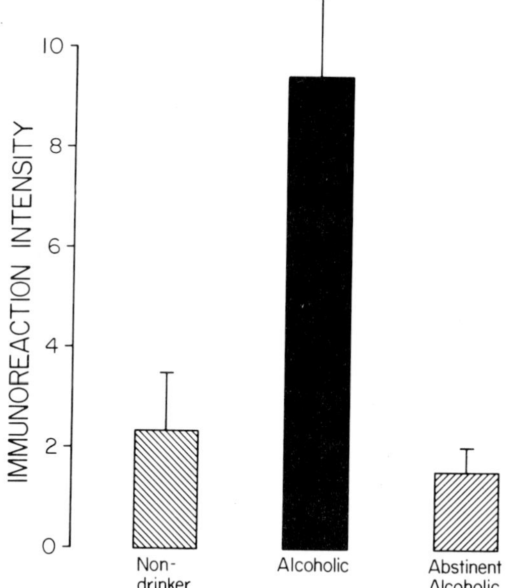

Fig. 2.2   Hepatic CYP2E1 levels in alcoholics and non-drinkers. CYP2E1 was quantitated by scanning of Western blots of percutaneous liver biopsies, using anti-CYP2E1 antibodies. Data from Tsutumi *et al.* (1989).

CYP2E1 cDNA probe indicated that CYP2E1 protein induction by "ethanol-like" agents may be regulated by post-translational events (Song *et al.* 1986), whereas other studies showed an increase in translatable CYP2E1 mRNA following treatment with ethanol in hamsters (Kubota *et al.* 1988) and in humans (Takahashi *et al.* 1993).

MEOS has a relatively high K_m for ethanol (8–10 mM compared with 0.2–2 mM for ADH) and thus normally ADH accounts for the bulk of ethanol oxidation at low blood ethanol levels (Fig. 2.3A), but not necessarily at high ethanol levels (Fig. 2.3B), especially during long-term use of alcohol (Fig. 2.3C), in view of the inducibility of the MEOS (Lieber and DeCarli 1968, 1970). Although data obtained with inhibitors are suggestive of MEOS involvement (Lieber and DeCarli 1970, 1972; Teschke *et al.* 1976; Matsuzaki *et al.* 1981), they cannot be considered conclusive, since the inhibitors are not sufficiently specific. However, increasing ethanol metabolism with rising ethanol concentrations was found not only in the presence of an ADH inhibitor but also in its absence, in isolated hepatocytes (Matsuzaki and Lieber 1975; Matsuzaki *et al.* 1981), in isolated perfused livers (Gordon 1968) and *in vivo* in man (Lereboullet *et al.* 1976; Feinman *et al.* 1978; Salaspuro and Lieber 1977,

1978), in rats (Feinman *et al.* 1978) and baboons (Salaspuro and Lieber 1977, 1978; Pikkarainen and Lieber 1980).

The fact that ethanol metabolism increases with rising ethanol concentrations well above the level needed to fully saturate the low K_m ADH suggests the involvement of a non-ADH pathway, at least in a species such as the rat devoid of the anodic high K_m ADH active with alcohol. Moreover, the acceleration of ethanol metabolism at higher ethanol concentrations explains that the disappearance of ethanol from the blood is not linear at high ethanol concentrations that fully saturate the ADH pathway (Lereboullet *et al.* 1976; Feinman *et al.* 1978; Salaspuro and Lieber 1977, 1978). Kinetic analysis *in vivo* indicated that ethanol elimination is best described by a two-compartment open model with parallel first-order and Michaelis-Menten elimination kinetics. The dose-dependency of the elimination rate was attributed to contributions of the ADH pathway at lower blood ethanol concentrations and of non-ADH first-order elimination pathways at higher blood ethanol concentrations (Fujimiya *et al.* 1989). The contribution of the first-order pathway increased with increases in the blood ethanol concentration and even exceeded that of the ADH pathway above 4.5 mg/ml of blood ethanol concentration. Finally, a mutant deermouse strain that lacks the hepatic low K_m ADH (ADH$^-$) nevertheless actively oxidizes ethanol (Burnett and Felder 1980; Shigeta *et al.* 1984; Alderman *et al.* 1987; Kato *et al.* 1987 a, b, 1988), and studies with stable isotopes indicated that this effect is mediated principally by the MEOS (Alderman *et al.* 1987). When ethanol is given parenterally, the MEOS rather than gastric ADH is the major pathway of ethanol oxidation in ADH$^-$ deermice, while both pathways contribute significantly to the metabolism of orally administered ethanol (Ito and Lieber 1993).

Role of catalase

Catalase is capable of oxidizing ethanol *in vitro* in the presence of an H_2O_2-generating system (Keilin and Hartree 1945), see Fig. 2.1. However, under physiologic conditions, catalase appears to play no major role and cannot account quantitatively for the ADH-independent pathway of ethanol metabolism. It is noteworthy that most patients with acatalasaemia are also asymptomatic (Moser and Moser 1992).

The catalase contribution might be enhanced if

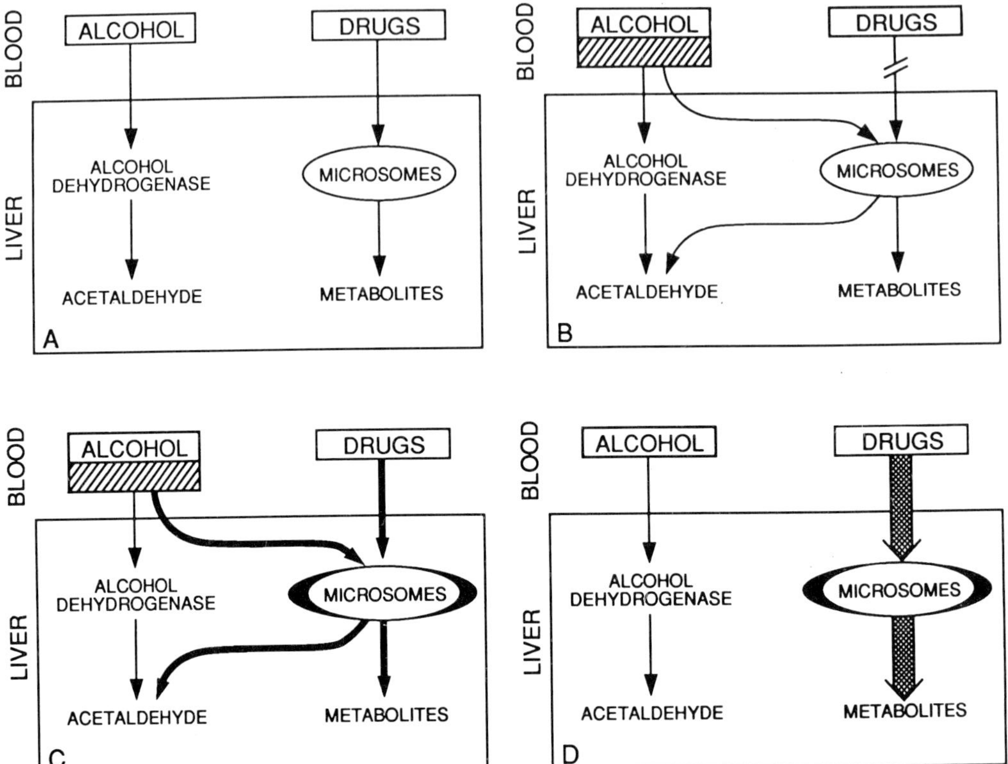

Fig. 2.3 Alcohol is metabolized by alcohol dehydrogenase, and drugs by microsomes (A). Microsomal drug metabolism is inhibited in the presence of high concentrations of ethanol, in part through competition for a common microsomal detoxification process (B). Microsomal induction after long-term alcohol consumption contributes to accelerated alcohol metabolism at high blood ethanol levels (C). Increased drug metabolism and activation of xenobiotics (due to microsomal induction) persist after cessation of long-term alcohol consumption (D). Hatching indicates high blood alcohol levels. Reproduced with permission from Lieber (1988).

significant amounts of H_2O_2 become available through β-oxidation of fatty acids such as octanoate, palmitate and oleate in peroxisomes (Handler and Thurman 1985). However, the peroxisomal enzymes do not oxidize short chain fatty acids such as octanoate and this phenomenon was observed only in the absence of ADH activity. Otherwise, the rate of ethanol metabolism is reduced by adding fatty acids (Williamson *et al.* 1969), and β-oxidation of fatty acids is inhibited by NADH produced from ethanol metabolism via ADH (Williamson *et al.* 1969). Similarly, the generation of reducing equivalents from ethanol by ADH in the cytosol inhibits H_2O_2 generation leading to significantly diminished rates of peroxidation of alcohols via catalase (Handler and Thurman 1990). Various other results have also indicated that peroxisomal fatty acid oxidation does not play a major role in ethanol metabolism (Inatomi *et al.* 1989). Furthermore, when

fatty acids were used by Handler and Thurman (1985) to stimulate alcohol oxidation, this effect was very sensitive to inhibition by aminotriazole, a catalase inhibitor. Therefore, if this mechanism were to play an important role *in vivo*, one would expect a significant inhibition of ethanol metabolism after aminotriazole administration *in vivo*, when physiologic amounts of fatty acids and other substrates for H_2O_2 generation are present. A number of studies, however, have shown that aminotriazole treatment has little, if any, effect on ethanol oxidation *in vivo*. Takagi *et al.* (1986) and Kato *et al.* (1987 a, b), have confirmed this relative lack of effect of aminotriazole on ethanol metabolism *in vivo*, while verifying its inhibitory effect on catalase-mediated ethanol peroxidation *in vitro*. Despite the considerable controversy that originally surrounded this issue, it is now agreed by the principal contenders involved that catalase cannot account for microsomal ethanol oxidation (Thurman and Brentzel 1977; Teschke *et al.* 1977).

Non-oxidative metabolism

The possible pathogenic role of a non-oxidative pathway of ethanol metabolism to form fatty acid ethyl esters was raised by Laposata and Lange (1986). The capacity of ethanol to form ethyl esters *in vivo* had been demonstrated by Goodman and Deykin (1963) and also by Lange (1982), who purified the enzyme (Mogelson and Lange 1984). Laposata and Lange (1986) found that in acutely intoxicated subjects, concentrations of fatty acid ethyl esters were significantly higher than in controls in pancreas, liver, heart and adipose tissue. Since this non-oxidative ethanol metabolism occurs in humans in the organs most commonly injured by alcohol abuse, and since some of these organs lack oxidative ethanol metabolism, Laposata and Lange (1986) postulated that fatty acid ethyl esters may have a role in the production of alcohol-induced injury. Further experiments are needed to verify this interesting hypothesis.

Alteration in metabolism of ethanol after chronic ethanol consumption

Regular drinkers tolerate large amounts of alcoholic beverages, mainly because of central nervous system adaptation, but also because of increased rates of blood alcohol clearance, that is metabolic tolerance (Kater *et al.* 1969; Ugarte *et al.* 1972).

ADH-related ethanol metabolism
ADH activity does not increase after chronic ethanol feeding; in fact, in some studies, there was actually a decrease in ADH activity in the liver (Lieber and DeCarli 1970; Brighenti and Pancaldi 1970; Salaspuro *et al.* 1981), and alcoholics may display decreased hepatic ADH activity in the presence (Zorzano *et al.* 1989) or even in the absence (Ugarte *et al.* 1967) of liver damage.

One mechanism that could contribute to the acceleration of ADH-dependent metabolism after chronic ethanol consumption involves enhanced ATPase activity (Bernstein *et al.* 1973) and the creation of a hypermetabolic state akin to hyperthy-

roidism (Israel *et al.* 1975; Bernstein *et al.* 1973). Oxygen consumption was also found to be increased in the livers of animals chronically treated with ethanol (Israel *et al.* 1973; Bernstein *et al.* 1973; Thurman *et al.* 1976), mimicking the effects of thyroxine (see also Chapter 19). It was proposed that this hypermetabolic state may in some aspects be similar to that found in the livers of animals treated with thyroid hormones, in which the hypermetabolic state appears to be associated with an increased hydrolysis of ATP by the Na^+-K^+-ATPase system (Ismail-Beigi and Edelman 1970, 1971) and a resulting lowering of the phosphorylation potential. Israel *et al.* (1975) used a low-fat diet in association with alcohol administration. Under the conditions used in this study, ethanol consumption did not result in liver changes comparable to those seen in human alcoholic liver injury, for example no fatty liver was observed. In contrast, under conditions that mimic the clinical situation with the development of fatty liver, chronic ethanol consumption was not found to be associated with increased ATPase activity (Gordon 1977).

Non-ADH-related acceleration of ethanol metabolism
Following chronic ethanol consumption, MEOS significantly increases in activity; the rise in MEOS activity might account for all of the increases in ethanol metabolism of hepatocytes isolated from ADH^- deermice (Alderman *et al.* 1989) and for a major fraction of the increase in blood ethanol clearance *in vivo* (Lieber and DeCarli 1972). That chronic ethanol feeding results in an increased activity of a non-ADH and non-catalase pathway in the liver was also shown in studies of liver microsomes, liver slices and in isolated hepatocytes. Ethanol oxidation was enhanced in isolated liver tissue by increasing the alcohol concentration employed *in vitro* from 10 to 30 mM. Of particular interest was the observation that this phenomenon was more pronounced in ethanol-fed rats than in their pair-fed controls (Teschke *et al.* 1977). To test whether or not MEOS is involved in this adaptive increase, ADH and catalase activities were inhibited by pyrazole and sodium azide, respectively. The activity of the non-ADH and non-catalase pathway was significantly higher in ethanol-fed rats than in controls. In addition, the difference between the two groups was more striking at 30 mM than at 10 mM. Similarly, when a relatively constant blood ethanol level is maintained through continuous infusion in the baboon, the acceleration of ethanol metabolism with

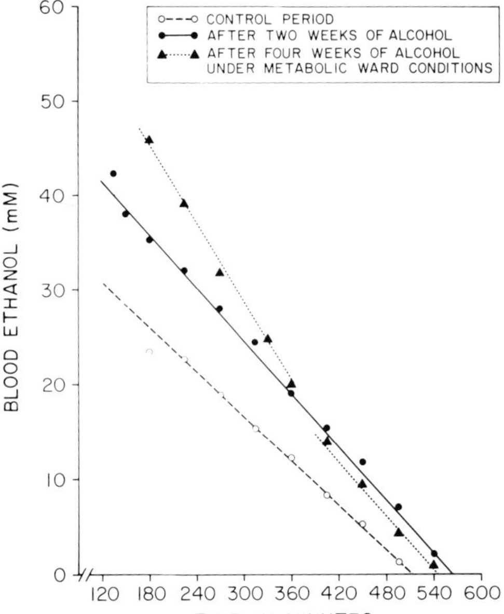

Fig. 2.4 The effect of chronic ethanol consumption on the blood ethanol elimination curve in a human volunteer. The dose of ethanol administration was 1.0 g/kg in the first experiment, 1.3 g/kg after 2 weeks of ethanol and 1.5 g/kg after 4 weeks of ethanol. Reproduced with permission from Salaspuro and Lieber (1978).

higher blood levels was more pronounced in ethanol-fed than in control animals (Pikkarainen and Lieber 1980). All these data indicate that a non-ADH pathway, most likely MEOS, represents a major mechanism for the acceleration of ethanol metabolism at high alcohol concentrations. A similar change was shown in human volunteers: alcohol consumption resulted in a progressive acceleration of blood alcohol clearance, particularly at high alcohol concentrations (Salaspuro and Lieber 1978) (Fig. 2.4).

Interactions of ethanol with drugs, other xenobiotics and vitamin A

Effects of other drugs on ethanol metabolism

The interaction of drugs such as phenobarbital with ethanol metabolism is complex. In addition to affecting liver weight and liver blood flow, barbiturates increase total hepatic MEOS activity (Lieber and DeCarli 1970) and enhance rates of blood ethanol clearance (Lieber and DeCarli 1970; Mezey and Robles 1974; Ruebner *et al.* 1975). Diabetics display accelerated ethanol metabolism in association with tolbutamide treatment (Carulli *et al.* 1971). Pretreatment with these drugs may accelerate ethanol metabolism, whereas the presence of the drug may have an inhibitory effect. Psychotropic medications such as chlorpromazine also influence serum ethanol concentrations by inhibiting ADH (Messiha 1980). Isoniazid may have a similar effect (Whitehouse *et al.* 1980). The mean ethanol elimination rate and mean blood acetate concentration were increased significantly after acute intake of glucocorticoids in healthy male students (Korri 1990).

In general, the drug effects are rather moderate; fructose is the only compound that produces a significant acceleration of ethanol metabolism via the ADH pathway (Lundquist and Wolthers 1958; Brown *et al.* 1972), and its effect is completely abolished by pyrazole (Berry 1971). In view of the extent of the fructose effect and the potential hepatotoxicity of the compound (Bode *et al.* 1973), its use is not recommended. Fructose solutions were not superior to placebo in alcohol detoxification (Iber 1987). Experimentally, oxygenation of the drinking water has been reported to accelerate ethanol elimination by 60 percent (Hyvarinen *et al.* 1978). By contrast, oxygen breathing was ineffective (Kinard *et al.* 1951). According to others, oxygen breathing (Larsen 1968) and increasing oxygen pressure (Mattie 1963) even slightly depressed rates of ethanol oxidation.

Effects of ethanol on other drugs and chemicals

Ethanol administration to volunteers under metabolic ward conditions resulted in a striking increase in the rate of blood clearance of meprobamate and pentobarbital (Misra *et al.* 1971). Similarly, increases in the metabolism of warfarin, phenytoin, tolbutamide, propranolol and rifampin have been linked to long-term ethanol consumption (Kater *et al.* 1969; Pritchard and Schneck 1977). The metabolic drug tolerance persists several days to weeks after the cessation of alcohol abuse, and the duration of recovery varies with each drug (Hetu and Joly 1985).

In contrast with the induction effect of the long-term consumption of ethanol, after short-term administration, inhibition of the hepatic metab-

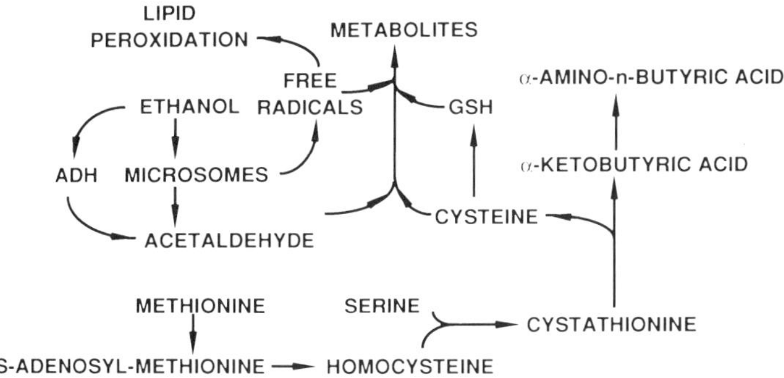

Fig. 2.5   Possible link between microsomal induction, enhanced free radical and acetaldehyde production, glutathione depletion and lipid peroxidation after chronic ethanol consumption.

olism of some drugs (e.g. methadone, tranquillizers and barbiturates) is seen (Lieber 1992) (Fig. 2.3B). These effects may be of clinical relevance, since approximately 50 percent of patients taking methadone are also alcohol abusers. One major mechanism of interaction is direct competition for a common metabolic process involving cytochrome P450, while another is competition for ADH (Lieber 1992). Ethanol can inhibit methanol metabolism, as increased blood methanol levels (from endogenous origin and/or derived from congeners) have been observed in alcoholics during detoxification (Roine *et al.* 1989; Jones and Sternebring 1992).

Aggravation of hepatotoxicity through enhanced ethanol metabolism

The proliferation of SER that results from chronic ethanol consumption in animals and humans (Iseri *et al.* 1966; Lane and Lieber 1966) is thought to be "adaptive", since it is associated with enhanced activity of the microsomal enzymes ("induction"). These enzymes are involved in liproprotein production, and thus enzyme induction may contribute to the increased capacity of the liver to secrete fat, as lipoproteins, into the bloodstream (Baraona *et al.* 1975) and to attenuate fat accumulation. A concomitant increase in drug metabolizing enzymes explains the enhanced metabolic tolerance of patients with alcoholism to a variety of drugs (*vide supra*).

Some injurious consequences may also ensue. Indeed, accelerated ethanol metabolism results in the enhanced production of acetaldehyde and exacerbation of its various toxic manifestations as illustrated in Fig. 2.1 and discussed in detail elsewhere.

The binding of acetaldehyde with cysteine or glutathione or both may contribute to a depression of liver glutathione (Shaw *et al.* 1981). In addition, rats chronically fed ethanol had significantly

increased rates of glutathione turnover without an increased oxidation (Vendemiale *et al.* 1984; Morton and Mitchell 1985). Acute ethanol administration inhibited glutathione synthesis and produced an increased loss from the liver (Speisky *et al.* 1985). Glutathione transferase activity (Kocak-Toker *et al.* 1985) was decreased by acute ethanol administration, and glutathione peroxidase after chronic treatment (Morton and Mitchell 1985). Glutathione offers one of the mechanisms for the scavenging of toxic free radicals (Fig. 2.5). Consistent with the increased glutathione turnover is the observation of a significant increase in alpha-aminobutyric acid (Fig. 2.5) after ethanol administration both in humans and in the baboon (Shaw and Lieber 1980). Although glutathione depletion is not necessarily sufficient to cause lipid peroxidation, it is generally agreed that it may favour the peroxidation produced by other factors. Glutathione is important in the protection of cells against electrophilic drug injury in general, and against reactive oxygen species in particular. Although it may not be an efficient antioxidant when acting alone, it has been shown to spare and potentiate vitamin E (Barclay 1988; see also Chapters 8 and 16).

Experimentally, glutathione depletion could in part be corrected, by the administration of the active form of methionine, namely *S*-adenosyl-L-methionine (Lieber *et al.* 1990), with an associated attenuation of hepatotoxicity of ethanol, as evidenced by a decreased leakage of hepatic enzymes into the bloodstream, including glutamic dehydrogenase, a mitochondrial enzyme. The toxic effect of acetaldehyde may also include enhanced peroxidation (Fig. 2.5). Increased microsomal activity may also enhance the oxygen requirements, as described in Chapter 8, thereby aggravating whatever hypoxia may be present.

Increased xenobiotic toxicity and carcinogenicity: Interactions with vitamin A

On occasion, the metabolites produced in the microsomes are more toxic than the precursor compound and, therefore, the induction produced by ethanol augments the toxicity of a number of agents. This pertains in particular to those substrates for which the ethanol-inducible CYP2E1, when compared with other P450s, displays an enhanced capacity for conversion to hepatotoxic metabolites. Indeed, much of the medical significance of MEOS and the ethanol-inducible CYP2E1 results not only from the oxidation of ethanol but also from the unusual and unique capacity of CYP2E1 to activate many xenobiotic compounds to toxic metabolites. This pertains, for instance, to carbon tetrachloride (CCl_4). It is known that CCl_4 exerts its toxicity after conversion to an active compound in the microsomes, and ethanol pre-treatment stimulates the toxicity of CCl_4 (Hasumura *et al.* 1974), with perivenular predominance, which can be explained by the selective presence and induction of CYP2E1 (Tsutsumi *et al.* 1989; Castillo *et al.* 1992; Takahashi *et al.* 1993; see also Chapter 16). Other organic compounds such as anaesthetics and industrial solvents – for example, benzene (Nakajima *et al.* 1987; Ingelman-Sundberg and Johansson 1984), bromobenzene (Hetu *et al.* 1983) and vinylidene chloride (Siegers *et al.* 1983) – also display a selective injurious action in association with chronic ethanol ingestion. Hepatic microsomal enflurane defluorination increases 10.5-fold 1 h after cessation of chronic treatment (Pantuck *et al.* 1985), and enflurane toxicity is increased (Tsutsumi *et al.* 1990). Animals pre-treated with ethanol develop potentiated zone 3 necrosis on exposure to halothane, especially when metabolism is rendered reductive (Takagi *et al.* 1983). It is noteworthy that halothane can be metabolized by various microsomal cytochrome P450s, including CYP2E1 (Gruenke *et al.* 1988).

Enhanced metabolism (and toxicity) pertains also to a variety of prescribed drugs, for example phenylbutazone (Beskid *et al.* 1980), and some "over the counter" medications, for example acetaminophen (paracetamol, *N*-acetyl-aminophenol) (Altomare *et al.* 1984a, b; see Chapter 16).

There is an association between ethanol abuse and an increased incidence of upper alimentary and respiratory tract cancers (Lieber *et al.* 1986). Many factors have been incriminated, including the effect of ethanol on the cytochrome P450-dependent activation of carcinogens (Garro and Lieber, 1990), and depressed hepatic levels of vitamin A, which were observed even when ethanol was given with diets containing large amounts of vitamin A (Sato and Lieber 1981). New hepatic enzyme pathways of retinol metabolism, inducible by either ethanol or drug administration, have been discovered (Leo and Lieber 1983; Leo *et al.* 1987). Hepatic vitamin A depletion is associated with lysosomal lesions (Leo *et al.* 1983) and decreased detoxification of NDMA (Leo *et al.* 1986). Although vitamin A deficiency might adversely affect the liver (Leo *et al.* 1983), an excess of vitamin A is also known to be hepatotoxic (Leo and Lieber 1988). Long-term ethanol consumption enhances this effect, resulting in striking morphologic and functional alterations of the mitochondria (Leo *et al.* 1982), along with hepatic necrosis and fibrosis (Leo and Lieber 1983). Hypervitaminosis A itself can induce fibrosis and even cirrhosis, as reviewed elsewhere (Leo and Lieber 1988; see also Chapter 16). Unlike retinoids, for which the case for interactive hepatotoxicity is well-established, the case for the possible interaction between β-carotene and liver disease, alcohol and/or drugs is virtually uncharted but cannot be excluded, since in subhuman primates enhanced toxicity of β-carotene has been observed in the presence of ethanol (Leo *et al.* 1992). Thus caution must also be exercised with β-carotene, in view of the possible existence of a defect in utilization and/or excretion associated with liver injury and/or alcohol abuse (Leo *et al.* 1993; Ahmed *et al.* 1994).

Effects of liver disease, circadian rhythm and other factors on ethanol metabolism

As discussed earlier, chronic ethanol consumption is associated with an increased rate of ethanol disappearance from the blood. In the presence of severe alcoholic liver disease, this acceleration vanishes, and on occasion there may be an actual reduction in blood alcohol clearance. This occurs, however, only with very severe liver disease shown to be associated with reduced liver ADH (Dow *et al.* 1975). In patients with cirrhosis, the rate of alcohol metabolism may be normal (Dacruz *et al.* 1975). In addition to the activity of the ethanol-metabolizing enzymes, the total hepatic mass is an important parameter which is not often measurable. Other key factors in ethanol metabolism *in vivo* include the availability of cofactors, and the capacity of the liver to dispose of the metabolic products (NADH and acetaldehyde). In addition to activation of MEOS, high ethanol concentrations diminish ADH activity (substrate inhibition) (Theorell *et al.* 1955; von Wartburg *et al.* 1964).

Another factor that is difficult to assess is that of *blood flow* (see Chapters 14 and 15). Chronic ethanol consumption tends to increase hepatic blood flow (Lieber *et al.* 1988). Acutely, the results depend on the dose used, some investigations showing no effect or even a decrease, whereas most studies have reported an increase as discussed elsewhere (Lieber 1992). The increase in portal blood flow after ethanol administration was attributed to a preportal vasodilatory effect of adenosine formed from acetate metabolism in extrahepatic tissues (Carmichael *et al.* 1988). In general, when unchanged or decreased flow was observed, this was associated with low blood ethanol levels. Conflicting reports on the effects of ethanol on hepatic haemodynamics may be related to the dose of alcohol administered (Jenkins *et al.* 1986). Such experiments are difficult to control, especially since very large doses of alcohol may also produce hypothermia (Nikki *et al.* 1971). Hypothermia, in turn, has been found to result in both a decrease in liver blood flow (Brauer *et al.* 1959) and a slowing of ethanol metabolism (Larsen 1971; Krarup and Larsen 1972).

Most studies also fail to mention the time of day that the experiments were carried out. Such information is important, in view of the *circadian variation* of ethanol metabolism (Wilson *et al.* 1956; Sturtevant *et al.* 1976; Pinkston and Soliman, 1979), which is particularly manifested and perhaps even altered in the alcoholic (Jones and Paredes 1974). Stress associated with the experimental conditions is rarely described, but it may significantly affect ethanol metabolism (Mezey *et al.* 1979).

Metabolic and forensic implications

Increased tolerance to alcohol is a key feature of chronic alcohol abuse (*vide supra*). However, at late stages, the development of severe liver disease may offset the adaptive increase in ethanol metabolism. Moreover, malnutrition, through the decrease in the activities of the ADH pathway, may also counteract the metabolic tolerance. The demonstration that the metabolic tolerance involves increased activity of the MEOS has a number of practical implications, which include the profound consequences on hormone and drug metabolism, the promotion of liver injury through enhanced activation of potentially toxic compounds and the increased generation of hepatotoxic metabolites of ethanol such as acetaldehyde (see Chapters 5 and 6). The energy wastage related to the activity of microsomal systems will be reviewed in Chapter 8.

Another consequence of the metabolic tolerance to ethanol pertains to forensic medicine. Because of the activity of the microsomal system, which has a higher K_m (8–10 mM or 37–46 mg/100 ml) than the bulk of hepatic ADH (K_m of 0.5–1.0 mM), the rate of ethanol disappearance from the bloodstream is significantly greater at higher than at lower ethanol concentrations. This is particularly evident after chronic ethanol consumption (Fig. 2.4). The observation of an acceleration of ethanol disappearance from the blood at high ethanol concentrations is of particular significance for the medico-legal application of blood alcohol measurements. Heretofore, a common procedure to determine retrospectively blood alcohol concentrations at any given time was to extrapolate linearly from a subsequent determination based on the assumption of a standard rate of metabolism. In view of the findings of the non-linear disappearance of ethanol and the adaptive increase after chronic consumption, conventional calculations should be applied with caution.

Summary

Ethanol oxidation, once thought to be a simple, one enzyme-mediated reaction, has now been shown to be a complex process affected by a variety of enzyme systems, nutritional status, the presence of liver disease, genetic factors and prior history of alcohol and drug use. Advances in our knowledge of hepatic metabolism of ethanol enable us to understand a number of metabolic alterations associated with the oxidation of alcohol that develop in the alcoholic. We have also gained better insight into various consequences of chronic ethanol consumption, including the metabolic tolerance to alcohol that develops in the alcoholic. The acceleration of blood ethanol clearance after chronic ethanol consumption is highest at high ethanol blood levels, which may have some forensic importance. The acute and chronic interactions between ethanol and drug metabolism are now better understood on the basis of the existence of an inducible non-ADH pathway of ethanol metabolism, namely the MEOS, involving a unique cytochrome P450, namely CYP2E1. In view of its relatively high K_m, MEOS is particularly active at high blood ethanol concentrations, and its role is greatest when induced by chronic ethanol consumption.

Acknowledgements

Original studies cited were supported, in part, by the Department of Veterans Affairs and DHHS Grants AA03508, AA07802, AA09479, AA05934 and AA07275. We thank Ms R. Cabell for skilfully typing the manuscript.

References

Ahmed, S., Leo, M.A. and Lieber, C.S. (1994). Interactions between alcohol and β-carotene in patients with alcoholic liver disease. *American Journal of Clinical Nutrition* **60**, 430–436.

Alderman, J., Takagi, T. and Lieber, C.S. (1987). Ethanol metabolizing pathways in deermice: Estimation of flux calculated from isotope effects. *Journal of Biological Chemistry* **262**, 7497–7503.

Alderman, J., Kato, S. and Lieber, C.S. (1989). The microsomal ethanol oxidizing system mediates metabolic tolerance to ethanol in deermice lacking alcohol dehydrogenase. *Archives of Biochemistry and Biophysics* **27**, 33–39.

Altomare, E., Leo, M.A. and Lieber, C.S. (1984a). Interaction of acute ethanol administration with acetaminophen metabolism and toxicity in rats fed alcohol chronically. *Alcoholism: Clinical and Experimental Research* **8**, 405–408.

Altomare, E., Leo, M.A., Sato, C., Vendemiale, G. and Lieber, C.S. (1984b). Interaction of ethanol with acetaminophen metabolism in the baboon. *Biochemical Pharmacology* **33**, 2207–2212.

Baraona, E., Pirola, R.C. and Lieber, C.S. (1975). Acute and chronic effects of ethanol on intestinal lipid metabolism. *Biochimica et Biophysica Acta* **388**, 19–28.

Baraona, E., Yokoyama, A., Ishii, H., Hernandez-Munoz, R., Takagi, T., Tsuchiya, M. and Lieber, C.S. (1991). Lack of alcohol dehydrogenase isoenzyme activities in the stomach of Japanese subjects. *Life Science* **49**, 1929–1934.

Barclay, L.R. (1988). The cooperative antioxidant role of glutathione with a lipid-soluble and a water-soluble antioxidant during peroxidation of liposomes initiated in the aqueous phase and in the lipid phase. *Journal of Biological Chemistry* **263**, 16138–16142.

Bernstein, J., Videla, L. and Israel, Y. (1973). Metabolic alterations produced in liver by chronic ethanol administration: Changes related to energetic parameters of the cell. *Biochemical Journal* **134**, 515–522.

Bernstein, J., Basillo, C. and Martinez, B. (1990). Ethanol sulfation by the pulmonary ethanol metabolizing system (PET). *Research Communications in Chemical Pathology and Pharmacology* **68**, 219–234.

Berres, H.H., Goslar, H.G. and Jaeger, K.H. (1970). Morphologische und histochemische Veranderungen in der Leber nach einmaliger Alkoholbelastung und nach Versuchen ihrer Beeinflussung. *Acta Histochemica* **35**, 173–185.

Berry, M.N. (1971). Effects of microsomal-metabolized drugs (MMD) on oxidation of ethanol, sorbitol or glycerol in rat. *Clinical Research* **19**, 471.

Beskid, M., Bialck, J., Dzieniszewski, J., Sadowski, J. and Tlalka, J. (1980). Effect of combined phenylbutazone and ethanol administration on rat liver. *Experimental Pathology* **18**, 487–491.

Bode, Ch., Goebell, H. and Stahler, M. (1970). Anderungen der Alkoholdehydrogenase Aktivitat in der Rattenleber durch Eiweissmangel und Athanol. *Zeitschrift fur die Gesamte Innere Medizin und Ihre Grenzgebiete* **152**, 111–124.

Bode, Ch., Buchwald, B. and Goebell, H. (1971). Inhibtion of ethanol breakdown due to protein deficiency in man. *German Medical Monthly* **1**, 149–151.

Bode, J.C. and Thiele, D. (1975). Hemmung des Athanolabbaus beim Menschen durch Fasten: Reversibilitat durch Fructose-Infusion. *Deutsche Medizinishe Wochenschrift* **100**, 1849–1851.

Bode, J.C., Bode, Ch., Rumpelt, H.J. and Zelder, O. (1973). Loss of hepatic adenosine phosphates and metabolic consequences following fructose or sorbitol administration in man and in the rat. In *Regulation of Hepatic Metabolism* (Edited by Lundquist, F. and Tygstrup, N.), pp. 267–284. Adademic Press, New York.

Bond, S.L. and Singh, S.M. (1990). Studies with cDNA probes on the *in vivo* effect of ethanol on expression of the genes of alcohol metabolism. *Alcohol and Alcoholism* **25**, 385–394.

Bosron, W.F., Li, T.-K., Dafeldecker, W.P. and Vallee, B.L. (1979). Human liver alcohol dehydrogenase: Kinetic and molecular properties. *Biochemistry* **18**, 1101–1105.

Bosron, W.F., Magnes, L.J. and Li, T.-K. (1983). Human liver alcohol dehydrogenase: ADH Indianapolis results from genetic polymorphism at the ADH2 gene locus. *Biochemical Genetics* **21**, 735–744.

Bosron, W.F., Ehrig, T. and Li, T.-K. (1993). Genetic factors in alcohol metabolism and alcoholism. *Seminars in Liver Disease* **13**, 126–135

Brauer, R.W., Holloway, R.J., Krebs, J.S. *et al.* (1959). The liver in hypothermia. *Annals of the New York Academy of Science* **80**, 395–423.

Brighenti, L. and Pancaldi, G. (1970). Effetto della somministrazione di alcool etilico su alcune attivita enzimatiche del fegato di ratto. *Bollettino – Societa Italiana Biologia Sperimentale* **46**, 1–5.

Brown, S.S., Forrest, J.A.H. and Roscoe, P. (1972). A controlled trial of fructose in the treatment of acute alcoholic intoxication. *Lancet* **ii**, 898–900.

Buehler, R., Hess. M. and von Wartburg. J.-P. (1982). Immunohistochemical localization of human liver alcohol dehydrogenase in liver tissue, cultured fibroblasts and hela cells. *American Journal of Pathology* **108**, 89–99.

Burnett, K.G. and Felder, M.R. (1980). Ethanol metabolism in peromyscus genetically deficient in alcohol dehydrogenase. *Biochemical Pharmacology* **28**, 1–8.

Caballeria, J., Frezza, M., Hernandez-Munoz, R., DiPadova, C., Korsten, M.A., Baraona, E. and Lieber, C.S. (1989a). The gastric origin of the first pass metabolism of ethanol in man: Effect of gastrectomy. *Gastroenterology* **97**, 1205–1209

Caballeria, J., Baraona, E., Rodamilans, M. and Lieber, C.S. (1989b). Effects of cimetidine on gastric alcohol dehydrogenase activity and blood ethanol levels. *Gastroenterology* **96**, 388–392.

Caballeria, J., Baraona, E., Deulofeu, R., Hernandez-Munoz, R., Rodes, J. and Lieber, C.S. (1991). Effects of H$_2$-receptor antagonists on gastric alcohol dehydrogenase activity. *Digestive Diseases and Sciences* **36**, 1673–1697.

Carmichael, F.J., Saldivida, V., Varghese, G.A., Israel, Y. and Orrego, H. (1988). Ethanol-induced increase in portal blood flow role of acetate and A$_1$- and A$_2$-adenosine receptors. *American Journal of Physiology* **255**, G417-G423.

Carulli, N., Manenti, F., Gallo, M. and Salviolli, G.F. (1971). Alcohol-drugs interaction in man: Alcohol and tolbutamide. *European Journal of Clinical Investigation* **1**, 421–424.

Castillo, T., Koop, D.R., Kamimura, S., Triadafilopoulos, G. and Tsukamoto, H. (1992). Role of cytochrome P-450 2E1 in ethanol-, carbon tetrachloride- and iron-dependent microsomal lipid peroxidation. *Hepatology* **16**, 992–996.

Chen, L., Sidner, R.A. and Lumeng, L. (1992). Distribution of alcohol dehydrogenase and the low K_m form of aldehyde dehydrogenase in isolated perivenous and periportal hepatocytes in rats. *Alcoholism: Clinical and Experimental Research* **16**, 23–29.

Conney, A.H. (1967). Pharmacological implications of microsomal enzyme induction. *Pharmacology Review* **19**, 317–366.

Cronholm, T., Jones, W.A. and Skagerberg, S. (1988). Mechanism and regulation of ethanol elimination in humans: Intermolecular hydrogen transfer and oxidoreduction *in vivo*. *Alcoholism: Clinical and Experimental Research* **12**, 683–686.

Crow, K.E., Cornell, N.W. and Veech, R.L. (1977). The rate of ethanol metabolism in isolated rat hepatocytes. *Alcoholism: Clinical and Experimental Research* **1**, 43–47.

Dacruz, A.G., Correia, J.P. and Menezes, L. (1975). Ethanol metabolism in liver cirrhosis and chronic alcoholism. *Acta Hepato-Gastroenterology* **22**, 369–374.

Di Padova, C., Worner, T.M., Julkunen, R.J.K. and Lieber, C.S. (1987). Effects of fasting and chronic alcohol consumption on the first pass metabolism of ethanol. *Gastroenterology* **92**, 1169–1173.

Di Padova, C., Roine, R., Frezza, M., Gentry, R.T., Baraona, E. and Lieber, C.S. (1992). Effects of ranitidine on blood alcohol levels after ethanol ingestion: Comparison with other H$_2$-receptor antagonists. *Journal of the American Medical Association* **267**, 83–86.

Domschke, S., Domschke, W. and Lieber, C.S. (1974). Hepatic redox state: Attenuation of the acute effects of ethanol induced by chronic ethanol consumption. *Life Science* **15**, 1327–1334.

Dow, J., Krasner, N. and Goldberg, A. (1975). Relation between hepatic alcohol dehydrogenase activity and the ascorbic acid in leucocytes of patients with liver disease. *Clinical Science and Molecular Medicine* **49**, 603–608.

Duester, G., Smith, M., Bilanchone, V. and Hatfield, G.W. (1986). Molecular analysis of the human class I alcohol dehydrogenase gene family and nucleotide sequence of the gene encoding the subunit. *Journal of Biological Chemistry* **261**, 2027–2033.

Edwards, J.A. and Price-Evans, D.A. (1967). Ethanol metabolism in subjects possessing typical and atypical liver alcohol dehydrogenase. *Clinical Pharmacology and Therapeutics* **8**, 824–829.

Faller, J. and Fox, I.H. (1982). Evidence for increased urate production by activation of adenine nucleotide turnover. *New England Journal of Medicine* **307**, 1598–1602.

Feinman, L., Baraona, E., Matsuzaki, S., Korsten, M. and Lieber, C.S. (1978). Concentration dependence of ethanol metabolism *in vivo* in rats and man. *Alcoholism: Clinical and Experimental Research* **2**, 381–385.

Frezza, M., Di Padova, C., Pozzato, G., Terpin, M., Baraona, M. and Lieber, C.S. (1990). High blood alcohol levels in women: Role of decreased gastric alcohol dehydrogenase activity and first pass metabolism. *New England Journal of Medicine* **322**, 95–99.

Fujimiya, T., Yamaoka, K. and Fukui, Y. (1989). Parallel first-order and Michaelis-Menten elimination kinetics of ethanol: Respective role of alcohol dehydrogenase (ADH), non-ADH and first-order pathways. *Journal of Pharmacology and Experimental Therapeutics* **249**, 311–317.

Garro, A.J. and Lieber, C.S. (1990). Alcohol and cancer. *Annual Review of Pharmacology and Toxicology* **30**, 219–249.

Goodman, D.W. and Deykin, D. (1963). Fatty acid ethyl ester formation during ethanol metabolism *in vivo*. *Proceedings of the Society for Experimental Biology* **113**, 65–67.

Gordon, E.R. (1968). The utilization of ethanol by the

isolated perfused rat liver. *Canadian Journal of Physiology and Pharmacology* **46**, 609–616.

Gordon, E.R. (1977). ATP metabolism in an ethanol induced fatty liver. *Alcoholism: Clinical and Experimental Research* **1**, 21–25.

Greenberger, N.J., Cohen, R.B. and Isselbacher, K.J. (1965). The effect of chronic ethanol administration on liver alcohol dehydrogenase activity in the rat. *Laboratory Investigation* **14**, 264–271.

Greenway, C.V. and Lautt, W.W. (1990). Acute and chronic ethanol on hepatic oxygen ethanol and lactate metabolism in cats. *American Journal of Physiology* **258**, G411–418.

Gruenke, L.D., Konopka, K., Koop, D.R. and Waskell, L.A. (1988). Characterization of halothane oxidation by hepatic microsomes and purified cytochromes P-450 using a gas chromatographic mass spectrometric assay. *Journal of Pharmacology and Experimental Therapeutics* **246**, 454–459.

Handler, J.A. and Thurman, R.G. (1985). Fatty acid-dependent ethanol metabolism. *Biochemical and Biophysical Research Communications* **133**, 44–51.

Handler, J.A. and Thurman, R.G. (1990). Redox interactions between catalase and alcohol dehydrogenase pathways of ethanol metabolism in the perfused rat liver. *Journal of Biological Chemistry* **265**, 1510–1515.

Harada, S., Agarwal, D.P. and Goedde, H.W. (1978). Human liver alcohol dehydrogenase isoenzyme variations: Improved separation methods using prolonged high voltage starch gel electrophoresis and isoelectric focusing. *Human Genetics* **40**, 215–220.

Haseba, T., Sato, S., Ishizaki, M., Yamamoto, I., Kurosu, M. and Watanabe, T. (1991). Intralobular and intracellular location of alcohol dehydrogenase (ADH) isozymes in mouse liver: Basic ADH (class I) and acidic ADH (class III). *Biomedical Research* **12**, 199–209.

Hasumura, Y., Teschke, R. and Lieber, C.S. (1974). Increased carbon tetrachloride hepatotoxicity, and its mechanism, after chronic ethanol consumption. *Gastroenterology* **66**, 415–422.

Hempel, J.D. and Pietruszko, R. (1979). Human stomach alcohol dehydrogenase: Isoenzyme composition and catalytic properties. *Alcoholism (NY)* **3**, 95–98.

Hernandez-Munoz, R., Caballeria, J., Baraona, E., Uppal, R., Greenstein, R. and Lieber, C.S. (1990). Human gastric alcohol dehydrogenase: Its inhibition by H_2-receptor antagonists, and its effect on the bioavailability of ethanol. *Alcoholism: Clinical and Experimental Research* **14**, 946–950.

Hetu, C. and Joly, J.-G. (1985). Differences in the duration of the enhancement of liver mixed-function oxidase activities in ethanol-fed rats after withdrawal. *Biochemical Pharmacology* **34**, 1211–1216.

Hetu, C., Dumont, A. and Joly, J.-G. (1983). Effect of chronic ethanol administration on bromobenzene liver toxicity in the rat. *Toxicology and Applied Pharmacology* **67**, 166–167.

Holmes, R.S. and VandeBerg, J.L. (1987). Baboon alcohol dehydrogenase isozymes: Phenotypic changes in liver following chronic consumption of alcohol. In *Current Topics in Biological and Medical Research*, pp. 1–20. Agriculture, Physiology and Medicine.

Horn, R.S. and Manthei, R.W. (1965). Ethanol metabolism in chronic protein deficiency. *Journal of Pharmacology and Experimental Therapeutics* **147**, 385–390.

Hyvarinen, J., Leakso, M., Sippel, H., Roine, R., Huopanienu, T., Leinonen, L. and Hytonen, V. (1978). Alcohol detoxification accelerated by oxygenated drinking water. *Life Sciences* **22**, 553–560.

Iber, F.L. (1987). Evaluation of an oral solution to accelerate alcoholism detoxification. *Alcoholism: Clinical and Experimental Research* **11**, 305–308.

Inatomi, N., Ito, D. and Lieber, C.S. (1990). Ethanol oxidation by deermice mitochondria under physiologic conditions. *Alcoholism: Clinical and Experimental Research* **14**, 130–133.

Ingelman-Sundberg, M. and Johansson, I. (1984). Mechanisms of hydroxyl radical formation and ethanol oxidation by ethanol-inducible and other forms of rabbit liver microsomal cytochromes P-450. *Journal of Biological Chemistry* **259**, 6447–6458

Iseri, O.A., Gottlieb, L.S. and Lieber, C.S. (1964). The ultrastructure of ethanol-induced fatty liver. *Federation Proceedings* **23**, 579.

Iseri, O.A., Lieber, C.S. and Gottlieb, L.S. (1966). The ultrastructure of fatty liver induced by prolonged ethanol ingestion. *American Journal of Pathology* **48**, 535–555.

Ismail-Beigi, F. and Edelman, I.S. (1970). Mechanism of thyroid calorigenesis: Role of active sodium transport. *Proceedings of the National Academy of Sciences, USA* **67**, 1071–1078.

Ismail-Beigi, F. and Edelman, I.S. (1971). The mechanism of the calorigenic action of thyroid hormone. *Journal of Genetics and Physiology* **57**, 710–722.

Israel, Y., Videla, L., MacDonald, A. and Bernstein, J. (1973). Metabolic alterations produced in the liver by chronic ethanol administration: Comparison between the effects produced by ethanol and by thyroid hormones. *Biochemical Journal* **134**, 523–529.

Israel, Y., Kalant, H., Orrego, H., Khanna, J.M., Videla, I. and Phillips, J.M. (1975). Experimental alcohol-induced hepatic necrosis: Suppression by propylthiouracil. *Proceedings of the National Academy of Sciences, USA* **72**, 1137–1141.

Ito, D. and Lieber, C.S. (1993). Ethanol metabolism in deermice: Role of extrahepatic alcohol dehydrogenase. *Alcoholism: Clinical and Experimental Research* **17**, 919–925.

Jauhonen, P., Baraona, E., Miyakawa, H. and Lieber C.S. (1982). Mechanism for selective perivenular hepatotoxicity of ethanol. *Alcoholism: Clinical and Experimental Research* **6**, 350–357.

Jauhonen, P., Baraona, E., Lieber, C.S. and Hassinen, I.E. (1985). Dependence of ethanol-induced redox shift on hepatic oxygen tensions prevailing *in vivo*. *Alcohol* **2**, 163–167.

Jeejeebhoy, K.N., Bruce-Robertson, A., Ho, J. and Sodtke, U. (1975). The effect of ethanol on albumin and fibrinogen synthesis *in vivo* and in hepatocyte suspension. In *Alcohol and Abnormal Protein Synthesis* (Edited by Rothschild, M.A., Oratz, M. and Schreiber, S.S.), p. 373. Pergamon Press, New York.

Jenkins, S.A., Baxter, J.N., Devitt, P., Taylor, I. and Shields, R. (1986). Effects of alcohol on hepatic haemodynamics in the rat. *Digestion* **34**, 236–242.

Jones, A.W. and Sternebring, B. (1992). Kinetics of ethanol and methanol in alcoholics during detoxification. *Alcohol and Alcoholism* **27**, 641–647.

Jones, B.M. and Paredes, A. (1974). Circadian variation of ethanol metabolism in alcoholics. *British Journal of Addiction* **69**, 3–10.

Jornvall, H., Hempel, J., Vallee, B.L., Bosron, W.F. and Li, T.-K. (1984). Human liver alcohol dehydrogenase: Amino acid substitution in the $\beta_2 \beta_2$ Oriental isozyme explains functional properties, establishes an active site structure, and parallels mutational exchanges in the yeast enzyme. *Proceedings of the National Academy of Sciences, USA* **81**, 3024–3028.

Jornvall, H., Hoog, J.-O., Bahr-Lindstrom, H. and Vallee, B.L. (1987). Mammalian alcohol dehydrogenases of separate classes: Intermediates between different enzymes and intraclass isozymes. *Proceedings of the National Academy of Sciences, USA* **84**, 2580–2584.

Julia, P., Farres, J. and Pares, X. (1987). Characterization of three isoenzymes of rat alcohol dehydrogenase: Tissue distribution and physical and enzymatic properties. *European Journal of Biochemistry* **162**, 179–189.

Julkunen, R.J.K., DiPadova, C. and Lieber, C.S. (1985a). First pass metabolism of ethanol: A gastrointestinal barrier against the systemic toxicity of ethanol. *Life Sciences* **37**, 567–573.

Julkunen, R.J.K., Tannenbaum, L., Baraona, E. and Lieber, C.S. (1985b). First pass metabolism of ethanol: An important determinant of blood levels after alcohol consumption. *Alcohol* **2**, 437–441.

Kater, R.M.H., Tobon, F. and Iber, F.L. (1969). Increased rate of tolbutamide metabolism in alcoholic patients. *Journal of the American Medical Association* **207**, 363–365.

Kato, S., Alderman, J. and Lieber, C.S. (1987a). Ethanol metabolism in alcohol dehydrogenase deficient deermice is mediated by the microsomal ethanol oxidizing system, not by catalase. *Alcohol and Alcoholism* **1**, 231–234 (suppl.).

Kato, S., Alderman, J. and Lieber, C.S. (1987b). Respective roles of the microsomal ethanol oxidizing system (MEOS) and catalase in ethanol metabolism by deermice lacking alcohol dehydrogenase. *Archives of Biochemistry and Biophysics* **254**, 586–591.

Kato, S., Alderman, J. and Lieber, C.S. (1988). *In vivo* role of the microsomal ethanol oxidizing system in ethanol metabolism by deermice lacking alcohol de-

hydrogenase. *Biochemistry and Pharmacology* **37**, 2706–2708.

Kato, S., Kawase, T., Alderman, J., Inatomi, N. and Lieber, C.S. (1990). Role of xanthine oxidase in ethanol-induced lipid peroxidation in rats. *Gastroenterology* **98**, 203–210.

Keilin, D. and Hartree, E.F. (1945). Properties of catalase: Catalysis of coupled oxidation of alcohols. *Biochemistry Journal* **39**, 293–301.

Kessler, B.J., Lieber, J.B., Bronfin, G.J. and Sass, M. (1954). The hepatic blood flow and splanchnic oxygen consumption in alcohol fatty liver. *Journal of Clinical Investigation* **33**, 1338–1345.

Kinard, F.W., McCord, W.M. and Aull, J.C. (1951). The failure of oxygen, oxygen–carbon dioxide, or pyruvate to alter alcohol metabolism. *Quarterly Journal on the Study of Alcohol* **12**, 179–183.

Kocak-Toker, N., Uysal, M., Aykac, G., Sivas, A., Yalcin, S. and Oz, H. (1985). Influence of acute ethanol administration on hepatic glutathione peroxidase and glutathione transferase activities in the rat. *Pharmacological Research Communications* **17**, 233–239.

Komori, M., Kikuchi, O., Sakuma, T., Funaki, J., Kitada, M. and Kamataki, T. (1992). Molecular cloning of monkey liver cytochrome P-450 cDNAs: Similarity of the primary sequences to human cytochromes P-450. *Biochimica et Biophysica Acta* **1171**, 141–146.

Koop, D.R. and Casazza, J.P. (1985). Identification of ethanol-inducible P-450 isozyme 3a as the acetone and acetol monooxygenase of rabbit microsomes. *Journal of Biological Chemistry* **260**, 13607–13612.

Koop, D.R., Morgan, E.T., Tarr, G.E. and Coon, M.J. (1982). Purification and characterization of a unique isozyme of cytochrome P-450 from liver microsomes of ethanol-treated rabbits. *Journal of Biological Chemistry* **257**, 8472–8480.

Korri, U.-M. (1990). The effect of glucocorticoids, beta-2-adrenoceptor agonists, theophylline and propranolol on the rate of ethanol elimination and blood acetate concentration in humans. *Alcohol and Alcoholism* **25**, 519–522.

Krarup, N. and Larsen, J.A. (1972). The effect of slight hypothermia on liver function as measured by the elimination rate of ethanol, the hepatic uptake and excretion of indocyanine green and bile formation. *Acta Physiologica Scandinavica* **84**, 396–407.

Kubota, S., Lasker, J.M. and Lieber, C.S. (1988). Molecular regulation of an ethanol-inducible cytochrome P-450IIE1 in hamsters. *Biochemical and Biophysical Research Communications* **150**, 304–310.

Lamboeuf, Y., De Saint Blanquat, G. and Derache, R. (1981). Mucosal alcohol dehydrogenase- and aldehyde dehyrogenase-mediated ethanol oxidation in the digestive tract of the rat. *Biochemistry and Pharmacology* **30**, 542–545.

Lamboeuf, Y., La Droitte, P. and De Saint Blanquat, G. (1983). The gastrointestinal metabolism of ethanol in the rat: Effect of chronic alcohol intoxication. *Archives Internationales de Pharmacodynamie et de Therapie* **261**, 157–169.

Lane, B.P. and Lieber, C.S. (1966). Ultrastructural alterations in human hepatocytes following ingestion of ethanol with adequate diets. *American Journal of Pathology* **49**, 593–603.

Lane, B.P. and Lieber, C.S. (1967). Effects of butylated hydroxytoluene on the ultrastructure of rat hepatocytes. *Laboratory Investigations* **16**, 341–348.

Lange, L.G. (1982). Nonoxidative ethanol metabolism: Formation of fatty acid ethyl esters by cholesterol esterase. *Proceedings of the National Academy of Science, USA* **79**, 3954–3957.

Laposata, E.A. and Lange, L.G. (1986). Presence of nonoxidative ethanol metabolism in human organs commonly damaged by ethanol abuse. *Science* **231**, 497–499.

Larsen, J.A. (1968). The effect of oxygen breathing at atmospheric pressure on the metabolism of glycerol and ethanol in cats. *Acta Physiologica Scandinavica* **73**, 186–195.

Larsen, J.A. (1971). The effect of cooling on liver function in cats. *Acta Physiologica Scandinavica* **81**, 197–207.

Lasker, J.M., Raucy, J., Kubota, S., Bloswick, B.P., Black, M. and Lieber, C.S. (1987). Purification and characterization of human liver cytochrome P-450-ALC. *Biochemistry and Biophysical Research Communications* **148**, 232–238.

Lefevre, A., Adler, H. and Lieber, C.S. (1970). Effect of ethanol on ketone metabolism. *Journal of Clinical Investigation* **49**, 1775–1782.

Leo, M.A. and Lieber, C.S. (1983). Hepatic fibrosis after long term administration of ethanol and moderate vitamin A supplementation in the rat. *Hepatology* **2**, 1–11.

Leo, M.A. and Lieber, C.S. (1988). Hypervitaminosis A: A liver lover's lament. *Hepatology* **8**, 412–417.

Leo, M.A., Arai, M., Sato, M. and Lieber, C.S. (1982). Hepatotoxicity of vitamin A and ethanol in the rat. *Gastroenterology* **82**, 194–205.

Leo, M.A., Sato, M. and Lieber, C.S. (1983). Effect of hepatic vitamin A depletion on the liver in men and rats. *Gastroenterology* **84**, 562–572.

Leo, M.A., Lowe, N. and Lieber, C.S. (1986). Interaction of drugs and retinol. *Biochemistry and Pharmacology* **35**, 3949–3953.

Leo, M.A., Kim, C.I. and Lieber, C.S. (1987). NAD$^+$-dependent retinol dehydrogenase in liver microsomes. *Biochemistry and Biophysics* **259**, 241–249.

Leo, M.A., Kim, C.I., Lowe, N. and Lieber, C.S. (1992). Interaction of ethanol with ß-carotene: Delayed blood clearance and enhanced hepatotoxicity. *Hepatology* **15**, 883–891.

Leo, M.A., Rosman, A. and Lieber, C.S. (1993). Differential depletion of carotenoids and tocopherols in liver disease. *Hepatology* **17**, 977–986.

Lereboullet, J., Barres, G. and Briard, J.P. (1976). La courbe d'alcoole'mie de Widmark est-elle toujours fiable? *Bulletin de L'Academie Nationale de Medicine* **160**, 312–315.

Li, T.-K. and Magnes, L.J. (1975). Identification of a distinctive molecular form of alcohol dehydrogenase in human livers with high activity. *Biochemical and Biophysical Research Communications* **63**, 202–208.

Lieber, C.S. (1984). Alcohol and the liver. In *Liver Annual* (Edited by Arias, I.M., Frenkel, M.S. and Wilson, J.H.P.), Vol IV, pp. 130–186. Excerpta Medica, Amsterdam.

Lieber, C.S. (1985). Alcohol and the liver: Metabolism of ethanol, metabolic effects and pathogenesis of injury. *Acta Medica Scandinavica* **703**, 11–55 (suppl.).

Lieber, C.S. (1987). Alcohol and the liver. In *Liver Annual* (Edited by Arias, I.M., Frenkel, M.S. and Wilson, J.H.P.), Vol VI, pp. 163–240. Excerpta Medica, Amsterdam.

Lieber, C.S. (1988). The influence of alcohol on nutritional status. *Nutrition Reviews* **46**, 241–245.

Lieber, C.S. (1992). *Medical and Nutritional Complications of Alcoholism: Mechanisms and Management*. Plenum Press, New York.

Lieber, C.S. (1994). Alcohol and the liver: 1994 update. *Gastroenterology* **106**, 1085–1105.

Lieber, C.S. and DeCarli, L.M. (1968). Ethanol oxidation by hepatic microsomes: Adaptive increase after ethanol feeding. *Science* **162**, 917–918.

Lieber, C.S. and DeCarli, L.M. (1970). Hepatic microsomal ethanol oxidizing system: *In vitro* characteristics and adaptive properties *in vivo*. *Journal of Biological Chemistry* **245**, 2505–2512.

Lieber, C.S. and DeCarli, L.M. (1972). The role of the hepatic microsomal ethanol oxidizing system (MEOS) for ethanol metabolism *in vivo*. *Journal of Pharmacology and Experimental Therapeutics* **181**, 279–287.

Lieber, C.S. and Pignon, J.-P. (1989). Ethanol and lipids. In *Human Plasma Lipoproteins: Chemistry, Physiology and Pathology* (Edited by Fruchart, J.C. and Shepherd, J.), pp. 245–280. Walter De Gruyter, Berlin.

Lieber, C.S. and Savolainen, M. (1984). Ethanol and lipids. *Alcoholism: Clinical and Experimental Research* **8**, 409–423.

Lieber, C.S. and Spritz, N. (1966). Effects of prolonged ethanol intake in man: Role of dietary, adipose, and endogenously synthesized fatty acids in the pathogenesis of the alcoholic fatty liver. *Journal of Clinical Investigation* **45**, 1400–1411.

Lieber, C.S., Jones, D.P., Losowsky, M.S and Davidson, C.S. (1962). Interrelation of uric acid and ethanol metabolism in man. *Journal of Clinical Investigation* **41**, 1863–1870.

Lieber, C.S., Spritz, N. and DeCarli, L.M. (1966). Role of dietary, adipose and endogenously synthesized fatty acids in the pathogenesis of the alcoholic fatty liver. *Journal of Clinical Investigation* **45**, 51–62.

Lieber, C.S., Garro, A., Leo, M.A., Mak, K.M. and

Worner, T.M. (1986). Alcohol and cancer. *Hepatology* **6**, 1005–1019.

Lieber, C.S., Lasker, J.M., DeCarli, L.M., Saeli, J. and Wojtowicz, T. (1988). Role of acetone, dietary fat, and total energy intake in the induction of the hepatic microsomal ethanol oxidizing system. *Journal of Pharmacology and Experimental Therapeutics* **247**, 791–795.

Lieber, C.S., Baraona, E., Hernandez-Munoz, R., Kubota, S., Sato, N., Kawano, S., Matsumura, T. and Inatomi, N. (1989). Impaired oxygen utilization: A new mechanism for the hepatotoxicity of ethanol in sub-human primates. *Journal of Clinical Investigation* **83**, 1682–1690.

Lieber, C.S., Casini, A., DeCarli, L.M., Kim, C., Lowe, N., Sasaki, R. and Leo, M.A. (1990). *S*-adenosyl-L-methionine attenuates alcohol-induced liver injury in the baboon. *Hepatology* **11**, 165–172.

Lumeng, L. and Crabb, D.W. (1984). Rate determining factors for ethanol metabolism in fasted and castrated male rats. *Biochemistry and Pharmacology* **33**, 2623–2628.

Lundquist, F. and Wolthers, H. (1958). The influence of fructose on the kinetics of alcohol elimination in man. *Acta Pharmacolology* **14**, 290–294.

Maly, I.P. and Sasse, D. (1985). Microquantitative determination of the distribution patterns of alcohol dehydrogenase activity in the liver of rat, guinea-pig and horse. *Histochemistry* **83**, 431–436.

Maly, I.P. and Sasse, D. (1987). The intra-acinar distribution patterns of alcohol-dehydrogenase activity in the liver of juvenile, castrated and testosterone-treated rats. *Biological Chemistry Hoppe-Seyler* **368**, 315–321

Maly, I.P. and Sasse, D. (1991). Intraacinar profiles of alcohol dehydrogenase and aldehyde dehydrogenase activities in human liver. *Gastroenterology* **101**, 1716–1723.

Matsuzaki, S. and Lieber, C.S. (1975). ADH-independent ethanol oxidation in the liver and its increase by chronic ethanol consumption. *Gastroenterology* **69**, 845.

Matsuzaki, S., Gordon, E. and Lieber, C.S. (1981). Increased alcohol dehydrogenase independent ethanol oxidation at high ethanol concentrations in isolated rat hepatocytes: The effect of chronic ethanol feedings. *Journal of Pharmacology and Experimental Therapeutics* **217**, 133–137.

Mattie, H. (1963). Elimination of ethanol in rats *in vitro* at different oxygen pressures. *Acta Physiologica et Pharmacologica* **12**, 1–11.

Meldolesi, J. (1967). On the significance of the hypertrophy of the smooth endoplasmic reticulum in liver cells after administration of drugs. *Biochemistry and Pharmacology* **16**, 125–131.

Messiha, F.S. (1980). Chlorpromazine and ethanol intoxication: An underlying mechanism. *Neurobehavioral Toxicology and Teratology* **7**, 185.

Mezey, E. and Potter, J.J. (1985). Effect of castration on the turnover of rat liver alcohol dehydrogenase. *Biochemistry and Pharmacology* **34**, 369–371.

Mezey, E. and Robles, E.A. (1974). Effects of phenobarbital administration on rates of ethanol clearance and on ethanol-oxidizing enzymes in man. *Gastroenterology* **66**, 248–253.

Mezey, E., Potter, J.J. and Kvetransky, R. (1979). Effect of stress by repeated immobilization on hepatic alcohol dehydrogenase and ethanol metabolism. *Biochemistry and Pharmacology* **28**, 657–663.

Misra, P.S., Lefevre, A., Ishii, H., Rubin, E. and Lieber, C.S. (1971). Increase of ethanol meprobamate and pentobarbital metabolism after chronic ethanol administration in man and in rats. *American Journal of Medicine* **51**, 346–351.

Miwa, G.T., Levin, W., Thomas, P.E. and Lu, A.Y.H. (1978). The direct oxidation of ethanol by catalase- and alcohol dehydrogenase-free reconstituted system containing cytochrome P-450. *Archives of Biochemistry and Biophysics* **187**, 464–475.

Mogelson, S. and Lange, L.G. (1984). Nonoxidative ethanol metabolism in rabbit myocardium: Purification to homogeneity of fatty acyl ethyl ester synthase. *Biochemistry* **23**, 4075–4081.

Moreno, A. and Pares, X. (1991). Purification and characterization of a new alcohol dehydrogenase from human stomach. *Journal of Biochemistry* **266**, 1128–1133.

Morgan, E.T., Koop, D.R and Coon, M.J. (1982). Catalytic activity of cytochrome P-450 isozyme 3a isolated from liver microsomes of ethanol-treated rabbits. *Journal of Biological Chemistry* **257**, 13951–13957.

Morgan, E.T., Koop, D.R. and Coon, M.J. (1983). Comparison of six rabbit liver cytochrome P-450 isozymes in formation of a reactive metabolite of acetaminophen. *Biochemical and Biophysical Research Communications* **112**, 8–13.

Morrison, G.R. and Brock, F.E. (1967). Quantitative measurement of alcohol dehydrogenase activity within the liver lobule of rats after prolonged alcohol ingestion. *Journal of Nutrition* **92**, 286–292.

Morton, S. and Mitchell, M.C. (1985). Effects of chronic ethanol feeding on glutathione turnover in the rat. *Biochemistry and Pharmacology* **34**, 1559–1563.

Moser, H.W. and Moser, A.B. (1992). Long chain fatty acids and peroxisomal disorders. In *Polyunsaturated Fatty Acids in Human Nutrition* (Edited by Bracco, U. and Deckelbaum R.J.), pp. 65–79. Nestec Ltd., Vevey/Raven Press, New York.

Nakajima, T., Okino, T. and Sato, A. (1987). Kinetic studies on benzene metabolism in rat liver – possible presence of three forms of benzene metabolizing enzymes in the liver. *Biochemical Pharmacology* **36**, 2799–2804.

Nikki, P., Vapaatalo, H. and Karppanen, H. (1971). Effect of ethanol on body temperature, postanaesthetic shivering and tissue monoamines in halothane-anaesthetized rats. *Annales Medicinae Experimentalis et Biologiae Fenniae* **49**, 157–161.

Ohnishi, K. and Lieber, C.S. (1977). Reconstitution of the microsomal ethanol-oxidizing system: Qualitative and quantitative changes of cytochrome P-450 after chronic ethanol consumption. *Journal of Biological Chemistry* **252**, 7124–7131.

Page, R.A., Kitson, K.E. and Hardman, M.J. (1991). The importance of alcohol dehydrogenase in regulation of ethanol metabolism in rat liver cells. *Biochemistry Journal* **278**, 659–665.

Panes, J., Caballeria, J., Guitart, R., Pares A., Soler, X., Rodamilans, M., Navasa, M., Pares, X., Bosch, J. and Rodes, J. (1993). Determinants of ethanol and acetaldehyde metabolism in chronic alcoholics. *Alcoholism: Clinical and Experimental Research* **17**, 48–53.

Pantuck, E.J., Pantuck, C.B., Ryan, D.E. and Conney, A.H. (1985). Inhibition and stimulation of enflurane metabolism in the rat following a single dose or chronic administration of ethanol. *Anesthesiology* **62**, 255–262.

Pares, X. and Vallee, B.L. (1981). New human liver alcohol dehydrogenase forms with unique kinetic characteristics. *Biochemical and Biophysical Research Communications* **98**, 122–130.

Pekkanen, L., Eriksson, K. and Silivonen, M.-L. (1978). Dietarily-induced changes in voluntary ethanol consumption and ethanol metabolism in the rat. *British Journal of Nutrition* **40**, 103–113.

Pestalozzi, D.M., Buhler, R., von Wartburg, J.P. and Hess, M. (1983). Immunohistochemical localization of alcohol dehydrogenase in the human gastrointestinal tract. *Gastroenterology* **85**, 1011–1016.

Pikkarainen, P. and Lieber, C.S. (1980). Concentration dependency of ethanol elimination rates in baboons: Effects of chronic alcohol consumption. *Alcoholism: Clinical and Experimental Research* **4**, 40–43.

Pikkarainen, P.H., Baraona, E., Jauhonen, P., Seitz, H. and Lieber, C.S. (1981) Contribution of oropharynx microflora and of lung microsomes to acetaldehyde in expired air after alcohol ingestion. *Journal of Laboratory and Clinical Medicine* **97**, 631–638.

Pinkston, J.N. and Soliman, K.F.A. (1979). Effect of light and fasting on the circadian variation of ethanol metabolism in the rat. *Journal of Interdisciplinary Cycle Research* **10**, 185–193.

Pritchard, J.F. and Schneck, D.W. (1977). Effects of ethanol and phenobarbital on the metabolism of propanolol by 9000g rat liver supernatant. *Biochemistry and Pharmacology* **26**, 2453–2454.

Qulali, M. and Crabb, D.W. (1992). Corticosterone induces rat liver alcohol dehydrogenase mRNA but not enzyme protein or activity. *Alcoholism: Clinical and Experimental Research* **16**, 427–431.

Rachmamin, G., MacDonald, J.A., Wahid, S., Clapp, J.J., Khanna, J.M. and Israel, Y. (1980). Modulation of alcohol dehydrogenase and ethanol metabolism by sex hormones in the spontaneously hypertensive rat: Effect of chronic ethanol administration. *Biochemistry Journal* **186**, 483–490.

Roine, R.P., Eriksson, C.J.P., Yilikahri, R., Pentitila, A. and Salaspuro, M. (1989). Methanol as a marker of alcohol abuse. *Alcoholism: Clinical and Experimental Research* **13**, 172–175.

Roine, R., Gentry, R.T., Hernandez-Munoz, R., Baraona, E. and Lieber, C.S. (1990). Aspirin increases blood alcohol concentrations in human after ingestion of ethanol. *Journal of the American Medical Association* **264**, 2406–2408.

Roine, R.P., Gentry, R.T., Lim, Jr., R.T., Baraona, E. and Lieber, C.S. (1991). Effect of concentration of ingested ethanol on blood alcohol levels. *Alcoholism: Clinical and Experimental Research* **15**, 734–738.

Roine, R.P., Hernandez-Munoz, R., Gentry, R.T., Baraona, E. and Lieber, C.S. (1992). H_2-antagonists and blood alcohol levels. *Digestive Diseases and Sciences* **37**, 891–896

Rothschild, M.A., Oratz, M., Mongelli, J. and Schreiber, S.S. (1971). Alcohol induced depression of albumin synthesis: Reversal by tryptophan. *Journal of Clinical Investigation* **50**, 1812–1818.

Ruebner, B.H., Krieger, R.I., Miller, J.L., Tsao, M. and Rorvik, M. (1975). Hepatic and metabolic effects of ethanol on rhesus monkeys. In *Alcohol Intoxication and Withdrawal II* (Edited by Gross, M.M.), pp. 395–405. Advances in Experimental Medicine and Biology Vol. 59. Plenum Press, New York.

Ryan, D.E., Ramathan, L., Iida, S., Thomas, P.E., Haniu, M., Shively, J.E., Lieber, C.S. and Levin, W. (1985). Characterization of a major form of rat hepatic microsomal cytochrome P-450 induced by isoniazid. *Journal of Biological Chemistry* **260**, 6385–6393.

Ryan, D.E., Koop, D.R., Thomas, P.E., Coon, M.J. and Levin, W. (1986). Evidence that isoniazid and ethanol induced the same microsomal cytochrome P-450 in rat liver, and isozyme homologous to rabbit liver cytochrome P-450 isozymes 3a. *Biochemistry and Biophysics* **246**, 633–644.

Salaspuro, M.P. and Lieber, C.S. (1977). Non-ADH pathway of alcohol metabolism: Its increase in activity at high ethanol concentrations and after chronic consumption. *Gastroenterology* **73**, A47.

Salaspuro. M.P. and Lieber, C.S. (1978). Non-uniformity of blood ethanol elimination: Its exaggeration after chronic consumption. *Annals of Clinical Research* **10**, 294–297.

Salaspuro, M.P., Shaw, S., Jayatilleke, E., Ross, W.A. and Lieber, C.S. (1981). Attenuation of the ethanol induced hepatic redox change after chronic alcohol consumption in baboons: Metabolic consequences *in vivo* and *in vitro*. *Hepatology* **1**, 33–38.

Sato, M. and Lieber, C.S. (1981). Hepatic vitamin A depletion after chronic ethanol consumption in baboons and rats. *Journal of Nutrition* **111**, 2015–2023.

Sato, N., Kamada, T., Kawano, S., Hayashi, N., Kishida, Y., Meren, H., Yoshihara, H. and Abe, H. (1983). Effect of acute and chronic ethanol consumption on hepatic tissue oxygen tension in rats. *Pharmacological and Biochemical Behavior* **18**, 443–447.

Seitz, H.K., Veith, S., Czygan, P., Bosche, J., Simon, B., Gugler, R. and Kommerell, B. (1984). *In vivo* interactions between H_2-receptor antagonists and ethanol metabolism in man and in rats. *Hepatology* **4**, 1231–1234.

Seitz, H.K., Egerer, G. and Simanowski, U.A. (1990). High blood alcohol levels in women. *New England Journal of Medicine* **323**, 58.

Shaw, S. and Lieber, C.S. (1980). Increased hepatic production of alpha-amino-*n*-butyric acid after chronic alcohol consumption in rats and baboons. *Gastroenterology* **78**, 108–113.

Shaw, S., Heller, E., Friedman, H., Baraona, E. and Lieber, C.S. (1977). Increased hepatic oxygenation following ethanol administration in the baboon. *Proceedings of the Society for Experimental Biology and Medicine* **156**, 509–513.

Shaw, S., Jayatilleke, E., Ross, W.A., Gordon, E.R. and Lieber, C.S. (1981). Ethanol induced lipid peroxidation: Potentiation by long-term alcohol feeding and attenuation by methionine. *Journal of Laboratory and Clinical Medicine* **98**, 417–424.

Shigeta, Y., Nomura, F., Iida, S., Leo, M.A., Felder, M.R. and Lieber, C.S. (1984). Ethanol metabolism *in vivo* by the microsomal ethanol oxidizing system in deermice lacking alcohol dehydrogenase (ADH). *Biochemistry and Pharmacology* **33**, 807–814.

Siegers, C.P., Heidbuchel, K. and Younes, M. (1983). Influence of alcohol, dithiocard and (+)-catechin on the hepatotoxicity and metabolism of vinylidene chloride in rats. *Journal of Applied Toxicology* **3**, 90–95.

Smith, M.M. and Dawson, A.G. (1985). Effect of triiodothyronine on alcohol dehydrogenase and aldehyde dehydrogenase activities in rat liver: Implication for the control of ethanol metabolism. *Biochemistry and Pharmacology* **34**, 2291–2296.

Smith, M., Hopkinson, D.A. and Harris, H. (1971). Developmental changes and polymorphism in human alcohol dehydrogenase. *Annals of Human Genetics (London)* **34**, 251–271.

Smith, T., DeMaster, E.G., Furne, J.K., Springfield, J. and Levitt, M.D. (1992). First-pass gastric mucosal metabolism of ethanol is negligible in the rat. *Journal of Clinical Investigation* **89**, 1801–1806.

Sokal, E.M., Collette, C. and Buts, J.P. (1993). Continuous increase of alcohol dehydrogenase activity along the liver plate in normal and cirrhotic human livers. *Hepatology* **17**, 202–205.

Song, B.J., Gelboin, H.V., Park, S.S. and Gonzales, F.J. (1986). Complementary DNA and protein sequences of ethanol-inducible rat and human cytochrome P-450s. *Journal of Biological Chemistry* **261**, 16689–16697.

Speisky, H., MacDonald, A., Giles, G., Orrego, H. and Israel, Y. (1985). Increased loss and decreased synthesis of hepatic glutathione after acute ethanol administration. *Biochemical Journal* **225**, 565–572.

Stamatoyannopoulos, G., Chen, S. and Fukui, M. (1975). Liver alcohol-dehydrogenase in Japanese: High population frequency of atypical form and its possible role in alcohol sensitivity. *American Journal of Human Genetics* **27**, 789–796.

Stone, C.L., Bosron, W.F. and Dunn, M.F. (1993). Amino acid substitutions at position 47 of human 11 and 22 alcohol dehydrogenases affect hydride transfer and coenzyme dissociation rate constants. *Journal of Biological Chemistry* **268**, 892–899.

Sturtevant, F.M., Sturtevant, R.P., Scheving, L.E. and Pauly, J.E. (1976). Chronopharmacokinetics of ethanol. II. Circadian rhythm in rate of blood level decline in a single subject. *Naunyn-Schmiedeberg's Archives of Pharmakology* **293**, 203–208.

Takagi, T., Ishii, H., Takahashi, H., Kato, S., Okuno, F., Ebihara, Y., Yamauchi, H., Nagata, Y., Tashiro, M. and Tsuchiya, M. (1983). Potentiation of halothane hepatotoxicity by chronic ethanol administration in rat: An animal model of halothane hepatitis. *Pharmacology, Biochemistry and Behavior* **18**, 461–465.

Takagi, T., Alderman, J., Gellert, J. and Lieber, C.S. (1986). Assessment of the role of non-ADH ethanol oxidation *in vivo* and in hepatocytes from deermice. *Biochemistry and Pharmacology* **35**, 3601–3606.

Takahashi, T., Lasker, M.M., Rosman, A.S. and Lieber, C.S. (1993). Induction of P450E1 in human liver by ethanol is due to a corresponding increase in encoding mRNA. *Hepatology* **17**, 236–245.

Teschke, R., Hasumura, Y., Joly, J.G., Ishii, H. and Lieber, C.S. (1972). Microsomal ethanol-oxidizing system (MEOS): Purification and properties of a rat liver system free of catalase and alcohol dehydrogenase. *Biochemical and Biophysical Research Communications* **49**, 1187–1193.

Teschke, R., Hasumura, Y. and Lieber, C.S. (1974). Hepatic microsomal alcohol oxidizing system: Solubilization, isolation and characterization. *Biochemistry and Biophysics* **163**, 404–415.

Teschke, R., Hasumura, Y. and Lieber, C.S. (1976). Hepatic ethanol metabolism: Respective roles of alcohol dehydrogenase, the microsomal ethanol oxidizing system and catalase. *Biochemistry and Biophysics* **175**, 635–643.

Teschke, R., Matsuzaki, S., Ohnishi, K., De Carli, L.M. and Lieber, C.S. (1977). Microsomal ethanol oxidizing system (MEOS): Current status of its characterization and its role. *Alcoholism: Clinical and Experimental Research* **1**, 7–15.

Teschke, R., Wannagat, F.-J., Lowendorf, F. and Strohmeyer, G. (1986). Hepatic alcohol-metabolizing enzymes after prolonged administration of sex hormones and alcohol in female rats. *Biochemistry and Pharmacology* **35**, 521.

Theorell, H. and Chance, B. (1951). Studies on liver alcohol dehydrogenase. II. The kinetics of the compounds of horse liver alcohol dehydrogenase and reduced diphosphopyridine nucleotide. *Acta Chemica Scandinavica* **5**, 1127–1144.

Theorell, H., Nygaard, A.P. and Bonnichsen, R. (1955).

Studies on liver alcohol dehydrogenase. III. The influence of pH and some anions on the reaction velocity constants. *Acta Chemica Scandinavica* **9**, 1148–1165.

Thompson, G.N. (1956). *Alcoholism*. Charles C. Thomas, Springfield, IL.

Thurman, R.G. and Brentzel, H.J. (1977). The role of alcohol dehydrogenase in microsomal ethanol oxidation and the adaptive increase in ethanol metabolism due to chronic treatment with ethanol. *Alcoholism: Clinical and Experimental Research* **1**, 33–38.

Thurman, R.G., McKenna, W.R. and McCaffrey, T.B. (1976). Pathways responsible for the adaptive increase in ethanol utilization following chronic treatment with ethanol: Inhibitor studies with the hemoglobin-free perfused rat liver. *Molecular Pharmacology* **12**, 156–166.

Tsutsumi, M., Lasker, J.M., Shimizu, M., Rosman, A.S. and Lieber, C.S. (1989). The intralobular distribution of ethanol-inducible P450IIE1 in rat and human liver. *Hepatology* **10**, 437–446.

Tsutsumi, R., Leo, M.A., Kim, C., Tsutsumi, M., Lasker, J.M., Lowe, N. and Lieber, C.S. (1990). Interaction of ethanol with enflurane metabolism and toxicity: Role of P450IIE1. *Alcoholism: Clinical and Experimental Research* **14**, 174–179.

Tsutsumi, M., Lasker, J.M., Takahashi, T. and Lieber, C.S. (1993). *In vivo* induction of hepatic P4502E1 by ethanol: Role of increased enzyme synthesis. *Archives of Biochemistry and Biophysics* **304**, 209–218.

Ugarte, G., Pino, M.E. and Insunza, I. (1967). Hepatic alcohol dehydrogenase in alcoholic addicts with and without hepatic damage. *American Journal of Digestive Diseases* **12**, 589–592.

Ugarte, G., Pereda, I., Pino, M.E. and Iturriaga, H. (1972). Influence of alcohol intake, length of abstinence and meprobamate on the rate of ethanol metabolism in man. *Quarterly Journal on the Studies of Alcohol* **33**, 698–705.

Vaananen, H., Salaspuro, M. and Lindros, K. (1984). The effect of chronic ethanol ingestion on ethanol metabolizing enzymes in isolated periportal and perivenous rat hepatocytes. *Hepatology* **4**, 862–866.

Vendemiale, G., Jayatilleke, E., Shaw, S. and Lieber, C.S. (1984). Depression of biliary glutathione excretion by chronic ethanol feeding in the rat. *Life Sciences* **34**, 1065–1073.

von Bahr-Lindstrom, H., von Hoog, J.-O., Heden, L.-O., Kaiser, R., Fleetwood, L., Larsson, K., Lake, M., Holmquist, B., Holmgren, A. and Hempel, J. (1986). cDNA and protein structure for the subunit of human liver alcohol dehydrogenase. *Biochemistry* **25**, 2465–2470.

von Wartburg, J.P. and Schurch, P.M. (1968). Atypical human liver alcohol dehydrogenase. *Annals of the New York Academy of Science* **151**, 936–946.

von Wartburg, J.P., Bethune, J.L. and Vallee, B.L. (1964). Human liver-alcohol dehydrogenase: Kinetic and physiochemical properties. *Biochemistry* **3**, 1175–1782.

von Wartburg, J.P., Papenberg, J. and Aebi, H. (1965). An atypical human alcohol dehydrogenase. *Canadian Journal of Biochemistry* **43**, 889–898.

Whitehouse, L.W., Paul, C.J. and Thomas, B.H. (1980). Isoniazid induced tolerance to ethanol in rabbits, guinea pig and rat. *Biopharmaceutics and Drug Disposition* **I**, 235–245.

Williamson, J.R., Scholz, R., Browning, E.T., Thurman, R.G. and Fukami, M.H. (1969). Metabolic effects of ethanol in perfused rat liver. *Journal of Biological Chemistry* **25**, 5044–5054.

Wilson, J.S., Korsent, M.A. and Lieber, C.S. (1986). The combined effects of protein deficiency and chronic ethanol administration on rat ethanol metabolism. *Hepatology* **6**, 823–829.

Wilson, R.H.L., Newman, E.J. and Newman, H.W. (1956). Diurnal variation in rate of alcohol metabolism. *Journal of Applied Physiology* **8**, 556–558.

Wrighton, S.A., Campanile, C., Thomas, P.E., Maines, S.L., Watkins, P.B., Parker, G., Mendez-Picon, G., Haniu, M., Shively, J.E., Levin, W. and Guzelian, P.S. (1986). Identification of a human liver cytochrome P-450 homologous to the major isosafrole-inducible cytochrome P-450 in the rat. *Molecular Pharmacology* **29**, 405–410.

Yang, C.S., Tu, Y.Y., Koop, D.R. and Coon, M.J. (1985). Metabolism of nitrosamines by purified rabbit liver cytochrome P-450 isozymes. *Cancer Research* **45**, 1140–1145.

Yasunami, M., Chen, C.-S. and Yoshida, A. (1991). A human alcohol dehydrogenase gene (ADH6) encoding an additional class of isozyme. *Proceedings of the National Academy of Sciences, USA* **88**, 7610–7614.

Yin, S.-J., Wang M.-F, Liao, C.-S., Chen, C.-M. and Wu, C.-W. (1990). Identification of a human stomach alcohol dehydrogenase with distinctive kinetic properties. *Biochemistry International* **22**, 829–835.

Yokoyama, H., Baraona, E. and Lieber, C.S. (1994). Molecular cloning of human class IV alcohol dehydrogenase. *Biochemical Biophysical Research Communications* **203**, 219–224.

Zorzano, A., Ruiz del Arbol, L. and Herrera, E. (1989). Effect of liver disorders on ethanol elimination and alcohol and aldehyde dehydrogenase activities in liver and erythrocytes. *Clinical Sciences* **76**, 51–57.

3 Pathological spectrum of alcoholic liver disease

Pauline de la M. Hall

Introduction

The morphological spectrum of alcoholic liver disease, which has traditionally included fatty change (steatosis), alcoholic hepatitis and cirrhosis (Galambos 1979; Beckett *et al.* 1961; Brunt *et al.* 1974), has been expanded in recent years to include features such as perivenular fibrosis (Van Waes and Lieber 1977), "alcoholic foamy degeneration" (Uchida *et al.* 1983) and occlusive venous lesions (Goodman and Ishak 1982). The chronic active hepatitis pattern of injury is now attributed, in many cases, to coexistent viral infection, usually hepatitis C (Brillanti *et al.* 1989; Lampertico *et al.* 1991; Takase *et al.* 1991).

Recent reviews by Ishak *et al.* (1991), French *et al.* (1993) and Hall (1994a,b) describe the histopathology of alcololic liver disease in considerable detail, while the criteria for the diagnosis of the various stages of liver injury have been described by international panels of liver pathologists: alcoholic hepatitis (Baptista *et al.* 1981), cirrhosis (Anthony *et al.* 1978) and benign, borderline and malignant lesions arising in chronic liver disease (Ferrell 1993). An unequivocal diagnosis of alcoholic liver disease requires both a history of alcohol ingestion, although not necessarily in vast amounts, and a liver biopsy showing features in keeping with an alcoholic aetiology. As discussed in detail by Zimmerman and Ishak in Chapter 11, a great variety of agents and disease states may result in liver injury that is morphologically indistinguishable from that associated with alcohol (non-alcoholic steatohepatitis or pseudoalcoholic liver disease).

The main purpose of this chapter is to illustrate the spectrum of alcohol-associated liver injury seen by electron microscopy and light microscopy, with a brief mention of clinical aspects in order to emphasize the generally poor correlation between the clinical features and the pattern and severity of liver injury. Some aspects of pathogenesis that are not covered elsewhere in this text, for example Mallory body formation, are included in this chapter. Finally, the prognostic significance of each of the main patterns of injury will be briefly considered.

Early alcohol-induced injury/ alcoholic steatosis

Human and animal studies have shown unequivocally that alcohol *per se* is a direct hepatotoxin, and that dietary manipulation does not prevent the alcohol-induced changes in the hepatocytes (Lieber and DeCarli 1974; Lieber *et al.* 1975, 1985; Rubin and Lieber 1967, 1968, 1974). Healthy, non-alcoholic volunteers given non-intoxicating doses of alcohol for only 2–4 days (Rubin and Lieber 1968) developed ultrastructural changes similar to those seen in the baboon model. The alcohol-associated changes include the accumulation of tiny membrane-bound fat droplets which gradually enlarge and fuse to become a single, large, non-membrane-bound droplet, proliferation of the smooth endoplasmic reticulum (SER) (see Fig. 3.1),

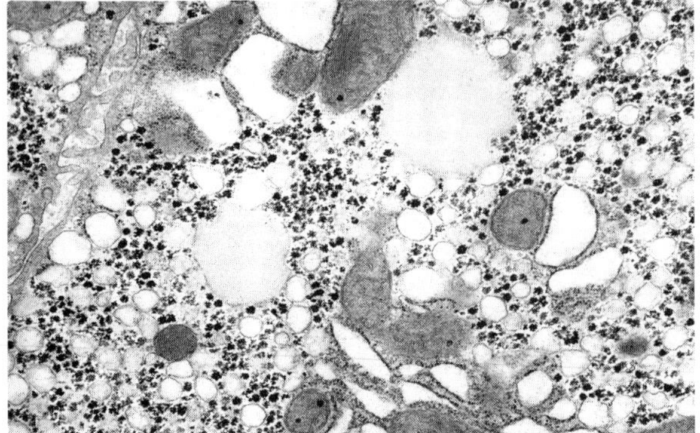

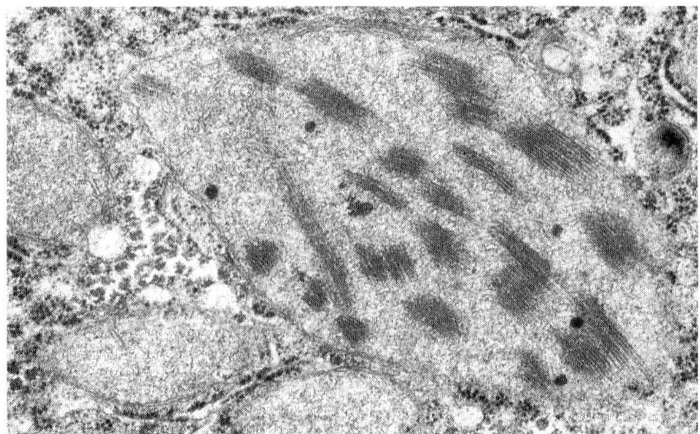

(a)

Fig. 3.1 Smooth endoplasmic reticulum (SER). Portion of a hepatocyte showing prominent SER, together with two fat droplets, mitochondria and glycogen granules. ×11,600.

and enlargement and distortion of the mitochondria with disrupted cristae and crystalline inclusions (Fig. 3.2; see also Plate 1). As discussed in detail in Chapter 2, the structural changes in the mitochondria are associated with considerable functional impairment.

As drinking continues, all of these changes become more pronounced; giant mitochondria 10–20 μ in diameter are frequently seen by light microscopy (Bruguera *et al.* 1977; Uchida *et al.* 1984). The giant or megamitochondria are often most pronounced in hepatocytes that exhibit microvesicular fatty change (Fig. 3.3). Giant mitochrondria are seen usually as globular, eosinophilic cytoplasmic inclusions that need to be differentiated from Mallory bodies, but they may be needle-shaped. Inagaki *et al.* (1989, 1992) confirmed that the eosinophilic globular bodies seen by light microscopy were indeed giant mitochondria by examining the same pieces of tissue by light microscopy and electron microscopy. Although giant mitochondria are nonspecific findings that occur in a variety of non-alcohol-associated liver diseases, Yokoo *et al.* (1978) suggest that their presence should be regarded as a diagnostic hint of recent heavy alcohol consumption.

The proliferation of SER has been confirmed by the isolation and chemical measurement of microsomes (Lane and Lieber 1966; Iseri *et al.* 1966). Alcohol and a variety of other drugs (e.g. phenytoin) have the ability to stimulate the cytochrome P450 enzyme system. Alcohol stimulates the alcohol-inducible isoenzymes and, in particular, the isoenzyme CYP2E1 (see Chapters 2 and 16). The structural counterpart of this phenomenon is pro-

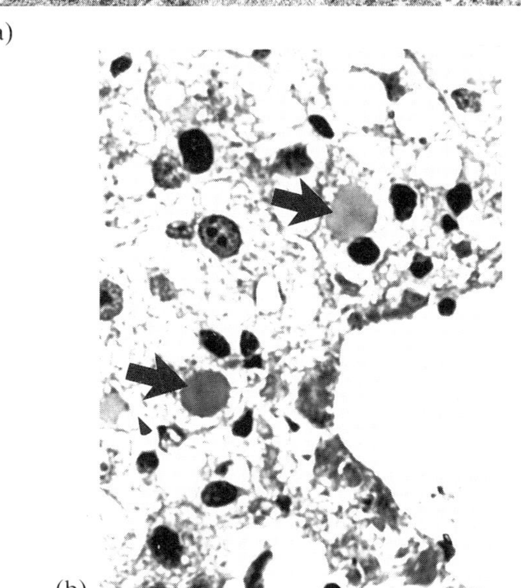

(b)

Fig. 3.2 Giant mitochondria. (a) Several normal mitochondria and a giant mitochondria, which contains numerous crystalline inclusions, are seen within the cytoplasm of a hepatocyte. ×22,200. (b) Liver showing mild fatty change and several giant mitochondria (arrows). Chromatrope aniline blue, ×600.

liferation of the SER (Fig. 3.1). The term "induction" is used to describe this process and the induced hepatocytes can sometimes be recognized by light microscopy by the presence of abundant "glassy" eosinophilic cytoplasm. The structural and functional changes relating to alcohol-mediated enzyme induction occur maximally in the zone 3 hepatocytes (McKinnon *et al.* 1994).

Macrovesicular steatosis

Steatosis is both the earliest manifestation of alcohol-associated liver injury and the most fre-

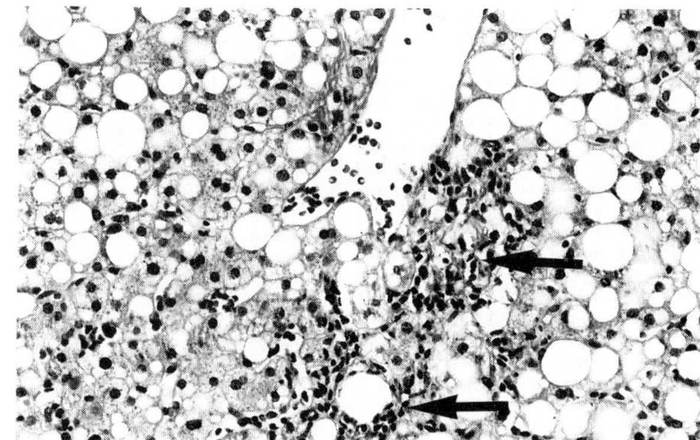

Fig. 3.3 Macrovesicular steatosis and lipogranulomata. Fatty liver showing a large lipogranulomata (arrows) in the region of a terminal hepatic venule. H&E, ×180.

quently seen pattern of injury. A study of patients presenting for treatment of chronic alcoholism revealed steatosis in 90 percent of the liver biopsies (Edmondson *et al.* 1967). Early/mild steatosis is seen in zone 3 (perivenular) hepatocytes (Fig. 3.3), however, when the liver injury is more severe, it can affect zone 2 and even zone 1 (periportal) hepatocytes. Although single, large macrovesicular fat droplets predominate, it is not unusual to see variable numbers of hepatocytes containing microvesicular fat droplets.

Fat is removed from hepatic tissue during routine processing and only empty spaces remain (Fig. 3.3). However, if a portion of the biopsy specimen is postfixed in osmium tetroxide, the fat is retained during processing and is seen as black droplets in unstained sections (Hall *et al.* 1980). This technique is invaluable in differentiating microvesicular steatosis from hydopic and ballooning degeneration. The presence and amount of fat, in both the hepatocytes and the Ito cells, can be assessed in haemotoxylin and eosin stained sections of the osmicated tissue and special stains, such as for collagen, can be performed (Hall *et al.* 1982).

At the simple fatty liver stage of injury the only inflammatory changes are those seen in association with lipogranulomata, which are usually perivenular in location (Christoffersen *et al.* 1971). Lipogranulomata usually comprise aggregated fat-laden macrophages with variable numbers of lymphocytes (Fig. 3.3). Occasionally, true epitheliod granulomata may be seen and serial sectioning may be required to demonstrate fat droplets within the epithelioid macrophages (Iversen *et al.* 1970). Lipo-

granulomata either disappear without sequelae or undergo varying degrees of fibrosis that may be seen as focal perivenular fibrosis.

Microvesicular steatosis (alcoholic foamy degeneration)

Uchida *et al.* (1983) introduced the term "alcoholic foamy degeneration" to describe microvesicular steatosis occurring in association with excessive alcohol consumption (at least 175 g/day for 2.7 to 44 years). A highly characteristic pattern of injury was seen in the liver (Fig. 3.4). The acinar architecture is essentially intact and the predominant feature is marked hepatocyte enlargement due to the massive accumulation of microvesicular (less than 1 μm) fat droplets surrounding centrally situated nuclei. Bile is seen in most cases both as plugs in dilated bile canaliculi and in the hepatocyte cytoplasm. Other changes include variable amounts of macrovesicular fatty change, giant mitochondria, hepatocyte dropout due to lysis, and small amounts of pericellular fibrosis in the perivenular regions. The pattern of injury can be easily differentiated from that of alcoholic hepatitis by the absence of hepatocyte necrosis, the lack of a neutrophil polymorph infiltrate and the sparsity – or more usually the absence – of Mallory bodies.

Microvesicular steatosis may also be seen in a wide range of apparently unrelated conditions,

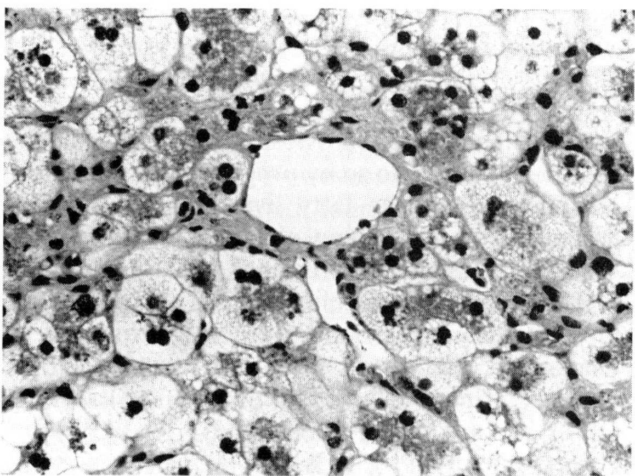

Fig. 3.4 Microvesicular steatosis (alcoholic foamy degeneration). Hepatocyte enlargement is due to the presence of myriads of tiny fat droplets. A terminal hepatic vein is seen (centre). The fatty change involves all zone 3 hepatocytes and extends into zone 2 (not shown). H&E, ×380.

Perivenular fibrosis

Nakano *et al.* (1982b) studied 10 patients with perivenular fibrosis, nine of whom continued to drink and showed progressive fibrosis over the next 2 years. A subsequent study by Worner and Lieber (1985) included 34 male drinkers and continued for up to 6 years. Fifteen patients showed perivenular fibrosis in the first biopsy. During the 1–4 year follow-up period, 13 of these patients showed progression in the amount of hepatic fibrosis: nine had more severe fibrosis, one had incomplete cirrhosis and three had developed established cirrhosis. In contrast, quantitative studies by Caulet *et al.* (1989) and Junge *et al.* (1991) failed to demonstrate perivenular fibrosis in livers showing alcoholic steatosis.

In general, there has been a slowly growing acceptance that perivenular fibrosis at the fatty liver stage indicates individuals at higher risk of progression to cirrhosis if they continue to drink (Nakano *et al.* 1982a,b; Worner and Lieber 1985). However, the possibility that alcoholic hepatitis is occurring at a subclinical level in drinkers who develop alcoholic cirrhosis is used to argue against this concept. Since some patients present clinically with established alcoholic cirrhosis without any clinical antecedents and others have the diagnosis of cirrhosis made as an unexpected finding at autopsy, it is likely that debate about the mode of progression of alcoholic liver injury to cirrhosis will continue.

Alcoholic hepatitis

Beckett *et al.* (1961) introduced the term *acute alcoholic hepatitis* to define a clinicopathological syndrome, but a wide range of clinical and biochemical abnormalities can accompany the pattern of liver injury described by Beckett (Brunt *et al.* 1974; Krasner *et al.* 1977; Morgan *et al.* 1978). The term *alcoholic hepatitis* is best restricted to a *morphological* pattern of alcohol-associated injury that is characterized by hepatocyte degeneration and necrosis accompanied by an infiltrate of neutrophil polymorphs (Baptista *et al.* 1981) (Fig. 3.7). Mallory bodies are usually present, and the neutrophil polymorph infiltrate frequently surrounds and sometimes extends into the hepatocytes that contain Mallory bodies (French and Burbridge 1979; Takahashi *et al.* 1987) (Fig. 3.8; see also Plate 2), but Mallory bodies are not obligatory for a diagnosis of alcoholic hepatitis. Other features that may be seen include fatty change, both macrovesicular and

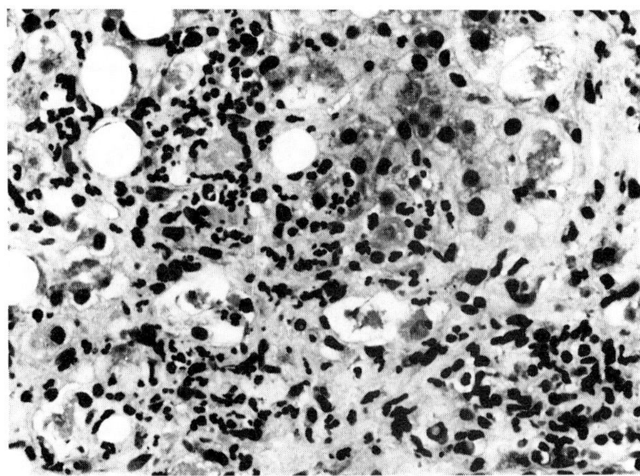

Fig. 3.7 Alcoholic hepatitis. Liver showing severe hepatocyte necrosis, a heavy infiltrate of neutrophil polymorphs, enlarged hepatocytes containing Mallory bodies and mild fatty change. H&E, ×200.

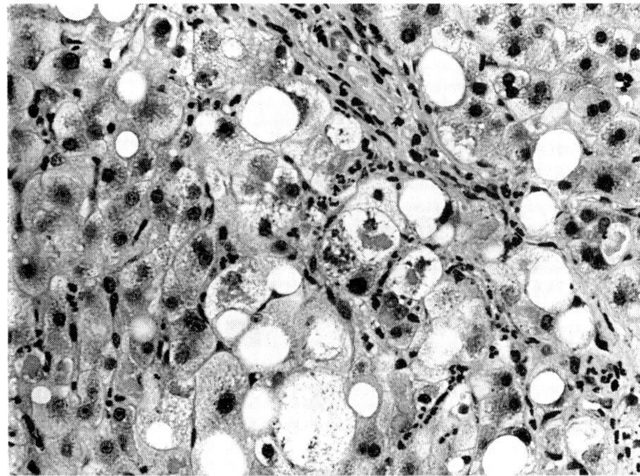

Fig. 3.8 Alcoholic hepatitis with Mallory bodies. Mallory bodies are seen in several enlarged hepatocytes together with a heavy infiltrate of neutrophil polymorphs. H&E, original magnification ×200.

microvesicular in type, sometimes with lipogranulomata; hepatocyte enlargement; apoptotic bodies (hepatocytes showing acidophilic necrosis); giant mitochondria, usually globular; a variable infiltrate of mononuclear cells (associated with the foci of hepatocyte necrosis and also in the portal tracts); cholestasis; siderosis; fibrosis, and Kupffer cell enlargement and proliferation. The Kupffer cells and portal tract macrophages may contain ceroid pigment, fat droplets and even stainable iron which has been released from necrotic hepatocyte. The extent of the fibrosis varies from patient to patient and ranges from minimal through perivenular/pericellular fibrosis in the zone 3 regions, to extensive pericellular fibrosis with the formation of fibrous septa and finally to established cirrhosis.

A recent Veterans Administration Cooperative Study (French *et al.* 1993) of 281 male alcoholic patients revealed 106 with acute alcoholic hepatitis diagnosed on liver biopsy. Moderate to severe fatty change was seen in 82 percent of the biopsies showing alcoholic hepatitis, and in 43 percent of those with alcoholic hepatitis and cirrhosis. Mallory bodies were present in 76 percent of patients with alcoholic hepatitis and in 95 percent of those with both alcoholic hepatitis and cirrhosis. Moderate to severe fibrosis was seen in 54 percent of those patients with alcoholic hepatitis and in 100 percent of those with cirrhosis. Cholestasis was found in 18 percent with alcoholic hepatitis, in 32 percent of patients with alcoholic hepatitis and cirrhosis, and in 15 percent of those whose livers showed inactive cirrhosis. The terms *alcoholic steatonecrosis* and *steatohepatitis* are sometimes used as synonyms for alcoholic hepatitis (Birschbach *et al.* 1974; see Chapter 11). The term *sclerosing hyaline necrosis* has been used to describe hepatocyte necrosis and fibrosis occurring in the perivenular region (Edmondson *et al.* 1963; Karasawa and Chedid 1976). This pattern of liver injury is now recognized as part of the spectrum of alcoholic hepatitis; French *et al.* (1993) reported sclerosing hyaline necrosis in 68 percent of their patients with alcoholic hepatitis. Early perivenular necrosis and fibrosis in alcoholic liver disease suggests selective injury in the zone 3 regions of the liver. Restriction of the early injury to these regions may reflect the relatively hypoxic state of this zone, which is the site of maximal metabolism of alcohol and some drugs, evidenced by the high levels of cytochrome P450, in particular the alcohol-metabolizing isoenzyme CYP2E1 (see Chapters 2, 17 and 19).

A chronic active hepatitis pattern of injury, characterized by the presence of piecemeal necrosis, is sometimes seen in liver biopsies that also show evidence of alcohol-related injury including alcoholic hepatitis (Goldberg *et al.* 1977; Hodges *et al.* 1982; Crapper *et al.* 1983). In many cases, this pattern of liver injury has been seen in association with a coexistent viral infection, frequently hepatitis C (Brillanti *et al.* 1989; Lampertico *et al.* 1991; Takase *et al.* 1991; see also Chapters 9 and 18). The possibility that alcohol *per se* can cause chronic active hepatitis remains controversial but is becoming less likely as more viruses are being identified.

In some cases of markedly cholestatic alcoholic hepatitis, an infiltrate of neutrophil polymorphs may be seen in and around bile duct walls, so-called "microscopic cholangitis" (Afshani *et al.* 1978). The clinical features, liver enzyme abnormalities and the histomorphology closely resemble the features of extrahepatic biliary obstruction which needs to be excluded by appropriate radiology.

Hepatocyte enlargement

Hepatocyte enlargement is often a prominent feature in alcoholic hepatitis (Fig. 3.9). The enlarged cells exhibit the features of ballooning degeneration, which is due to the accumulation of lipids and proteins, including Mallory bodies, with a proportional amount of water retention (Baraona *et al.* 1977) (see Fig. 3.10). Protein retention has been attributed, at least in part, to the toxic effects of acetaldehyde and acetone on the microtubule-mediated secretion of albumin and transferin (Baraona *et al.* 1977; Matsuda *et al.* 1979, 1983). Microtubules help maintain the architecture of the normal hepatocyte and alterations in their structure and function may also contribute to ballooning (Berman *et al.* 1983). Impaired secretion of hepatic glycoproteins by the Golgi apparatus also contributes to the retention of proteins (Matsuda *et al.* 1979, 1991). Studies of alcohol-treated rats have shown that 50 percent of the accumulated secretory

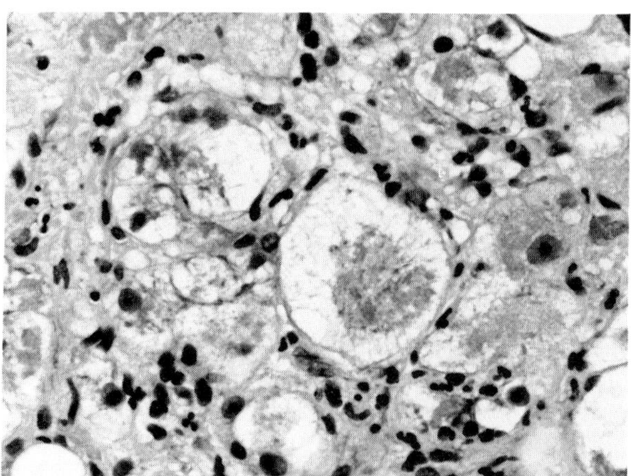

Fig. 3.9 Alcoholic hepatitis with enlarged hepatocytes. Mallory bodies are seen in hepatocytes which exhibit marked ballooning degeneration. An infiltrate of neutrophil polymorphs surrounds these cells. H&E, ×420.

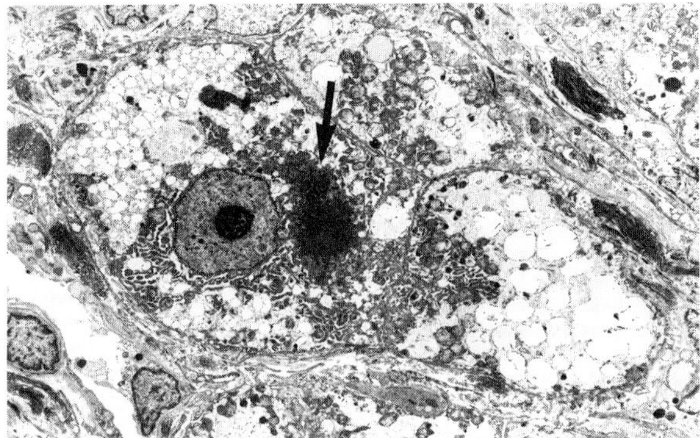

Fig. 3.10 Hepatocyte enlargement. The hepatocyte contains numerous fat droplets and Mallory bodies (arrow). ×1670.

proteins are located in the Golgi apparatus, with the remainder equally distributed in the SER, RER and cytosol (Volentine *et al.* 1986).

Ballooning degeneration is often most pronounced in hepatocytes that contain Mallory bodies (see Figs 3.7–3.10). The enlarged cells otherwise appear to be empty and show little or no immunostaining for the intermediate filaments – cytokeratins 8 and 18 – normally demonstrated in the cytoplasm of hepatocytes by the antibody CAM5.2 (French *et al.* 1993). Preisegger *et al.* (1991), using a panel of monoclonal antibodies directed against different cytokeratin polypeptide components, suggested that the "empty cell" phenomenon is due to a diminution of the cytokeratin network rather than altered antigenic determinants. Studies in both humans and animal models indicate that hepatocyte enlargement contributes to portal hypertension in alcoholic liver disease (Orrego *et al.* 1981; Blendis *et al.* 1982; Israel *et al.* 1982; Vidins *et al.* 1985; Tarao *et al.* 1989; Sato *et al.*1989; Valla *et al.* 1989; see also Chapter 19). For example, Vidins *et al.* (1985) showed that the surface area of hepatocytes was significantly increased in alcoholic liver disease (563 ± 32 μm compared with 301 ± 26 μm in normal livers), with a significant inverse correlation between hepatocyte size and sinusoidal area suggesting sinusoidal compression. Patients in whom the sinusoidal area was reduced to less than 20 percent of normal showed an inverse correlation between the portal pressure and the sinusoidal area. Okanoue *et al.* (1988) performed serial liver biopsies and intrahepatic portal vein pressure measurements on 12 patients, and found reductions in both hepatocyte size and portal pressure in those with mild fibrosis; with severe fibrosis, the intrahepatic pressure

remained elevated despite the reduction in hepatocyte size. These results support the hypothesis that hepatocyte enlargement makes a significant contribution to portal hypertension and, in addition, demonstrate that abstinence from alcohol may reduce portal pressure at least in the early stages of liver injury.

However, some animal studies failed to support the role of hepatocyte enlargement in portal hypertension (Mastai *et al.* 1989; Huet *et al.* 1990) and the hypothesis remains controversial.

Mallory bodies

Mallory (1911) described amorphous, eosinophilic, intracytoplasmic inclusions in alcoholic liver disease. Initially, these inclusions were thought to be pathognomonic of alcohol-induced liver injury and the term *alcoholic hyalin* was coined. However, since morphologically and biochemically identical cytoplasmic inclusions are now recognized in a great variety of unrelated, non-alcoholic liver diseases, the term alcoholic hyalin is no longer meaningful and should be abandoned (for a review, see Hall 1994a; for a detailed discussion see Chapter 11). Mallory bodies appear to be an entirely non-specific manifestation of hepatocyte injury.

Mallory bodies can usually be recognized in haematoxylin and eosin-stained sections as irregularly shaped, eosinophilic cytoplasmic inclusions (see Figs 3.7–3.9); however, immunohistochemical stains, using a variety of antibodies to the various components of the Mallory bodies, will not only confirm their presence but will often reveal small Mallory bodies that were not apparent in the routinely stained sections (Ray 1987; Yoshioka *et al.* 1989). Anti-ubiquitin is a useful, but non-specific marker for Mallory bodies (Vyberg and Leth 1991) (Fig. 3.11; see also Plate 3). Van Eyken *et al.* (1988) have demonstrated the variable expression of bile duct cytokeratins K7 and K19 in Mallory bodies and adjacent hepatocytes (Fig. 3.12)

Yokoo *et al.* (1972) described, using electron microscopy, three morphologically distinct forms of Mallory bodies: type I, bundles of filaments in parallel arrays; type II, clusters of randomly orientated fibrils; type III, granular or amorphous substance containing only scattered remains of fibrils. The Mallory bodies seen in alcoholic liver disease are usually type II (Fig. 3.13). Mallory body filaments, after removal of non-filamentous material by detergent extraction, consist of filamentous rods

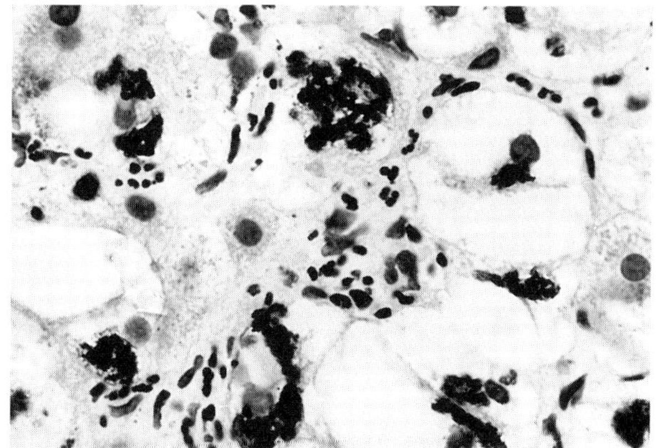

Fig. 3.11 Mallory bodies. Large Mallory bodies can be clearly seen in a liver stained immunohistochemically using a ubiquitin antibody. PAP, ×470.

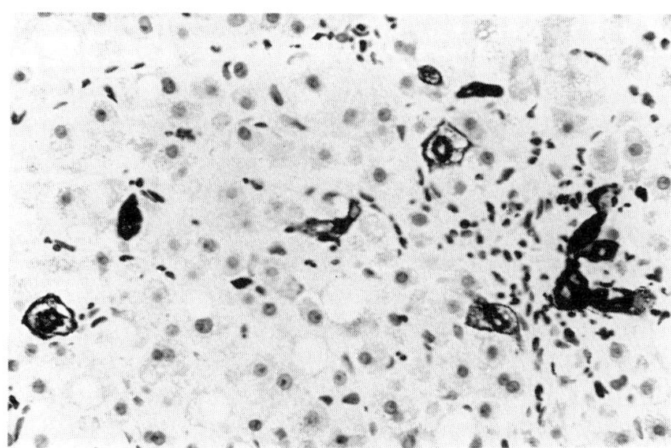

Fig. 3.12 "Pre-Mallory bodies". The presence of abnormal (biliary-type) cytokeratin is demonstrated in several hepatocytes using an antibody to cytokeratin 19. A bile duct (right) also stains positively. PAP, ×220.

10 nm in width (Franke *et al.* 1979; French 1981; Denk *et al.* 1982; Denk and Lackinger 1986).

The isolation of Mallory bodies in a purified fraction has made chemical analysis possible (French *et al.* 1972). Mallory body protein, which occurs in humans with alcoholic hepatitis, is composed of five major polypeptides of 56, 50, 47, 43, and 30 kDa (Tinberg 1981; French 1983). Some of the polypeptides are of similar size to normal hepatocyte keratins, while the smaller components may represent degradation products (see review by Worman 1990).

Immunological studies have shown that Mallory bodies are composed of intermediate filaments

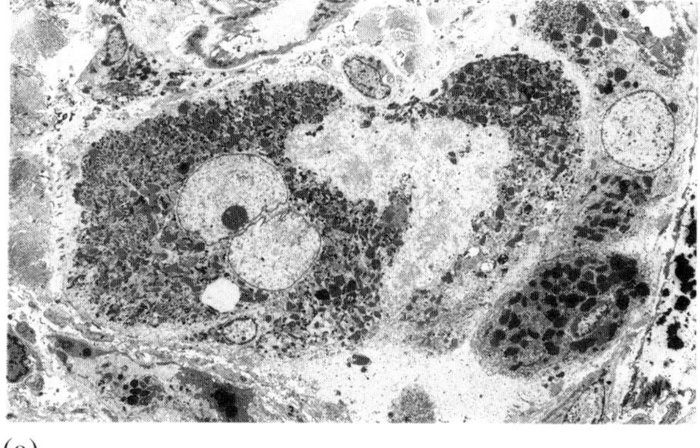

(a)

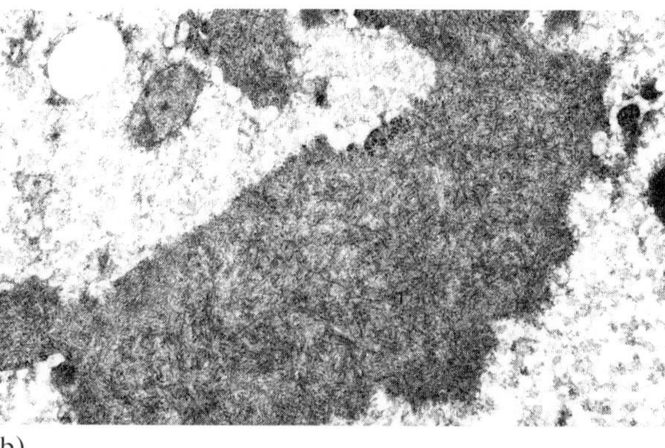

(b)

Fig. 3.13 Mallory body. (a) Hepatocyte containing a large, degenerate (type III) Mallory body situated to the right of the nucleus. ×1120. (b) Mallory body (type II) comprising a mass of randomly oriented filaments. ×12,000.

which are similar, but not entirely identical, to the cytokeratins of the normal hepatocyte (Franke *et al.* 1979; Kimoff and Haung 1981; French 1983). Morton *et al.* (1981) developed a monoclonal antibody which demonstrated the presence of certain unique antigenic determinants in Mallory bodies; they also showed that Mallory bodies from both alcoholic and non-alcoholic liver disease share a common antigenic determinant. Hazen *et al.* (1986) have developed a monoclonal antibody that, by immunofluoresence microscopy, recognizes Mallory bodies but not intermediate filaments in normal hepatocytes. The results of this study and of similar studies by Katsuma *et al.* (1987) and Ray (1987) have led to the suggestion that some "masked" epitopes of normal intermediate filaments are exposed during the formation of Mallory bodies. Worman (1990), in summarizing the resuts of a number of recent studies states "all of these data suggest that Mallory bodies are composed of intermediate filament proteins and likely arise from the disruption of pre-existing normal cellular intermediate filament networks".

The pathogenesis of Mallory body formation remains to be elucidated. Current hypotheses include direct and indirect mechanisms of injury of the intermediate filaments (cytokeratin) of the hepatocyte.

Direct injury of existing or newly formed intermediate filaments

Worman (1990) speculated that alcohol or its metabolites could injure intermediate filaments, which are constantly undergoing assembly, disassembly and rearrangement, in hepatocytes that are regenerating following an episode of alcoholic hepatitis.

Microtubular failure

Griseofulvin, a known antimicrotubular agent, reliably induces Mallory body production in mice (Denk *et al.* 1975). Acohol or acetaldehyde might have a similar effect and result in a decrease in polymerized hepatocyte microtubules (Denk *et al.* 1979; Denk and Lackinger 1986; French 1981, 1983; French *et al.* 1987). A reduction in the amount of hepatocyte microtubules has been reported in alcoholic liver disease in humans (Matsuda *et al.* 1979). At present, it is uncertain whether hepatocytes *in vivo* are exposed to concentrations of acetaldehyde high enough to cause polymerization of microtubules (Baraona *et al.* 1984).

Vitamin A deficiency

Many disorders associated with intermediate filament derangement and Mallory body formation are associated with vitamin A deficiency (Denk *et al.* 1979; Denk and Lackinger 1986). Hepatic vitamin A levels are low in griseofulvin-treated mice (Denk *et al.* 1979), and vitamin A deficiency in these mice can induce Mallory body formation (Akeda *et al.* 1986). Conflicting results have been obtained in human studies. Leo and Lieber (1983) were unable to show a correlation between low vitamin A levels and the presence of Mallory bodies, but Ray *et al.* (1988), using sensitive immunohistochemical techniques, showed a significant inverse correlation between serum vitamin A and the amount of cytokeratin antigen in hepatocytes. Thus vitamin A deficiency could be a trigger for the aggregation of cytokeratin filaments.

Preneoplasia

Mallory bodies have been observed in hepatocellular carcinomas in humans (Keeley *et al.* 1972; Nakanuma and Ohta 1984) and in rats treated with diethylnitrosamine (Borenfreund and Bendich 1978). That Mallory bodies were located in "enzyme-altered" cells led to the suggestion that Mallory body formation might be a preneoplastic change. However, in humans with alcoholic liver disease, there is a poor correlation between the presence of Mallory bodies in non-neoplastic cells and the frequency of subsequent tumours (Nakanuma and Ohta 1985). Clearly, the "preneoplastic hypothesis" cannot be invoked to account for the development of Mallory bodies in the many and varied non-neoplastic diseases with which they are associated (see Chapter 11).

Autoimmune damage to intermediate filament network

As discussed by Bird and MacSween in Chapter 6, a wide spectrum of immunological responses has been reported in association with alcoholic liver disease. Mallory bodies could initiate an immune response that contributes to hepatocyte injury in alcoholic hepatitis; alternatively antibodies against intermediate filament subunits or filament-associated proteins might be responsible for the disruption of the intermediate filament networks seen in this condition. Although antibodies against intermediate filaments (Zauli *et al.* 1985) and microtubules (Kurki *et al.* 1983) have been described, they are not present in the majority of patients with alcoholic hepatitis (for further discussion see review by Worman 1990).

Abnormal intermediate filament metabolism

Abnormalities in the degradation of intermediate filament protein subunits might be responsible for the cytoskeletal disturbances seen in alcoholic hepatitis (Irie *et al.* 1984; Denk and Lackinger 1986; Ohta *et al.* 1988). Ohta *et al.* (1988) have demonstrated the presence of the polypeptide ubiquitin on both the cytokeratin filaments and Mallory bodies, but it is not yet clear whether abnormalities in the ubiquitin-dependent degradation pathway are primary or secondary phenomena (Denk *et al.* 1989).

Mallory bodies resemble Lewy bodies of Parkinson's disease, the neurofibrillary tangles and plaques of Alzheimer's disease in several respects. All these structures are morphologically similar (both light and electron microscopically) and share similar histochemical and immunohistochemical properties (Ohta *et al.* 1988; Preisegger *et al.* 1992).

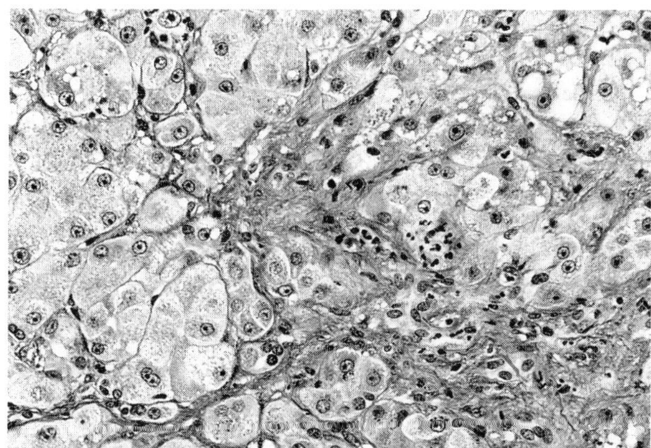

Fig. 3.14 Pericellular fibrosis. The liver shows focal pericellular fibrosis and a focal infiltrate of neutrophil polymorphs. Sirius red, ×230.

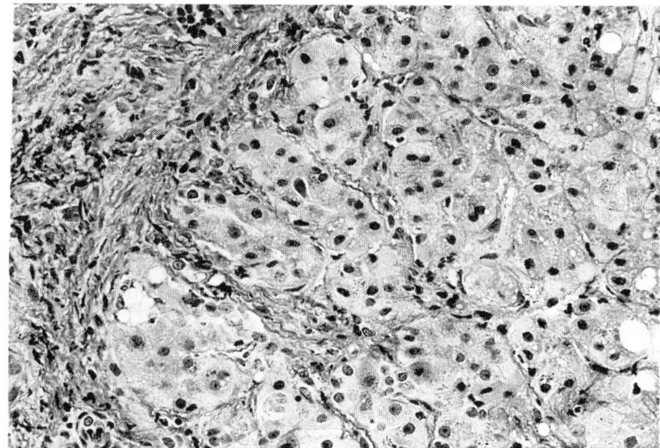

Fig. 3.15 Pericellular fibrosis. The liver shows extensive pericellular fibrosis which extends through the parenchyma. Sirius red, ×190.

Hepatic fibrosis

The pathophysiology of hepatic fibrosis is reviewed by Maher and Friedman in Chapter 4. The patterns of hepatic fibrosis, perivenular fibrosis at the fatty liver stage of injury (Van Waes and Lieber 1977; Nakano *et al.* 1982a,b; Worner and Lieber 1985) (see Fig. 3.5) and perivenular and pericellular or "chicken-wire" fibrosis seen in association with alcoholic hepatitis (Figs 3.14 and 3.15; see also Plates 4 and 5), although non-specific, are highly characteristic of alcohol-related liver.

Several Japanese studies have reported pericellular fibrosis, often termed "alcoholic fibrosis", appar-

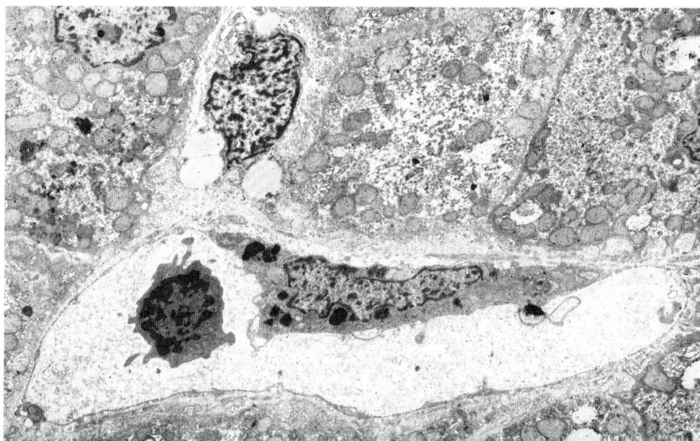

Fig. 3.16 Ito cell. An Ito cell is seen in the space of Disse with a portion of a hepatocyte on either side (top). A lymphocyte and a Kupffer cell are seen within a sinusoid. ×2470.

ently occurring in the absence of alcoholic hepatitis (Karasawa *et al.* 1980; Takada *et al.* 1982; Ohnishi and Okuda 1985). The role of coexistent hepatitis C virus infection in the development of "alcoholic fibrosis" requires further evaluation.

Pericellular fibrosis is thought to develop as a result of cytokine-mediated stimulation and transformation of the Ito (fat-storing) cells situated in the space of Disse (Fig. 3.16) into transitional cells, myofibroblasts and fibroblasts which are responsible for the deposition of collagen in the perisinusoidal space (Nakano *et al.* 1982a, b; Mak *et al.* 1984; Mak and Lieber 1988). Ito cells, in a ratio of about 1:20 hepatocytes, can be demonstrated in sections of normal human liver using an anti-α-smooth muscle actin antibody (personal observation). In alcoholic hepatitis and alcoholic cirrhosis, both the number of positively stained cells and the intensity of staining per cell are greatly increased (Fig. 3.17; see also Plate 6). Numerous α-smooth muscle actin-containing cells are also seen in fibrous tissue septa (Yamaoka *et al.* 1993). The presence of α-smooth muscle actin has been used as a marker for "activation" of Ito cells in studies of rat liver, both in tissue sections and in Ito cell cultures (Ramadori *et al.* 1990; Rockey *et al.* 1992; see also Chapter 6). The development of fibrosis in the perivenular region is partially explained by the proliferation of myofibroblasts, which are normally located in this region of the liver (Bhathal 1972; Nakano *et al.* 1982a). Immunohistochemical studies have demonstrated both desmin and vimentin intermediate filaments as well as α-smooth muscle actin in myofibroblasts (Skalli *et al.* 1989).

A reduction in hepatic vitamin A, which is associ-

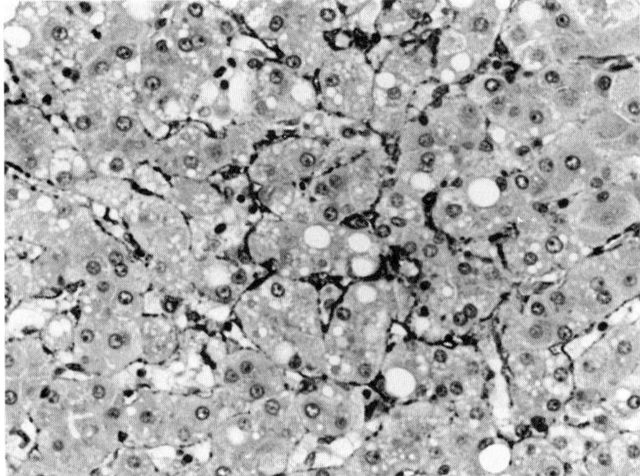

Fig. 3.17 Ito cells. Liver from a patient with alcoholic liver disease stained with an α-smooth muscle actin antibody. The positively stained cells are "activated" Ito cells. PAP, ×220.

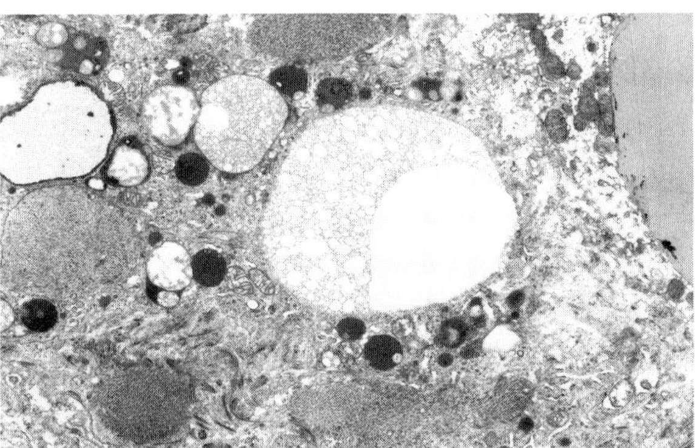

Fig. 3.18 Multivesicular lysosomes. Hepatocyte containing two multivesicular lysosomes. Large masses of collagen are seen in the space of Disse (top, bottom and left). ×4400.

ated with the formation of multivesiculate lysosomes in hepatocytes (Leo *et al*. 1983) (see Fig. 3.18), may contribute to the transformation of Ito cells into collagen-producing cells (see Chapter 4).

The process of *capillarization of the sinusoids* described by Schaffner and Popper (1963) is today explained by the deposition in the space of Disse of various types of collagen and basal lamina-like material, produced predominantly by transformed Ito cells (Hahn *et al*. 1980; Mak *et al*. 1984; Minato *et al*. 1983; Okanoue *et al*. 1983), but also to a lesser

extent by the sinusoidal endothelial cells (Clement *et al*. 1986). The deposition of extracellular matrix proteins has been demonstrated in tissue sections by immunogold techniques (Burt *et al*. 1988). The deposition of collagenous and non-collagenous proteins in the space of Disse is thought to interfere with the normal exchange of oxygen and nutrients between the blood and the hepatocytes (Le Bail *et al*. 1990); thus this process may contribute to hepatocyte dysfunction and hepatocyte injury in alcoholic liver disease.

Defenestration of the hepatic sinusoids is discussed in detail in Chapter 15. Several studies have suggested that there is a relationship between alcohol-induced changes in the "porosity" of the endothelial lining of the sinusoids and the presence of pericellular fibrosis (Mak and Lieber 1984; Brouwer *et al*. 1988; Horn *et al*. 1986, 1987); while the results of a morphometric study by Sztark *et al*. (1986) suggested that changes in the sinusoidal barrier may precede and contribute to the development of hepatic fibrosis (see Chapters 4, 14 and 15).

Occlusive venous lesions

Partial occlusion of hepatic venules and veins in association with "sclerosing hyaline necrosis" was described by Edmondson *et al*. (1963). It is of interest that in 1969 Reynolds and colleagues described 28 patients with portal hypertension occurring in the absence of cirrhosis but in association with central hyaline sclerosis accompanied by variable degrees of venous occlusion. More recently, a retrospective review of 200 autopsy cases of alcoholic liver disease by Goodman and Ishak (1982) revealed three types of venous lesions:

1. Lymphocytic phlebitis, characterized by the presence of a mononuclear cell infilrate in the vein walls. This lesion was seen in 16.7 percent of livers showing alcoholic hepatitis and in 4.3 percent of cirrhotic livers.
2. Phlebosclerosis, characterized by perivenular fibrosis and variable obliteration of the lumen of the terminal hepatic venules. This lesion was found to some degree in all livers showing the feature of alcoholic hepatitis, and sometimes also involved the larger intercalated veins (interlobular veins).
3. Veno-oclusive lesions, characterized by fibrointimal hyperplasia with varying degrees of occlusion of the lumen of the vein (Fig. 3.19; see also Plate 7). This process, which usually affec-

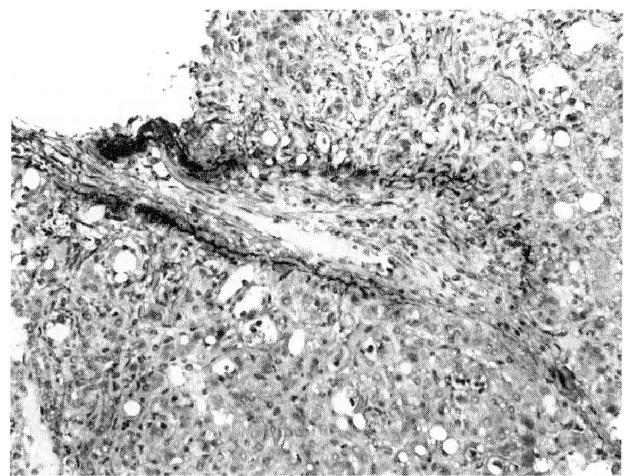

Fig. 3.19 Veno-occlusive lesion. Terminal hepatic venule showing prominent fibrointimal proliferation. The liver exhibited alcoholic hepatitis (not shown). Verhoeff-Van Gieson, ×90.

ted terminal hepatic venules, sometimes intercalated veins and occasionally the portal veins, was seen in 52.1 percent of patients with alcoholic hepatitis and 74.1 percent of those with cirrhosis. Almost 50 percent of the patients with alcoholic hepatitis without cirrhosis had portal hypertension, and 81.8 percent of those patients had marked phebosclerosis and some degree of veno-occlusive change.

However, another retrospective review, which included 256 liver biopsies and 51 autopsy livers from patients with alcoholic liver disease, revealed veno-occlusive lesions in only 9.8 percent of the biopsied livers and in 22 percent of the autopsy livers (Burt and MacSween 1986). This study confirmed the universal finding of phlebosclerosis in alcoholic hepatitis and cirrhosis; the severity of the phlebosclerosis increased with progressive liver injury and the authors speculated that the venous lesions may be implicated in the evolution of liver injury.

Pathogenesis

The pathogenesis of alcoholic hepatitis is unclear. The pattern of liver injury is that of an acute process which is characterized by hepatocyte necrosis and an infiltrate of neutrophil polymorphs. Alcohol and/or its metabolites are assumed to cause the acute hepatocyte injury despite the following observations:

only a small proportion of drinkers develop alcoholic hepatitis; the association is with chronic and not acute alcohol consumption; in most cases, there is a lack of association with binge drinking; and the wide variety of agents and diseases associated with a similar pattern of liver injury in the absence of alcohol (see Chapter 12). As discussed in Chapter 12, non-alcoholic steatohepatitis (pseudoalcoholic liver disease) is usually less severe and progresses to cirrhosis more slowly than the similar pattern of liver injury in drinkers. Perhaps chronic alcohol ingestion makes the liver more susceptible to injury by the agents that are aetiologically associated with the pseudoalcoholic form of liver injury. This suggestion could explain the failure of alcohol *per se* to result in alcoholic hepatitis in the various animal models (see Chapter 17). Future studies in humans and animal models could be designed to test the hypothesis that so-called alcoholic hepatitis in drinkers is not due to alcohol *per se*, but that alcohol exacerbates liver injury by other agents. Only a low dose of alcohol may be required to potentiate injury in susceptible individuals who are exposed to other agents/disease states, for example drugs such as methotrexate (see Chapter 18), diabetes mellitus and obesity (see Chapter 12). In such cases, the liver injury could then be regarded as alcohol-associated rather than alcoholic liver disease.

Clinical aspects and prognosis

Alcoholic hepatitis may be seen in liver biopsies from drinkers who are asymptomatic (French and Burbridge 1979). Seventeen percent of liver biopsies from people presenting for treatment of alcoholism revealed alcoholic hepatitis (Bhathal *et al.* 1975). A liver biopsy study by Hislop *et al.* (1983) showed alcoholic hepatitis superimposed on established cirrhosis at the time of initial presentation in 39 percent of patients, suggesting that previous alcohol-induced liver injury may have been asymptomatic. Thus the concept of "acute alcoholic hepatitis" as a syndrome that can be diagnosed purely on the basis of clinical and biochemical features has virtually been abandoned. However, most patients have nonspecific gastrointestinal symptoms, hepatomegaly and raised liver enzymes (Brunt *et al.* 1974; Morgan and Sherlock 1977; Hislop *et al.* 1983). About 25 percent of patients with extensive hepatocyte necrosis present with the clinical features of liver failure or hepatic encephalopathy (Brunt *et al.* 1974; Morgan and Sherlock 1977).

Liver biopsy changes that correlate with a poor prognosis include active and extensive hepatocyte necrosis with widespread pericellular fibrosis (Nassrallah *et al.* 1980), architectural disturbance with the formation of fibrous tissue septa, widespread veno-occlusive lesions (Goodman and Ishak 1982) and severe cholestasis (Nissenbaum *et al.* 1990). The number of Mallory bodies was suggested to have prognostic significance (Christoffersen *et al.* 1973; Harinasuta and Zimmerman 1971; Boitnott and Maddrey 1981), but the poor outcome in these cases probably reflects the severity of the hepatocyte injury rather than the Mallory bodies *per se*.

Using light microscopy, Chedid *et al.* (1986) investigated the significance of giant mitochondria, in sections of liver biopsies from 202 patients with alcoholic hepatitis. The patients with alcoholic hepatitis and giant mitochondria were thought to belong to a subgroup who had mild clinical features, a low incidence of cirrhosis and a good long-term survival .

Controversy persists about the prognostic significance of perivenular fibrosis at the fatty liver stage of alcoholic liver disease; however, there is general agreement that the presence of perivenular and pericellular fibrosis in liver biopsies showing alcoholic hepatitis indicates that progression to cirrhosis is likely, particularly in those patients who continue to drink (Nasrallah *et al.* 1980). The natural history of alcoholic hepatitis is one of progression, over a variable period of time, to cirrhosis. In most cases, this progression is associated with continued drinking; for example, Sorensen *et al.* (1984) reported that 50 percent of patients with alcoholic hepatitis who continued to drink, progressed to cirrhosis in 10–13 years. However, progression to cirrhosis has also been recorded despite apparent abstinence (Galambos 1972).

The highest mortality rate for patients with alcoholic hepatitis is in the first year after diagnosis irrespective of the presence or absence of cirrhosis (Orrego *et al.* 1987). Three variables that independently increase the risk of cirrhosis are the severity of the liver injury in the initial biopsy, continued drinking and female gender (Pares *et al.* 1986; see also Chapter 7).

It is not the purpose of this chapter to discuss the treatment of alcoholic hepatitis, but the reader is referred to recent reviews that discuss clinical features, management and prognosis (Maddrey 1988, 1990; Sherlock 1990; Schenker and Halff 1993; Mezey 1993; see also Chapter 19).

Alcoholic cirrhosis

The standardized criteria for the morphological diagnosis of cirrhosis (Anthony *et al.* 1978) should be strictly adhered to because of the prognostic implications of this diagnosis, as well as to facilitate meaningful comparisons of the prevalence of alcoholic cirrhosis, and the risk of the complication of hepatocellular carcinoma, in different parts of the world. It is also always important to differentiate septal fibrosis (Gerber and Popper 1972) that is seen in the evolution of cirrhosis from an established micronodular cirrhosis, but particularly when the effects of therapeutic modalities are being evaluated.

Micronodular cirrhosis

The features that are considered essential for the diagnosis of cirrhosis are generalized involvement of the liver by concurrent parenchymal necrosis, regeneration and fibrosis resulting in disorganization of the acinar architecture. Anthony *et al.* (1978) defined cirrhosis as "a diffuse process characterized by fibrosis and the conversion of normal liver architecture into structurally abnormal nodules".

Alcoholic cirrhosis is usually of the micronodular type (Baptista *et al.* 1981), but the cirrhotic process may become macronodular particularly if the patient becomes abstinent (Fauerholdt *et al.* 1983; Rubin *et al.* 1962). Macroscopically, the micronodular cirrhotic liver is usually smaller than normal and has a uniformly and finely nodular capsular and cut

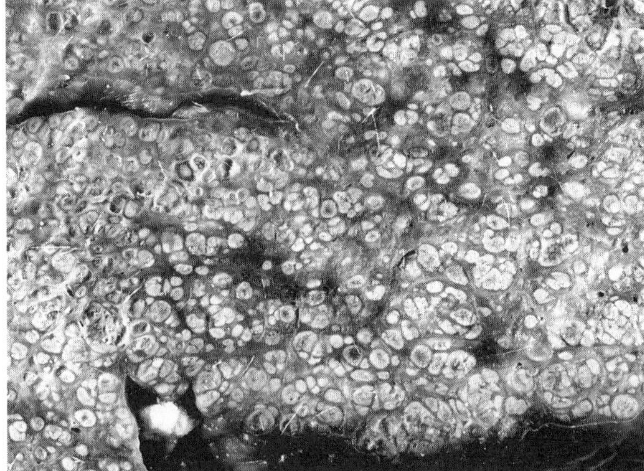

Fig. 3.20 Micronodular cirrhosis. Liver showing the classical appearance of a micronodular cirrhosis. The pallor of the regenerative nodules is due to fatty change.

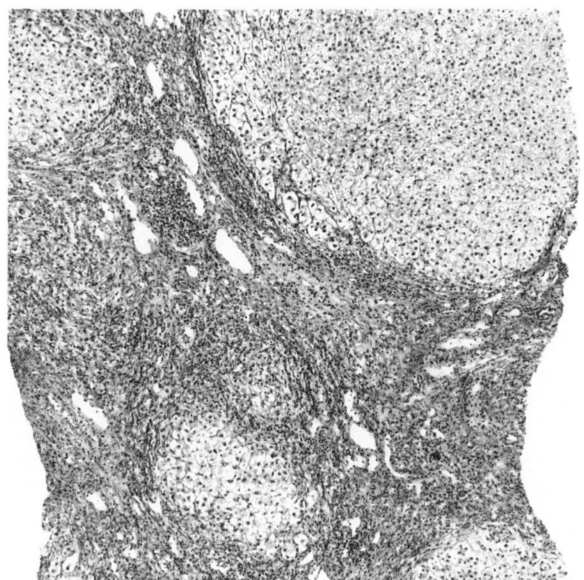

Fig. 3.21 Micronodular cirrhosis. The liver shows established micronodular cirrhosis, and also focal pericellular fibrosis within the regenerative nodules. Sirius red, ×50.

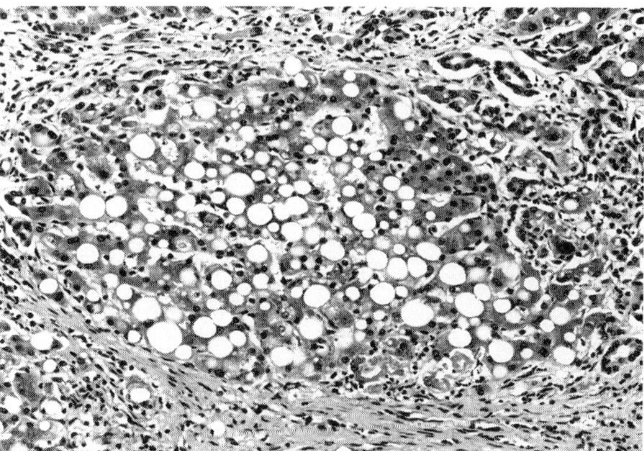

Fig. 3.22 Micronodular cirrhosis and steatosis. Autopsy liver from a patient who continued to drink until dying suddenly from bleeding varices. The liver shows moderately severe macrovesicular steatosis superimposed on an established cirrhosis. H&E, ×100.

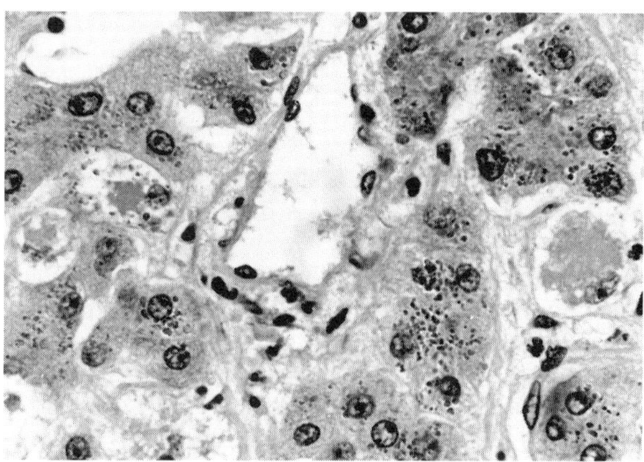

Fig. 3.23 Persistent Mallory bodies. The patient, a 37-year-old woman, underwent liver transplant for liver failure due to alcoholic cirrhosis. She had abstained from alcohol for 4 months prior to transplantation. Mallory bodies are seen in several hepatocytes on either side of a terminal hepatic venule. H&E, ×400.

surface (Fig. 3.20). In some cases, where drinking has continued, the liver may be rather enlarged and yellow due to fatty change; while the finding of a dark brown cirrhotic liver in a drinker is highly suggestive of coexistent haemochromatosis. The regenerative nodules of a micronodular cirrhosis are remarkably uniform in appearance and measure 1–3 mm in diameter. It is easy to diagnose an established cirrhosis on needle biopsy samples of liver because of the small size of the nodules (Fig. 3.21; see also Plate 8). Sometimes, biopsy tissue from a cirrhotic liver will fragment, resulting in a number of small nodules of hepatocytes that are wholly or partially surrounded by fibrous tissue, which is highly suggestive of cirrhosis (Anthony *et al.* 1978).

Characteristically in micronodular cirrhosis there is widespread loss of the normal acinar architecture, and the terminal hepatic venules and hepatic vein branches are no longer recognizable due to their incorporation into the bands of fibrous tissue that surround the regenerative nodules. Shunts develop between pre-existing and newly-formed vessels.

The presence of fatty change and active alcoholic hepatitis, which is usually most pronounced at the periphery of the regenerative nodules, is highly suggestive of continued drinking (Fig. 3.22). The observation that fatty change is rarely seen in alco-

holic cirrhosis was probably based on post mortem findings in patients who had been hospitalized for some weeks prior to death. Mallory bodies, however, may persist for many months after the cessation of alcohol (Fig. 3.23). Excess stainable iron is frequently seen in the hepatocytes in alcoholic liver disease (Fig. 3.24). Jakobovits *et al.* (1979) reported mild siderosis in 57 percent and marked siderosis in 7 percent of their cases. The differentiation of alco-

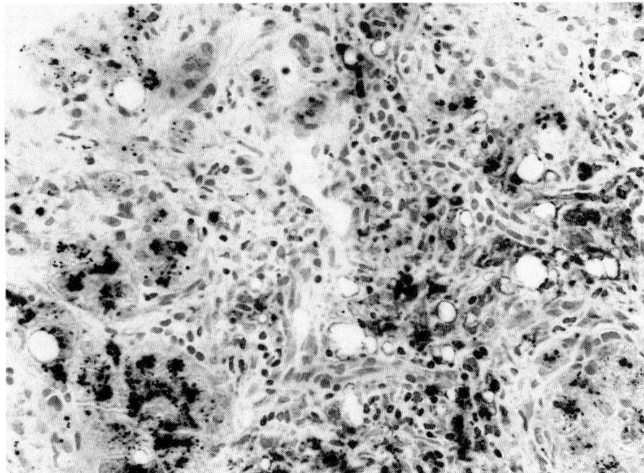

Fig. 3.24 Alcoholic siderosis? Liver from a 50-year-old man with alcoholic cirrhosis. Occasional periportal hepatocytes contain large amounts of iron. Heavy iron deposition is also seen in portal tract macrophages (centre). Perls' method for iron, ×230.

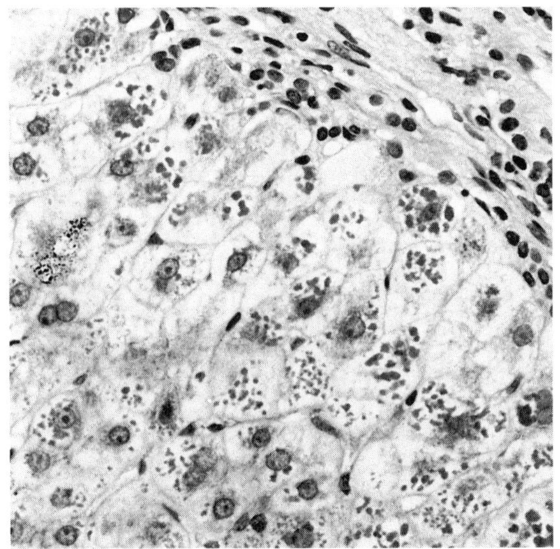

Fig. 3.25 Alpha-1-antitrypsin (AAT) droplets. Alcoholic cirrhotic liver showing numerous PAS-positive, diastase-resistant droplets in hepatocytes at the edge of a regenerative nodule. D/PAS, ×360.

holic siderosis from genetic haemochromatosis occurring in drinkers is of paramount importance because of the therapeutic implications, and is discussed in detail by Powell *et al.* in Chapter 12. Occasionally, high-grade siderosis is an unexpected finding in the liver biopsy. A methodology has been developed and validated which allows the retrieval of any remaining tissue from the paraffin block and chemical measurement of the hepatic iron concentration (Williams *et al.*, manuscript in preparation), thus permitting calculation of the hepatic iron index (Bassett *et al.* 1986).

The secondary accumulation of either alpha-1-antitrypsin droplets (Pariente *et al.* 1981) or copper (Berresford *et al.* 1980) manifests as diastase-resistant/PAS-positive droplets which are seen maximally in hepatocytes at the periphery of the regenerative nodules (Fig. 3.24). The exact nature of these cytoplasmic inclusions can be determined immunohistochemically in the case of alpha-1-antitrypsin or by an orcein or rhodanine stain for copper.

Oncocytic hepatocytes are frequently seen in alcoholic cirrhosis; the oncocytic appearance is due to the presence of large numbers of mitochondria, which result in a deeply and uniformly eosinophilic cytoplasm (Lefkowitch *et al.* 1980; Gerber and Thung 1981). Immunohistochemical stains may be required to differentiate these oncocytic cells from the "ground glass" cells of chronic hepatitis B virus infection (Hadziyannis *et al.* 1973).

Regeneration – "stem cells"

Regenerating hepatocytes seen in association with both acute and chronic liver injury of any aetiology often exhibit an abnormal architecture (so-called lobular or acinar disarray) and can be seen as two-cell-thick plates and as small acinar or gland-like structures (Fig 3.25). Bile is often secreted into the central lumina of these regenerative acini. This regenerative process is due to the division of uninjured hepatocytes and mitotic figures are often numerous.

After severe acute hepatic injury, large numbers of small epithelial cells and proliferating ductules are seen in the portal and periportal regions; in chronic injury, the proliferating ductules are seen in the bands of fibrous tissue that surround the regenerative nodules in a cirrhotic liver (Uchida and Peters 1983; see Fig. 3.26). In addition, regenerating hepatocytes may exhibit a ductal configuration, sometimes termed "ductal metaplasia" (Fig. 3.27). As discussed by Van Eyken *et al.* in Chapter 10, these features may represent the proliferation of "stem cells", with the subsequent differentiation into cells with the morphological and histochemical features of either biliary epithelial cells or hepatocytes (De Vos and Desmet 1992; Sigal *et al.* 1992; Ray 1987) (see Figs 3.28 and 3.29). The relationship

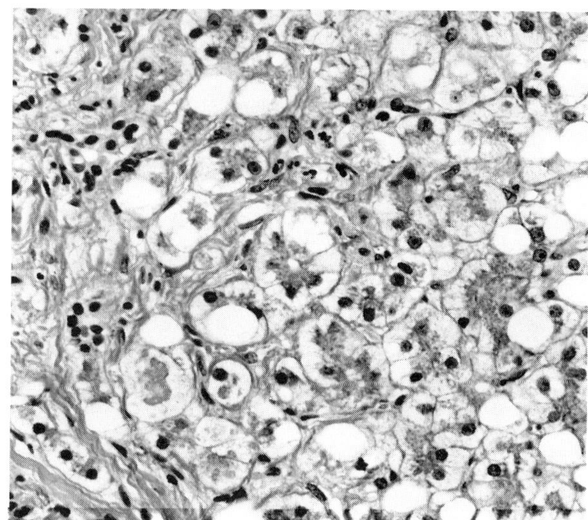

Fig. 3.26 Acinar regeneration. Liver showing alcoholic hepatitis with focal hepatocyte necrosis, a mild neutrophil polymorph infiltrate, Mallory bodies and fatty change. Acinar regeneration is a prominent feature (centre). The biopsy was performed several weeks after the patient was admitted to hospital with alcoholic hepatitis. H&E, ×270.

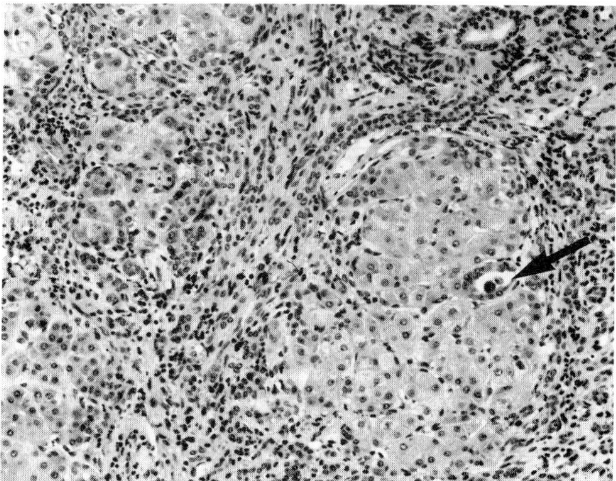

Fig. 3.27 Ductular proliferation. Liver biopsy, performed after some months of abstinence, showing micronodular cirrhosis and proliferating ductules (top right) both at the edge and within (arrow) a regenerative nodule. H&E, ×100.

between the groups of cells showing ductal metaplasia and the regenerative acini composed of differentiated hepatocytes is as yet unclear although the features seen in Fig. 3.30 suggest that the ductal cells may differentiate into hepatocytes.

Macronodular cirrhosis

In macronodular cirrhosis, the much larger nodules – generally ranging in size from 3 mm to 3 cm – often contain terminal hepatic venules and portal tracts (Fig. 3.31; see also Plate 9a). Macronodular cirrhosis may be suspected but cannot be confidently diagnosed by needle biopsy, because of the large size of the nodules. The biopsy specimens from cirrhotic livers often fragment along the bands of fibrous tissue that surround the regenerative nodules; helpful criteria for the diagnosis have been described (Anthony *et al.* 1978; Scheuer and Lefkowich 1994).

A study of 209 autopsy livers (about 50 percent of the cases were drinkers) found a mixed pattern of macronodular and micronodular cirrhosis in 43 percent indicating that a mixed pattern of cirrhosis is not uncommon (Rubin *et al.* 1962).

Fauerholdt *et al.* (1983), who for the purpose of their study defined "macroregenerative" nodules as nodules greater than 1.5 mm in diameter, found a 90

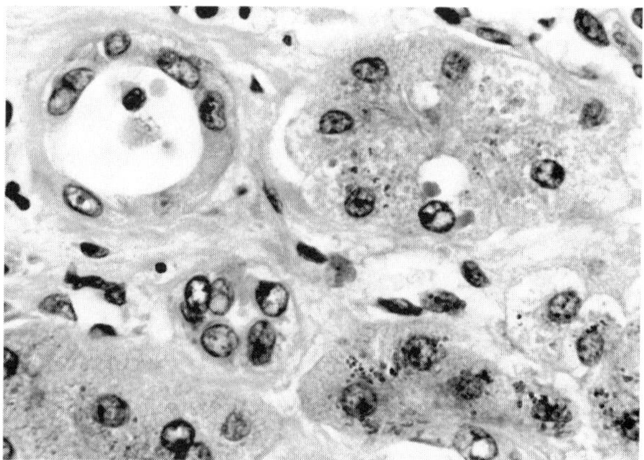

Fig. 3.28 "Ductal metaplasia". Cirrhotic liver containing several "ductules" composed of cells with features suggesting a transition between biliary-type cells and hepatocytes. H&E, ×450.

percent conversion rate from micronodular to macronodular cirrhosis, occurring with a median time interval of 2.25 years following the initial liver biopsy diagnosis of cirrhosis. The conversion rate was similar in men and women, and was faster in patients who became abstinent. One of the problems with this study is that the initial needle biopsy, due to sampling error, may have missed the macrono-

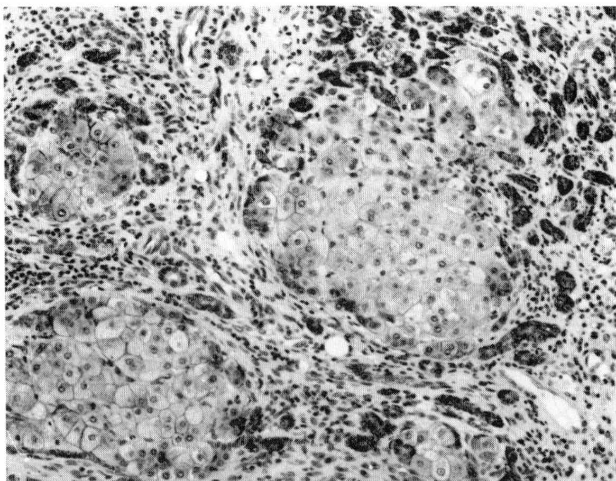

Fig. 3.29 Ductal proliferation. Alcoholic cirrhotic liver after 4 months of abstinence showing marked ductal proliferation (demonstrated by the antibody BerEP4), particularly at the periphery of the regenerative nodules. PAP, ×100.

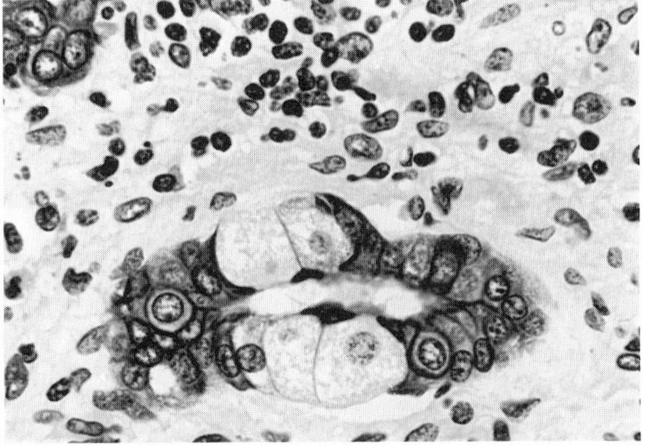

Fig. 3.30 "Stem cells". "Ductule" composed partially of cells with biliary epithelial features (stained positively by an antibody to cytokeratin 19) and partially by cells with the appearance of hepatocytes. Numerous small, positively stained epithelial cells ("stem cells") are also seen within the adjacent fibrous tissues. PAP, ×470.

dules that were already present, while the subsequent autopsy examination of the liver was unlikely to miss the larger nodules.

Gluud *et al.* (1987), in a serial liver biopsy study of 106 men with alcohol-related micronodular cirrhosis followed for a median time of 31 months, demon-

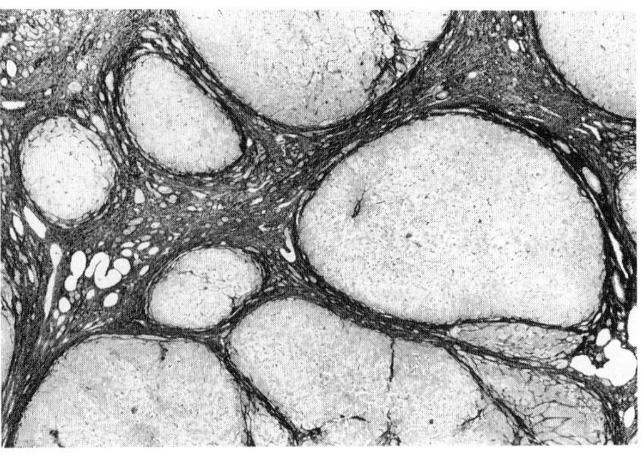

Fig. 3.31 Macronodular cirrhosis. "Native" liver showing macroregenerative nodules in which rudimentary portal tracts are apparent. The patient, who had been abstinent for several years, received a liver transplant for alcoholic cirrhosis. Sirius red, ×20.

strated the development of hyperplastic nodules (defined as nodules greater than 1.5 mm in diameter, which is the maximal diameter of the normal acinus) in 44 percent. The prevalence of the development of "hyperplastic" nodules was inversely related to the amount of alcohol consumed during the follow-up period: 57 percent in abstainers, 58 percent in those who consumed small amounts (< 50 g/day), 32 percent in moderate drinkers (51–100 g/day) and 18 percent in heavy drinkers (> 100 g/day). Alcohol has an inhibitory effect on hepatocyte regeneration (Duguay *et al.* 1982; Dalke *et al.* 1990). The development of macroregenerative nodules following abstinence may be a reflection of unimpaired hepatocyte regeneration.

It is readily apparent, from the studies mentioned above, that the use of varying criteria for the diagnosis of macronodular cirrhosis make it difficult to compare results. In addition, nodules which are detected by radiologic techniques in cirrhotic livers, and removed surgically – by local resection, partial hepatectomy or during liver transplantation – are often difficult to classify, with opinions on any one case ranging from benign/regenerative, through atypical/dysplastic to malignant (well-differentiated hepatocellular carcinoma). The lack of standardized criteria for hepatocellular lesions arising in chronic liver disease prompted a multinational panel of liver pathologists to propose the standardization of nomenclature and histological criteria for the diagnosis of such lesions as outlined below (Ferrell *et al.* 1993).

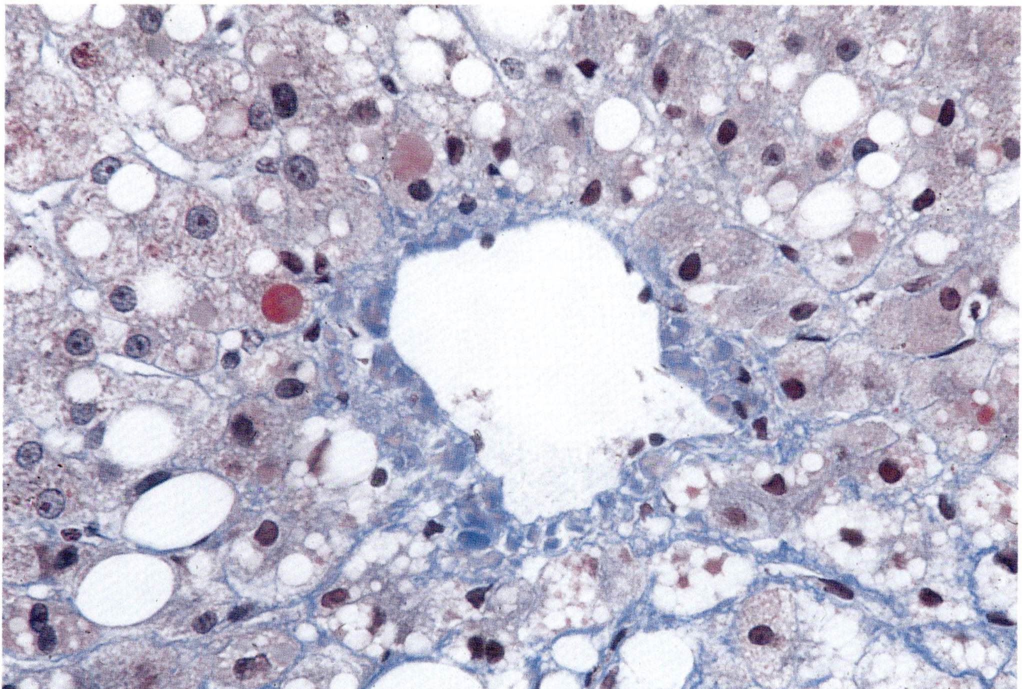

Plate 1 Giant mitochondria. Liver showing mild fatty change and several giant mitochondria (pink globules seen top left). Chromotrope-aniline blue, objective ×40.

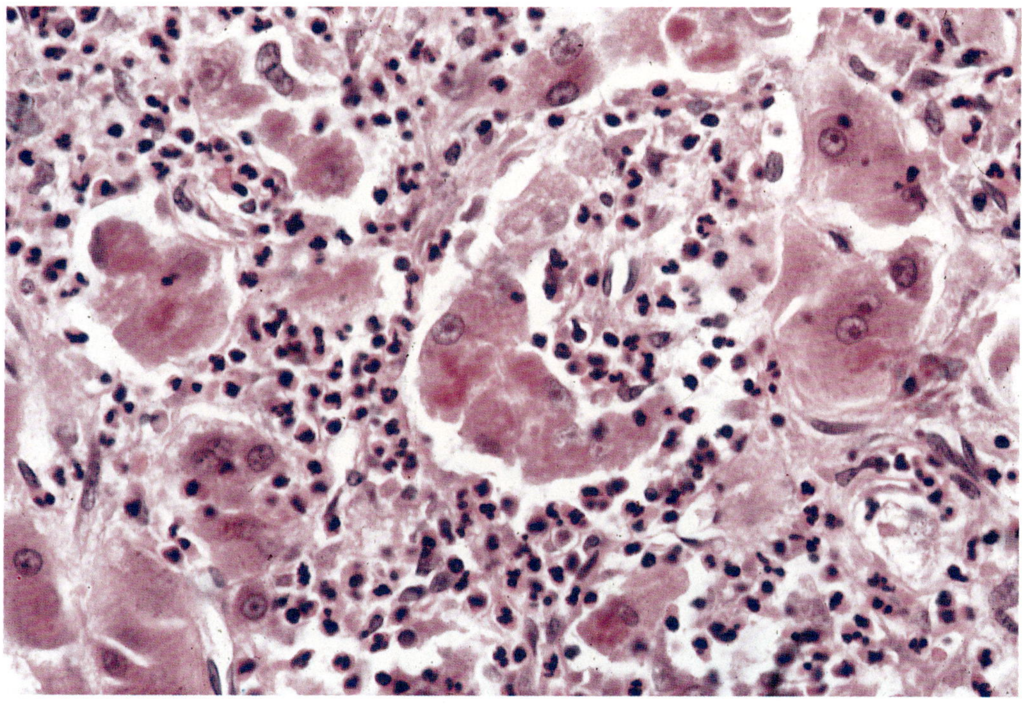

Plate 2 Alcoholic hepatitis with Mallory bodies. Mallory bodies are seen in several enlarged hepatocytes together with a heavy infiltrate of neutrophil polymorphs. H&E, objective ×40.

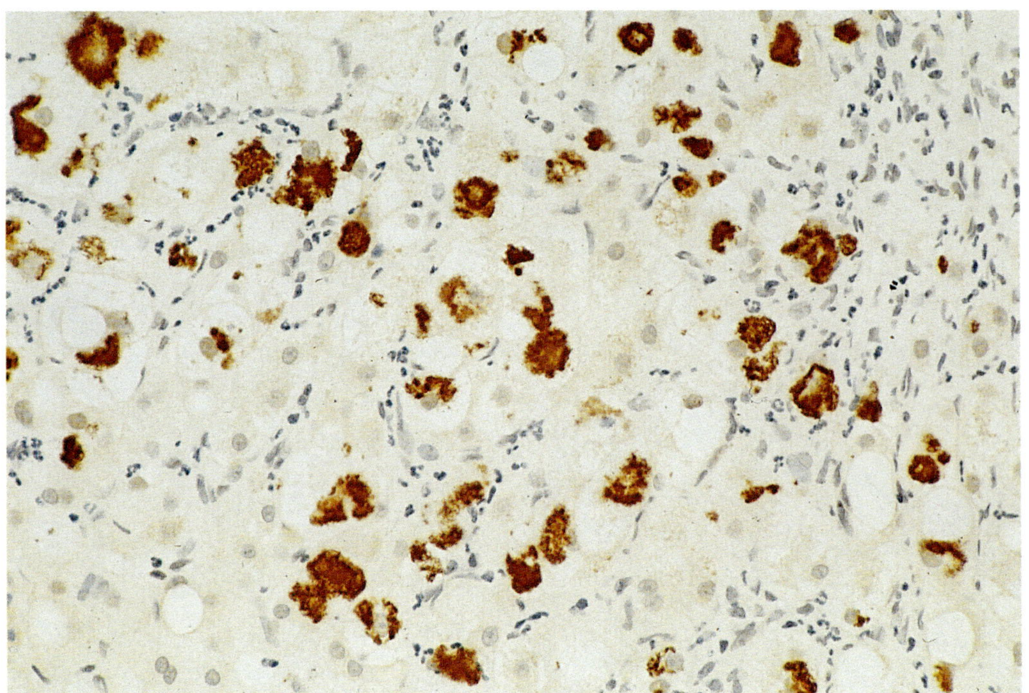

Plate 3 Mallory bodies. Large Mallory bodies can be seen clearly in a liver stained immunohisto-chemically using an antibody to ubiquitin. PAP, objective ×25.

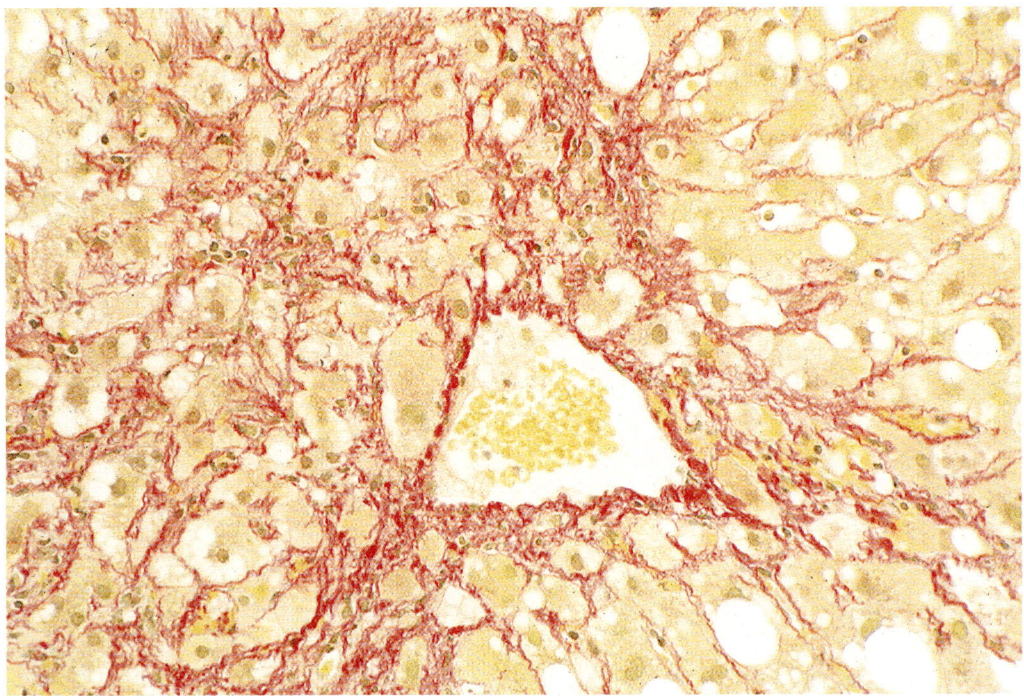

Plate 4 Pericellular fibrosis. The liver shows prominent pericellular fibrosis localized to the zone 3 region. Sirius red, objective ×25.

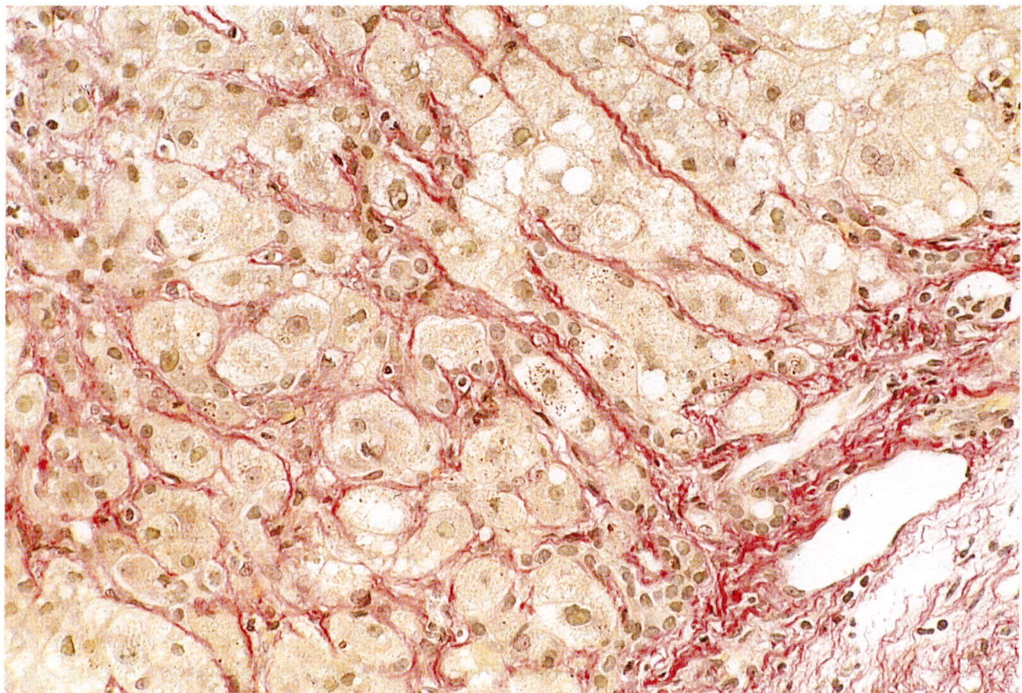

Plate 5 Pericellular fibrosis. Extensive pericellular fibrosis extending through the liver acinus. Also mild fatty change, Mallory bodies and cholestasis. Sirius red, objective ×25.

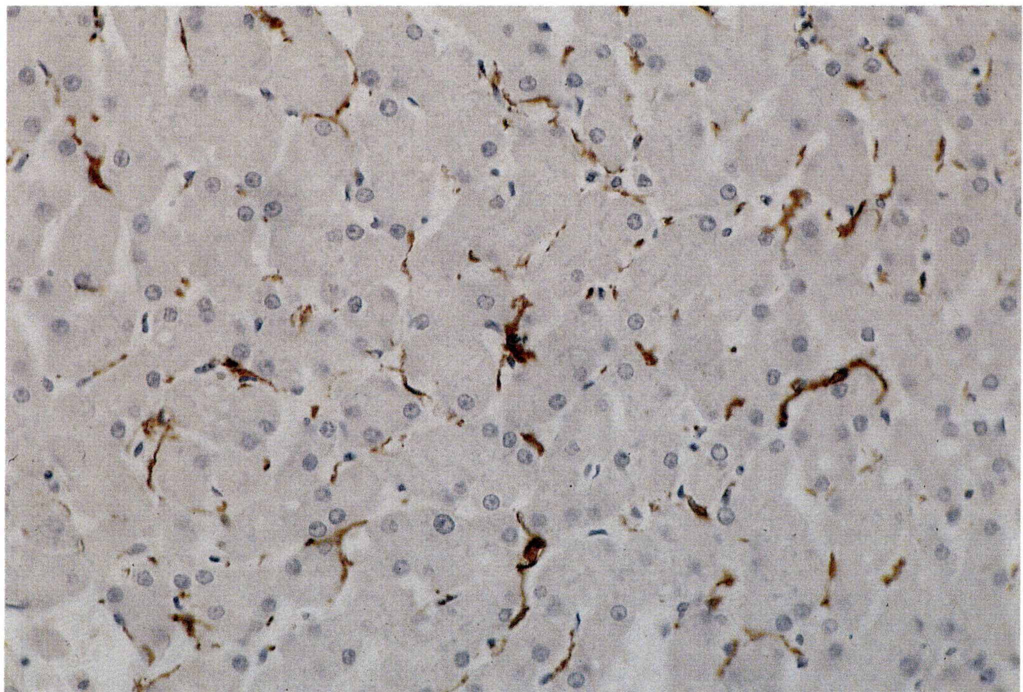

Plate 6 Ito cells. Liver stained with an α-smooth muscle actin antibody to demonstrate numerous "activated" Ito cells in a liver biopsy from a patient with alcoholic liver disease. PAP, objective ×25.

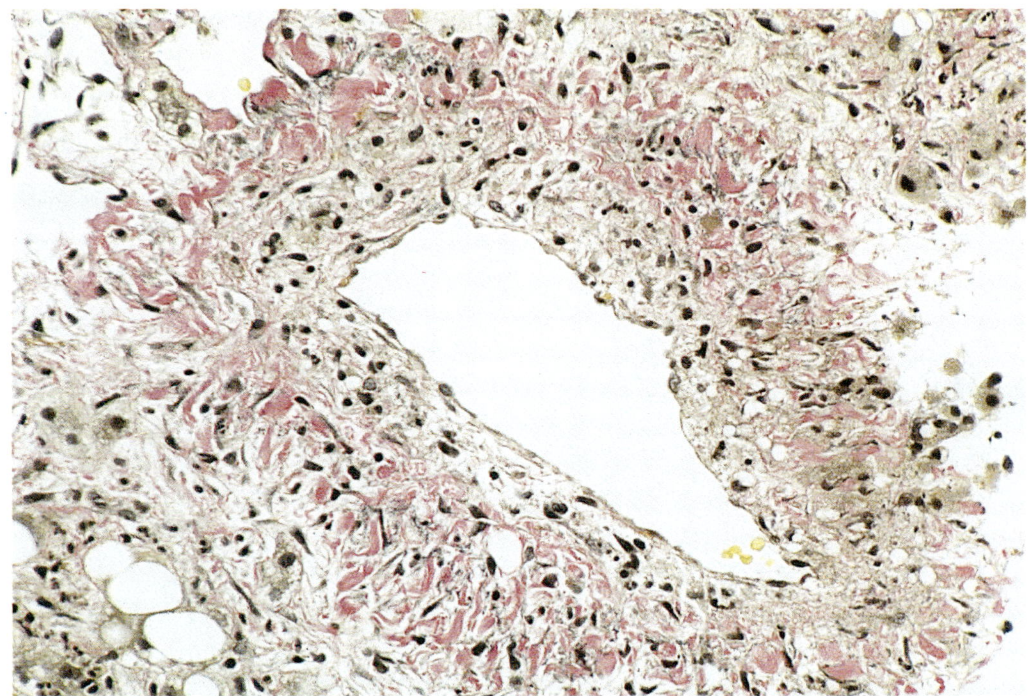

Plate 7 Veno-occlusive lesion. Terminal hepatic venule showing prominent fibrointimal proliferation. The liver exhibited alcoholic hepatitis (not shown). Verhoeff–Van Gieson, objective ×25.

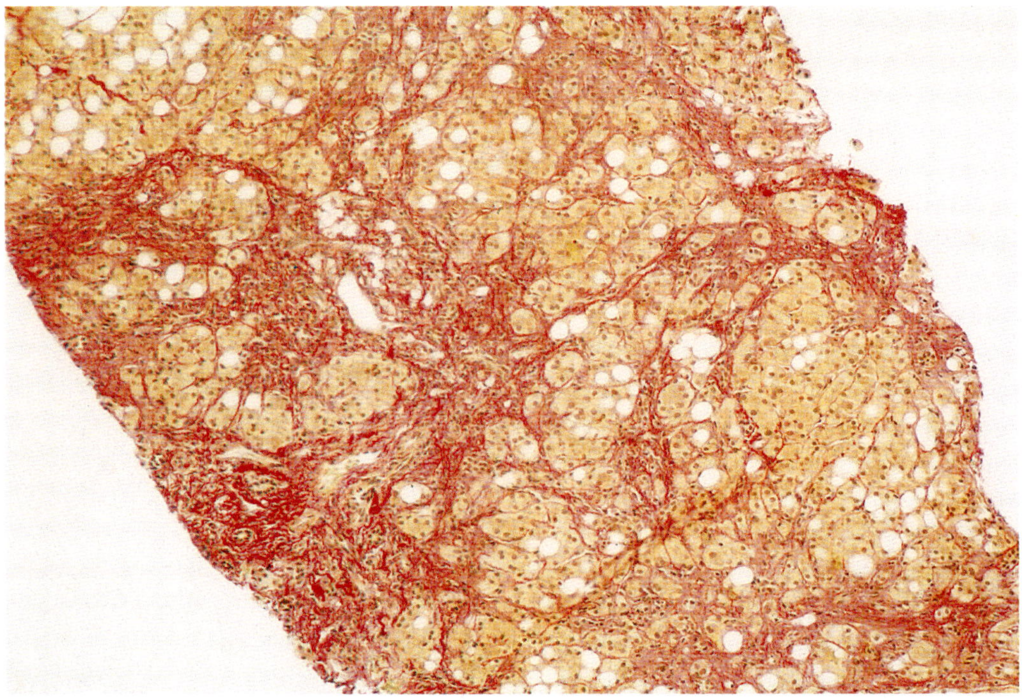

Plate 8 Micronodular cirrhosis. The liver shows established micronodular cirrhosis, and also focal pericellular fibrosis within the regenerative nodules. Sirius red, objective ×10.

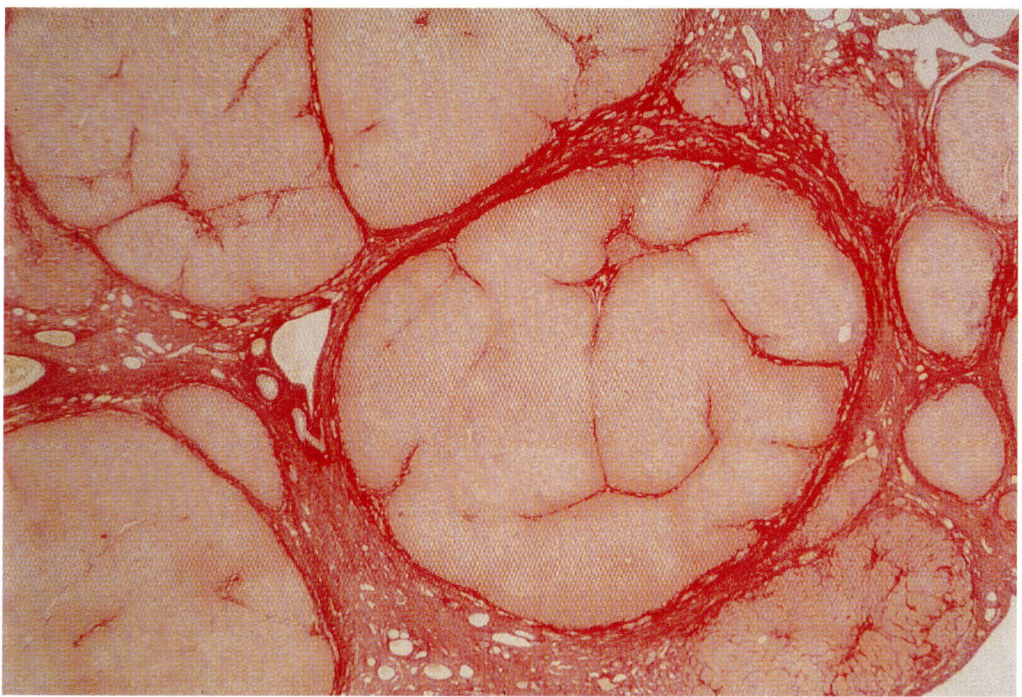

Plate 9a Macronodular cirrhosis. "Native" liver showing macroregenerative nodules in which rudimentary portal tracts are apparent. The patient, who had been abstinent for several years, received a liver transplant for alcoholic cirrhosis. Sirius red, objective ×2.5

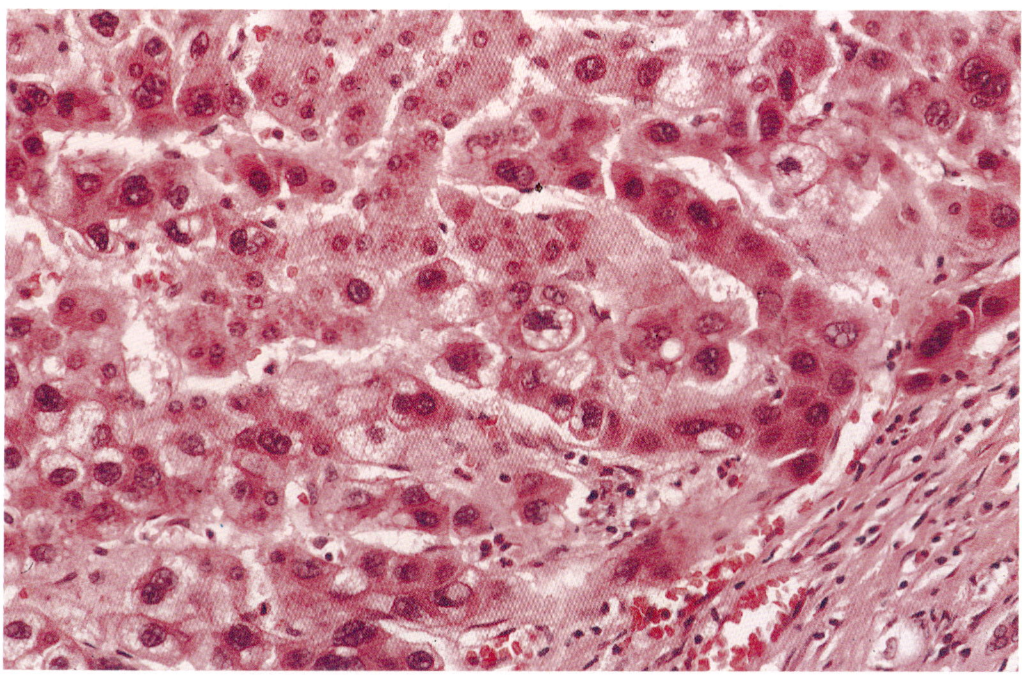

Plate 9b Hepatocellular carcinoma. Moderately differentiated, trabecular hepatocellular carcinoma which developed in association with alcoholic cirrhosis. H&E, objective ×40.

Macroregenerative nodules

Such nodules are defined as measuring 0.8 cm or more in diameter with an essentially intact reticulin framework and liver cell plates no greater than two cells thick. Intranodal portal zones are are usually present, and when well-developed show features typical of portal tracts (Fig. 3.32). The component hepatocytes and their nuclei may be enlarged, so-called large cell dysplasia (Crawford 1990), but the normal cytoplasmic to nuclear ratio is maintained (Fig. 3.32). Synonyms for the term macroregenerative nodule include adenomatous hyperplasia (Edmondson 1976), type I macroregenerative nodule (Furuya *et al.* 1988) and large regenerative nodule (Eguchi *et al.* 1992).

Borderline nodules

Borderline nodules can contain decreased amounts of reticulin, liver cell plates up to three cells in thickness, groups of cells showing "small-cell dysplasia" (Crawford 1990), Mallory bodies and a few groups of hepatocytes exhibiting "pseudoglandular" differentiation. The edges of such nodules can be irregular; however, the histological features are not sufficient for a diagnosis of malignancy. In previous publications this type of nodule has been termed a type II macroregenerative nodule (Furuya *et al.* 1988), adenomatous hyperplasia and atypical adenomatous hyperplasia (Eguchi *et al.* 1992), and grade I hepatocellular carcinoma (Edmondson and Steiner 1954; Craig *et al.* 1989).

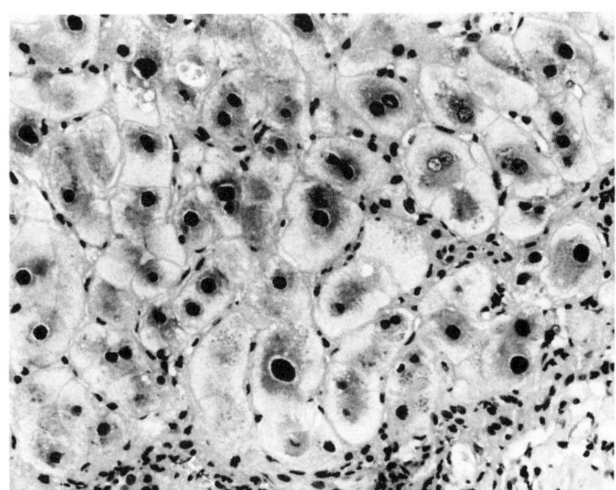

Fig. 3.32 "Large cell" dysplasia. A group of large hepatocytes, from within a regenerative nodule in a cirrhotic liver, showing large pleomorphic nuclei. H&E, ×170.

The term "borderline" for lesions of uncertain or low malignant potential, is widely accepted by histopathologists and hopefully will become widely used for hepatic nodules that until now have been difficult to characterize. Borderline nodules may progress to or predispose to hepatocellular carcinoma. Such nodules may also be seen in tissue adjacent to carcinomas (Crawford 1990; Terada *et al.* 1993).

Hepatocellular carcinoma

Well-differentiated hepatocellular carcinomas are usually composed of uniformly thick cell plates (three or more cells) lined by endothelial cells (Fig. 3.33; see also Plate 9b). Isolated trabecular fragmants often appear to "float" in dilated sinusoidal spaces. Glandular structures resembling acini may also be seen. A reticulin stain will usually show little or no sinusoidal collagen. Other features that may be present include Mallory bodies, other types of eosinophilic, proteinaceous cytoplasmic inclusions, fatty change, clear-cell change, and bile production. The tumour cells show local invasion into the adjacent cirrhotic liver.

Hepatocellular carcinoma develops in about 5–10 percent of patients with alcoholic cirrhosis (Lee 1966; Hislop *et al.* 1982). As discussed above, there may be a progression from micronodular cirrhosis to macronodular cirrhosis (i.e. macroregenerative nodules) with the subsequent development of borderline nodules and then unequivocal malignancy (Arakawa *et al.* 1986; Wada *et al.* 1988; Sakamoto *et al.* 1991). In other cases, hepatocellar carcinomas have developed in benign-appearing regenerative nodules (Takayama *et al.* 1990; Sakamoto *et al.* 1991).

On rare occasions, hepatocellular carcinomas have been reported in the livers of drinkers in the absence of cirrhosis (Lieber *et al.* 1981; MacSween 1981). Alcohol may act as a promoter or co-carcinogen by inducing a variety of cytochrome P450 isoenzymes, thus increasing the metabolism of numerous potentially carcinogenic agents (Lieber *et al.* 1981; see also Chapter 2).

The role of the hepatitis B virus in the pathogenesis of hepatocellular carcinoma in alcoholic liver disease remains controversial, with some studies (Brechot *et al.* 1982; Ohnishi *et al.* 1982) supporting a role for this virus and others (Walter *et al.* 1988) refuting this association. On the other hand, a number of recent studies have shown that co-existent hepatitis C virus infection increases the risk of developing hepatocellular carcinoma in alcoholic liver disease (Bruix *et al.* 1989; Nalpas *et al.* 1991;

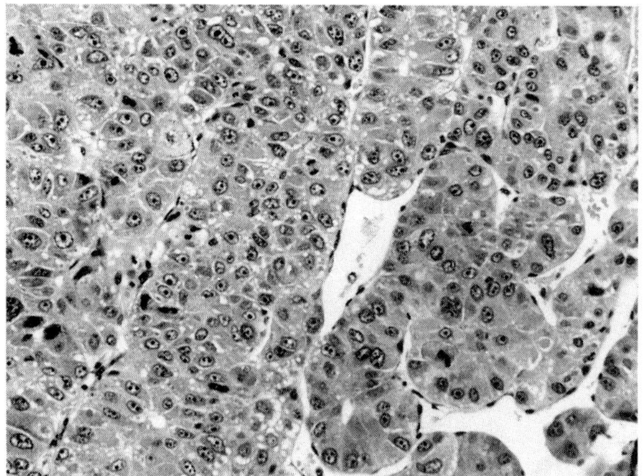

Fig. 3.33 Hepatocellular carcinoma. Well-differentiated, trabecular hepatocellular carcinoma which developed in association with alcoholic cirrhosis. H&E, ×130.

Ikeda *et al.* 1993; Yamauchi *et al.* 1993; see also Chaper 9).

Reversibility and prognosis of cirrhosis

Cirrhosis, diagnosed by the internationally accepted criteria of Anthony *et al.* (1978), is generally regarded as an irreversible process. Some animal studies of carbon tetrachloride-induced cirrhosis have reported reversibility of the process following withdrawal of the toxin (Perez-Tamayo 1979). However, in the alcohol/"low-dose" carbon tetrachloride rat model for cirrhosis (Hall *et al.* 1991), cessation of alcohol-feeding and carbon tetrachloride exposure was associated with the persistence of the cirrhotic process and, in some animals, the development of macroregenerative nodules (personal observation).

Follow-up liver biopsies that show an apparent disappearance of the cirrhotic process have probably sampled macroregenerative nodules that have developed in association with abstinence from alcohol.

Alcoholic cirrhosis, especially if decompensated, is associated with an increase in mortality compared with age- and sex-matched controls, and with each advancing decade of age mortality increases by 55 percent (Bouchier *et al.* 1992). Abstinence from alcohol can improve the survival of patients with alcoholic cirrhosis. Powell and Klatskin (1968) reported that 63 percent of cirrhotic patients who stopped drinking survived for 5 years compared with 41 percent who continued to drink. Borowsky

et al. (1981) also showed that continued drinking is associated with poor survival of alcoholic cirrhotics, particularly those with decompensated cirrhosis who continue to drink heavily. Abstinence may prolong the survival of patients with alcoholic cirrhosis but, as discussed above, the subsequent development of a macroregenerative cirrhosis may be associated with an increased risk of developing hepatocellular carcinoma.

The role of liver biopsy in the diagnosis of liver disease in drinkers

The diagnostic value of the liver biopsy relates to:

1. Confirmation of clinically suspected alcoholic liver disease.
2. Assessment of the stage and severity of liver injury.
3. Diagnosis of coexistent liver disease.
4. Diagnosis of non-alcoholic liver disease in drinkers.
5. Evaluation of therapy.

As discussed earlier, the provisional diagnosis of alcoholic hepatitis and/or alcoholic cirrhosis may be made on clinical grounds but requires morphological confirmation. In particular, the presence of cirrhosis should be confirmed by liver biopsy, since the clinical features of portal hypertension can be seen in the absence of cirrhosis. For example, portal hypertension may occur in association with alcoholic hepatitis (see review by Hall 1991); such patients have a better prognosis than those with established cirrhosis, particularly if they abstain from alcohol (Pares *et al.* 1986).

Levin *et al.* (1979) performed liver biopsies on 145 consecutive patients who were drinking at least 80 g alcohol daily for prolonged periods; alcoholic liver disease was confirmed in only 80 percent of those in whom it was clinically suspected. Important coexistent diseases seen in the liver biopsies of drinkers include acute and chronic drug-related injury (see Chapters 2 and 16), acute viral hepatitis (Feller *et al.* 1985), chronic viral hepatitis (see Chapter 9), genetic haemochromatosis (see Chapter 12) and, particularly in South Africa, changes related to porphyria cutanea tarda (see Chapter 13).

Conclusion

The spectrum of histopathological injury in alcohol-related liver disease is entirely non-specific, with identical patterns of injury being seen in drug-related injury (Hall 1994b), non-alcoholic steatohepatitis and other types of pseudoalcoholic liver disease (see Chapter 11). Thus, before ascribing any of the various patterns of liver injury to alcohol, it is necessary to obtain the alcohol history for the particular patient. Nevertheless, a variety of histological features – fatty liver with perivenular fibrosis, microvesicular steatosis, giant mitochondria, hepatocyte necrosis with a neutrophil polymorph infiltrate ± Mallory bodies, peiricellular fibrosis, micronodular cirrhosis with fatty change and/or alcoholic hepatitis, and low-grade iron deposition in hepatocytes with a random distribution throughout the acini – are suggestive of alcohol-associated liver injury.

While it is generally accepted that alcohol, alcohol metabolites and the various metabolic (see Chapter 2) and immunologic (see Chapters 4–6) disturbances that occur in association with chronic alcohol ingestion are responsible for alcoholic liver injury, it is also possible that alcohol may be contributing to liver injury by making the hepatocytes more susceptible to injury by other agents/disease states (see Chapters 12, 13, 16 and 18).

Acknowledgement

Several of my studies referred to in this manuscript, were supported by the National Health and Medical Research Council of Australia and the University Research Budget, Flinders University of South Australia.

References

Afshani, P., Littenberg, G.D., Wollman, J. and Kaplowitz, N. (1978). Significance of microscopic cholangitis in alcoholic liver disease. *Gastroenterology* **75**, 1045–1050.

Akeda, S., Fujita, K., Kosada, Y. and French, S.W. (1986). Mallory body formation and amyloid deposition in the liver of aged mice fed a vitamin A deficient diet for a prolonged period. *Laboratory Investigation* **54**, 228–233.

Anthony, P.P., Ishak, K.G., Nayak, N.C., Poulsen, H.E., Scheuer, P.J. and Sobin, L.H. (1978). The morphology of cirrhosis: Recommendations on definition, nomenclature, and classification by a working group sponsored by the World Health Organization. *Journal of Clinical Pathology* **31**, 395–414.

Arakawa, M., Kage, M., Sugihara, S., Nakashima, T., Suenaga, M. and Okuda, K. (1986). Emergence of malignant lesions within an adenomatous hyperplasia nodule in a cirrhotic liver. *Gastroenterology* **91**, 198–208.

Baptista, A., Bianchi, L., de Groote, J., Desmet, V.J., Gedigk, P., Korb, G. MacSween, R.N.M., Popper, H., Poulsen, H., Scheuer, P.J., Schmid, M., Thaler, H. and Wepler, W. (1981). Alcoholic liver disease: Morphological manifestations. Review by an Internal Group. *Lancet* **i**, 707–711.

Baraona, E., Leo, M.A., Borowsky, S.A. and Lieber, C.S. (1977). Pathogenesis of alcohol-induced accumulation of protein in the liver. *Journal of Clinical Investigation* **60**, 546–554.

Baraona, E., Finkelman, F. and Lieber, C.S. (1984). Reevaluation of the effects of alcohol consumption on rat microtubules: Effects of feeding status. *Research Communications in Chemical Pathology and Pharmacology* **44**, 265–278.

Bassett, M.L., Halliday, J.W. and Powell, L.W. (1986). Value of hepatic iron measurements in early haemochromatosis and determination of the critical iron level associated with fibrosis. *Hepatology* **6**, 24–29.

Beckett, A.G., Livingstone, A.V. and Hill, K.R. (1961). Acute alcoholic hepatitis. *British Medical Journal* **2**, 1113–1119.

Berman, W.J., Gill, J., Jennett, R.B., Tuma, D., Sorrell, M.F. and Rubin, E. (1983). Ethanol, hepatocellular organelles, and microtubules: A morphometric study *in vivo* and *in vitro*. *Laboratory Investigation* **48**, 760–767.

Berresford, P.A., Sunter, J.P., Harrison, V. and Lesna, M. (1980). Histological demonstration and frequency of intrahepatic copper in patients suffering from alcoholic liver disease. *Histopathology* **4**, 637–643.

Bhathal, P.S. (1972). Presence of modified fibroblasts in cirrhotic livers in man. *Pathology* **4**, 139–144.

Bhathal, P.S., Wilkinson, P., Clifton, S., Rankin, J.G. and Santamaria, J.N. (1975). The spectrum of liver diseases in alcoholism. *Australian and New Zealand Journal of Medicine* **5**, 49–57.

Birschbach, H.R., Harinasuta, U. and Zimmerman, H.J. (1974). Alcoholic steatonecrosis. *Gastroenterology* **66**, 1195–1202.

Blendis, L.M., Orrego, H., Crossley, I.R., Blake, J.E., Medline, A. and Israel, Y. (1982). The role of hepatocyte enlargement in hepatic pressure in cirrhotic and noncirrhotic alcoholic liver disease. *Hepatology* **2**, 539–546.

Boitnott, J.K. and Maddrey, W.C. (1981). Alcoholic liver disease. I. Interrelationships among histologic features and the histologic effects of prednisolone therapy. *Hepatology* **1**, 599–612.

Borenfreund, E. and Bendich, A. (1978). *In vitro* demonstration of Mallory body formation in liver cells from rats fed diethylnitrosamine. *Laboratory Investigation* **38**, 295–303.

Borowsky, S.A., Strome, S. and Lott, E. (1981). Continued heavy drinking and survival in alcoholic cirrhosis. *Gastroenterology* **80**, 1405–1409.

Bouchier, I.A.D., Hislop, W.S. and Prescott, R.J. (1992). A prospective study of alcoholic liver disease and mortality. *Journal of Hepatology* **16**, 290–297.

Brechot, C., Nalpas, B., Courouce, A.-M., Duhamel, G., Callard, P., Carnot, F., Tiollais, P. and Berthelot, P. (1982). Evidence that hepatitis B virus has a role in liver-cell carcinoma in alcoholic liver disease. *New England Journal of Medicine* **306**, 1384–1387.

Brillanti, S., Barbara, L., Miglioli, M. and Bonino, F. (1989). Hepatitis C virus: A possible cause of chronic hepatitis in alcoholics. *Lancet* **ii**, 1390–1391.

Brouwer, A., Wisse, E. and Knook, D.L. (1988). Sinusoidal endothelial cells and perisinusoidal fat-storing cells. In *The Liver: Biology and Pathobiology* (Edited by Arias, I.M., Jakoby, W.B., Popper, H., Schachter, D. and Shafritz, D.A.), 2nd edn, pp. 665–682. Raven Press, New York.

Bruguera, M., Bertran, A., Bombi, J.A. and Rodes, J. (1977). Giant mitochondria in hepatocytes: A diagnostic hint for alcoholic liver disease. *Gastroenterology* **73**, 1383–1387.

Bruix, J., Barrera, J.M., Calvet, X., Ercilla, G., Costa, J. Sanchez-Topias, J.M., Ventura, M., Vall, M., Bruguera, M., Bru, C., Castillo, R. and Rodes, J. (1989). Prevalence of antibodies to hepatitis C in Spanish patients with hepatocellular carcinoma and hepatic cirrhosis. *Lancet* **ii**, 1004–1006.

Brunt, P.W., Kew, M.C., Scheuer, P.J. and Sherlock, S. (1974). Studies in alcoholic liver disease in Britain. I. Clinical and pathological patterns related to natural history. *Gut* **15**, 52–58.

Burt, A.D. and MacSween, R.N.M. (1986). Hepatic vein lesions in alcoholic liver disease: Retrospective biopsy and necropsy study. *Journal of Clinical Pathology* **39**, 63–67.

Burt, A.D., Griffiths, M., MacSween, R.N.M., Schuppan, D. and Voss, B. (1988). Identification of extracellular matrix proteins in human liver biopsies using an immunogold technique. *Hepatology* **8**, 334 A, 1302.

Caulet, S., Fabre, M., Schoevaert, D., Lesty, C., Meduri, G. and Martin, E. (1989). Quantitative study of centrolobular hepatic fibrosis in alcoholic disease before cirrhosis. *Virchows Archives A* **416**, 11–17.

Chedid, A., Mendenhall, C.L., Tosch, T., Chen, T., Rabin, L., Garcia-Pont, P., Goldberg, S.J., Kiernan, T., Seeff, L.B., Sorrell, M. *et al.* (1986). Significance of megamitochondria in alcoholic liver injury. *Gastroenterology* **90**, 1858–1864.

Chedid, A., Mendenhall, C.L., Gartside, P., French, S.W., Chen, T., Rabin, L. and the Veterans Administrative Cooperative Study Group (1991). Prognostic factors in alcoholic liver disease. *American Journal of Gastroenterology* **86**, 210–216.

Christoffersen, P., Braendstrup, O., Juhl, E. and Poulsen, H. (1971). Lipogranulomas in human liver biopsies with fatty change: A morphological, biochemical and clinical investigation. *Acta Pathologica et Microbiologica Scandinavica* **79**, 150–158.

Christoffersen, P., Eghoje, K. and Juhl, E. (1973). Mallory bodies in liver biopsies from chronic alcoholics: A comparative morphological, biochemical and clinical study of two groups of chronic alcoholics with and without Mallory bodies. *Scandinavian Journal of Gastroenterology* **8**, 341–346.

Clement, B., Grimaud, J.-A., Campion, J.-P., Deugnier, Y. and Guillouzo, A. (1986). Cell types involved in collagen and fibronectin production in normal and fibrotic human liver. *Hepatology* **6**, 225–234.

Craig, J., Peters, R. and Edmonson, J. (1989). Tumours of the liver and intrahepatic bile ducts: Fascicle 26. In *Atlas of Tumour Pathology*, pp. 145–169. Armed Forces Institute of Pathology, Washington, DC.

Crapper, R.M., Bhathal, P.S. and Mackay, I.R. (1983). Chronic active hepatitis in alcoholic patients. *Liver* **3**, 327–337.

Crawford, J.M. (1990). Pathologic assessment of liver cell dysplasia and benign liver tumours: Differentiation from malignant tumours. *Seminars in Diagnostic Pathology* **7**, 115–128.

Dalke, D.D., Sorrell, M.F., Casey, C.A. and Tuma, D.J. (1990). Chronic ethanol administration impairs receptor-mediated endocytosis of epidermal growth factor by rat hepatocytes. *Hepatology* **12**, 1085–1091.

Denk, H. and Lackinger, E. (1986). Cytoskeleton in liver disease. *Seminars in Liver Disease* **6**, 199–211.

Denk, H., Gschnait, F. and Wolff, K. (1975). Hepatocellular hyalin (Mallory bodies) in long-term griseofulvin-treated mice: A new experimental model for the study of hyalin formation. *Laboratory Investigation* **32**, 773–776.

Denk, H., Franke, W.W., Kerjaschki, D. and Eckerstorfer, R. (1979). Mallory bodies in experimental animals and man. *International Review of Experimental Pathology* **20**, 77–121.

Denk, H., Krepler, R., Lackinger, E., Artlieb, U. and Franke, W.W. (1982). Immunological and biochemical characterization of the keratin-related component of Mallory bodies: A pathological pattern of hepatocyte cytokeratins. *Liver* **2**, 165–175.

Denk, K., Zatloukal, K. and Preisegger, K.-H. (1989). Ubiquitin: A common denominator in intermediate filament pathology of brain and liver? *Hepatology* **10**, 514–515.

De Vos, R. and Desmet, V. (1992). Ultrastructural characteristics of novel epithelial cell types identified in human pathologic liver specimens with chronic ductular reaction. *American Journal of Pathology* **140**, 1441–1450.

Dufour, M.C. (1993). Chronic liver disease and cirrhosis. In *Digestive Diseases in the United States: Epidemiology* and Impact (Edited by Everhart, J.). Government Printing Office, Washington, DC.

Dufour, M.C., Stinson, F.S. and Caces, M. F. (1993). Trends in cirrhosis morbidity and mortality: United States, 1979–1988. *Seminars in Liver Disease* **13**, 109–125.

Duguay, L., Coutu, D., Hetu, C. and Joly, J.-G. (1982). Inhibition of liver regeneration by chronic alcohol administration. *Gut* **23**, 8–13.

Edmondson, H.A. (1976). Benign epithelial tumours and tumour-like lesions of the liver. In *Hepatocellular Carcinoma* (Edited by Okuda, K. and Peters, R.L.), pp. 309–330. John Wiley, New York.

Edmondson, H.A. and Steiner, P. (1954). Primary carcinoma of the liver: A study of 100 cases among 48,900 necropsies. *Cancer* **1**, 462 503.

Edmondson, H.A., Peters, R.L., Reynolds, T.B. and Kuzuma, O.T. (1963). Sclerosing hyaline necrosis of the liver in the chronic alcoholic. *Annals of Internal Medicine* **59**, 646–673.

Edmondson, H.A., Peters, R.L., Frankel, H.H. and Borowsky, S. (1967). The early stage of liver injury in the alcoholic. *Medicine* **46**, 119–129.

Eguchi, A., Nakashima, O., Okudaira, S., Sugihara, S. and Kojiro, M. (1992). Adenomatous hyperplasia in the vicinity of small hapatocellular carcinoma. *Hepatology* **15**, 843–848.

Fauerholdt, L., Schlichting, P., Christensen, E., Poulsen, H., Tygstrup, N., Jahl, E. and the Copenhagen Study Group for Liver Diseases (1983). Conversion of micronodular cirrhosis into macronodular cirrhosis. *Hepatology* **3**, 928–931.

Feller, A., Uchida, T. and Rakela, J. (1985). Acute viral hepatitis superimposed on alcoholic liver cirrhosis. *Liver* **5**, 239–246.

Ferrell, L.D., Crawford, J.M., Dhillon, A.P., Scheuer, P.J. and Nakanuma, Y. (1993). Proposal for standardized criteria for the diagnosis of benign, borderline, and malignant hepatocellular lesions arising in chronic advanced liver disease. *American Journal of Surgical Pathology* **17**, 1113–1123.

Flejou, J.F., Degott, C., Kharsa, G., Soulier, A., Rueff, B. and Potet, F. (1987). La steatose spongiocytaire alcoolique: Etude de trois cas. *Gastroenterologie Clinique Bioligica* **11**, 165–168.

Franke, W.F., Denk, H., Schmid, E., Osborne, M. and Weber, K. (1979). Ultrastructural, biochemical and immunologic characterization of Mallory bodies in livers of griseofulvin-treated mice: Fimbriated rods of filaments containing prekeratin-like polypeptides. *Laboratory Investigation* **40**, 207–220.

French, S.W. (1981). The Mallory body: Structure, composition and pathogenesis. *Hepatology* **1**, 76–83.

French, S.W. (1983). Present understanding of the development of Mallory's body. *Archives of Pathology and Laboratory Medicine* **107**, 445–450.

French, S.W. (1989). Biochemical basis for alcohol-induced liver injury. *Clinical Biochemistry* **22**, 41–49.

French, S.W. and Burbridge, E.J. (1979). Alcoholic hepatitis: Clinical, morphological and therapeutic agents. In *Progress in Liver Disease* (Edited by Popper, H. and Schaffner, F.), Vol. VI, pp. 557–580. Grune and Stratton, New York.

French, S.W., Ihrig, T.J. and Norum, M.L. (1972). A method of isolation of Mallory bodies in a purified fraction. *Laboratory Investigation* **26**, 240–244.

French, S.W., Katsuma, Y., Ray, M.B. and Swierenga, S.H.H. (1987). Cytoskeletal pathology induced by ethanol. In *Alcohol and the Cell* (Edited by Rubin, E.), pp. 262–276. Annals of the New York Academy of Science, New York.

French, S.W., Nash, J., Shitabata, P., Kachi, K., Hara, C., Chedid, A., Mendenhall, C.L. and the Veterans Administration Coooperative Study Group (1993). Pathology of alcoholic liver disease. *Seminars in Liver Disease* **13**, 154–169.

Furuya, K., Nakamura, M., Yamamoto, Y., Togei, K. and Otsuka, H. (1988). Macroregenerative nodule of the liver: A clinicopathological study of 345 autopsy cases of chronic liver disease. *Cancer* **61**, 99–105.

Galambos, J.T. (1972). Natural history of alcoholic hepatitis. III. Histological changes. *Gastroenterology* **63**, 1026–1035.

Galambos, J.T. (1979). *Cirrhosis*. W.B. Saunders, Philadelphia, PA.

Galambos, J.T. (1985). Epidemiology of alcoholic liver disease in the United States of America. In *Alcoholic Liver Disease* (Edited by Hall, P.), pp. 230–249. Edward Arnold, London.

Gerber, M.A. and Popper, H. (1972). Relation between central canals and portal tracts in alcoholic hepatitis: A contribution to the pathogenesis of cirrhosis in alcoholics. *Human Pathology* **3**, 199–207.

Gerber, M.A. and Thung, S.N. (1981). Hepatic oncocytes: Incidence, staining characteristics, and ultrastructural features. *American Journal of Clinical Pathology* **75**, 498–503.

Glover, S.C., McPhie, J.L. and Brunt, P.W. (1977). Cholestasis in acute alcoholic liver disease. *Lancet* **ii**, 1305–1307.

Gluud, C., Christoffersen, P., Eriksen, J., Wantzin, P., Knudsen, B.B. and the Copenhagen Study Group for the Liver (1987). Influence of alcohol on hyperplastic nodules in alcoholic men with micronodular cirrhosis. *Gastroenterology* **93**, 256–260.

Goldberg, S.J., Mendenhall, C.L., Connell, A.M. and Chedid, A. (1977). "Non-alcoholic" chronic hepatitis in the alcoholic. *Gastroenterology* **72**, 598–604.

Goodman, Z.D. and Ishak, K.G. (1982). Occlusive venous lesions in alcoholic liver disease: A study of 200 cases. *Gastroenterology* **83**, 786–796.

Hadziyannis, S., Gerber, M.A., Vissoulis, C. and Popper, H. (1973). Cytoplasmic hepatitis B antigen in "ground-glass" hepatocytes of carriers. *Archives of Pathology* **96**, 327–330.

Hahn, E., Wick, G., Pencev, D. and Temple, R. (1980). Distribution of basement membrane proteins in normal and fibrotic human liver: Collagen type IV, laminin and fibronectin. *Gut* **21**, 63–71.

Hall, P. de la M. (Ed.) (1985). *Alcoholic Liver Disease: Pathobiology, Epidemiology and Clinical Aspects.* Edward Arnold, London.

Hall, P. de la M. (1991). Pathologic features of alcohol liver disease. In *Portal Hypertension* (Edited by Okuda, K. and Benhamou, J.-P.), pp. 41–68. Springer-Verlag, Tokyo.

Hall, P. de la M. (1994a). Alcoholic liver disease. In *Pathology of the Liver* (Edited by MacSween, R.N.M., Anthony, P.P., Scheuer, P.J., Portmann, B.C. and Burt, A.D.), 3rd edn. Churchill Livingstone, Edinburgh, in press.

Hall, P. de la M. (1994b). Histopathological spectrum of drug-induced liver injury. In *Drug-induced Liver Disease* (Edited by Farrell, G.C.), pp. 115–151. Churchill Livingstone, Edinburgh.

Hall, P., Gormley, B.M., Jarvis, L.R. and Smith, R.D. (1980). A staining method for the detection and measurement of fat droplets in hepatic tissue. *Pathology* **12**, 605–608.

Hall, P., Smith, R.D. and Gormley, R.D. (1982). "Routine" stains on osmicated resin embedded hepatic tissue. *Pathology* **14**, 73–74.

Hall, P. de la M., Plummer, J.L., Ilsley, A.H. and Cousins, M.J. (1991). Hepatic fibrosis and cirrhosis after chronic administration of alcohol and "low-dose" carbon tetrachloride vapour in the rat. *Hepatology* **13**, 815–819.

Harinasuta, U. and Zimmerman, H.J. (1971). Alcoholic steatonecrosis. I. Relationship between severity of hepatic disease and presence of Mallory bodies in the liver. *Gastroenterology* **60**, 1036–1046.

Hautekeete, M.L., Degott, C. and Benhamou, J.-P. (1990). Microvesicular steatosis of the liver. *Acta Clinica Belgica* **45**, 311–326.

Hazen, R., Denk, H., Franke, W.W., Lackinger, E. and Schiller D.L. (1986). Change in cytokeratin organization during the development of Mallory bodies as revealed by a monoclonal antibody. *Laboratory Investigation* **54**, 543–553.

Hislop, W.S., Masterton, N., Bouchier, I.A.D. and Hopwood, D. (1982). Cirrhosis and primary liver cell carcinoma in Tayside: A five year study. *Scottish Medical Journal* **27**, 29–36.

Hislop, W.S., Bouchier, I.A.D., Allan, J.G., Brunt, P.W., Eastwood, M., Finlayson, N.D.C., James, O., Russell, R.I. and Watkinson, G. (1983). Alcoholic liver disease in Scotland and Northeastern England: Presenting features in 510 patients. *Quarterly Journal of Medicine* **206**, 232–243.

Hodges, J.R., Millward-Sadler, G.H. and Wright, R. (1982). Chronic active hepatitis: The spectrum of disease. *Lancet* **i**, 550–552.

Horn, T., Lyon, H. and Christoffersen, P. (1986). The "blood–hepatocyte barrier": A light microscopical transmission and scanning electron microscopic study. *Liver* **6**, 233–245.

Horn, T., Christoffersen, P. and Henriksen, J.H. (1987). Alcoholic liver injury: Defenestration in non-cirrhotic livers. A scanning electron microscopic study. *Hepatology* **7**, 77–82.

Huet, P., Mastai, R., Dagenais, M. and Cote, J. (1990). Even the French *foie gras de canard* does not induce portal hypertension. *Hepatology* **12**, 1455–1457.

Ikeda, K., Saitoh, S., Koida, I., Arase, Y., Tsubota, A., Chayama, K., Kumada, H. and Kawanishi, M. (1993). Multivariate analysis of risk factors for hepatocellular carcinogenesis: A prospective observation of 795 patients with viral and alcoholic cirrhosis. *Hepatology* **18**, 47–53.

Inagaki, T., Koike, M., Ikuta, K., Kobayashi, S., Suzuki, M., Kato, K. and Kato, K. (1989). Ultrastructural identification and clinical significance of light microscopic giant mitochondria and alcoholic liver injuries. *Gastroenterologica Japonica* **24**, 46–53.

Inagaki, T., Kobayashi, S., Ozeki, N., Suzuki, M., Fukuzawa, Y., Shimizu, K., Kato, K. and Kato, K. (1992). Ultrastructural identification of light microscopic giant mitochondria in alcoholic liver disease. *Hepatology* **15**, 46–53.

Irie, T., Benson, N.C. and French, S.W. (1984). Electron microscopic study of the *in vitro* calcium-dependent degradation of Mallory bodies and intermediate filaments in hepatocytes. *Laboratory Investigation* **50**, 303–312.

Iseri, O.A., Lieber, C.S. and Gottlieb, L.S. (1966). The ultrastructure of fatty liver induced by prolonged ethanol ingestion. *American Journal of Pathology* **48**, 535–555.

Ishak, K.G., Zimmerman, H.J. and Ray, M.B. (1991). Alcoholic liver disease: Pathology, pathogenesis and clinical aspects. *Alcoholism: Clinical and Experimental Research* **15**, 45–46.

Israel, Y., Orrego, H., Coleman, J.C. and Britton, R.S. (1982). Alcohol-induced hepatomegaly: Pathogenesis and role in the production of portal hypertension. *Federation Proceedings* **41**, 2472–2477.

Iversen, K., Christoffersen, P. and Poulsen, H. (1970). Epithelioid granulomas in liver biopsies. *Scandinavian Journal of Gastroenterology* **7**, 61–67 (Suppl.).

Jakobovits, A.W., Morgan, M.Y. and Sherlock, S. (1979). Hepatic siderosis in alcoholics. *Digestive Diseases and Science* **24**, 305–310.

Junge, J., Horn, T., Vyberg, M., Christoffersen, P. and Svendsen, L.B. (1991). The pattern of fibrosis in the acinar zone 3 areas in early alcoholic liver disease. *Journal of Hepatology* **12**, 83–86.

Karasawa, T. and Chedid, A. (1976). Sclerosing hyaline necrosis in noncirrhotic chronic alcoholic hepatitis. *American Journal of Clinical Pathology* **66**, 802–809.

Karasawa, T., Kushida, T., Shikata, T. and Kaneda, H. (1980). Morphologic spectrum of liver disease among chronic alcoholics: A comparison between Tokyo, Japan and Cincinnati, U.S.A. *Acta Pathologica Japonica* **30**, 505–514.

Katsuma, Y., Swierenga, S.H., Khettry, U., Marceau, N. and French, S.W. (1987). Changes in the cytokeratin intermediate filament cytoskeleton association in mouse and human liver. *Hepatology* **7**, 1215–1223.

Keegan, A.D. and Batey, R. (1993). Computer assisted quantitation of terminal hepatic vein connective tissue in the rat. *Pathology* **24**, 275–279.

Keeley, A.F., Iseri, O.A. and Gottlieb, L.S. (1972). Ultrastructure of hyaline cytoplasmic inclusions in a human hepatoma: Relationship to Mallory's alcoholic hyalin. *Gastroenterology* **62**, 280–293.

Kimoff, R.J. and Haung, S. (1981). Immunocytochemical and immunoelectron microscopic studies of Mallory bodies. *Laboratory Investigation* **45**, 491–503.

Krasner, N., Davis, M., Portmann, B. and Williams, R. (1977). Changing patterns of alcoholic liver disease in Great Britain: Relation to sex and signs of autoimmunity. *British Medical Journal* **1**, 1497–1500.

Kurki, P., Miettinen, A., Salaspuro, M., Virtanen, I. and Stenman, S. (1983). Cytoskeleton antibodies in chronic active hepatitis, primary biliary cirrhosis and alcoholic liver disease. *Hepatology* **3**, 297–302.

Lampertico, P., Colombo, M., Rumi, M.G., Annoni, G., Romeo, R., Donato, M.F. and Del Ninno, E. (1991). Hepatitis C virus (HCV)-related chronic hepatitis in Italian alcoholic patients. *Hepatology* **14**, 654, 211A.

Lane, B.P. and Lieber, C.S. (1966). Ultrastructural alterations in human hepatocytes following ingestion of ethanol with adequate diets. *American Journal of Pathology* **49**, 593–603.

Le Bail, B., Bioulac-Sage, P., Senuita, R., Quinton, A., Saric, J. and Ballabaud, C. (1990). Fine structure of hepatic sinusoids and sinusoidal cells in disease. *Journal of Electron Microscopic Technique* **14**, 257–282.

Lee, F.I. (1966). Cirrhosis and hepatoma in alcoholics. *Gut* **7**, 77–85.

Lefkowitch, J.H., Arborgh, B.A. and Scheuer, P.J. (1980). Oxyphilic granular hepatocytes: Mitochondrion-rich liver cells in hepatic disease. *American Journal of Clinical Pathology* **74**, 432–441.

Leo, M.A., Sato, M. and Lieber, C.S. (1983). Effect of hepatic vitamin A depletion on the liver in humans and rats. *Gastroenterology* **84**, 562–572.

Levensen, H., Greensite, F., Hoefs, J., Friloux, L. and Applegate, G. (1991). Fatty infiltration of the liver: Quantification with phase-contrast MR imaging at 1.5 T *vs* biopsy. *American Journal of Roentgenology* **156**, 307–312.

Levin, D.M., Baker, A.L., Riddell, R.H., Rochman, H. and Boyer, J.L. (1979). Non-alcoholic liver disease: Overlooked causes of liver injury in patients with heavy alcohol consumption. *American Journal of Medicine* **66**, 429–434.

Lieber, C.S. and DeCarli, L.M. (1974). An experimental model of alcohol feeding and liver injury in the baboon. *Journal of Medical Primatology* **3**, 153–163.

Lieber, C.S., DeCarli, L.M. and Rubin, E. (1975). Sequential production of fatty liver, hepatitis, and cirrhosis in sub-human primates fed ethanol with adequate diets. *Proceedings of the National Academy of Sciences, USA* **72**, 437–441.

Lieber, C.S., Seitz, H.K., Garro, A.J. and Worner, T.M. (1981). Alcohol as a co-coarcinogen. In *Frontiers in Liver Disease* (Edited by Berk, P.D. and Chalmers, T.C.), pp. 320–335. Thieme-Stratton, New York.

Lieber, C.S., Leo, M.A., Mak, K.M., DeCarli, L.M. and Sato, S. (1985). Choline fails to prevent liver fibrosis in ethanol-fed baboons but causes toxicity. *Hepatology* **5**, 561–572.

MacSween, R.N.M. (1981). Alcohol and cancer. *British Medical Bulletin* **38**, 31–33.

Maddrey, W.C. (1988). Alcoholic hepatitis: Clinicopathologic features and therapy. *Seminars in Liver Disease* **8**, 91–102.

Maddrey, W.C. (1990). Alcoholic hepatitis: Pathogenesis and approaches to treatment. *Scandinavian Journal of Gastroenterology* **25**, 118–130 (suppl.).

Mak, K.M and Lieber, C.S. (1984). Alterations in endothelial fenestrations in liver sinusoids of baboons fed alcohol: A scanning electron microscopic study. *Hepatology* **4**, 389–391.

Mak, K.M. and Lieber, C.S. (1988). Lipocytes and transitional cells in alcoholic liver disease: A morphometric study. *Hepatology* **8**, 1027–1033.

Mak, K.M., Leo, M.A. and Lieber, C.S. (1984). Alcoholic liver injury in baboons: Transformation of lipocytes to transitional cells. *Gastroenterology* **87**, 188–200.

Mallory, F.B. (1911). Cirrhosis of the liver: Five different types of lesions from which it may arise. *Bulletin of Johns Hopkins Hospital* **22**, 69–75.

Mastai, R., Huet, M.P., Brault, A. and Belgiorno, J. (1989). The rat liver microcirculation in alcohol-induced hepatomegaly. *Hepatology* **10**, 941–945.

Matsuda, Y., Baraona, E., Salaspuro, M. and Lieber, C.S. (1979). Effects of ethanol on microtubules and Golgi apparatus: Possible role in altered hepatic secretion of plasma proteins. *Laboratory Investigation* **41**, 455–463.

Matsuda, Y., Takada, A., Kanayama, R. and Takase, S. (1983). Changes in hepatic microtubules and secretory proteins in human alcoholic liver disease. *Pharmacology, Biochemistry and Behaviour* **18**, 479–482 (suppl. 1).

Matsuda, Y., Takada, A., Takase, S. and Sato, H. (1991). Accumulation of glycoproteins in the Golgi apparatus of hepatocytes of alcoholic liver injuries. *American Journal of Gastroenterology* **86**, 854–860.

McGill, D.B., Rakela, J., Zinsmeister, A.R. and Ott, B.J. (1990). A 21-year experience with major haemorrhage after percutaneous liver biopsy. *Gastroenterology* **99**, 1396–1400.

McKinnon, R.A., Hall, P. de la M., Gonzalez, F.J. and McManus, M.E. (1994). Localization of human cytochrome P-4502EI mRNA in alcoholic liver disease by *in situ* hybridisation. In preparation.

Mezey, E. (1993). Treatment of alcoholic liver disease. *Seminars in Liver Disease* **13**, 210–216.

Minato, Y., Hasumura, Y. and Takeuchi, J. (1983). The role of fat-storing cells in Disse space fibrogenesis in alcoholic liver disease. *Hepatology* **3**, 559–566.

Morgan, M.Y. (1985). Epidemiology of alcoholic liver disease in the United Kingdom. In *Alcoholic Liver Disease* (Edited by Hall, P.), pp. 193–229. Edward Arnold, London.

Morgan, M.Y. and Sherlock, S. (1977). Sex-related differences among 100 patients with alcoholic liver disease. *British Medical Journal* **1**, 939–941.

Morgan, M.Y., Sherlock, S. and Scheuer, P.J. (1978). Acute cholestasis, hepatic failure, and fatty liver in the alcoholic. *Scandinavian Journal of Gastroenterology* **13**, 299–303.

Morton, J.A., Bastin, J., Fleming, K.A., McMichael, A., Burns, J. and McGee, J.O'D. (1981). Mallory bodies in alcoholic liver disease: Identification of cytoplasmic filament/cell membrane and unique antigenic determinants by monoclonal antibodies. *Gut* **22**, 1–7.

Nakano, M., Worner, T.M. and Lieber, C.S. (1982a). Ultrastructure of initial stages of perivenular fibrosis in alcohol-fed baboons. *American Journal of Pathology* **106**, 145–155.

Nakano, M., Worner, T.M. and Lieber, C.S. (1982b). Perivenular fibrosis in alcoholic liver injury: Ultrastructure and histologic progression. *Gastroenterology* **83**, 777–785.

Nakanuma,Y. and Ohta, G. (1984). Small hepatocellular carcinoma containing many Mallory bodies. *Liver* **4**, 128–133.

Nakanuma, Y. and Ohta, G. (1985). Is Mallory body formation a preneoplastic change? A study of 181 cases of liver bearing hepatocellular carcinoma and 82 cases of cirrhosis. *Cancer* **55**, 2400–2404.

Nalpas, B., Driss, F., Pol, S., Hamelin, B., Duhamel, G., Courouce, A.M., Tiollais, P. and Brechot, C. (1991). Association between HCV and HBV infection in hepatocellular carcinoma and alcoholic liver disease: A study of 146 chronic alcoholics. *Journal of Hepatology* **12**, 70–74.

Nasrallah, S.M., Nassar, V.H. and Galambos, J.T. (1980). Importance of terminal hepatic venule thickening. *Archives of Pathology and Laboratory Medicine* **104**, 84–86.

Nissenbaum, M., Chedid, A., Mendenhall, C., Gartside, P. and the Veterans Administration Cooperative Study Group (1990). Prognostic significance of cholestatic alcoholic hepatitis. *Digestive Diseases and Sciences* **35**, 891–896.

Oda, M., Azuma, T., Nishizaki, Y., Komatsu, H., Tsukada, N., Watanabe, M., Nakamura, M. and Tsuchiya, M. (1989). Alterations of hepatic sinusoids in liver cirrhosis: Their involvement in the pathogenesis of portal hypertension. *Journal of Gastroenterology and Hepatology* **4**, 111–113 (suppl. 1).

Ohnishi, K. and Okuda, K. (1985). Epidemiology of alcoholic liver disease in Japan. In *Alcoholic Liver Disease* (Edited by Hall, P.) pp. 167–183. Edward Arnold, London.

Ohnishi, K., Iida, S., Iwama, S., Goto, N., Nomura, F., Takashi, M., Mishima, A., Kono, K., Kimura, K., Musha, H., Kototo, K. and Okuda, K. (1982). The effect of chronic habitual alcohol intake on the development of liver cirrhosis and hepatocellular carcinoma. *Cancer* **49**, 672–677.

Ohta, M., Marceau, N., Perry, G., Manetto, V., Gambetti, P., Autilio-Gambetti, L., Metuzals, J., Kawahara, H., Cadrin, M. and French, S.W. (1988). Ubiquitin is present on the cytokeratin intermediate filaments and Mallory bodies of hepatocytes. *Laboratory Investigation* **59**, 848–856.

Okanoue, T., Burbrige, E.J. and French, S.W. (1983). The role of the Ito cell in perivenular and intralobular fibrosis in alcoholic hepatitis. *Archives of Pathology and Laboratory Medicine* **107**, 459–463.

Okanoue, T., Sawa, Y., Kanaoka, H., Ohta, Y., Kachi, K., Kagawa, K. and Takino, T. (1988). Clinical and experimental studies of the pathophysiology of portal hypertension. *Hepatology* **8**, 1388 (abstract).

Orrego, H., Blendis, L.M., Crossley, I.R., Medline, A., MacDonald, A., Ritchie, S. and Israel, Y. (1981). Correlation of intrahepatic pressure with collagen in the Disse space and hepatomegaly in humans and in the rat. *Gastroenterology* **80**, 546–556.

Orrego, H., Blake, J.E., Blendis, L.M. and Medline, A. (1987). Prognosis of alcoholic cirrhosis in the presence and absence of alcoholic hepatitis. *Gastroenterology* **92**, 208–214.

Pares, A., Caballeria, J., Bruguera, M., Torres, M. and Rodes, J. (1986). Histological course of alcoholic hepatitis: Influence of abstinence, sex and extent of hepatic damage. *Journal of Hepatology* **2**, 33–42.

Pariente, E.-A., Degott, C., Martin, J.-P., Feldmann, G., Potet, F. and Benhamou, J.-P. (1981). Hepatocyte PAS-positive-diastase-resistent inclusions in the absence of alpha-1-antitrypsin deficiency – high prevalence in alcoholic cirrhosis. *American Journal of Clinical Pathology* **76**, 299–302.

Perez-Tamayo, R. (1979). Cirrhosis in the liver: A reversible disease? In *Pathology Annual* (Edited by Sommers, C. and Rosen, P.P.), Vol. 14, Part 2, pp. 183–213. Appleton-Century-Croft, New York.

Popper, H. and Lieber, C.S. (1980). Histogenesis of alcoholic fibrosis and cirrhosis in the baboon. *American Journal of Pathology* **98**, 695–716.

Powell, W.J., Jr. and Klatskin, G. (1968). Duration of survival in patients with Laennec's cirrhosis. *American Journal of Medicine* **44**, 406–420.

Preisegger, K.H., Zatloukal, K., Spurej, G. and Denk, H. (1991). Changes in cytokeratin filament organization in human and murine Mallory body-containing livers as revealed by a panel of monoclonal antibodies. *Liver* **11**, 300–309.

Preisegger, K.H., Zatloukal, K., Spurej, G., Riegelnegg, D. and Denk, H. (1992). Common epitopes of human and murine Mallory bodies and Lewy bodies as revealed by a neurofilament antibody. *Laboratory Investigation* **66**, 193–199.

Ramadori, G., Veit, T., Schwogler, S., Dienes, H.P., Knittel, T., Rieder, H. and Meyer zum Buschenfelde, K.H. (1990). Expression of the gene of the alpha smooth muscle-actin isoform in rat liver and in rat fat-storing (Ito) cells. *Virchows Archives B* **59**, 349–357.

Ray, M.B. (1987). Distribution patterns of cytokeratin antigen determinants in alcoholic and nonalcoholic liver diseases. *Human Pathology* **18**, 61–66.

Ray, M.B., Mendenhall, C.L., French, S.W., Gartside, P.S. and the Veterans Administrative Cooperative Study Group (1988). Serum vitamin A deficiency and increased intrahepatic expression of cytokeratin antigen in alcoholic liver disease. *Hepatology* **8**, 1019–1026.

Reynolds, T.B., Hidemura, R., Michel, H. and Peters, R. (1969). Portal hypertension without cirrhosis in alcoholic liver disease. *Annals of Internal Medicine* **70**, 496–506.

Rockey, D.C., Boyles, J.K., Gabbiani, G. and Friedman, S.L. (1992). Rat hepatic lipocytes express smooth muscle actin upon activation *in vivo* and in culture. *Journal of Submicroscopic Cytological Pathology* **24**, 193–203.

Rosmorduc, O., Rachardet, J.P., Lageron, A., Munz, C., Callard, P. and Beaugrand, M. (1992). Severe hepatic steatosis: A cause of sudden death in the alcoholic patient. *Gastroenterologie Clinique Biologica* **16**, 801–804.

Rubin, E. and Lieber, C.S. (1967). Early fine structural changes in the human liver induced by alcohol. *Gastroenterology* **52**, 1–13.

Rubin, E. and Lieber, C.S. (1968). Alcohol-induced hepatic injury in nonalcoholic volunteers. *New England Journal of Medicine* **278**, 869–876.

Rubin, E. and Lieber, C.S. (1974). Fatty liver, alcoholic hepatitis and cirrhosis produced by alcohol in primates. *New England Journal of Medicine* **298**, 128–135.

Rubin, E., Krus, S. and Popper, H. (1962). Pathogenesis of postnecrotic cirrhosis in alcoholics. *Archives of Pathology* **73**, 288–299.

Sakamoto, M., Hirohashi, S. and Shimosato, Y. (1991). Early stages of multi-step hepatocarcinogenesis: Adenomatous hyperplasia and early hepatocellular carcinoma. *Human Pathology* **22**, 172–178.

Sato, H., Takase, S. and Takada, A. (1989). Changes in liver and spleen volume in alcoholic liver disease. *Journal of Hepatology* **8**, 150–157.

Schaffner, F. and Popper, H. (1963). Capillarization of hepatic sinusoids in man. *Gastroenterology* **44**, 239–242.

Schenker, S. and Halff, G.A. (1993). Nutritional therapy of alcoholic liver disease. *Seminars in Liver Disease* **13**, 196–209.

Scheuer, P.J. and Lefkowitch, J.H. (1994). *Liver Biopsy Interpretation*, 5th edn. W.B. Saunders, Philadelphia, PA.

Sherlock, S. (1990). Alcoholic hepatitis. *Alcohol and Alcoholism* **25**, 189–196.

Sigal, S.H., Brill, S., Fiorino, A.S. and Reid, L.M. (1992). The liver as a stem cell and lineage system. *American Journal of Physiology* **263**, G139–148.

Skalli, O., Schurch, W., Seemayer, T. *et al.* (1989). Myofibroblasts from diverse pathological settings are heterogeneous in their content of actin isoforms and intermediate filament proteins. *Laboratory Investigation* **60**, 275–285.

Sorensen, T.I.A. (1989). Alcohol and liver injury: Dose-related or permissive effect? *Liver* **9**, 189–197.

Sorensen, T.I.A., Orholm, M., Bentsen, K.D., Hoybye, G., Eghoje, K. and Christoffersen, P. (1984). Prospective evaluation of alcohol abuse and alcoholic liver injury in men as predictors of development of cirrhosis. *Lancet* **ii**, 241–244.

Sztark, F., Latry, P., Quinton, A., Balabaud, C. and Bioulac-Sage, P. (1986). The sinusoidal barrier in alcoholic patients without fibrosis: A morphometric study. *Virchows Archives A* **409**, 385–393.

Takada, A., Nei, J., Matsuda, Y. and Kanayama, R. (1982). Clinicopathological study of alcoholic fibrosis. *American Journal of Gastroenterology* **77**, 660–666.

Takahashi, T., Kamimura, T. and Ichida, F. (1987). Ultrastructural findings on polymorphonuclear leukocyte infiltration and acute hepatocellular damage in alcoholic hepatitis. *Liver* **7**, 347–358.

Takase, S., Takada, N., Enomoto, N., Yasuhara, M. and Takada, A. (1991). Different types of chronic hepatitis in alcoholic patients: Does chronic hepatitis induced by alcohol exist? *Hepatology* **13**, 876–881.

Takayama, T., Makuuchi, M., Hirohashi, S. *et al.* (1990). Malignant transformation of adenomatous hyperplasia to hepatocellular carcinoma. *Lancet* **336**, 1150–1153.

Tarao, K., Hoshino, H., Motohashi, I., Iimori, K., Tamai, S., Ito, Y., Takagi, S. *et al.* (1989). Changes in liver and spleen volume in alcoholic liver fibrosis of man. *Hepatology* **9**, 589–593.

Terada, T., Terasaki, S. and Nakanuma, Y. (1993). A clinicopathological study of adenomatous hyperplasia of the liver in 209 consecutive cirrhotic livers examined by autopsy. *Cancer* **72**, 1551–1556.

Thaler, H. (1988). Fatty change. *Balliere's Clinical Gastroenterology* **2**, 453–462.

Tinberg, H.M. (1981). Intermediate filaments: Immunochemical composition of major polypeptides of alcoholic hyalin. *FEBS Letters* **125**, 53–56.

Uchida, T. and Peters, R.L. (1983). The nature and origin of proliferated bile ductules in alcoholic liver disease. *American Journal of Clinical Pathology* **79**, 326–333.

Uchida, T., Kao, H., Quispe-Sjogren, M. and Peters, R.L. (1983). Alcoholic foamy degeneration – a pattern of acute alcoholic injury of the liver. *Gastroenterology* **84**, 683–692.

Uchida, T., Kronberg, I. and Peters, R.L. (1984). Giant mitochondria in alcoholic liver disease: Their identification, frequency and pathological significance. *Liver* **4**, 29–38.

Valla, D., Flejou, J.F., Lebrec, D., Bernuau, J., Rueff, B., Salzmann, J.L. and Benhamou, J.-P. (1989). Portal hypertension and ascites in acute hepatitis: Clinical, hemodynamic and histological correlations. *Hepatology* **10**, 482–487.

Van Eyken, P., Sciot, R. and Desmet, V.J. (1988). A cytokeratin immunohistochemical study of alcoholic liver disease: Evidence that hepatocytes can express "bile duct-type" cytokeratins. *Histopathology* **13**, 605–617.

Van Waes, L. and Lieber, C.S. (1977). Early perivenular sclerosis in alcoholic fatty liver: An index of progressive liver injury. *Gastroenterology* **73**, 646–650.

Vidins, E.J., Britton, R.S., Medline, A., Blendis, L.M., Israel, Y. and Orrego, H. (1985). Sinusoidal calibre in alcoholic and nonalcoholic liver disease: Diagnostic and pathogenic implications. *Hepatology* **5**, 408–414.

Volentine, G.D., Tuma, D.J. and Sorrell, M.F. (1986). Subcellular location of secretory proteins retained in the liver during the ethanol-induced inhibition of hepatic protein secretion in the rat. *Gastroenterology* **90**, 158–165.

Vyberg, M. and Leth, P. (1991). Ubiquitin: An immunohistochemical marker of Mallory bodies and alcoholic liver disease. *APMIS Supplement* **23**, 46–52.

Wada, K., Kondo, F. and Kondo, Y. (1988). Large regenerative nodules and dysplastic nodules in cirrhotic livers: A histopathologic study. *Hepatology* **6**, 1684–1688.

Walter, E., Blum, H.E., Meir, P., Huonker, M., Schmid, M., Mair, K.-P., Offensperger, W.-B., Offensperger, S. and Gerok, W. (1988). Hepatocellular carcinoma in alcoholic liver disease: No evidence for a pathogenic role of hepatitis B virus infection. *Hepatology* **8**, 745–748

Worman, H.J. (1990). Cellular intermediate filament networks and their derangement in alcoholic hepatitis. *Alcoholism: Clinical and Experimental Research* **14**, 789–804.

Worner, T.M. and Lieber, C.S. (1985). Perivenular fibrosis as precursor lesion of cirrhosis. *Journal of the American Medical Association* **253**, 627–630.

Yamaoka, K., Nouchi, T., Marumo, F. and Sato, C. (1993). Alpha-smooth-muscle actin expression in normal and fibrotic human livers. *Digestive Diseases and Sciences* **38**, 1473–1479.

Yamauchi, M., Nakahara, M., Maezawa, Y., Satoh, S., Nishikawa, F. and Ohata, M. (1993). Prevalence of hepatocellular carcinoma in patients with alcoholic liver disease and prior exposure to hepatitis C. *American Journal of Gastroenterology* **88**, 39–43.

Yokoo, H., Minick, O.T., Batti, F. and Kent, G. (1972). Morphologic variants of alcoholic hyalin. *American Journal of Pathology* **69**, 25–40.

Yokoo, H. Singh, K.S. and Hawasli, A.H. (1978). Giant mitochondria in alcoholic liver disease. *Archives of Pathology and Laboratory Medicine* **102**, 213–214.

Yoshioka, K., Kakumu, S. and Tahara, H. (1989). Occurrence of immunohistologically detected small Mallory bodies in liver disease. *American Journal of Gastroenterology* **84**, 535–539.

Zauli, D., Crespi, C., Dall'Amore, P., Bianchi, F.B., Fusconi, M., Zerbini, M. and Pisi, E. (1985). Relationship between cytoskeleton and smooth muscle antibodies (SMA) in chronic liver disease (CLD). *Journal of Hepatology* **1**, 5155 (Suppl.).

Part III
Pathogenesis of Alcoholic Liver Disease

4 Pathogenesis of hepatic fibrosis

Jacquelyn J. Maher and Scott L. Friedman

Introduction

Hepatic fibrosis is a serious form of liver injury that occurs in association with prolonged and excessive alcohol intake. Fibrosis is characterized by deposition of connective tissue around the terminal hepatic venules (perivenular fibrosis), around the hepatocytes (pericellular fibrosis) and in the later stage of hepatic injury by broad bands that surround regenerative nodules of hepatocytes. Fibrosis, particularly when seen in association with alcoholic hepatitis, is ominous because of its propensity to lead to cirrhosis. This end-stage lesion is believed to be irreversible, with no effective therapy on the horizon (Brenner and Alcorn 1990). Cirrhosis represents the ninth leading cause of death in the United States, with the majority of cases attributable to alcohol abuse (Grant *et al.* 1988). In Japan, as many as two-thirds of cirrhosis-related deaths are attributable to alcohol (Parrish *et al.* 1991). Indeed, surveys from around the world (Grant *et al.* 1988; Parrish *et al.* 1991; Corrao *et al.* 1992; Savolainen *et al.* 1992) document that death from cirrhosis is directly related to per capita alcohol consumption. The aetiologic role of alcohol in promoting hepatic fibrosis is supported by studies using experimental animals as models (Lieber *et al.* 1975; Van Waes and Lieber 1977; Nakano *et al.* 1982; Tsukamoto *et al.* 1986). Given the widespread nature of alcoholic fibrosis and the lack of an effective means to treat it, current research efforts are directed towards identification of the mechanism(s) whereby alcohol ingestion leads to extracellular matrix deposition in the liver. The following summarizes our current understanding of the cellular pathophysiology of hepatic fibrosis in alcohol-associated liver injury.

Histology and biochemistry of alcoholic fibrosis

Alcoholic fibrosis begins with deposition of connective tissue around the terminal hepatic venules (Van Waes and Lieber 1977; Nakano and Lieber 1982; Worner and Lieber 1985). As the lesion progresses, thin strands of fibrous material extend to surround zone 3 hepatocytes, creating a "chicken wire" pattern visible by special stains (e.g. sirius red or trichrome stains). With ongoing injury, central–central and central–central–portal bridging and nodular regeneration ensue, resulting in destruction of hepatic acinar architecture and the eventual development of cirrhosis. There is limited evidence that alcoholic fibrosis is reversible at the pre-cirrhotic stage (Marbet *et al.* 1987). Once cirrhosis is established, however, a return to normal hepatic architecture is highly unlikely.

The connective tissue which is deposited in liver following prolonged ethanol exposure represents a complex mixture of collagens, non-collagenous glycoproteins and proteoglycans (Galambos and Shapira 1973; Rojkind and Martinez-Palomo 1976; Rojkind *et al.* 1979; Hahn *et al.* 1980a, b; Murata *et al.* 1984; Tsutsumi *et al.* 1993). These extracellular matrix proteins are all present in the subendothelial space of normal liver, but are produced in excess in the setting of chronic liver injury. Specific proteins which have been shown to accumulate in alcoholic human liver include collagen types I, III, IV and V (Rojkind and Martinez-Palomo 1976; Rojkind *et al.* 1979; Murata *et al.* 1984; Tsutsumi *et al.* 1993) as well as laminin (Hahn and Schuppan 1985) and sulphated proteoglycans (Galambos and Shapira 1973). The overall composition of the fibrotic matrix in alcoholic liver injury is similar to that in non-alcoholic liver injury (Rojkind *et al.* 1979), suggesting a common mechanism of fibrogenesis among diseases of diverse aetiology. In alcoholic liver disease, alterations in hepatic collagen have been studied extensively. With the onset of alcohol-associated fibrosis, total hepatic collagen increases in a linear fashion (Tsutsumi *et al.* 1993). The proportion of specific collagen subtypes, however, changes dramatically as fibrosis progresses. In the early stages of alcoholic fibrosis, there is a pronounced increase in type IV collagen, a non-fibril-forming collagen which is a component of the normal hepatic extracellular matrix (Tsutsumi *et al.* 1993). The increase in type IV collagen reaches an early plateau, however, while total hepatic collagen continues to rise as fibrosis progresses to cirrhosis. In the most advanced stages of fibrosis and cirrhosis, "interstitial" or "fibril-forming" collagens (types I and III) clearly predominate (Rojkind *et al.* 1979; Murata *et al.* 1984). Together these findings indicate that alcoholic fibrosis is characterized by a change in the hepatic extracellular matrix from one rich in basement membrane collagen to one rich in fibrillar collagen.

Liver cells implicated as effectors of alcoholic fibrosis

Histologic studies of alcoholic liver fibrosis have implicated mesenchymal cells as the main producers of hepatic collagen. Serial liver biopsies in both alcohol-fed baboons (Mak *et al.* 1984) and human alcoholics (Minato *et al.* 1983; Okanoue *et al.* 1983; Horn *et al.* 1986; Mak and Lieber 1988) demonstrate a progressive increase in the number of mesenchymal liver cells within areas of connective tissue deposition. The precise identity of these cells has been debated; most investigators now believe that they represent hepatic lipocytes (Ito cells). Lipocytes, also known as fat-storing, perisinusoidal or stellate cells, were first recognized by Kupffer, who

identified the cells using a gold chloride-staining technique (Kupffer 1876). Kupffer, who termed the cells *sternzellen* (star-cells) because of their shape, thought the cells were phagocytic. However, Ito (1951) subsequently distinguished these cells from the resident macrophage population bearing Kupffer's name. In 1971, Wake definitively established that lipocytes were the same cell type as Kupffer's *sternzellen*.

Lipocytes are located in normal liver in the subendothelial space of Disse, situated between the luminal surface of hepatocytes and the anti-luminal surface of sinusoidal endothelial cells (Fig. 4.1). They are approximately as numerous as Kupffer cells, or about 4–6 lipocytes per 100 hepatocytes (Bronfenmajer *et al.* 1966). The cells are distributed equally throughout zones 1–3 of the hepatic acinus, although some morphometric studies have noted a slight perivenular predominance (Giamperi *et al.* 1981; Jezequel *et al.* 1990). Several characteristic features of lipocytes facilitate their identification both *in vivo* and following isolation. These cells are the primary depot for hepatic and total body retinoids (vitamin A), which are stored within cytoplasmic droplets around the nucleus. Almost all the vitamin A is in the form of retinyl esters, primarily retinyl palmitate (Blaner *et al.* 1985). The retinoid-containing fat droplets are readily apparent by electron microscopy. The retinoids emit a characteristic rapidly fading blue–green fluorescence when intact cells or frozen sections of unfixed tissue are excited by 328 nm wavelength light which permits recognition of the cells by light microscopy (Friedman *et al.* 1985). Lipocytes express vimentin, an intermediate filament characteristic of mesenchyme, and in most species also contain desmin, a myogenic filament (Rockey *et al.* 1992). The expression of desmin has led to the suggestion that lipocytes may be contractile. Indeed, activated lipocytes also express a smooth muscle-specific isoform of α actin (Ramadori *et al.* 1990; Rockey *et al.* 1992) both *in vivo* and in culture (see pp. 74–75).

Chronic alcohol ingestion provokes a striking change in lipocyte morphology. The cells elongate, lose much of their cytoplasmic lipid, and display increased rough endoplasmic reticulum which becomes dilated (see Table 4.1). Although these modified cells are still recognized as lipocytes, some prefer to call them "transitional cells" (Mak *et al.* 1984; Mak and Lieber 1988), designating their transition from a vitamin A-storing to a myofibroblastic phenotype. Accompanying these changes *in vivo* is the appearance of collagen fibrils outside the

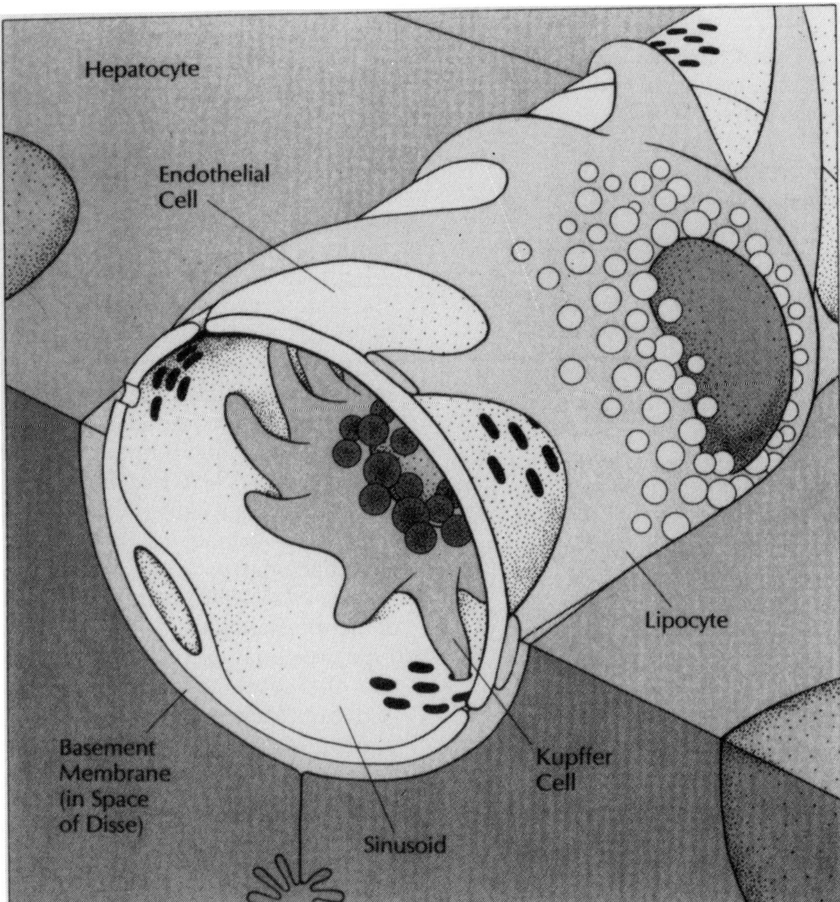

Fig. 4.1 Schematic representation of lipocytes in normal liver. Lipocytes are localized in the perisinusoidal space of normal liver between hepatocytes and sinusoidal endothelial cells. They are recognized by their abundant cytoplasmic lipid droplets which serve as reservoirs of vitamin A. As shown here, lipocytes encircle sinusoidal endothelial cells with their stellate cytoplasmic processes. Endothelial cells are also surrounded on their abluminal side by extracellular matrix proteins, which occupy the space of Disse. A Kupffer cell is illustrated within the sinusoidal lumen. Reproduced with permission from Friedman and Bissell (1990).

plasma membrane of lipocytes. Lipocytes are capable of producing large amounts of interstitial collagens, when exposed to appropriate fibrogenic stimuli (see pp. 77–79). Some investigators have noted that transitional cells are distributed widely throughout zone 3 in alcoholic liver disease (Horn *et al.* 1986; Mak and Lieber 1988), whereas fibrosis begins quite locally around the terminal hepatic venule. This suggests that morphologic activation is a prerequisite to fibrosis, but that additional signals may supervene to provoke collagen production (French *et al.* 1988).

While lipocytes are the predominant mesenchy-

mal cell in the hepatic parenchyma, they are not the only fibroblast-like cells in liver. "Fibroblasts", which lack retinoid, have been identified in normal liver around portal triads; their relationship to lipocytes is uncertain. In addition, Bhunchet and Wake (1992) have described "second-layer cells" in a non-alcohol rodent model of liver injury which migrate from large vessels and lack lipocyte-specific markers. Like portal "fibroblasts", their relationship to lipocytes and role in alcoholic fibrogenesis is uncertain.

Hepatic myofibroblasts (Savolainen *et al.* 1984b; Takase *et al.* 1988) are mesenchymal liver cells

Table 4.1 Characteristics of quiescent and activated lipocytes

	Quiescent	Activated
Cytoplasmic retinoid	Abundant	Sparse
Nuclear membrane	Regular	Convoluted
Endoplasmic reticulum	Flattened	Dilated
Contractile filaments	+	+++
Smooth muscle α actin	–	++
Extracellular collagen	–	++
Dense bodies	++	++
Pinocytic vesicles	++	++
Vimentin	++	++
Desmin	++	++

which may represent a highly activated form of lipocyte. They are elongated in shape and, like both lipocytes and transitional cells, they contain cytoplasmic filaments, dense bodies and pinocytic vesicles. Hepatic myofibroblasts have a convoluted nuclear membrane, whereas lipocytes and transitional cells do not; in addition, hepatic myofibroblasts stain negatively for the intermediate filament protein desmin, whereas both lipocytes and transitional cells stain positively. Hepatic myofibroblasts are localized preferentially in the perivenous zones of the liver, where alcoholic fibrogenesis begins. Although some contend that myofibroblasts are a distinct population of liver cells, it is our belief that they represent lipocytes that have gone beyond the stage of transitional cells to assume a proliferative, collagen-producing phenotype. Indeed, "activation" of lipocytes from a quiescent to a fibrogenic phenotype is the cellular event which represents the hallmark of alcohol-associated fibrogenesis. The following section reviews the cellular pathophysiology of lipocyte activation in alcoholic liver disease.

Lipocyte activation in hepatic fibrogenesis

Characteristics of lipocyte activation

Activation of lipocytes into myofibroblast-like cells is a central event in both alcoholic and non-alcoholic liver injury. Some of the morphologic features of lipocyte activation, loss of vitamin A and acquisition of dilated rough endoplasmic reticulum (RER), have been described in the previous section. The full spectrum of activation, however, includes a wide variety of morphologic and functional changes that contribute to hepatic fibrogenesis and perhaps to portal hypertension as well. Our current understanding of lipocyte activation *in vivo* has been greatly aided by the recognition that activation can be provoked by culturing cells on uncoated plastic or a type I collagen substratum. Virtually all the features of activation noted in culture parallel those that have been identified *in vivo*. With time in culture on uncoated plastic, lipocytes will spread (Friedman *et al.* 1989), lose intracellular retinoid (Bachem *et al.* 1992), proliferate (Friedman *et al.* 1989) and begin to express α smooth muscle actin (Ramadori *et al.* 1990; Rockey *et al.* 1992). Coincident with these changes is an increase in the extracellular matrix components typically identified in fibrotic liver, including fibril-forming collagens (Geerts *et al.* 1989; Friedman *et al.* 1989) and sulphated proteoglycans (Schafer *et al.* 1987; Arenson *et al.* 1988). Lipocytes also produce a large number of other matrix components, including laminin (Maher *et al.* 1988), tenascin (Ramadori *et al.* 1991), entactin (Ramadori 1992), undulin (Knittel *et al.* 1992), cellular fibronectin (Ramadori *et al.* 1992) and the cytokine-binding molecules decorin and biglycan (Meyer *et al.* 1992).

As noted, culture-induced activation is clearly dependent on the composition of the extracellular milieu and/or the ability of cells to spread. For example, when cultured cells are maintained on a basement membrane-like gel akin to the subendothelial matrix of normal liver, they remain compact and do not acquire features of activation (Friedman *et al.* 1989). Interestingly, quiescence can also be preserved if the cells are prevented from adhering by growing in suspension (Friedman *et al.* 1994). In either of these models, activation can be initiated if cells are transferred to uncoated plastic from their quiescence-preserving environment.

Contractility, another feature of lipocyte activation, has recently been studied in detail. Lipocytes plated on a variety of substrata exhibit features of contraction, including an intracellular influx of calcium after treatment with contractile agonists (Pinzani *et al.* 1992a) and wrinkling of deformable membranes (Kawada *et al.* 1992). Contractility is clearly activation-dependent, as quiescent cells in early culture do not exhibit this type of activity (Rockey *et al.* 1993). Lipocytes activated *in vivo* or in culture are strongly contractile, coincident with expression of smooth muscle α actin (Rockey *et al.* 1993). These interesting findings suggest that with progressive injury *in vivo*, lipocytes could restrict intrahepatic flood flow, either by distorting acinar architecture via shortening of fibrotic bands or through a perisinusoidal sphincter-like constriction. Such activities could underlie, at least in part, the elevated portal pressures observed in progressive alcoholic fibrosis.

In addition to elaborating matrix proteins, lipocytes may also accelerate matrix remodelling during liver injury through the secretion of matrix proteinases. Activated lipocytes from rat (Arthur *et al.* 1989) and human (Iredale *et al.* 1992) liver produce a collagenase with the ability to degrade type IV collagen, a constituent of the normal hepatic subendothelial matrix. Moreover, proteinase activity may be further modulated by lipocytes through their secretion of a specific inhibitor, TIMP-1 (tissue inhibitor of metalloproteinase) (Iredale *et al.* 1992). The roles played by metalloproteinases and their inhibitors *in vivo* in alcoholic liver injury and fibrosis are an area of active, ongoing investigation.

Mechanisms of lipocyte activation

Evidence to date suggests that the basic process of lipocyte activation is similar among all forms of liver injury, including that caused by alcohol. Those mediators that have been shown to induce lipocyte activation in culture are included within this section. The subsequent section reviews compounds relevant to alcohol that may promote hepatic fibrogenesis.

The ability of lipocytes to be activated depends on the interplay of stimulation from the extracellular matrix and soluble mediators (cytokines). As noted previously, uncoated plastic or a type I collagen substratum will facilitate activation, as will other matrix components including laminin and heparin sulphate proteoglycan (Friedman *et al.* 1989). Recently, a cellular isoform of fibronectin has been shown to activate lipocytes beyond that induced by type I collagen (Jarnagin *et al.* 1993). Interestingly, in a rat model of bile duct obstruction, this fibronectin isoform is produced in the early stages of injury by sinusoidal endothelial cells; whether a similar event occurs in alcoholic liver injury is unknown. Early subendothelial (pericellular) fibrosis is a central feature of alcoholic liver injury, however, and appears to predict progression to cirrhosis (Worner and Lieber 1985). Thus, elucidation of mechanisms underlying this early fibronectin deposition could have important clinical consequences.

Based on culture studies, lipocyte activation in culture may be either provoked or accelerated by exposing the cells to conditioned medium from hepatic macrophages (Kupffer cells) (Friedman and Arthur 1989). A role for Kupffer cells *in vivo* is attractive to postulate, given that macrophage infiltration is prominent and immediately precedes lipocyte activation (Johnson *et al.* 1992). Several studies have shown that lipocyte proliferation, matrix synthesis and retinoid release are stimulated by Kupffer cell-conditioned medium (Shiratori *et al.* 1986a; Friedman and Arthur 1989; Armendariz-Borunda *et al.* 1989; Zerbe and Gressner 1988). Moreover, stimulatory activity is greater when Kupffer cells are isolated from injured rather than normal liver (Shiratori *et al.* 1986a; Armendariz-Borunda *et al.* 1989).

An increasing number of well-characterized cytokines has been shown to affect lipocyte activation. Such cytokines may be autocrine or paracrine. In each case, cytokines must bind to their own receptor to exert their relevant action. Thus, current work examines not only the sources and effects of cytokines during activation, but also the modulation of cytokine receptors. This methodical consideration of the many levels of cytokine regulation has greatly advanced our understanding of the specific features of activation, as listed below (see Table 4.2).

1. *Proliferation.* Several mitogens stimulate lipocyte proliferation in culture; among these, platelet-derived growth factor (PDGF) is the most potent (Friedman and Arthur 1989; Pinzani *et al.* 1989), although mitogenesis has also been reported in response to epidermal growth factor (EGF)/ transforming growth factor α (TGFα) (Bachem *et al.* 1989), interleukin-1 (Matsuoka *et al.* 1989), tumour necrosis factor α (TNFα) (Matsuoka *et al.* 1989) and basic fibroblast growth factor (bFGF) (Pinzani *et al.* 1989). An important requirement for the lipocyte to respond to PDGF is the induction of its receptors, which are not expressed on normal (quiescent) cells but are rapidly upregulated following activation in culture and *in vivo* (Friedman and Arthur 1989). It is not known whether receptors for other mitogens are also induced during activation.

2. *Fibrogenesis.* Stimulation of matrix synthesis by lipocytes has been ascribed primarily to the actions of transforming growth factor β-1 (TGFβ-1). Both Kupffer cells (Matsuoka and Tsukamoto 1990; Meyer *et al.* 1990) and lipocytes (Bachem *et al.* 1992) represent local sources of this cytokine. *In vivo*, increased TGBβ-1 gene

Table 4.2   Characteristics of lipocyte activation and their provocative stimuli

	Provocative stimuli	
Characteristics of activation	*Soluble*	*Matrix*
Proliferation	Kupffer cell medium PDGF EGF/TGFα IL-1 TNFα bFGF IGF-I	Fibril-forming collagens
Fibrogenesis	Kupffer cell medium TGFβ Acetaldehyde Lipid aldehydes	Fibril-forming collagens
Contraction	Serum Endothelin-1 Thrombin Angiotensin II Prostaglandin E2	
Retinoid release	Kupffer cell medium PDGF	
Matrix degradation	—	Fibril-forming collagens
Cytokine release (M-CSF, MCP-1, ET, TGFβ)	PDGF bFGF IL-1 TNFα	Fibril-forming collagens

expression in consistently identified in fibrotic liver (Nakatsukasa *et al.* 1990; Milani *et al.* 1991; Castilla *et al.* 1991). In culture, lipocyte activation is similarly accompanied by increased TGFβ-1 production (Bachem *et al.* 1992) and gene expression. Concurrent with these changes, there is increased TGFβ-1 binding activity with downregulation of receptor mRNA expression (Friedman *et al.* 1994).

3. *Contraction.* As noted, lipocytes acquire the ability to contract upon activation. Studies in cultured cells consistently show that endothelin is a potent contractile agonist (Rockey *et al.* 1993). Moreover, production of endothelin-1 by lipocytes increases with activation, suggesting that autocrine-mediated contraction could occur *in vivo* during injury (Housset *et al.* 1993). In contrast to other cytokine receptors, minimal change in expression of either the A or B type endothelin receptors has been observed (Housset *et al.* 1993), which are present even on quiescent cells. Thus, the development of a contractile phenotype during lipocyte activation does not simply result from induction of receptors for a contractile agonist, unlike the mechanism underlying cellular proliferation. The importance of other contractile agonists in lipocyte contraction is less settled; experiments using primary rat lipocytes show no activity of thrombin, PDGF, TGFβ-1 or angiotensin (Rockey *et al.* 1993), whereas some responsiveness to angiotensin II and thrombin has been reported in passaged human lipocytes (Pinzani *et al.* 1992a).

4. *Retinoid release.* The release of retinoid by lipocytes during culture-induced activation occurs predominantly as loss of free retinol, reflecting intracellular hydrolysis of retinyl esters. Retinyl ester hydrolysis is associated with an increase in bile-salt independent hydrolase activity (Friedman *et al.* 1993). These findings may explain the decreased hepatic vitamin A content measured in patients with alcoholic liver disease (Sato and Lieber 1981). A major unresolved question is whether retinoid release by lipocytes is required

in order for activation to occur and, if so, whether efforts to prevent retinoid release could be exploited to develop new anti-fibrotic therapies.

5. *Matrix degradation.* Mechanisms underlying the modulation of matrix proteinases and their inhibitors are still unknown, although data from other tissues suggest that cytokines and retinoids are likely to play important roles.

6. *Cytokine release by lipocytes.* An important concept has emerged that lipocytes are not only targets for cytokines, but also elaborate factors which may amplify inflammatory and fibrotic responses. Specifically, lipocytes elaborate both macrophage colony-stimulating factor (M-CSF) (Pinzani *et al.* 1992b) and monocyte chemotactic peptide-1 (MCP-1) (Marra *et al.* 1993). Moreover, expression of these cytokines increases *in vivo* with progressive injury. The data provide an important mechanism whereby early lipocyte activation could provoke or accelerate inflammatory cell infiltration, thus establishing a positive stimulatory loop between these two cell types. Lipocytes also secrete insulin-like growth factor I (IGF-I) (Pinzani *et al.* 1990), which might serve as an autocrine mitogen during cellular activation.

Putative mediators of lipocyte activation in alcoholic liver disease

It is clear from the discussion above that lipocytes can be activated by either humoral or matrix-related extracellular signals or both. Thus, although lipocyte activation represents the final common pathway to fibrogenesis in many types of liver injury, the signals that provoke activation may differ depending upon the inciting agent. In alcoholic liver disease, three classes of compounds have been implicated as mediators of fibrogenesis: acetaldehyde, lipid aldehydes and TGFβ-1. Neutrophil chemoattractants such as 19-hydroxy 20-hydroperoxy-arachidic acid or IL-8 may also play an indirect role in hepatic fibrogenesis, by causing neutrophils to release matrix-degrading proteinases. These proteinases may activate lipocytes indirectly by altering their interactions with the surrounding extracellular matrix. Kupffer cells and lipocytes themselves can elaborate type IV collagenases. It remains uncertain, however, whether ethanol ingestion provokes collagenase production by these cells.

Acetaldehyde, lipid aldehydes and TGF-1 are each produced in the liver in response to chronic ethanol feeding. These compounds have been proposed as mediators of hepatic fibrogenesis based on their ability to provoke collagen synthesis by lipocytes in culture. The data in support of their activity are mixed; although each compound enhances collagen synthesis by lipocytes under restricted culture conditions, none of them provokes activation of otherwise quiescent lipocytes. This leaves some uncertainty about their respective roles in alcoholic fibrogenesis *in vivo*.

Acetaldehyde

Acetaldehyde, the first product of ethanol oxidation, was first demonstrated to influence collagen synthesis in experiments using fibroblasts from extrahepatic sources. Brenner and Chojkier (1987) showed that human foreskin fibroblasts, when incubated with 200 μM acetaldehyde for 24 h, increased their collagen synthesis and gene expression by two- to three-fold. This led to similar experiments with lipocytes; Moshage *et al.* (1990) demonstrated that when acetaldehyde was added to lipocytes in late (14 days) primary or passaged culture, synthesis of type I collagen also increased two- to three-fold. Acetaldehyde exerts its effect on lipocytes by enhancing transcription of the the pro-α1(I) collagen gene (Casini *et al.* 1991). The effect can be inhibited by cycloheximide, indicating that it is dependent upon protein synthesis (Casini *et al.* 1991). Moreover, stimulation of collagen synthesis and gene expression is achieved at an equilibrium concentration of acetaldehyde of approximately 50 μM (Moshage *et al.* 1990; Casini *et al.* 1991), a dose which is comparable to that measured in the venous circulation of human alcoholics (Korsten *et al.* 1975). Not all studies support the notion that acetaldehyde stimulates collagen synthesis by lipocytes. Shiratori and colleagues (1986b) noted that when lipocytes from normal rat liver were incubated with acetaldehyde in early primary culture (18 h), collagen synthesis was not increased. By contrast, when acetaldehyde was added to lipocytes from rats that had been treated *in vivo* with CCl_4, collagen synthesis was enhanced as early as 2 days after plating. Proteoglycan production by lipocytes is also unaffected by acetaldehyde when added at early culture intervals (Gressner and Althaus, 1988). Together these findings suggest that quiescent lipocytes (mimicked *in vitro* by early primary culture) are not inherently responsive to acetaldehyde, but acquire this feature upon late primary culture or upon subculture. Studies from our laboratory have attempted to define the event(s) which render lipocytes responsive to acetaldehyde in culture. To date, we have been unable to link responsiveness to acetaldehyde to other features of activation, including spreading, proliferation and baseline collagen production (Maher *et al.* 1994a). The fact that lipocytes respond to the fibrogenic effects of acetaldehyde only under certain culture conditions suggests that its role as a fibrogenic mediator *in vivo* may be limited (see below).

Lipid aldehydes

Oxidation of ethanol and acetaldehyde can lead to the production of reactive oxygen intermediates. Particularly important is the formation of hydroxyl (·OH) radicals, which can interact with cellular elements (lipids, proteins and DNA) and cause irreversible cell injury. Research to date has focused primarily on the interaction of hydroxyl radicals with polyunsaturated lipids; this leads to a repetitive cycle of lipid peroxidation, with formation of lipid aldehydes as by-products. The lipid aldehydes malondialdehyde and 4-hydroxynonenal (4-HNE) have been measured as indices of lipid peroxidation in the liver after ethanol feeding (Kawase *et al.* 1989; Kamimura *et al.* 1992). They increase significantly when ethanol is administered in combination with a diet that is either high in polyunsaturated fat (Kamimura *et al.* 1992) or low in vitamin E (Kawase *et al.* 1989). Like acetaldehyde, lipid aldehydes stimulate collagen synthesis when added to lipocytes in passaged culture (Parola *et al.* 1993).

Studies from our laboratory indicate that lipocytes require activation before becoming responsive to the fibrogenic effects of lipid aldehydes (Maher *et al.* 1994b). Thus, *in vivo*, lipid aldehydes may enhance hepatic fibrosis but are unlikely to initiate it. Further study is required to determine whether lipid peroxidation in human alcoholics represents an important mechanism of hepatic fibrogenesis.

TGFβ-1

TGFβ-1 is a macrophage-derived cytokine that enhances extracellular matrix synthesis and gene expression when added to lipocytes in primary and passaged culture (Matsuoka *et al.* 1989; Weiner *et al.* 1990; Meyer *et al.* 1990; Armendariz-Borunda *et al.* 1992). Kupffer cells represent a local source of TGFβ-1 in liver (Matsuoka and Tsukamoto 1990; Meyer *et al.* 1990; Milani *et al.* 1991) and, after prolonged ethanol feeding, their production of TGFβ-1 is increased (Matsuoka and Tsukamot 1990). Matsuoka and Tsukamoto (1990) showed that conditioned medium from Kupffer cells isolated from ethanol-fed rats enhances lipocyte collagen production, and that the increase can be blocked by an antibody against TGFβ-1. Ethanol feeding also increases TGFβ-1 mRNA in Kupffer cells, indicating that the mechanism of its upregulation is pre-translational. It remains uncertain whether the signal that provokes upregulation of TGFβ-1 derives from hepatocytes or from another hepatic or extrahepatic source.

It is of interest that TGFβ-1, like both acetaldehyde and lipid aldehydes, has a greater effect on activated than on quiescent lipocytes in culture. This cytokine enhances collagen synthesis by only 50 percent in lipocytes in early primary culture (Matsuoka *et al.* 1989), whereas in late primary or passaged culture it enhances collagen synthesis by 3-fold or more (Weiner *et al.* 1990; Armendariz-Borunda *et al.* 1992). This phenomenon appears to occur also *in vivo*, as Kupffer cell-derived TGFβ-1 exerts a much greater effect on lipocytes from ethanol-fed rats than on cells from normal rat liver (Matsuoka and Tsukamoto 1990). This suggests that ethanol feeding provokes lipocyte activation independently of TGFβ-1, which enables them to respond more readily to this fibrogenic mediator, possibly via increased binding activity (Friedman *et al.* 1994).

Matrix-degrading proteinases

Perturbation of the hepatic extracellular matrix can provoke lipocyte activation by altering cell-matrix interactions which normally maintain these cells in a quiescent state *in vivo* (see above). Neutrophils contain a 92 kDa type IV collagenase (gelatinase) (Hibbs *et al.* 1985), which is released into the extracellular milieu upon degranulation. Hepatocytes oxidizing ethanol secrete at least one chemoattractant for neutrophil polymorphs (19 hydroxy 20-hydroperoxy-arachidic acid) (Roll *et al.* 1992); another chemoattractant, interleukin-8 (IL-8), is present in the plasma of patients with alcoholic hepatitis (Hill *et al.* 1993; Sheron *et al.* 1993) and may derive from hepatocytes (Thornton *et al.* 1992; Shiratori *et al.* 1993a, b). These compounds are of interest to alcoholic fibrogenesis in that they provoke degranulation as well as migration of neutrophils. Release of collagenase during degranulation facilitates the migration of neutrophils through the hepatic extracellular matrix. Whether collagenase secretion also promotes fibrogenesis remains speculative.

Collagenases can be produced not only by neutrophils recruited to the liver during alcoholic hepatitis, but also by Kupffer cells and by activated lipocytes (Arthur *et al*. 1989; Iredale *et al*. 1992). Thus matrix degradation could play a role in alcoholic liver fibrosis even in the absence of overt hepatic inflammation. The role of collagenases as mediators of lipocyte activation in alcoholic liver disease is currently under investigation.

A working model of lipocyte activation

Lipocyte activation can be conceptually divided into at least two stages, initiation and perpetuation (Fig. 4.2). Initiation refers to the early events which render the cells susceptible to proliferative, fibrogenic and contractile stimuli. Perpetuation encompasses those responses which can only occur after the cell has already been made responsive to specific extracellular stimuli. For example, a major element of initiation is the induction of receptors for PDGF. Once receptors are present, proliferation may be perpetuated in the presence of PDGF. Similarly it appears likely that acetaldehyde is a perpetuating rather than initiating stimulus to fibrogenesis (Friedman and Bissell 1990).

Identification of initiating stimuli in alcoholic fibrosis is a major focus of current research efforts. Candidates include as yet uncharacterized paracrine mediators from Kupffer cells, and products of liver cell injury (particularly reactive oxygen species and acetaldehyde–protein adducts). Early disruption of the subendothelial extracellular matrix by collagenases could play a role in the initiation of injury, with replacement by cellular fibronectin from endothelial cells initially and then from lipocytes. As lipocytes become activated, they may accelerate matrix re-

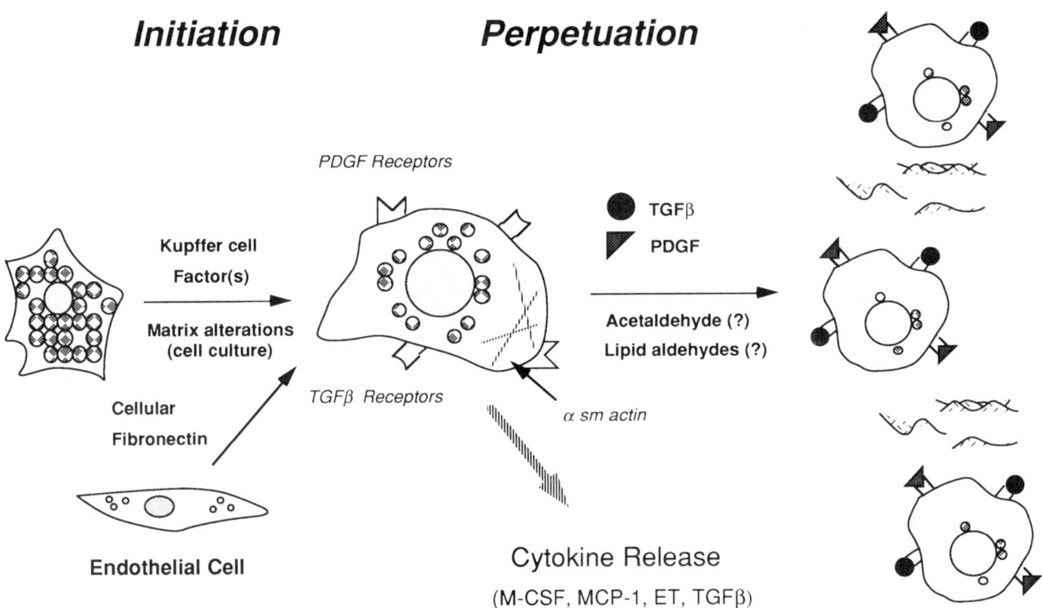

Fig. 4.2 Proposed model of lipocyte activation. Activation is divisible into two stages, termed "initiation" and "perpetuation". During initiation, lipocytes acquire certain characteristics which render them susceptible to mitogens and fibrogenic mediators. Among these are expression of receptors for PDGF and TGFβ. Lipocytes also begin to express smooth muscle α-actin during initiation, which may facilitate their responsiveness to contractile mediators. The stimuli which provoke initiation may be soluble (e.g. factors secreted by Kupffer cells) or insoluble (in the form of altered cell–matrix interactions, as occurs in culture on plastic or fibrillar collagen substrata). Cellular fibronectin, produced by sinusoidal endothelial cells in primary culture, also initates activation. The second phase of activation ("perpetuation") is characterized by the interaction of lipocytes with specific mitogens and fibrogenic mediators. It is at this stage that alcohol metabolites such as acetaldehyde and lipid aldehydes may exert their effects. Of note is that lipocytes acquire the ability to produce cytokines during activation. This may enhance the activation process directly (autocrine stimulation of lipocytes by TGFβ-1) or indirectly (by activating inflammatory cells to produce additional fibrogenic mediators).

modelling via enhanced proteinase activity against the normal matrix, and by replacing this normal subendothelial matrix with one rich in fibril-forming (e.g. type I) collagen, itself a potential activating stimulus. At present, it is not certain how all those events relate temporally to one another, but this paradigm provides a working framework for incorporating recent insights made using the cell-culture model.

A major unresolved question is what determines when this activation cascade becomes irreversible. Clinically, it is documented that fibrosis can be reversed in the alcoholic patient who becomes abstinent, yet frank cirrhosis with nodule formation is unlikely to regress even if drinking ceases. The simple answer is that reversal will not occur once the organ is no longer able to resorb the excess extracellular matrix. It is uncertain, however, how this irreversibility is expressed at the cellular level. Specifically, does the bulk of matrix become inaccessible to proteinases because of its thickness, or is matrix degradative activity simply exhausted as injury persists? Continued elucidation of the cellular responses by lipocytes and other resident liver cells using modern culture, molecular and biochemical techniques is likely to yield an answer in the coming years.

Does alcoholic fibrosis occur in the absence of alcoholic hepatitis?

There is continued debate whether alcoholic hepatitis always precedes fibrosis. In some measure, the issue depends upon whether mediators from inflammatory cells are necessary to provoke lipocyte activation, or whether other cells (e.g. hepatocytes, sinusoidal endothelial cells) can produce these stimuli. Hepatocytes can elaborate putative fibrogenic mediators such as acetaldehyde and lipid aldehydes, which suggests that alcoholic fibrosis may occur via a direct hepatocyte–lipocyte communication without the need for inflammatory cells as intermediates. Indeed, serial biopsies of baboons drinking alcohol suggest that these animals progress from steatosis to hepatic fibrosis and cirrhosis in the absence of alcoholic hepatitis (Van Waes and Lieber 1977). In rats, alcoholic fibrosis can be induced by feeding ethanol in conjunction with a diet rich in polyunsaturated fat (Tsukamoto *et al.* 1986). Fibrosis in these animals, however, is accompanied by neutrophilic and monocytic infiltration of the liver (Tsukamoto *et al.* 1986). Studies of human alcoholics are mixed in their

conclusions regarding the role of inflammation in hepatic fibrogenesis. Okanoue and colleagues (1983), who examined lipocyte morphology in patients with alcoholic liver disease, found activated cells only in the liver biopsies that showed the features of alcoholic hepatitis. Others have reported that activation occurs in the presence of steatosis alone (Minato *et al.* 1983; Mak *et al.* 1984; Mak and Lieber 1988), while still others suggest that activation can occur in the absence of alcoholic hepatitis but is more pronounced in its presence (Horn *et al.* 1986). These inconsistencies emphasize the difficulty one encounters in predicting pathophysiologic mechanisms based on static histologic observations. The fact that alcoholics with hepatic fibrosis do not always have concomitant alcoholic hepatitis does not exclude a role for inflammatory cells in the fibrogenic process. Kupffer cells, for example, may serve as important sources of fibrogenic cytokines or matrix-degrading proteinases (see above), but because they are normal residents of liver they may be overlooked as inflammatory intermediates. Circulating neutrophils could also elaborate fibrogenic mediators or proteinases during bouts of alcoholic hepatitis, but be inapparent in a liver biopsy because of the intermittent nature of the hepatic injury. In a similar context, the inflammatory process may be subclinical even though mediators are present and cellular alterations are underway. Given that hepatocyte-derived compounds such as acetaldehyde and lipid aldehydes perpetuate, but do not initate, lipocyte activation in culture, it is unlikely that these compounds by themselves will provoke alcoholic fibrogenesis *in vivo*.

Cofactors that enhance the risk of hepatic fibrosis in alcoholics

Only 10–15 percent of persons who consume alcohol to excess actually develop hepatic fibrosis (Lelbach 1976). Moreover, although there appears to be a threshold of alcohol consumption that leads to acquisiton of liver disease (on average 80 g of ethanol daily), in individual patients the severity of liver injury is not dose-dependent (Marbet *et al.* 1987; Corrao *et al.* 1992). These observations suggest that genetic or environmental cofactors or both act in conjunction with ethanol to promote hepatic fibrogenesis. Several histocompatibility antigens, including HLA-A1, A9, A28, B13, B15, BW35 and B40, have been noted with increased frequency in patients with alcoholic cirrhosis (Melendez *et al.*

1979; Bell and Nordhagen 1980; Doffoel *et al.* 1986; Monteiro *et al.* 1988); none of these, however, have been confirmed upon repeated testing (Scott *et al.* 1977; Faizallah *et al.* 1982; Mills *et al.* 1988). Others have proposed that hepatic fibrogenesis is facilitated by derangements in alcohol or acetaldehyde metabolism caused by genetic polymorphisms in the alcohol-metabolizing enzymes alcohol dehydrogenase (ADH) or aldehyde dehydrogenase (ALDH). ADH polymorphisms can cause up to 20-fold differences in ethanol elimination rates among various ethnic groups (Bosron and Li 1986; Bosron *et al.* 1988). Despite this, there is only limited evidence that such polymorphisms enhance the incidence of liver injury (Day *et al.* 1991). Interestingly, it appears that persons with the most rapid rates of ethanol elimination are at risk of end-organ damage, suggesting that liver injury is caused by ethanol metabolites rather than the parent compound *per se*. In a similar fashion, persons having impaired oxidation of acetaldehyde due to inheritance of the ALDH2^2 allele may be at greater risk of developing alcoholic fibrosis than persons with normal ALDH activity. Individuals homozygous for ALDH2^2 experience a disulfiram reaction upon ethanol ingestion, and often have such an aversion to alcohol that abuse is not a risk. Inviduals heterozygous for ALDH2^2, however, occasionally drink to excess. Enomoto *et al.* (1991) conducted a survey in which the incidence of liver injury in alcoholic patients heterozygous for ALDH2^2 was compared with that in alcoholics with a normal ALDH phenotype. They found that of seven patients with an abnormal ALDH phenotype who drank 80 g or more of ethanol daily, all exhibited signs of liver injury. Moreover, these individuals contracted alcoholic hepatitis and fibrosis at a cumulative dose of ethanol which was only half that in the control population. These findings are of interest in view of the connection between acetaldehyde and hepatic fibrogenesis (see above).

The collagen gene itself has been proposed as a target of polymorphisms which predispose patients to alcoholic fibrosis (Weiner *et al.* 1988). Data in support of this notion are limited, however, and have been challenged by more recent studies (Bashir *et al.* 1992). To date there is no firm evidence linking fibrosis to abnormalities in the collagen gene.

Several environmental cofactors have been postulated to contribute to the risk of hepatic fibrosis in alcoholics. Malnutrition, for example, which often portends a poor outcome in patients with alcoholic hepatitis (Mendenhall *et al.* 1984), may also play a role in alcoholic fibrogenesis. The role of malnutrition in human alcoholic liver disease has been the subject of great debate; although hepatic fibrosis can develop in ethanol-fed animals despite a nutritionally adequate diet, malnutrition may indeed contribute to alcoholic fibrogenesis in humans. There is evidence that a reduced intake of antioxidants (such as vitamin E) or an increased intake of pro-oxidants (such as polyunsaturated fat) in combination with ethanol abuse enhances liver injury in experimental animals and may indeed be profibrogenic (Kawase *et al.* 1989; Tsukamoto *et al.* 1986; Kamimura *et al.* 1992). There is also evidence in humans, albeit limited, that alcoholics who consume large amounts of polyunsaturated fat have an increased incidence of alcoholic cirrhosis (Nanji and French 1986). Given the current interest in oxidant stress and lipid peroxidation as putative mechanisms of alcoholic fibrogenesis, further study regarding interactions between diet and ethanol consumption is warranted.

Alcoholics with cirrhosis are more likely to be seropositive for the hepatitis C virus (35.9 percent) than those without cirrhosis (17.7 percent) (Nalpas *et al.* 1991). This has led to the hypothesis that concomitant infection with hepatitis C places alcoholics at higher risk of developing hepatic fibrosis. Investigators from Japan attribute the rising death rate from cirrhosis in men between 24 and 85 years of age to a synergistic effect of viral hepatitis and alcoholism (Parrish *et al.* 1991); others, however, suggest that although alcoholics with antibodies against hepatitis C have an increased risk of cirrhosis, the increase is additive rather than synergistic (Corrao *et al.* 1992). Hepatitis B has also been examined as a potential synergistic agent in the pathogenesis of alcoholic cirrhosis. As with hepatitis C, alcoholics who are seropositive for hepatitis B often have an increased incidence of cirrhosis; hepatitis B infection, however, does not appear to enhance the risk of alcoholic fibrosis (Chevillotte *et al.* 1983; Corrao *et al.* 1992).

A recent study examined whether cigarette smoking and coffee drinking increase the risk of cirrhosis in alcoholics (Klatsky and Armstrong 1992). Alcoholics who smoke more than one pack of cigarettes per day have a three-fold higher incidence of hepatic fibrosis than non-smoking alcoholics (Klatsky and Armstrong 1992). Coffee drinkers, however, have a reduced incidence of alcoholic fibrosis, with persons drinking four or more cups of coffee per day having a five-fold lower risk of cirrhosis than those who do not drink coffee. The effect of coffee consumption is not related to caffeine, as tea drinking did not enhance the development of alcoholic cirrhosis. Thus, it appears that cigarette smoking increases the risk of alcoholic cirrhosis, whereas coffee drinking may protect against it.

Diagnosis of alcoholic fibrosis

Liver biopsy represents the most accurate method for assessing hepatic fibrosis. Although attempts have been made to quantitate fibrosis non-invasively using serum assays for procollagen peptides, such assays have not found broad clinical application. The rationale underlying the use of procollagen peptides as markers of fibrosis is that collagens are secreted as precursor molecules which undergo cleavage after secretion into the extracellular space. Several assays have been developed which measure the *N*- or *C*-terminal propeptides of collagen types I, III and IV in patient sera (Raedsch *et al.* 1982; Risteli and Risteli 1987; Rohde *et al.* 1979; Risteli *et al.* 1981; Savolainen *et al.* 1984a; Schuppan *et al.* 1986a). Additional assays have been introduced which measure proteolytic fragments of laminin (Risteli *et al.* 1981; Pick-Kober *et al.* 1985) and hyaluronate (Frebourg *et al.* 1986). Some studies suggest that the level of procollagen peptides in serum correlate well with the degree of hepatic fibrosis (Sato *et al.* 1986; Torres-Salinas *et al.* 1986; Schuppan *et al.* 1986b); several others, however, indicate that procollagen peptides are poor predictors of hepatic fibrosis (Niemela *et al.* 1983; Nouchi *et al.* 1987; Bentsen *et al.* 1987). Procollagen peptides in serum could fail to mirror collagen levels in the liver for several reasons. First, propeptides in serum may derive from collagen produced outside the liver, resulting in a falsely high estimate of hepatic fibrosis. Alternatively, procollagen peptides produced in the liver may be eliminated before reaching the serum, resulting in artifactually low estimates of hepatic fibrosis. There is, for example, substantial biliary excretion of procollagen peptides which increases in cirrhosis (Raedsch *et al.* 1983). In addition, procollagen peptides can be endocytosed and degraded by sinusoidal endothelial cells before they reach the systemic circulation (Bentsen *et al.* 1988; Smedsrod 1988). Finally, there is evidence that some collagen molecules are assembled into fibrils without ever losing their propieces (Fleischmajer *et al.* 1986; Sakakibara *et al.* 1986; Davis and Madri 1987). These propieces could instead be released upon degradation of mature collagen, creating some confusion as to whether propeptides are in

fact indicators of collagen synthesis or breakdown. Together, these multiple pathways of procollagen peptide metabolism cast doubt on the reliability of serum assays for the detection of hepatic fibrosis.

Procollagen peptides are more likely to be elevated in serum when collagen synthesis and perhaps collagen degradation are active (e.g. in active *vs* inactive cirrhosis). This is supported by studies demonstrating that procollagen peptides are highest during the inflammatory phases of both alcoholic (Niemela *et al.* 1983; Annoni *et al.* 1989) and nonalcoholic (McCullough *et al.* 1987) liver disease. For this reason, propeptide levels may correlate with prognosis. However, until the true utility of serum assays for extracellular matrix proteins is established, they are likely to remain as research tools.

Summary

Hepatic fibrosis represents a severe, potentially irreversible consequence of chronic alcohol abuse for which no effective treatment has been identified. Prolonged exposure to high doses of ethanol is definitely a prerequisite for developing alcoholic fibrosis, although genetic or environmental cofactors may enhance the risk in certain individuals. At the cellular level, alcoholic fibrosis is initiated by activation of hepatic lipocytes, mesenchymal cells which reside in the hepatic perisinusoidal space. In response to ethanol, lipocytes transform from quiescent, vitamin A-storing cells to proliferating, matrix-producing myofibroblasts. Several compounds including acetaldehyde, lipid aldehydes and TGFβ-1 have been implicated as mediators of fibrogenesis in alcoholic liver disease. These compounds enhance collagen synthesis by lipocytes *in vitro*, but only under specific conditions of culture. Of note is that none of these mediators initiates activation of lipocytes from a quiescent to a fibrogenic phenotype.

The fact that alcohol metabolites and TGFβ-1 appear to enhance, rather than initiate, alcoholic fibrogenesis has provoked speculation regarding alternative mechanisms of fibrogenesis in the setting of ethanol abuse. Two attractive hypotheses are that lipocyte activation can be initiated either by Kupffer cell-derived mediators (independent of TGFβ-1) or by matrix-degrading proteinases released by Kupffer cells or by neutrophils recruited to the liver during episodes of alcoholic hepatitis. Future studies should determine whether these mechanisms are operative in alcoholic liver disease.

References

Annoni, G., Colombo, M., Cantaluppi, M.C., Khlat, B., Lampertico, P. and Rojkind, M. (1989). Serum type III procollagen peptide and laminin (Lam-P1) detect alcoholic hepatitis in chronic alcohol abusers. *Hepatology* **9**, 693–697.

Arenson, D.M., Friedman, S.L. and Bissell, D.M. (1988). Formation of extracellular matrix in normal rat liver: Lipocytes as a major source of proteoglycan. *Gastroenterology* **95**, 441–447.

Armendariz-Borunda, J., Greenwel, P. and Rojkind, M. (1989). Kupffer cells from CCl₄-treated rat livers induce skin fibroblast and liver fat-storing cell proliferation in culture. *Matrix* **9**, 150–158.

Armendariz-Borunda, J., Katayama, K. and Seyer, J.M. (1992). Transcriptional mechanisms of type I collagen gene expression are differentially regulated by interleukin-1 beta, tumor necrosis factor alpha, and transforming growth factor beta in Ito cells. *Journal of Biological Chemistry* **267**, 14316–14321.

Arthur, M.J.P., Friedman, S.L., Roll, F.J. and Bissell, D.M. (1989). Lipocytes from normal rat liver release a neutral metalloproteinase that degrades basement membrane (type IV) collagen. *Journal of Clinical Investigation* **84**, 1076–1085.

Bachem, M.G., Riess, U. and Gressner, A.M. (1989). Liver fat storing cell proliferation is stimulated by epidermal growth factor/transforming growth factor alpha and inhibited by transforming growth factor beta. *Biochemical and Biophysical Research Communications* **162**, 708–714.

Bachem, M.G., Meyer, D., Melchior, R., Sell, K.M. and Gressner, A.M. (1992). Activation of rat liver perisinusoidal lipocytes by transforming growth factors derived from myofibroblast like cells. *Journal of Clinical Investigation* **89**, 19–27.

Bashir, R., Day, C.P., James, O.F., Ogilvie, D.J., Sykes, B. and Bassendine, M.F. (1992). No evidence for involvement of type I collagen structural genes in "genetic predisposition" to alcoholic cirrhosis. *Journal of Hepatology* **16**, 316–319.

Bell, H. and Nordhagen, R. (1980). HLA antigens in alcoholics, with special reference to alcoholic cirrhosis. *Scandinavian Journal of Gastroenterology* **15**, 453–456.

Bentsen, K.D., Horn, T., Risteli, J. *et al.* (1987). Serum aminoterminal type III procollagen peptide and the 7S domain of type IV collagen in patients with alcohol abuse: Relation to ultrastructural fibrosis in the acinar zone 3 and to serum hyaluronan. *Liver* **7**, 339–346.

Bentsen, K.D., Boesby, S., Kirkegaard, P. *et al.* (1988). Is the aminoterminal propeptide of type III procollagen degraded in the liver? A study of type III procollagen peptide in serum during liver transplantation in pigs. *Journal of Hepatology* **6**, 144–150.

Bhunchet, E. and Wake, K. (1992). Role of mesenchymal cell populations in porcine serum-induced rat liver fibrosis. *Hepatology* **16**, 1452–1473.

Blaner, W.S., Hendriks, H.F.J., Brouwer, A., DeLeeuw, A.M., Knook, D.L. and Goodman, D.S. (1985). Retinoids, retinoid-binding proteins, and retinyl palmitate hydrolase distributions in different types of rat liver cells. *Journal of Lipid Research* **26**, 1241–1251.

Bosron, W.F. and Li, T.-K. (1986). Genetic polymorphism of human liver alcohol and aldehyde dehydrogenases, and their relationship to alcohol metabolism and alcoholism. *Hepatology* **6**, 502–510.

Bosron, W.F., Lumeng, L. and Li, T.-K. (1988). Genetic polymorphism of enzymes of alcohol metabolism and susceptibility to alcoholic liver disease. *Molecular Aspects of Medicine* **10**, 147–158.

Brenner, D.A. and Alcorn, J.M. (1990). Therapy for hepatic fibrosis. *Seminars in Liver Disease* **10**, 75–83.

Brenner, D.A. and Chojkier, M. (1987). Acetaldehyde increases collagen gene transcription in cultured human fibroblasts. *Journal of Biological Chemistry* **262**, 17690–17695.

Bronfenmajer, S., Schaffner, F. and Popper, H. (1966). Fat-storing cells (lipocytes) in human liver. *Archives of Pathology* **82**, 447–453.

Casini, A., Cunningham, M., Rojkind, M. and Lieber, C.S. (1991). Acetaldehyde increases procollagen type I and fibronectin gene transcription in cultured rat fat-storing cells through a protein synthesis-dependent mechanism. *Hepatology* **13**, 758–765.

Castilla, A., Prieto, J. and Fausto, N. (1991). Transforming growth factors β–1 and α in chronic liver disease: Effects of interferon-α therapy. *New England Journal of Medicine* **324**, 933–940.

Chevillotte, G., Durbec, J.P., Gerolami, A., Berthezene, P., Bidart, J.M. and Camatte, R. (1983). Interaction between hepatitis B virus and alcohol consumption in liver cirrhosis: An epidemiologic study. *Gastroenterology* **85**, 141–145.

Corrao, G., Carle, F., Lepore, A.R., Zepponi, E., Galatola, G. and Di Orio, F. (1992). Interaction between alcohol consumption and positivity for antibodies to hepatitis C virus on the risk of liver cirrhosis: A case-control study. *European Journal of Epidemiology* **8**, 634–639.

Davis, B.H. and Madri, J.A. (1987). Type I and type III procollagen peptides during hepatic fibrogenesis. An immunohistochemical and ELISA serum study in the CCl₄ rat model. *American Journal of Pathology* **126**, 137–147.

Day, C.P., Bashir, R., James, O.F., Bassendine, M.F., Crabb, D.W., Thomasson, H.R., Li, T.-K. and Edenberg, H.J. (1991). Investigation of the role of polymorphisms at the alcohol and aldehyde dehydrogenase loci in genetic predisposition to alcohol-related end-organ damage. *Hepatology* **14**, 798–801.

Doffoel, M., Tongio, M.M., Gut, J.-P., Ventre, G., Charrault, A., Vetter, D., Ledig, M., North, M.L.,

Mayer, S. and Bockel, R. (1986). Relationships between 34 HLA-A, HLA-B and HLA-DR antigens and three serological markers of viral infections in alcoholic cirrhosis. *Hepatology* **6**, 457–463.

Enomoto, N., Takase, S., Takada, N. and Takada, A. (1991). Alcoholic liver disease in heterozygotes of mutant and normal aldehyde dehydrogenase-2 genes. *Hepatology* **13**, 1071–1075.

Faizallah, R., Woodrow, J.C., Krasner, N.K., Walker, R.J. and Morris, A.I. (1982). Are HLA antigens important in the development of alcohol-induced liver disease? *British Medical Journal* **285**, 533–534.

Fleischmajer, R., Olsen, B.R., Timpl, R. *et al.* (1986). Collagen fibril formation during embryogenesis. *Proceedings of the National Academy of Sciences, USA* **80**, 3354–3358.

Frebourg, T., Delpech, B., Bercoff, E. , Senant, P., Deugnier, Y. and Bourneille, J. (1986). Serum hyaluronate in liver diseases: Study by enzymoimmunological assay. *Hepatology* **6**, 392–395.

French, S.W., Miyamoto, K., Wong, K., Jui, L. and Briere, L. (1988). Role of the Ito cell in liver parenchymal fibrosis in rats fed alcohol and a high fat-low protein diet. *American Journal of Pathology* **132**, 73–85.

Friedman, S.L. (1990). Acetaldehyde and alcoholic fibrogenesis – fuel to the fire but not the spark. *Hepatology* **12**, 609–612.

Friedman, S.L. and Arthur, M.J.P. (1989). Activation of cultured rat hepatic lipocytes by Kupffer cell conditioned medium. *Journal of Clinical Investigation* **84**, 1780–1785.

Friedman, S.L. and Bissell, D.M. (1990). Hepatic fibrosis: New insights into pathogenesis. *Hospital Practice* **25**, 43–50.

Friedman, S.L., Roll, J.F., Boyles, J. and Bissell, D.M. (1985). Hepatic lipocytes: The principal collagen-producing cells of normal rat liver. *Proceedings of the National Academy of Sciences, USA* **82**, 8681–8685.

Friedman, S.L., Roll, F.J., Boyles, J., Arenson, D.M. and Bissell, D.M. (1989). Maintenance of differentiated phenotype of cultured rat hepatic lipocytes by basement membrane matrix. *Journal of Biological Chemistry* **264**, 10756–10762.

Friedman, S.L., Wei, S. and Blaner, W.S. (1993). Retinol release by activated rat hepatic lipocytes – regulation by Kupffer cell conditioned medium and PDGF. *American Journal of Physiology* **264**, G947-G952.

Friedman, S.L., Yamasaki, G. and Wong, L.S. (1994). Modulation of TGFβ receptors in rat hepatic lipocytes during liver injury: Enhanced binding but reduced gene expression accompany cellular activation in culture and *in vivo*. *Journal of Biological Chemistry* **269**, 10551–10558.

Galambos, J.T. and Shapira, R. (1973). Natural history of alcoholic hepatitis. IV. Glycosaminoglycuronans and collagen in the hepatic connective tissue. *Journal of Clinical Investigation* **52**, 2952–2962.

Geerts, A., Vrijsen, R., Rauterberg, J., Burt, A.,

Schellinck, P. and Wisse, E. (1989). *In vitro* differentiation of fat-storing cells parallels marked increase of collagen synthesis and secretion. *Journal of Hepatology* **9**, 59–68.

Giamperi, M.P., Jezequel, A.M. and Orlandi, F. (1981). The lipocytes in normal human liver. *Digestion* **22**, 165–169.

Grant, B.F., Dufour, M.C. and Harford, T.C. (1988). Epidemiology of alcoholic liver disease. *Seminars in Liver Disease* **8**, 12–25.

Gressner, A.M. and Althaus, M. (1988). Effects of ethanol, acetaldehyde, and lactate on proteoglycan synthesis and proliferation of cultured rat liver fat-storing cells. *Gastroenterology* **94**, 797–807.

Hahn, E.G. and Schuppan, D. (1985). Ethanol and fibrogenesis in the liver. In *Alcohol Related Liver Diseases in Gastroenterology* (Edited by Seitz, H.K. and Kommerell, B.), pp.124–153. Springer-Verlag, Berlin.

Hahn, E., Wick, G., Pencev, D. and Timpl, R. (1980a). Distribution of basement membrane proteins in normal and fibrotic human liver: Collagen type IV, laminin and fibronectin. *Gut* **21**, 63–71.

Hahn, E.G., Timpl, R., Nakano, M. and Lieber, C.S. (1980b). Distribution of hepatic collagens, elastin and structural glycoproteins during the development of alcoholic liver injury in baboons. *Gastroenterology* **79**, 1024.

Hibbs, M.S., Hasty, K.A., Seyer, J.M., Kang, A.H. and Mainardi, C.L. (1985). Biochemical and immunological characterization of the secreted forms of human neutrophil gelatinase. *Journal of Biological Chemistry* **260**, 2493–2500.

Hill, D.B., Marsano, L.S. and McClain, C.J. (1993). Increased plasma interleukin-8 concentrations in alcoholic hepatitis. *Hepatology* **18**, 576–580.

Horn, T., Junge, J. and Christoffersen, P. (1986). Early alcoholic liver injury: Activation of lipocytes in acinar zone 3 and correlation to degree of collagen formation in the Disse space. *Journal of Hepatology* **3**, 333–340.

Housset, C.N., Rockey, D.C. and Bissell, D.M. (1993). Endothelin receptors in rat liver: Lipocytes as a contractile target for endothelin-1. *Proceedings of the National Academy of Sciences, USA* **90**, 9266–9270.

Iredale, J.P., Murphy, G., Hembry, R.M., Friedman, S.L. and Arthur, M.J.P. (1992). Human hepatic lipocytes synthesize and release TIMP-1, an important regulator of matrix metalloproteinase activity. *Journal of Clinical Investigation* **90**, 282–287.

Ito, T. (1951). Cytological studies on stellate cells of Kupffer and fat storing cells in the capillary wall of the human liver. *Acta Anatomica Nippon* **48**, 2.

Jarnagin, W.R., Rockey, D.C. and Bissell, D.M. (1993). Fibronectin splicing in rat hepatic fibrogenesis: A possible role in lipocyte activation. *Gastroenterology* **104**, 923A.

Jezequel, A.M., Ballardini, G., Mancini, R., Paolucci, F., Binchi, R.B. and Orlandi, F. (1990). Modulation of extracellular matrix components during dimethylnitrosamine-induced cirrhosis. *Journal of Hepatology* **11**, 206–214.

Johnson, S.J., Hines, J.E. and Burt, A.D. (1992). Macrophage and perisinusoidal cell kinetics in acute liver injury. *Journal of Pathology* **166**, 351–358.

Kamimura, S., Gaal, K., Britton, R.S., Bacon, B.R., Triadafilopoulos, G. and Tsukamoto, H. (1992). Increased 4-hydroxynonenal levels in experimental alcoholic liver disease: Association of lipid peroxidation with liver fibrogenesis. *Hepatology* **16**, 448–453.

Kawada, N., Klein, H. and Decker, K. (1992). Eicosanoid-mediated contractility of hepatic stellate cells. *Biochemical Journal* **285**, 367–371.

Kawase, T., Kato, S. and Lieber, C.S. (1989). Lipid peroxidation and antioxidant defense systems in rat liver after chronic ethanol feeding. *Hepatology* **10**, 815–821.

Klatsky, A.L. and Armstrong, M.A. (1992). Alcohol, smoking, coffee, and cirrhosis. *Journal of Epidemiology* **136**, 1248–1257.

Knittel, T., Armbrust, T., Schwogler, S., Schuppan, D. and Ramadori, G. (1992). Distribution and cellular origin of undulin in rat liver. *Laboratory Investigation* **67**, 779–787.

Korsten, M.A., Matsuzaki, S., Feinman, L. and Lieber, C.S. (1975). High blood acetaldehyde levels after ethanol administration: Difference between alcoholic and nonalcoholic subjects. *New England Journal of Medicine* **292**, 386–389.

Kupffer, C. (1876). Ueber sternzellen der leber: Briefliche mittheilung an Professor Waldeyer. *Arch Mikr Anat* **12**, 353–358.

Lelbach, W.K. (1976). Epidemiology of alcoholic liver disease. In *Progress in Liver Disease* (Edited by Popper, H. and Schaffner, F.), Vol. V, pp. 494–513. Grune and Stratton, New York.

Lieber, C.S., DeCarli, L. and Rubin, E. (1975). Sequential production of fatty liver, hepatitis and cirrhosis in sub-human primates fed ethanol and adequate diets. *Proceedings of the National Academy of Sciences, USA* **72**, 437–441.

Maher, J.J., Friedman, S.L., Roll, F.J. and Bissell, D.M. (1988). Immunolocalization of leminin in normal rat liver and biosynthesis of leminin by hepatic lipocytes in primary culture. *Gastroenterology* **94**, 1053–1062.

Maher, J.J., Zia, S. and Tzagarakis, C. (1994a). Acetaldehyde-induced stimulation of collagen synthesis and gene expression is dependent on conditions of cell culture: studies with rat lipocytes and fibroblasts. *Alcohol: Clinical and Experimental Research*, **18**, 403–409.

Maher, J.J., Tzagarakis, C. and Gimenez, A. (1994b). Malondialdehyde stimulates collagen production by hepatic lipocytes only upon activation in primary culture. *Alcohol and Alcoholism*, **29**, 605–610.

Mak, K.M. and Lieber, C.S. (1988). Lipocytes and transitional cells in alcoholic liver disease: A morphometric study. *Hepatology* **8**, 1027–1033.

Mak, K.M., Leo, M.A. and Lieber, C.S. (1984). Alcoholic liver injury in baboons: Transformation of lipocytes to transitional cells. *Gastroenterology* **87**, 188–200.

Marbet, U.A., Bianchi, L., Meury, U. and Stalder, G.A. (1987). Long-term histological evaluation of the natural history and prognostic factors of alcoholic liver disease. *Journal of Hepatology* **4**, 364–372.

Marra, F., Valente, A.J., Pinzani, M. and Abboud, H.E. (1993). Cultured human liver fat-storing cells produce monocyte chemotactic protein-1: Regulation by proinflammatory cytokines. *Journal of Clinical Investigation* **92**, 1674–1680.

Matsuoka, M. and Tsukamoto, H. (1990). Stimulation of hepatic lipocyte collagen production by Kupffer cell-derived transforming growth factor β: Implication for a pathogenetic role in alcoholic liver fibrogenesis. *Hepatology* **11**, 599–605.

Matsuoka, M., Pham, N.-T. and Tsukamoto, H. (1989). Differential effects of interleukin-1 alpha, tumor necrosis factor alpha, and transforming growth factor beta 1 on cell proliferation and collagen formation by cultured fat-storing cells. *Liver* **9**, 71–78.

McCullough, A.J., Stassen, W.N., Wiesner, R.H. and Czaja, A.J. (1987). Serum type III procollagen peptide concentrations in severe chronic active hepatitis: Relationship to cirrhosis and disease activity. *Hepatology* **7**, 49–54.

Melendez, M., Vargas-Tank, L., Fuentes, C., Armas-Merino, R., Castillo, D., Wolffe, C., Wegman, M.E. and Soto, J. (1979). Distribution of HLA histocompatibility antigens, ABO blood groups and Rh antigens in alcoholic liver disease. *Gut* **20**, 288–290.

Mendenhall, C.L., Anderson, S., Weesner, R.E., Goldberg, S.J. and Crolic, K.A. (1984). Protein-calorie malnutrition associated with alcoholic hepatitis. *American Journal of Medicine* **76**, 211–222.

Meyer, D.H., Bachem, M.G. and Gressner, A.M. (1990). Modulation of hepatic lipocyte proteoglycan synthesis and proliferation by Kupffer cell-derived transforming growth factors type $\beta 1$ and α. *Biochemical and Biophysical Research Communications* **171**, 1122–1129.

Meyer, D.H., Krull, N., Dreher, K.L. and Gressner, A.M. (1992). Biglycan and decorin gene expression in normal and fibrotic rat liver: Cellular localization and regulatory factors. *Hepatology* **16**, 204–216.

Milani, S., Herbst, H., Schuppan, D., Riecken, E.O. and Stein, H. (1989). Cellular localization of laminin gene transcripts in normal and fibrotic human liver. *American Journal of Pathology* **134**, 1175–1182.

Milani, S., Herbst, H., Schuppan, D., Stein, H. and Surrenti, C. (1991). Transforming growth factors beta-1 and beta-2 are differentially expressed in fibrotic liver disease. *American Journal of Pathology* **139**, 1221–1229.

Mills, P.R., MacSween, R.N.M., Dick, H.M. and Hislop, W.S. (1988). Histocompatibility antigens in patients with alcoholic liver disease in Scotland and northeastern England: Failure to show an association. *Gut* **29**, 146–148.

Minato, Y., Hasumura, Y. and Takeuchi, J. (1983). The role of fat-storing cells in Disse space fibrogenesis in alcoholic liver disease. *Hepatology* **3**, 559–566.

Monteiro, E., Alves, P., Santos, M.L., Quintas, I., Baptista, A., Galvao-Teles, A. and Gavaler, J.S. (1988). Histocompatibility antigens: Markers of susceptibility to and protection from alcoholic liver disease in a Portuguese population. *Hepatology* **8**, 455–458.

Moshage, H., Casini, A. and Lieber, C.S. (1990). Acetaldehyde selectively stimulates collagen production in cultured rat liver fat-storing cells but not in hepatocytes. *Hepatology* **12**, 511–518.

Murata, K., Kudo, M., Onuma, F. and Motoyama, T. (1984). Changes of collagen types at various stages of human liver cirrhosis. *Hepato-gastroenterology* **31**, 158–161.

Nakano, M. and Lieber, C.S. (1982). Ultrastructure of initial stages of perivenular fibrosis in alcohol-fed baboons. *American Journal of Pathology* **106**, 145–155.

Nakano, M., Worner, T.M. and Lieber, C.S. (1982). Perivenular fibrosis in alcoholic liver injury: Ultrastructure and histologic progression. *Gastroenterology* **83**, 777–785.

Nakatsukasa, H., Nagy, P., Evarts, R.P., Hsia, C.-C., Marsden, E. and Thorgeirsson, S.S. (1990). Cellular distribution of transforming growth factor-beta 1 and procollagen types I, III and IV transcripts in carbon tetrachloride-induced rat liver fibrosis. *Journal of Clinical Investigation* **85**, 1833–1843.

Nalpas, B., Driss, F., Pol, S., Hamelin, B., Housset, C., Brechot, C. and Berthelot, P. (1991). Association between HCV and HBV infection in hepatocellular carcinoma and alcoholic liver disease. *Journal of Hepatology* **12**, 70–74.

Nanji, A.A. and French, S.W. (1986). Dietary factors and alcoholic cirrhosis. *Alcohol: Clinical and Experimental Research* **10**, 271–273.

Niemela, O., Risteli, L., Sotaneimi, E.A. and Risteli, J. (1983). Aminoterminal propeptide of type III procollagen in serum in alcoholic liver disease. *Gastroenterology* **85**, 254–259.

Niemela, O., Risteli, L., Sotaniemi, E.Z. and Risteli, J. (1985). Type IV collagen and laminin-related antigens in human serum in alcoholic liver disease. *European Journal of Clinical Investigation* **15**, 132–137.

Nouchi, T., Worner, T.M., Sato, S. and Lieber, C.S. (1987). Serum procollagen type III *N*-terminal peptides and laminin P1 peptide in alcoholic liver disease. *Alcoholism (NY)* **11**, 287–291.

Okanoue, T., Burbige, E.J. and French, S.W. (1983). The role of the Ito cell in perivenular and intralobular fibrosis in alcoholic hepatitis. *Archives of Pathology and Laboratory Medicine* **107**, 459–463.

Parola, M., Pinzani, M., Casini, A., Albano, E., Poli, G., Gentiline, A., Gentiline, P. and Dianzani, M.U. (1993). Stimulation of lipid peroxidation or 4-hydroxynonenal treatment increases procollagen alpha 1 (I) gene expression in human liver fat-storing cells.

Biochemical and Biophysical Research Communications **194**, 1044–1050.

Parrish, K.M., Higuchi, S., Muramatsu, T., Stinson, F.S. and Harford, T.C. (1991). A method for estimating alcohol-related liver cirrhosis mortality in Japan. *International Journal of Epidemiology* **20**, 921–926.

Pick-Kober, K.H., Negwer, A. and Gressner, A.M. (1985). Determination of laminin in serum by a competetive radioimmunoassay directed against the pepsin-resistant fragment P1. *Clinical Chemistry and Clinical Biochemistry* **23**, 572–573.

Pinzani, M., Gesualdo, L., Sabbah, G.M. and Abboud, H.E. (1989). Effects of platelet-derived growth factor and other polypeptide mitogens on DNA synthesis and growth of cultured rat liver fat-storing cells. *Journal of Clinical Investigation* **84**, 1786–1793.

Pinzani, M., Abboud, H.E. and Aron, D.C. (1990). Secretion of insulin-like growth factor-I and binding proteins by rat liver fat-storing cells: Regulatory role of platelet-derived growth factor. *Endocrinology* **127**, 2343–2349.

Pinzani, M., Failli, P., Ruocco, C., Casini, A., Milani, S., Baldi, E., Giotti, A. and Gentilini, P. (1992a). Fat-storing cells as liver-specific pericytes: Spatial dynamics of agonist-stimulated intracellular calcium transients. *Journal of Clinical Investigation* **90**, 642–646.

Pinzani, M., Abboud, H.E., Gesualdo, L. and Abboud, S.L. (1992b). Regulation of macrophage colony-stimulating factor in liver fat-storing cells by peptide growth factors. *American Journal of Physiology* **262**, C876–881.

Raedsch, R., Stiehl, A., Waldherr, R., Mall, G., Gmelin, K., Goetz, R., Walker, S., Czgan, P. and Kommerell, B. (1982). Procollagen-type III peptide serum concentrations in chronic persistent and chronic active hepatitis and in cirrhosis of the liver and their diagnostic value. *Zeitschrift fur Gastroenterologie* **20**, 738–743.

Raedsch, R., Stiehl, A., Sieg, A., Walker, S. and Kommerell, B. (1983). Biliary excretion of procollagen type III peptide in healthy humans and in patients with alcoholic cirrhosis of the liver. *Gastroenterology* **85**, 1265–1270.

Ramadori, G. (1992). Pathogenesis of liver fibrosis: Synthesis of collagen and non-collagen proteins in cell culture and *in vivo*. *Zeitschrift fur Gastroenterologie* **1**, 17–20 (Suppl.).

Ramadori, G., Veit, T., Schwogler, S., Dienes, H.P., Knittel, T., Rieder, H. and Meyer zum Buschenfelde, K.H. (1990). Expression of the gene of the alpha smooth muscle-actin isoform in rat liver and in rat fat-storing (Ito) cells. *Virchows Archives B* **59**, 349–357.

Ramadori, G., Schwogler, S., Veit, T., Rieder, H., Chiquet-Ehrismann, R., Mackie, E.J. and Meyer zum Buschenfelde, K.H. (1991). Tenascin gene expression in rat liver and in rat liver cells: *In vivo* and *in vitro* studies. *Virchows Archives B* **60**, 145–153.

Ramadori, G., Knottel, T., Odenthal, M., Schwogler, S., Neubauer, K. and Meyer zum Buschenfelde, K.H.

(1992). Synthesis of cellular fibronectin by rat liver fat-storing (Ito) cells: Regulation by cytokines. *Gastroenterology* **103**, 1313–1321.

Risteli, L. and Risteli, J. (1987). Analysis of extracellular matrix proteins in biological fluids. *Methods in Enzymology* **145**, 391–411.

Risteli, J., Rohde, H. and Timpl, R. (1981). Sensitive radioimmunoassays for 7S collagen and laminin: Application to serum and tissue studies of basement membranes. *Analytical Biochemistry* **113**, 372–378.

Rockey, D.C., Boyles, J.K., Gabbiani, G. and Friedman, S.L. (1992). Rat hepatic lipocytes express smooth muscle actin upon activation *in vivo* and in culture. *Journal of Submicroscopic Cytology and Pathology* **24**, 193–203.

Rockey, D.C., Housset, C.N. and Friedman, S.L. (1993). Activation-dependent contractility of rat hepatic lipocytes in culture and *in vivo*. *Journal of Clinical Investigation* **92**, 1795–1804.

Rohde, H., Vargas, L., Hahn, E., Kalbfeisch, E., Bruegera, M. and Timpl, R. (1979). Radioimmunoassay for type III procollagen peptide and its application to human liver disease. *European Journal of Clinical Investigation* **9**, 451–459.

Rohde, H., Langer, I., Krieg, T. and Timpl, R. (1983). Serum and urine analysis of the aminoterminal procollagen peptide type III by radioimmunoassay with antibody Fab fragments. *Collagen and Related Research* **3**, 371–379.

Rojkind, M. and Martinez-Palomo, A. (1976). Increase in type I and type III collagens in human alcoholic liver cirrhosis. *Proceedings of the National Academy of Sciences, USA* **73**, 539–543.

Rojkind, M., Giambrone, M.-A. and Biempica, L. (1979). Collagen types in normal and cirrhotic liver. *Gastroenterology* **76**, 710–719.

Roll, F.J., Perez, H.D. and Serhan, C.N. (1992). Characterization of a novel arachidonic acid-derived neutrophil chemoattractant. *Biochemical and Biophysical Research Communications* **186**, 269–276.

Sakakibara, K., Ooshima, A., Igarashi, S. and Sakakibara, J. (1986). Immunolocalization of type III collagen and procollagen in cirrhotic human liver using monoclonal antibodies. *Virchows Archives A* **409**, 37–46.

Sato, M. and Lieber, C.S. (1981). Hepatic vitamin A depletion after chronic ethanol consumption in baboons and rats. *Journal of Nutrition* **111**, 2015–2023.

Sato, S., Nouchi, T., Worner, T.M. and Lieber, C.S. (1986). Fab radioimmunoassay of serum procollagen-III-peptides detects liver fibrosis in alcoholics. *Journal of the American Medical Association* **256**, 1471–1473.

Saunders, J.B., Haines, A., Portmann, B., Wodak, A.D., Powell-Jackson, P.R., Portman, B., Davis, M. and Williams, R. (1982). Accelerated development of alcoholic cirrhosis in patients with HLA-B8. *Lancet* **1**, 1381–1484.

Savolainen, E.-R., Goldberg, B., Leo, M.A., Velez, M. and Lieber, C.S. (1984a). Diagnostic value of serum procollagen peptide measurements in alcoholic liver disease. *Alcoholism (NY)* **8**, 384–389.

Savolainen, E.-R., Leo, M.A., Timpl, R. and Lieber, C.S. (1984b). Acetaldehyde and lactate stimulate collagen synthesis of cultured baboon liver myofibroblasts. *Gastroenterology* **87**, 777–787.

Savolainen, V.T., Penttila, A. and Karhunen, P.J. (1992). Delayed increases in liver cirrhosis mortality and frequency of alcoholic liver cirrhosis following an increment and redistribution of alcohol consumption in Finland: Evidence from mortality statistics and autopsy survey covering 8533 cases in 1968–1988. *Alcohol: Clinical and Experimental Research* **16**, 661–664.

Schafer, S., Zerbe, O. and Gressner, A.M. (1987). The synthesis of proteoglycans in fat storing cells of rat liver. *Hepatology* **7**, 680–687.

Schuppan, D., Besser, M., Schwarting, R. and Hahn, E.G. (1986a). Radioimmunoassay for the carboxy-terminal cross-linking domain of type IV (basement membrane) procollagen in body fluids: Characterization and application to collagen type IV metabolism in fibrotic liver disease. *Journal of Clinical Investigation* **78**, 241–248.

Schuppan, D., Dumont, J.M., Kin, K.Y. *et al.* (1986b). Serum concentration of the aminoterminal procollagen type III peptide in the rat reflects early formation of connective tissue in experimental liver cirrhosis. *Journal of Hepatology* **3**, 27–37.

Scott, B.B., Rajah, S.M. and Losowsky, M.S. (1977). Histocompatibility antigens in chronic liver disease. *Gastroenterology* **72**, 122–125.

Sheron, N., Bird, G., Koskinas, J., Portmann, B., Ceska, M., Lindley, I. and Williams, R. (1993). Circulating and tissue levels of the neutrophil chemotaxin interleukin-8 are elevated in severe acute alcoholic hepatitis, and tissue levels correlate with neutrophil infiltration. *Hepatology* **18**, 41–46.

Shiratori, Y., Geerts, A., Ichida, T., Kawase, T. and Wisse, E. (1986a). Kupffer cells from CCl4-induced fibrotic livers stimulate proliferation of fat-storing cells. *Journal of Hepatology* **3**, 294–303.

Shiratori, Y., Ichida, T., Kawase, T. and Wisse, E. (1986b). Effect of acetaldehyde on collagen synthesis by fat-storing cells isolated from rats treated with carbon tetrachloride. *Liver* **6**, 246–251.

Shiratori, Y., Takada, H., Hikiba, Y., Okano, K., Niwa, Y., Matsumura, M., Komatsu, Y. and Omata, M. (1993a). Increased release of KC/gro protein, intercrine cytokine family, from the hepatocytes of chronically ethanol fed rats. *Biochemical and Biophysical Research Communications* **197**, 319–325.

Shiratori, Y., Takada, H., Hikiba, Y., Nakata, R., Okano, K., Komatsu, Y., Niwa, Y., Matsumura, M., Shiina, S., Omata, M. and Kamii, K. (1993b). Production of chemotactic factor, interleukin-8, from hepatocytes exposed to ethanol. *Hepatology* **18**, 1477–1482.

Smedsrod, B. (1988). Aminoterminal propeptide of type III procollagen is cleared from the circulation by receptor-mediated endocytosis in liver endothelial cells. *Collagen and Related Research* **8**, 375–388.

Takase, S., Leo, M.A., Nouchi, T. and Lieber, C.S. (1988). Desmin distinguishes cultured fat-storing cells from myofibroblasts, smooth muscle cells and fibroblasts in the rat. *Journal of Hepatology* **6**, 267–276.

Thornton, A.J., Ham, J. and Kunkel, S.L. (1992). Kupffer cell-derived cytokines induce the synthesis of a leukocyte chemotactic peptide, interleukin-8, in human hepatoma and primary hepatocyte cultures. *Hepatology* **15**, 1112–1122.

Torres-Salinas, M., Pares, A., Caballeria, J., Jimenez, W., Heredia, D., Brugera, M. and Rodes, J. (1986). Serum procollagen type III peptide as a marker of hepatic fibrogenesis in alcoholic hepatitis. *Gastroenterology* **90**, 1241–1246.

Tsukamoto, H., Towner, S.J., Ciofalo, L.M. and French, S.W. (1986). Ethanol-induced liver fibrosis in rats fed high fat diet. *Hepatology* **6**, 814–822.

Tsutsumi, M., Urashima, S., Matsuda, Y., Takase, S. and Takada, A. (1993). Changes in type IV collagen content in livers of patients with alcoholic liver disease. *Hepatology* **17**, 820–827.

Van Waes, L. and Lieber, C.S. (1977). Early perivenular sclerosis in alcoholic fatty liver: An index of progressive liver injury. *Gastroenterology* **73**, 646–650.

Wake, K. (1971). "Sternzellen" in the liver: Perisinusoidal cells with special reference to storage of vitamin A. *American Journal of Anatomy* **132**, 429–462.

Weiner, F.R., Eskreis, D.S., Compton, K.V., Orrego, H. and Zern, M.A. (1988). Haplotype analysis of a type I collagen gene and its association with alcoholic cirrhosis in man. *Molecular Aspects of Medicine* **10**, 159–168.

Weiner, F.R., Giambrone, M.A., Czaja, M.J., Shah, A., Annoni, G., Takahashi, S., Eghbali, M. and Zern, M.A. (1990). Ito-cell gene expression and collagen regulation. *Hepatology* **11**, 111–117.

Worner, T.M. and Lieber, C.S. (1985). Perivenular fibrosis as precursor lesion of cirrhosis. *Journal of the American Medical Association* **254**, 627–630.

Zerbe, O. and Gressner, A.M. (1988). Proliferation of fat storing cells is stimulated by secretions of Kupffer cells from normal and injured liver. *Experimental Molecular Pathology* **49**, 87–101.

5 The role of acetaldehyde adducts in liver injury

Dean J. Tuma and Michael F. Sorrell

Introduction

Most of the alcohol absorbed by the body is eliminated via oxidative metabolism. The organ responsible for the majority of alcohol (ethanol) metabolism is the liver. Since the liver is also a major target organ of alcohol-induced toxicity, many of the derangements of hepatic structure and function have been attributed to the products of alcohol oxidation. In this regard, a considerable body of evidence has been obtained that implicates an active role of acetaldehyde, the first metabolite of ethanol oxidation, in mediating the hepatotoxicity of alcohol (Lieber 1988; Jennett *et al.* 1990). For every mole of alcohol that is oxidized, 1 mole of acetaldehyde is generated in the liver. Thus, when large quantities of alcohol are consumed, an equally large amount of acetaldehyde is produced. Although the liver has a very efficient mechanism to detoxify acetaldehyde (via oxidation to acetate), significant amounts of this reactive aldehyde accumulate in the liver during ethanol metabolism and these amounts are even further elevated in alcoholics (Nuutinen *et al.* 1984). Since acetaldehyde is a chemically reactive molecule, the covalent binding of this aldehyde to hepatic proteins has been proposed as a key event leading to alcoholic liver injury (Sorrell and Tuma 1985; Tuma and Sorrell 1985). This chapter focuses on recent developments in the chemistry of acetaldehyde–protein adduct formation, targets of adduct formation in the liver, functional consequences of acetaldehyde-modified proteins and potential relationships of adducts to liver injury.

Chemistry of acetaldehyde–protein interactions

Because of the electrophilic nature of the carbonyl carbon, acetaldehyde is a reactive compound and is able to react with a variety of nucleophilic groups (O'Donnell 1982). It appears that the ε-amino group of internal lysine residues and the α-amino group of N-terminal amino acids of proteins are the major nucleophilic groups that participate in acetaldehyde binding, resulting in the formation of two types of reaction products which have been classified as unstable and stable adducts (Donohue *et al.* 1983a; Tuma *et al.* 1987, 1991b).

Unstable adducts are characterized by their ability to readily dissociate when exposed to conditions such as dialysis, gel filtration, treatment with weak acids or bases or by simple dilution (Donohue *et al.* 1983a; Tuma and Sorrell 1985). Although unstable binding to thiol, hydroxyl and imidazole groups is possible, it appears that Schiff bases, resulting from the reaction of the carbonyl carbon with amino groups, are the most important unstable protein adducts that are formed (Donohue *et al.* 1983a; Tuma *et al.* 1987). These unstable Schiff base adducts can be stabilized and, therefore, made de-

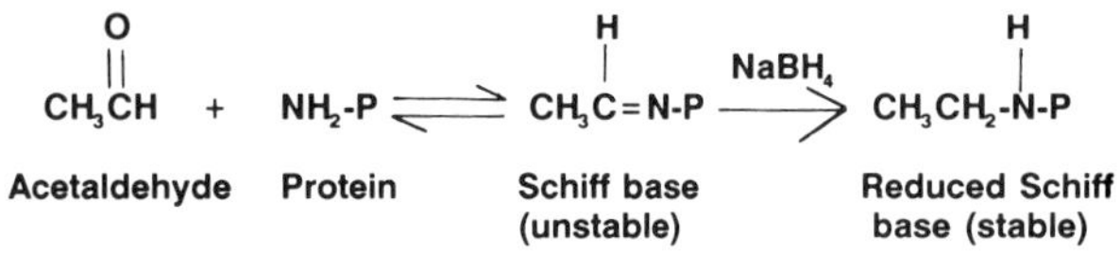

$$CH_3CH + NH_2\text{-P} \rightleftharpoons CH_3C{=}N\text{-P} \xrightarrow{NaBH_4} CH_3CH_2\text{-N-P}$$

Acetaldehyde   Protein   Schiff base   Reduced Schiff
                           (unstable)   base (stable)

Fig. 5.1 The stabilization of Schiff base acetaldehyde–protein adducts by sodium borohydride reduction.

tectable by converting them to secondary amines (specifically *N*-ethyl derivatives) by treatment with a strong reducing agent (e.g. sodium borohydride) (Fig. 5.1). The direct role of unstable adducts in toxicity is probably limited; however, unstable adducts probably serve as precursors or intermediates in the formation of stable adducts (Tuma *et al.* 1991b).

Stable adducts are essentially irreversible products characterized by their resistance to various treatments, including exhaustive dialysis, gel filtration and mild acid or base hydrolysis (Donohue *et al.* 1983a; Tuma and Sorrell 1985; Tuma *et al.* 1987). These adducts form when acetaldehyde reacts with proteins under physiological conditions (pH 7.4 and 37°C) and are not dependent upon the presence of a reducing agent for their formation (Donohue *et al.* 1983a; Tuma and Sorrell 1985; Tuma *et al.* 1987). Because of their stability and irreversibility, stable adducts are the most likely candidates to produce toxic effects, and the understanding of the chemistry of their formation is an essential part of evaluating their role in hepatotoxicity.

Studies to date have indicated that unstable Schiff base adducts probably serve as intermediates in the formation of stable adducts (Tuma *et al.* 1991b; Hoffmann *et al.* 1993), suggesting that the stabilization of Schiff bases represents the key event in stable adduct formation. One such stabilization process involves a cyclization reaction which takes place when a Schiff base is generated on the α-amino group of a *N*-terminal amino acid of a protein. This cyclic adduct has been identified to be 2-methyl-imidazolidin-4-one (San George and Hoberman 1986) (Fig. 5.2). Although this cyclic product may be an important stable adduct that could potentially be produced in the liver, proteins such as actin (Xu *et al.* 1989) and calmodulin (Jennett *et al.* 1989a) which have blocked *N*-terminal amino acids can still stably bind considerable amounts of acetaldehyde. Moreover, other studies have indicated that the ε-amino group of internal lysine residues can also participate in stable binding (Tuma *et al.* 1987, 1991b; Gross *et al.* 1994; Lin *et al.* 1993b). There-

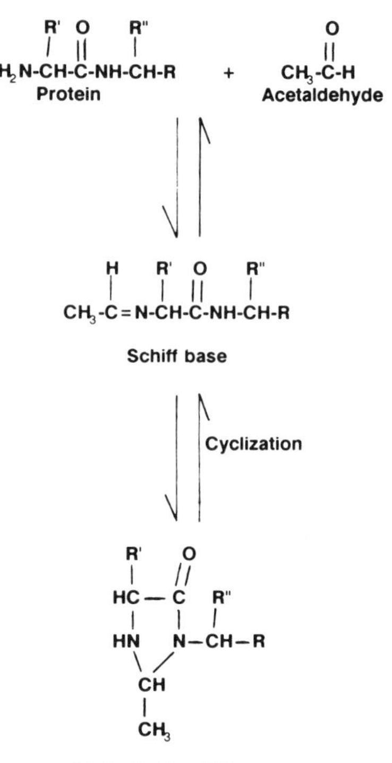

Fig. 5.2 The formation of a stable acetaldehyde–protein adduct on the α-amino group of a *N*-terminal amino acid of a protein. R' and R'' represent the side chains of the first and second amino acid residues of the protein, respectively. R represents the remainder of the polypeptide chain.

fore, the stabilization of Schiff bases of internal lysines probably plays an important role in the overall formation of most stable acetaldehyde–protein adducts.

Two possibly important stabilization reactions of lysine Schiff bases could involve additions across the double bond, either by reduction or by nucleophilic addition of a thiol group (Fig. 5.3). It was proposed initially that reduction and subsequent formation of *N*-ethyllysine residues could be the major mechanism of stabilization (Sorrell and Tuma 1985; Tuma and Sorrell 1985), since Schiff bases were readily stabilized by reducing agents such as cyanoborohydride (Donohue *et al.* 1983a; Tuma *et al.* 1987) and since ascorbic acid, a physiological reducing agent, increased the formation of stable adducts (Tuma *et al.* 1984, 1987). This mechanism was especially attractive since excessive reducing equivalents are generated during ethanol oxidation in the liver and would be readily available to reduce Schiff bases (Sorrell and Tuma 1985; Tuma and Sorrell 1985).

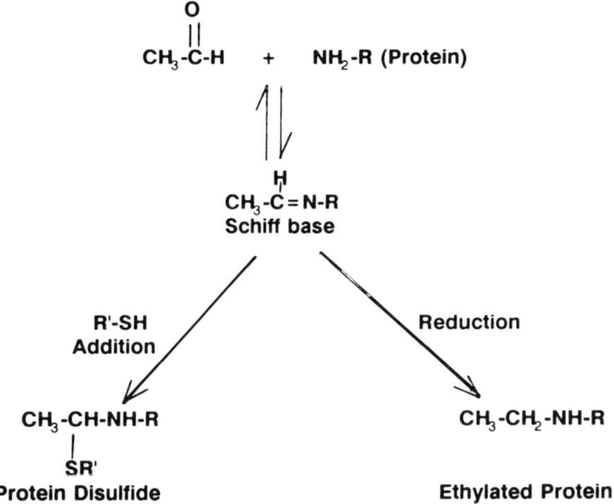

Fig. 5.3 Stable acetaldehyde–protein adduct formation via stabilization of Schiff bases by reduction or thiol addition. R represents the polypeptide chain and R'-SH represents any biological thiol compound.

$$CH_3\text{-}CH = CH\text{-}CH = N\text{------}(Protein)$$

Fig. 5.4 Crotonaldehyde Schiff base adduct with proteins.

However, analysis of reaction products by HPLC revealed that stable adducts formed in the absence of strong reducing agents, such as cyanoborohydride, were distinctly different than the ethylated amino groups generated under reductive conditions (Tuma *et al.* 1987). These findings were also confirmed by immunochemical methods, using a monoclonal antibody that specifically recognizes *N*-ethyllysine epitopes. Stable adducts formed under non-reducing conditions were not recognized by this antibody (Klassen *et al.* 1994). It was also reported that the mechanism of increased stable adduct formation by ascorbate did not involve the classical reduction of Schiff bases, indicating that alternate mechanisms must be operative in the ascorbate-induced increase in stable binding (Tuma *et al.* 1987). The addition of thiol groups across the double bond was also suggested as a possible stabilization mechanism (Sorrell and Tuma 1985; Tuma and Sorrell 1985), since the amino acid, cysteine, which contains an amino group and a thiol group, readily forms stable adducts (thiazolidine derivatives) when reacted with aldehydes, including acetaldehyde (Cederbaum and Rubin 1976). However, polylysine and proteins, lacking free thiol groups, are still able to form considerable amounts of stable adducts with acetaldehyde (Tuma *et al.* 1987, 1991b; Jennett *et al.* 1990). Thus, it appears that stabilization of Schiff bases by either reduction or thiol addition does not represent primary mechan-

isms of stable adduct formation under physiological conditions.

Recent studies from our laboratory have shown that the reaction of acetaldehyde with polylysine or proteins results in the formation of both fluorescent and non-fluorescent stable adducts (Hoffmann *et al.* 1993). In addition, the presence of sodium cyanoborohydride, which reduces Schiff bases, in the reaction mixtures prevented the generation of fluorescent products, indicating that Schiff bases serve as intermediates in fluorescent adduct formation. Because of their fluorescent properties, these stable adducts are likely to be highly conjugated products. Similar types of products have also been identified by Kikugawa and co-workers (1985, 1988, 1989), who demonstrated that monofunctional aldehydes can react with simple amines or polypeptides and form various advanced fluorescent and non-fluorescent adducts. These authors proposed that such products are generated via repeated aldol and Michael condensation reactions. Taken together, these findings suggest that the initial reaction of a Schiff base involves an amine-catalysed aldol condensation reaction with another molecule of acetaldehyde, resulting in the formation of a crotonaldehyde Schiff base derivative (Fig. 5.4). Because of the presence of the conjugated double bond system, this product, whose formation could conceivably be the rate-limiting reaction in stable adduct formation, would be relatively reactive and would be available to undergo further reactions. One or more molecules of acetaldehyde, as well as other aldehydes or other reactive compounds present in cellular systems, reacting with this crotonaldehyde Schiff base, would be expected to produce a wide variety of advanced, conjugated products with proteins. In addition, such a reaction scheme would also explain the cross-linking of membrane proteins that has been reported to occur in the presence of acetaldehyde (Gaines *et al.* 1977).

In conclusion, the chemistry of stable acetaldehyde–protein adducts has proven to be more complicated than originally anticipated with the possibility of multiple products forming under various conditions. Further studies, with their emphasis on structural determinations of adducts, are needed to resolve the chemistry of stable adduct formation.

Protein targets of acetaldehyde binding

Different proteins vary in their ability to form stable adducts with acetaldehyde (Tuma *et al.* 1984; Mauch *et al.* 1986). Since lysine residues are major targets of acetaldehyde binding, proteins containing many lysines might be expected to be most reactive with acetaldehyde. However, not all lysine residues in proteins are equally reactive with acetaldehyde. This phenomenon was clearly evident in work from our laboratory, investigating the acetaldehyde binding properties of the important cytoskeletal protein, tubulin. In summary of these studies (Jennett *et al.* 1987, 1989b; Smith *et al.* 1989), tubulin, isolated from either bovine brain or rat liver, exhibited rather unique acetaldehyde binding properties as compared to other proteins. When acetaldehyde–tubulin reaction mixtures were submitted to SDS-polyacrylamide gel electrophoresis to separate the α- and β-chains of the heterodimeric protein, the α-chain was found to be the preferential site of stable adduct formation. The α-chain formed 2–3 times more stable adducts than the β-chain, despite the fact that the two subunits contain essentially equal numbers of lysine residues. This selective binding was most pronounced at low acetaldehyde concentrations (25–100 μM). Furthermore, tubulin had to be in its depolymerized form (free dimer as opposed to its polymerized form, microtubules) and in its native state (undenatured) in order to preferentially form stable adducts on its α-subunit. Competition binding studies revealed that α-tubulin could effectively compete with β-tubulin and albumin for stable binding, especially at low concentrations of acetaldehyde. On the other hand, unstable adducts with tubulin did not preferentially form with the α-chain.

Additional studies showed that the free tubulin dimer was much more reactive with acetaldehyde than polymerized tubulin; depending upon reaction conditions (time and acetaldehyde concentrations), the dimer bound 20–100 percent more acetaldehyde than microtubules (Smith *et al.* 1989, 1992). The free tubulin dimer also bound 2–3 times more acetaldehyde on its α-chain as on its β-chain, whereas microtubules exhibited an equal distribution of stable adducts between the two subunits (Smith *et al.* 1989, 1992). These results were consistent with the previous findings of Sternlicht and co-workers (Sherman *et al.* 1983; Szasz *et al.* 1986), who reported that the α-chain of tubulin contains a highly reactive lysine residue that is accessible when tubulin is in the depolymerized state but not in microtubules. These same workers identified lysine-394 as an unusually nucleophilic region of the α-tubulin polypeptide, and this residue was proposed to be critical to overall tubulin structure and function (Szasz *et al.* 1986). Therefore, lysine residues of tubulin can be divided into two general classes with regard to their reactivity towards acetaldehyde – those of normal reactivity (bulk lysines) and the highly reactive lysine located in the α-subunit (Jennett *et al.* 1990; Tuma *et al.* 1991c). This increased reactivity of specific lysine residues with carbonyl groups most probably resides in the particular microenvironment of these lysines in the three-dimensional structure of the protein (Acharya *et al.* 1983; Neglia *et al.* 1985; Watkins *et al.* 1985; Szasz *et al.* 1986). The enhanced nucleophilicity of certain lysines in proteins is thought to involve a lowered pKa induced by the local environment. A lower pKa would make a larger fraction of the unprotonated form of the reactive lysine available as a nucleophile at physiological pH (Neglia *et al.* 1985; Szasz *et al.* 1986). An additional explanation of enhanced reactivity could also involve the participation of neighbouring amino acids in the catalysis of stable adduct formation with lysine residues (Acharya *et al.* 1983; Watkins *et al.* 1985). This latter explanation could account for the increased stable binding of acetaldehyde to specific lysines on α-tubulin, since unstable adducts did not exhibit α-chain selective binding (Tuma *et al.* 1991c). Regardless, by virtue of containing highly reactive lysine residues, α-tubulin may be a selective target of stable acetaldehyde binding in cell systems, especially the liver, during ethanol oxidation. As will be discussed later in more detail, this conclusion is consistent with the known damaging effects of ethanol on the microtubule system in the liver and the ethanol-induced impairments of hepatic protein trafficking pathways (Jennett *et al.* 1990; Tuma *et al.* 1991c).

Alpha tubulin is not the only protein with highly reactive lysine residues. Actin in its G-form (Xu *et al.* 1989), RNase (Mauch *et al.* 1987) and cilia dynein (Sisson *et al.* 1991) have all been shown to exhibit enhanced reactivity to acetaldehyde. In addition, the key calcium-binding regulatory protein, calmodulin, dramatically increases in reactivity towards acetaldehyde in the presence of calcium (Jennett *et al.* 1989a). Calmodulin contains certain lysine residues whose reactivities towards electrophiles are very sensitive to calcium-induced conformational changes (Giedroc *et al.* 1987). Competition-binding studies demonstrated that calmodulin can successfully compete with other proteins for a limited amount of acetaldehyde, and this effect was a sensitive function of the calcium concentration (Jennett *et al.* 1989a). Therefore, analogous to the situation with α-tubulin, reactive lysines in calmodulin are also dependent upon the conformation of the protein. Thus, it appears that some proteins, such as tubulin and calmodulin, are likely to be more reactive than other proteins in forming stable acetaldehyde adducts in cellular systems because of specific structural features that depend upon the primary amino acid sequence and conformational factors. Overall, these considerations raise the possibility that proteins with "reactive" lysines are selective targets for stable acetaldehyde adduct formation in the hepatocyte during ethanol oxidation.

Binding of metabolically derived acetaldehyde to hepatic proteins

Although *in vitro* acetaldehyde binding experiments with purified proteins and identification of potential protein targets of acetaldehyde adduct formation are very important and useful in gaining basic information about the chemistry of acetaldehyde–protein interactions, verification that metabolically derived acetaldehyde reacts with liver proteins during alcohol oxidation to form stable adducts is a key element in evaluating the role of acetaldehyde adducts in alcoholic liver injury. In this regard, a considerable body of evidence exists that indicates that acetaldehyde–protein adducts form in the liver during the metabolism of alcohol.

In vitro studies showed that alcohol oxidation in cell-free liver homogenates (Donohue *et al.* 1983b) and in liver slices (Medina *et al.* 1985) resulted in the generation of acetaldehyde which, subsequently, reacted with hepatic proteins to form both unstable and stable acetaldehyde–protein adducts. In addition, it appeared that unstable adducts were formed initially, and then were stabilized during more prolonged incubation to form stable products. The use of classic inhibitors of various enzymes along the oxidative pathway of ethanol metabolism showed predictable effects on acetaldehyde binding; pyrazole decreased and cyanamide increased acetaldehyde levels and subsequent unstable and stable

adduct formation (Donohue *et al.* 1983b; Medina *et al.* 1985).

Israel *et al.* (1986) and Niemela *et al.* (1987) have reported the presence of circulating antibodies that specifically reacted against acetaldehyde–protein adducts in mice chronically treated with alcohol as well as in alcoholic subjects, indicating that stable adducts form and exist *in vivo* as a result of alcohol consumption. These antibodies recognized acetaldehyde-generated epitopes independent of the carrier protein. Subsequent to these studies, other groups have also detected circulating antibodies to acetaldehyde adducts in chronically alcohol-fed rats (Worrall *et al.* 1989) and in alcoholic subjects (Hoerner *et al.* 1988; Worrall *et al.* 1990; Koskinas *et al.* 1992). Especially high titres of these anti-adduct antibodies were seen in the sera of patients with alcoholic hepatitis (Niemela *et al.* 1987; Koskinas *et al.* 1992).

More direct evidence for the formation of acetaldehyde adducts *in vivo* during alcohol consumption was provided by studies which took advantage of the finding that acetaldehyde–protein adducts can elicit a distinct humoral response and can generate antibodies which specifically recognized acetaldehyde-generated epitopes independent of carrier proteins (Israel *et al.* 1986). By using such specific antibodies directed against acetaldehyde–protein adducts, many groups have demonstrated the presence of adducts in the liver of rats (Behrens *et al.* 1988; Lin *et al.* 1988; Worrall *et al.* 1991), guinea-pigs (Yokoyama *et al.* 1991) and humans (Niemela *et al.* 1991) chronically consuming alcohol. In addition, adducts with haemoglobin and plasma proteins have been detected *in vivo* in experimental animals (Peterson and Scott 1989; Peterson *et al.* 1990) and humans (Peterson and Polizzi 1987; Lin *et al.* 1990; Niemela *et al.* 1990a) following alcohol intake.

Although it appears that acetaldehyde adduct formation in the liver as a result of alcohol consumption has been well established, the chemical nature or structures of these adducts, their subcellular distribution and the identity of specific protein targets are still uncertain. The work to date reported in the literature has yielded variable results and inconclusive information. For example, in chronically alcohol-fed rats, Lin *et al.* (1988) and Lin and Lumeng (1989) reported that a single cytosolic 37 kDa protein (recent evidence suggests that this protein is an aldehyde reductase: Lin *et al.* 1993a) was the predominant adduct found in the liver, whereas Behrens *et al.* (1988) identified cytochrome

P4502E1 in microsomes as the major target and Worrall *et al.* (1991) found numerous cytosolic proteins that formed adducts with acetaldehyde. In guinea-pigs, Yokoyama *et al.* (1991) reported adduct formation with numerous cytosolic and microsomal proteins. In human alcoholics, Niemela *et al.* (1991) suggested that numerous cytosolic and mitochondrial proteins formed adducts in the liver; in contrast, Koskinas *et al.* (1992) suggested that a 200 kDa cytosolic protein was the major acetaldehyde adduct formed.

Because all these studies (described above) used an antibody directed against acetaldehyde–protein adducts in order to assay for and identify adducts in the liver, it appears that antigen preparation for immunization and production of specific antibodies are critical concerns; variations in these procedures probably explain the variable and conflicting results reported in the literature. At the present time, specific information on the characterization of the various antibody preparations used to detect adducts, in terms of what actual antigens (epitopes) are being recognized, is lacking. Furthermore, a variety of methods has been employed to prepare adducts for use as antigens, but in general most studies have treated various carrier proteins with high acetaldehyde concentrations in the presence of the strong reducing agent, sodium cyanoborohydride, to generate antigens for antibody production (Behrens *et al.* 1988; Lin *et al.* 1988; Niemela *et al.* 1991; Worrall *et al.* 1991). Under these reaction conditions, *N*-ethyllysine residues in proteins would be by far the most predominant product formed (Tuma *et al.* 1987). However, recent studies from our laboratory have shown that a monoclonal antibody that specifically recognizes *N*-ethyllysine epitopes on proteins did not detect the presence of acetaldehyde adducts in livers from ethanol-fed rats, whereas a polyclonal antiserum to non-reduced adducts (adducts prepared in the absence of a reducing agent and lacking *N*-ethyllysine epitopes) did recognize adducts in liver cytosolic preparations of ethanol-fed rats (Klassen *et al.* 1992, 1994). These results strongly suggest that non-reduced rather than reduced adducts predominate in the livers of alcohol-fed animals.

Although the stable binding of metabolically derived acetaldehyde to hepatic proteins during ethanol metabolism is well established, further work is needed to characterize adduct formation and reconcile the conflicting reports in the literature concerning the nature, subcellular distribution and identity of acetaldehyde–protein adducts. It appears that the development of well-characterized monoclonal and polyclonal antibodies to specifically defined acetaldehyde-generated epitopes on proteins would shed light on these problems and help clarify the role of adducts in the development of alcohol-induced liver injury.

Functional consequences of acetaldehyde adducts and their role in liver injury

Although the ability of acetaldehyde to bind to proteins and the formation of acetaldehyde–protein adducts in the liver during ethanol oxidation have been well established and well described, the functional consequences of adducts and their role in liver injury remain to be clarified. Correlation of adduct formation with impaired function of a specific protein and with cellular dysfunction are essential steps in evaluating the role of adducts in alcohol-induced hepatocellular damage.

Extensive formation of Schiff bases (unstable adducts) could potentially modify the function of proteins. Such alterations could include the displacement of pyroxidal phosphate from its binding site on proteins (Lumeng 1978) and interference with the activity of certain enzymes, especially those forming Schiff base–enzyme complexes as intermediates in their catalytic activity (Grazi *et al.* 1963). However, since Schiff bases are readily reversible, these effects would be relatively transient and the possibility of permanent dysfunction is doubtful. Furthermore, since Schiff bases readily undergo dissociation, it would take very high concentrations of acetaldehyde to produce extensive Schiff-base formation. This factor, in view of the low concentrations of acetaldehyde in the liver during ethanol metabolism (Nuutinen *et al.* 1984), would argue against a direct role of Schiff bases in alcoholic liver injury. Therefore, it is likely that Schiff base adducts must be stabilized before any significant alterations of protein function would be manifested and be relevant to the development of liver injury.

Stable acetaldehyde–protein adducts are logical candidates to serve as mediators of alcoholic liver injury. These adducts are not readily reversible and their presence in the liver would persist, even when all of the acetaldehyde has been metabolized. Consistent with a role of stable adducts in the development of liver damage are the findings of Niemela *et al.* (1991), who reported the localization of stable adducts in the perivenous region of the liver, where alcoholic liver injury starts and predominates, in humans consuming excessive amounts of alcohol. One possibility by which stable adducts could cause toxicity may involve the altered biological properties of adducted proteins.

Early studies from our laboratory indicated that the activity of enzymes with lysine residues essential for catalytic activity was inhibited by the stable binding of acetaldehyde to a much greater extent than enzymes lacking essential lysines (Mauch *et al.* 1986). More detailed studies on the model enzyme, ribonuclease A, using [^{13}C] proton-decoupled NMR spectroscopy, demonstrated that enzyme inhibition by acetaldehyde is a direct consequence of stable adduct formation with a reactive lysine residue at the active site (Mauch *et al.* 1987). To what extent enzyme inhibition of stable adducts contributes to alcoholic liver injury is unknown, but any enzyme with a lysine residue that is both reactive and catalytically important should be subject to inhibition by adduct formation. Long-term inhibition of critical enzyme systems by irreversible active site adducts could lead to impaired cellular functions; however, this contention must still be proven experimentally. The cross-linking of membrane proteins (Gaines *et al.* 1977), altered function of regulatory proteins such as calmodulin (Jennett *et al.* 1989a) and impaired cilia motion (Sisson *et al.* 1991) are examples of other alterations thought to be a result of stable acetaldehyde binding to reactive and essential lysine residues of specific proteins.

Some other examples of altered biological properties of adducted proteins include: accelerated low-density lipoprotein catabolism (Kesaniemi *et al.* 1987), inhibited activity of O^6-methylguanine transferase (Espina *et al.* 1988), decreased prostaglandin binding to hepatic plasma membranes (Buko and Zavodnik 1990), altered DNA methylation (Garro *et al.* 1991) and impaired histone binding to DNA (Niemela *et al.* 1990b). The functional consequences of these alterations at the cellular level and their role in liver injury have not been established.

Studies from our laboratory which demonstrated impaired tubulin function by stable adducts are especially important because they can be related to specific alcohol-induced functional impairments at the hepatocellular level which potentially could lead to liver damage. Furthermore, substoichiometric binding of acetaldehyde to tubulin leads to major changes in tubulin function. A detailed description of these studies will be summarized below.

As previously discussed, α-tubulin is a preferential target protein of stable acetaldehyde binding because it contains a highly reactive lysine (HRL) residue. In addition, the binding of acetaldehyde to the HRL was associated with a marked impairment of tubulin function which is to polymerize and form microtubules, an integral component of the cellular cytoskeleton. However, when bulk lysines were modified, but not the HRL, no effects on tubulin polymerization were observed (Smith *et al.* 1989; Tuma *et al.* 1991c). Furthermore, when low concentrations of acetaldehyde (<50 μM) were used to generate stable adducts to HRL residues, an adduct on only 1 of 20 tubulin molecules was sufficient to totally block polymerization (Tuma *et al.* 1991c; Smith *et al.* 1992). In a copolymerization assay, HRL adducts, in addition to being themselves assembly-incompetent, also interfered with the polymerization of normal (unadducted) tubulin. Bulk lysine adducts did not alter assembly and were incorporated normally into the growing microtubules (Tuma *et al.* 1991c; Smith *et al.* 1992). Overall, these findings indicate that substoichiometric amounts of acetaldehyde bound to HRL of tubulin can markedly inhibit microtubule formation via direct interference of tubulin dimer–dimer interactions, and that adducted HRL tubulin can interfere with the assembly of normal (unadducted) tubulin. These studies further suggest that low concentrations of acetaldehyde could generate sufficient levels of HRL tubulin adducts in the hepatocyte to alter microtubule structure and function.

Evidence linking the role of tubulin adducts to altered function at the cellular level is derived from studies demonstrating the disordering effects of alcohol on hepatic protein trafficking (Tuma and Sorrell 1988; Tuma *et al.* 1991a). In these studies, alcohol-induced impairments of several protein trafficking pathways, including protein secretion, plasma membrane assembly and receptor- and fluid-phase endocytosis, were reported, and evidence was presented that supported the role of acetaldehyde as a mediator of these defects in protein trafficking. Since microtubules play a central role in directing protein trafficking (Omsted and Borisy 1983), and since altered microtubule structures have been observed in the livers of ethanol-fed rats (Lieber 1991), alterations of tubulin polymerization by adduct formation to HRL of tubulin could very well be the underlying basis for defective protein trafficking in the liver. Furthermore, altered microtubule function could lead to considerable hepatocellular disorganization with cellular protein retention, ballooning of the cell and other structural changes (Tuma and Sorrell 1988; Lieber 1991), events which could progress to produce severe liver damage in the alcoholic. In addition to tubulin, actin, another component of the hepatocyte cytoskeleton, can also be a preferential target of acetaldehyde binding (Xu *et al.* 1989). In view of previous findings that cytoskeleton damage is a critical event leading to cell injury and necrosis (Rungger-Brandle and Gabbiani 1983; Lemasters *et al.* 1987), acetaldehyde adducts to cytoskeletal elements may be a key contributing factor in the pathogenesis of alcoholic liver damage.

Another important cellular process which may be modified as a result of altered function of adducted proteins is extracellular matrix production by the liver; such a defect could potentially lead to hepatic fibrosis. Fibrosis is one of the important histologic features of alcoholic liver disease and is characterized by marked accumulation of extracellular matrix components, especially collagen, in the perisinusoidal space (Maher 1990). Stable acetaldehyde adducts may play a direct role in fibrogenesis, as suggested by studies showing that adducts increase collagen gene transcription in fibroblasts (Brenner and Chojkier 1987), in activated Ito cells (Casini *et al.* 1991) and in hepatocytes (Niemela *et al.* 1990b). The role of adduct-stimulated collagen production in the overall mechanism of alcoholic hepatic fibrosis has not been clarified but does represent an attractive possibility.

Another intriguing mechanism by which stable adducts could induce liver injury involves immunological events. The demonstration that acetaldehyde adducts elicit a distinct humoral response and the demonstration of circulating anti-adduct antibodies in humans and mice following chronic alcohol exposure (Israel *et al.* 1986; Niemela *et al.* 1987) suggests a possible role of the immune system in the pathogenesis of alcoholic liver damage. Stable adducts may be recognized as neo-antigens by the immune system, thus triggering potentially harmful immune responses. Since earlier studies suggested that alcoholic liver disease might have an autoimmune basis (Zetterman and Sorrell 1981), stable acetaldehyde adducts represent logical candidates to serve as antigens to trigger immune responses. In addition to the numerous studies demonstrating the presence of anti-adduct antibodies in the sera of alcoholics (Niemela *et al.* 1987; Hoerner *et al.* 1988; Worrall *et al.* 1990; Koskinas *et al.* 1992) and ethanol-fed animals (Israel *et al.* 1986; Worrall *et al.* 1989). Terabayashi and Kolber (1990) showed that acetaldehyde-modified spleen cells could generate a

cytotoxic T-cell response in synergetic hosts. These studies clearly demonstrated that cell-associated acetaldehyde adducts could also modify a cellular immune response. These effects of stable adducts on the immune system have been given increased pathophysiologic relevance by the studies of Yokoyama *et al.* (1993), who reported that experimental hepatitis could be induced in guinea pigs by feeding alcohol to animals that had been previously immunized with acetaldehyde adducts. Future studies in this exciting area of research should clarify the role of stable acetaldehyde adducts and the immune system in the pathogenesis of alcoholic liver disease.

Conclusion

Since the original hypothesis implicating a role of stable acetaldehyde–protein adducts in the pathogenesis of alcohol-induced liver damage was formulated (Sorrell and Tuma 1985; Tuma and Sorrell 1985), a considerable body of evidence has accumulated in support of this proposal; however, further experimental proof of it is still required for its complete verification. Before a definite conclusion can be made that acetaldehyde–protein adducts are involved in liver injury, more information on the chemistry of the adducts and improved methods of adduct detection are required. In addition, the identification of target proteins and the subcellular distribution of adducts and a rigorous correlation of the presence of adducts with altered function of target proteins and modified cellular processes are necessary. Finally, innovative approaches to prove causal effects of adducts in the liver injury process remain the most challenging goals. This area will probably be a fertile area of future research and provide valuable information concerning the hepatotoxicity of alcohol.

References

Acharya, A.S., Sussman, L.G. and Manning, J.M. (1983). Schiff base adducts of glyceraldehyde with hemoglobin. *Journal of Biological Chemistry* **258**, 2296–2302.

Behrens, U.J., Hoerner, M., Lasker, J.M. and Lieber, C.S. (1988). Formation of acetaldehyde adducts with ethanol-inducible P450IIE1 *in vivo*. *Biochemical and Biophysical Research Communications* **154**, 584–590.

Brenner, D.A. and Chojkier, M. (1987). Acetaldehyde

increases collagen gene transcription in cultured human fibroblasts. *Journal of Biological Chemistry* **262**, 17690–17695.

Buko, V.U. and Zavodnik, I.B. (1990). Effect of acetaldehyde on binding of prostaglandins by receptors of liver plasma membranes. *Alcohol and Alcoholism* **25**, 483–487.

Casini, A., Cunningham, M., Rojkind, M. and Lieber, C.S. (1991). Acetaldehyde increases procollagen type I and fibronectin gene transcription in cultured rat fat-storing cells through a protein synthesis-dependent mechanism. *Hepatology* **13**, 758–765.

Cederbaum, A.I. and Rubin, E. (1976). Protective effect of cysteine on the inhibition of mitochondrial functions by acetaldehyde. *Biochemical Pharmacology* **25**, 963–973.

Donohue, T.M., Tuma, D.J. and Sorrell, M.F. (1983a). Acetaldehyde adducts with proteins: Binding of [^{14}C]acetaldehyde to serum albumin. *Archives of Biochemistry and Biophysics* **220**, 239–246.

Donohue, T.M., Tuma, D.J. and Sorrell, M.F. (1983b). Binding of metabolically derived acetaldehyde to hepatic proteins *in vitro*. *Laboratory Investigation* **49**, 226–229.

Espina, N., Lima, V., Lieber, C.S. and Garro, A.J. (1988). *In vitro* and *in vivo* inhibitory effect of ethanol and acetaldehyde on O^6-methylguanine transferase. *Carcinogenesis* **9**, 761–766.

Gaines, K.C., Salhany, J.M., Tuma, D.J. and Sorrell, M.F. (1977). Reaction of acetaldehyde with human erythrocyte membrane proteins. *FEBS Letters* **75**, 115–119.

Garro, A.J., McBeth, D.L., Lima, V. and Lieber, C.S. (1991). Ethanol consumption inhibits fetal DNA methylation in mice: Implications for the fetal alcohol syndrome. *Alcoholism: Clinical and Experimental Research* **15**, 395–398.

Giedroc, D.P., Puett, D., Sinha, S.K. and Brew, K. (1987). Calcium effect on calmodulin lysine reactivities. *Archives of Biochemistry and Biophysics* **252**, 136–144.

Grazi, E., Melochi, H., Martinez, G., Wood, W.A. and Horecker, B.L. (1963). Evidence for Schiff base formation in enzymatic aldol condensations. *Biochemical and Biophysical Research Communications* **10**, 4–10.

Gross, M.D., Hays, R., Gapstur, S.M., Chaussee, M. and Potter, J.D. (1994). Evidence for the formation of multiple types of acetaldehyde–hemoglobin adducts. *Alcohol and Alcoholism* **29**, 31–41.

Hoerner, M., Behrens, U.J., Worner, T.M., Blacksberg, I., Braly, L.F., Schaffner, F. and Lieber, C.S. (1988). The role of alcoholism and liver disease in the appearance of serum antibodies against acetaldehyde adducts. *Hepatology* **8**, 569–574.

Hoffmann, T., Meyer, R.J., Sorrell, M.F. and Tuma, D.J. (1993). Reaction of acetaldehyde with proteins: Formation of stable fluorescent adducts. *Alcoholism: Clinical and Experimental Research* **17**, 69–74.

Israel, Y., Hurwitz, E., Niemela, O. and Arnon, R. (1986). Monoclonal and polyclonal antibodies against acetaldehyde-containing epitopes in acetaldehyde–protein adducts. *Proceedings of the National Academy of Sciences, USA* **83**, 7923–7927.

Jennett, R.B., Sorrell, M.F., Johnson E.L. and Tuma, D.J. (1987). Covalent binding of acetaldehyde to tubulin: Evidence for preferential binding to the α-chain. *Archives of Biochemistry and Biophysics* **256**, 10–18.

Jennett, R.B., Saffari-Fard, A., Sorrell, M.F., Smith S.L. and Tuma, D.J. (1989a). Increased covalent binding of acetaldehyde to calmodulin in the presence of calcium. *Life Sciences* **45**, 1461–1466.

Jennett, R.B., Sorrell, M.F., Saffari-Fard, A., Ockner, J.L. and Tuma, D.J. (1989b). Preferential covalent binding of acetaldehyde to the α-chain of purified rat liver tubulin. *Hepatology* **9**, 57–62.

Jennett, R.B., Tuma, D.J. and Sorrell, M.F. (1990). Effects of acetaldehyde on hepatic proteins. In *Progress in Liver Diseases* (Edited by Popper, H. and Schaffner, F.), Vol. IX, pp. 325–333. W.B. Saunders, Philadelphia, PA.

Kesaniemi, Y.A., Kervinen, K. and Miettinen, T.A. (1987). Acetaldehyde modification of low density lipoprotein accelerates its catabolism in man. *European Journal of Clinical Investigation* **17**, 29–36.

Kikugawa, K., Takayanagi, K. and Watanabe, S. (1985). Polylysines modified with malonaldehyde, hydroperoxylinoleic acid and monofunctional aldehydes. *Chemical and Pharmaceutical Bulletin* **33**, 5437–5444.

Kikugawa, K., Iwata, A. and Beppu, M. (1988). Formation of cross-links and fluorescence in polylysine, soluble proteins and membrane proteins by reaction with 1-butanal. *Chemical and Pharmaceutical Bulletin* **36**, 685–692.

Kikugawa, K., Kato, T. and Iwata, A. (1989). A tetrameric dialdehyde formed in the reaction of butyraldehyde and benzylamine: A possible intermediate component for protein cross-linking induced by lipid oxidation. *Lipids* **24**, 962–969.

Klassen, L.W., Sorrell, M.F., Tuma, D.J. and Thiele, G.M. (1992). Antigenic specificity of RT1.1: A monoclonal antibody specific for reduced acetaldehyde protein adducts. *Alcoholism: Clinical and Experimental Research* **16**, 632.

Klassen, L.W., Tuma, D.J., Sorrell, M.F., McDonald, T.L., DeVasure, J.M. and Thiele, G.M. (1994). Detection of reduced acetaldehyde protein adducts using a unique monoclonal antibody. *Alcoholism: Clinical and Experimental Research* **18**, 164–171.

Koskinas, J., Kenna, J.G., Bird, G.L., Alexander, G.J.M. and Williams, R. (1992). Immunoglobulin A antibody to a 200-kilodalton cytosolic acetaldehyde adduct in alcoholic hepatitis. *Gastroenterology* **103**, 1860–1867.

Lemasters, J.J., DiGuiseppi, J., Nieminen, A.-L. and Herman, B. (1987). Blebbing, free Ca^{2+} and mitochondrial membrane potential preceding cell death in hepatocytes. *Nature, London* **325**, 78–81.

Lieber, C.S. (1988). Metabolic effects of acetaldehyde. *Biochemical Society Transactions* **16**, 241–247.

Lieber, C.S. (1991). Hepatic, metabolic and toxic effects of ethanol: 1991 update. *Alcoholism: Clinical and Experimental Research* **15**, 573–592.

Lin, R.C. and Lumeng, L. (1989). Further studies on the 37 kD liver protein–acetaldehyde adduct that forms *in vivo* during chronic alcohol ingestion. *Hepatology* **10**, 807–814.

Lin, R.C., Smith, R.S. and Lumeng, L. (1988). Detection of a protein–acetaldehyde adduct in the liver of rats fed alcohol chronically. *Journal of Clinical Investigation* **81**, 615–619.

Lin, R.C., Lumeng, L., Shahidi, S., Kelly, T. and Pound, D.C. (1990). Protein–acetaldehyde adducts in serum of alcoholic patients. *Alcoholism: Clinical and Experimental Research* **14**, 438–443.

Lin, R.C., Fillenworth, M.J. and Lumeng, L. (1993a). Identification of the 37 kD liver protein that forms acetaldehyde adduct in alcohol-fed rats. *Alcoholism: Clinical and Experimental Research* **17**, 477.

Lin, R.C., Shahidi, S., Kelly, T.J., Lumeng, C. and Lumeng, L. (1993b). Measurement of hemoglobin–acetaldehyde adduct in alcoholic patients. *Alcoholism: Clinical and Experimental Research* **17**, 669–674.

Lumeng, L. (1978). The role of acetaldehyde in mediating the deleterious effect of ethanol on pyridoxal 5′ phosphate metabolism. *Journal of Clinical Investigation* **62**, 286–293.

Maher, J.J. (1990). Hepatic fibrosis caused by alcohol. *Seminars in Liver Disease* **10**, 66–74.

Mauch, T.J., Donohue, T.M., Zetterman, R.K., Sorrell, M.F. and Tuma, D.J. (1986). Covalent binding of acetaldehyde selectively inhibits the catalytic activity of lysine-dependent enzymes. *Hepatology* **6**, 263–269.

Mauch, T.J., Tuma, D.J. and Sorrell, M.F. (1987). The binding of acetaldehyde to the active site of ribonuclease: Alterations in catalytic activity and effects of phosphate. *Alcohol and Alcoholism* **22**, 103–112.

Medina, V.A., Donohue, T.M., Sorrell, M.F. and Tuma, D.J. (1985). Covalent binding of acetaldehyde to hepatic proteins during ethanol oxidation. *Journal of Laboratory and Clinical Medicine* **105**, 5–10.

Neglia, C.I., Cohen, H.J., Garber, A.R., Thorpe, S.R. and Baynes, J.W. (1985). Characterization of glycated proteins by ^{13}C NMR spectroscopy. *Journal of Biological Chemistry* **260**, 5406–5410.

Niemela, O., Klajner, F., Orrego, H., Vidins, E., Blendis, L. and Israel, Y. (1987). Antibodies against acetaldehyde-modified protein epitopes in human alcoholics. *Hepatology* **7**, 1210–1214.

Niemela, O., Israel, Y., Mizoi, Y., Fukunaga, T. and Eriksson, C.J.P. (1990a). Hemoglobin–acetaldehyde adducts in human volunteers following acute ethanol ingestion. *Alcoholism: Clinical and Experimental Research* **14**, 838–841.

Niemela, O., Mannermaa, R.-M. and Oikarinen, J. (1990b). Impairment of histone H′ DNA binding by adduct formation with acetaldehyde. *Life Sciences* **47**, 2241–2249.

Niemela, O., Juvonen, T. and Parkkila, S. (1991). Immunohistochemical demonstration of acetaldehyde-modified epitopes in human liver after alcohol consumption. *Journal of Clinical Investigation* **87**, 1367–1374.

Nuutinen, H.U., Salaspuro, M.P., Valle, M. and Lindros, K.O. (1984). Blood acetaldehyde concentration gradient between hepatic and antecubital venous blood in ethanol-intoxicated alcoholics and controls. *European Journal of Clinical Investigation* **14**, 306–311.

O'Donnell, J.P. (1982). The reaction of amines with carbonyls: Its significance in the nonenzymatic metabolism of xenobiotics. *Drug Metabolism Reviews* **13**, 123–159.

Omsted, J.B. and Borisy, G.G. (1983). Microtubules. *Annual Review of Biochemistry* **42**, 507–540.

Peterson, C.M. and Polizzi, C.M. (1987). Improved method for acetaldehyde in plasma and hemoglobin-associated acetaldehyde: Results in teetotalers and alcoholics reporting for treatment. *Alcohol* **4**, 477–480.

Peterson, C.M. and Scott, B.K. (1989). Studies of whole blood associated acetaldehyde as a marker for alcohol intake in mice. *Alcoholism: Clinical and Experimental Research* **13**, 845–848.

Peterson, C.M., Scott, B.K., Sun, G.Y. and Sun, A.Y. (1990). A comparative blinded study in miniature swine of whole blood-, hemoglobin-, platelet-, plasma-, and lymphocyte-associated acetaldehyde as markers for ethanol intake. *Alcoholism: Clinical and Experimental Research* **14**, 717–720.

Rungger-Brandle, E. and Gabbiani, G. (1983). The role of cytoskeleton and cytocontractile elements in pathologic processes. *American Journal of Pathology* **110**, 361–392.

San George, R.C. and Hoberman, H.D. (1986). Reaction of acetaldehyde with hemoglobin. *Journal of Biological Chemistry* **261**, 6811–6821.

Sherman, G., Rossenberry, T.L. and Sternlicht, H. (1983). Identification of lysine residues essential for microtubule assembly *Journal of Biological Chemistry* **258**, 2148–2156.

Sisson, J.H., Tuma, D.J. and Rennard, S.I. (1991). Acetaldehyde-mediated cilia dysfunction in bovine bronchial epithelial cells. *American Journal of Physiology* **260**, L29-L36.

Smith, S.L., Jennett, R.B., Sorrell, M.F. and Tuma, D.J. (1989). Acetaldehyde substoichiometrically inhibits bovine neurotubulin polymerization. *Journal of Clinical Investigation* **84**, 337–341.

Smith, S.L., Jennett, R.B., Sorrell, M.F. and Tuma, D.J. (1992). Substoichiometric inhibition of microtubule formation by acetaldehyde–tubulin adducts. *Biochemical Pharmacology* **44**, 65–72.

Sorrell, M.F. and Tuma, D.J. (1985). Hypothesis: Alcoholic liver injury and the covalent binding of acetaldehyde. *Alcoholism: Clinical and Experimental Research* **9**, 306–309.

Szasz, J., Yaffe, M.B., Elzinga, M., Blank, G.S. and Sternlicht, H. (1986). Microtubule assembly is dependent on a cluster of basic residues in the α-tubulin. *Biochemistry* **25**, 4572–4582.

Terabayashi, H. and Kolber, M.A. (1990). The generation of cytotoxic T lymphocytes against acetaldehyde-modified syngeneic cells. *Alcoholism: Clinical and Experimental Research* **14**, 893–899.

Tuma, D.J. and Sorrell, M.F. (1985). Covalent binding of acetaldehyde to hepatic proteins: Role in alcoholic liver injury. In *Aldehyde Adducts in Alcoholism* (Edited by Collins, M.A.), pp. 3–17. Alan R. Liss, New York.

Tuma, D.J. and Sorrell, M.F. (1988). Effects of ethanol on protein trafficking in the liver. *Seminars in Liver Disease* **8**, 69–80.

Tuma, D.J., Donohue, T.M., Medina, V.A. and Sorrell, M.F. (1984). Enhancement of acetaldehyde–protein adduct formation by L-ascorbate. *Archives of Biochemistry and Biophysics* **234**, 377–381.

Tuma, D.J., Newman, M.R., Donohue, T.M. and Sorrell, M.F. (1987). Covalent binding of acetaldehyde to proteins: Participation of lysine residues. *Alcoholism: Clinical and Experimental Research* **11**, 579–584.

Tuma, D.J., Casey, C.A. and Sorrell, M.F. (1991a). Effects of alcohol on hepatic protein metabolism and trafficking. *Alcohol and Alcoholism* **1**, 297–303 (Suppl.).

Tuma, D.J., Hoffmann, T. and Sorrell, M.F. (1991b). The chemistry of acetaldehyde-protein adducts. *Alcohol and Alcoholism* **1**, 271–276 (Suppl.).

Tuma, D.J., Smith, S.L. and Sorrell, M.F. (1991c). Acetaldehyde and microtubules. *Annals of the New York Academy of Sciences* **625**, 786–792.

Watkins, N.G., Thorpe, S.R. and Baynes, J.W. (1985). Glycation of amino groups in protein. *Journal of Biological Chemistry* **260**, 10629–10636.

Worrall, S., DeJersey, J., Shanley, B.C. and Wilce, P.A. (1989). Ethanol induces the production of antibodies to acetaldehyde-modified epitopes in rats. *Alcohol and Alcoholism* **24**, 217–223.

Worrall, S., DeJersey, J., Shanley, B.C. and Wilce, P.A. (1990). Antibodies against acetaldehyde-modified epitopes: Presence in alcoholics, non-alcoholic liver disease and control subjects. *Alcohol and Alcoholism* **25**, 509–517.

Worrall, S., DeJersey, J., Shanley, B.C. and Wilce, P.A. (1991). Detection of stable acctaldehyde-modified proteins in the livers of ethanol-fed rats. *Alcohol and Alcoholism* **26**, 437–444.

Xu, D.S., Jennett, R.B., Smith, S.L., Sorrell, M.F. and Tuma, D.J. (1989). Covalent interactions of acetaldehyde with the actin/microfilament system. *Alcohol and Alcoholism* **24**, 281–289.

Yokoyama, H., Ishii, H., Nagata, S., Kato, S. and Tsuchiya, M. (1991). Evidence for acetaldehyde adducts formation in hepatic microsomes and cytosol of guinea pig after chronic ethanol administration. *Research Communications in Substances of Abuse* **12**, 173–180.

Yokoyama, H., Ishii, H., Nagata, S., Kato, S., Kamegaya, K. and Tsuchiya, M. (1993). Experimental hepatitis induced by ethanol after immunization with acetaldehyde adducts. *Hepatology* **17**, 14–19.

Zetterman, R.K. and Sorrell, M.F. (1981). Immunologic aspects of alcoholic liver disease. *Gastroenterology* **81**, 616–624.

6 Pathogenesis of alcoholic liver disease: Immune mechanisms

George L.A. Bird and Roderick N.M. MacSween

Introduction

Whereas the pathogenesis of alcoholic fatty liver is largely explicable on a biochemical basis, the pathogenesis of alcoholic hepatitis and cirrhosis remains incompletely understood. A number of general observations on the characteristic features of alcoholic hepatitis and cirrhosis suggest that immune factors could play a role in promoting liver injury. These include the observation that – as in autoimmune diseases in general – there is a variation in *individual* susceptibility and women are more vulnerable. In unremittingly heavy drinkers the incidence of cirrhosis is between 10 and 50 percent (Lelbach 1975; Hislop *et al.* 1983; Fleming and McGee 1984) and women develop cirrhosis more rapidly in spite of a similar cumulative intake of alcohol (Saunders *et al.* 1982). Furthermore, there is no well-defined dose–effect relationship of alcohol on the liver, and long-term prospective studies have shown that over a threshold level of daily alcohol intake the severity of liver injury bears no relationship to the cumulative alcohol consumption (Marbet *et al.* 1987). Thus, even at the highest alcohol intake levels the incidence of cirrhosis may be less than 50 percent. In patients with alcoholic hepatitis there may be clinical and laboratory evidence of liver damage pro-gressing for a period of 2–4 weeks after cessation of alcohol ingestion (Reynolds *et al.* 1989). Accordingly, it has been suggested that immune mechanisms might be important in the perpetuation of liver injury.

A large number of immunologic abnormalities have been reported in alcoholic liver disease, but it is difficult to determine whether these are the result rather than the cause of the liver injury. Many of the reported abnormalities could represent epiphenomena arising from liver dysfunction itself, or could be secondary to the clinical complications, such as malnutrition and infection. However, studies concentrating on patients with progressive and continuing liver damage (i.e. alcoholic hepatitis and active cirrhosis) have provided the most compelling evidence for a role of immune-mediated mechanisms in producing hepatocyte injury. In particular, recent evidence linking activation of the cytokine cascade with the severity of liver disease has underlined the possible role of immune-mediated tissue injury in the development of alcoholic hepatitis and cirrhosis.

Humoral abnormalities in alcoholic liver disease

Serum immunoglobulin

A polyclonal hypergammaglobulinaemia is seen in almost all patients with alcoholic liver disease, irrespective of histological type, and is characterized by a variable increase in IgG, IgM and IgE and disproportionate increases in IgA levels (Bailey *et al.* 1976; Van Epps *et al.* 1976; Iturriaga *et al.* 1977). However, raised serum IgA is also seen in a small proportion of alcohol abusers with no evidence of liver dysfunction (Drew *et al.* 1984). Interest has focused in particular on IgA because positive correlations have been demonstrated between serum levels and both the severity of liver damage and the average daily alcohol consumption (Iturriaga *et al.* 1977; Van de Wiel *et al.* 1985).

Although the mechanisms responsible for the hypergammaglobulinaemia observed not only in alcoholic liver disease but also in other forms of liver disease of widely differing aetiology have not been established, several studies have suggested that high levels of circulating immunoglobulins are secondary to an increase in immunoglobulin synthesis rather than decreased catabolism (Drew *et al.* 1984; Kalsi *et al.* 1983; McKeever *et al.* 1985). Absolute numbers of circulating B-cells are not increased in patients with alcoholic cirrhosis (Thomas *et al.* 1976), but cultured peripheral blood lymphocytes have enhanced spontaneous secretion of IgG and IgA (Holdstock *et al.* 1982; Rodriguez *et al.* 1984; Giron *et al.* 1992). However, immunoglobulin synthesis by peripheral blood lymphocytes may not be a wholly accurate reflection of total immunoglobulin synthesis as indicated by plasma levels (Drew *et al.* 1984). Increased synthesis of immunoglobulins may be explained either by a normal immune response due to excessive antigenic stimulation or a hyperactive immune response to altered regulation of B-cells as a consequence of changes within T-cell subsets.

Increased antigenic stimulation could arise from the following mechanisms:

1. *Alcohol-induced changes in the permeability of the gastrointestinal mucosa* giving rise to increased absorption of dietary, bacterial or other antigens (Baraona *et al.* 1974). Patients with alcoholic liver disease have increased circulating levels of antibodies to dietary and bacterial proteins originating within the gastrointestinal tract (Triger *et al.* 1972; Bjorneboe *et al.* 1972; Prytz *et al.* 1976; Mutchnik and Kerin 1981). Of particular interest is the observation that the number of positive reactions to *Escherichia coli* O-antigens correlates with serum IgA levels in patients with alcoholic liver disease and that serum IgA levels fall significantly in those patients who abstain from alcohol (Staun-Olsen *et al.* 1983). Further evidence of direct B-cell activation comes from *in vitro* studies in which lymphocytes from normal controls have been shown to increase immunoglobulin synthesis after pre-incubation with sera from patients with alcoholic cirrhosis (Holdstock *et al.* 1982; Rodriguez *et al.* 1984).

An increased antigen load could be secondary to damage to the mucosa of the gut, allowing greater permeability to macromolecules. Intestinal ultrastructural damage from alcohol has been demonstrated in man and in animal models (Baraona *et al.* 1974; Millan *et al.* 1980). Increased permeability to the low molecular weight probes polyethylene glycol 400 and chromium 51 EDTA has been shown in humans following alcohol ingestion (Robinson *et al.* 1981; Bjarnsson *et al.* 1984).

2. *Impaired clearance of gut-derived antigens entering the liver via the portal circulation.* The diseased liver may fail to sequester and inactivate gut-derived antigens due to impaired Kupffer cell function or because of intrahepatic shunting of blood away from Kupffer cells (Triger *et al.* 1979; Pomier-Layrargues *et al.* 1980). Furthermore, the presence of portal hypertension with an established collateral circulation may allow blood to bypass the liver (Webb *et al.* 1980), although a correlation between the degree of portal hypertension and hypergammaglobulinaemia, or levels of *E. coli* antibody, has not been demonstrated (Pomier-Layrargues *et al.* 1980).

3. *Local release of antigenic material from the damaged liver or the formation of neo-antigens* by the action of alcohol and its metabolites on hepatocytes and other macromolecules. Immunoglobulin synthesis could be enhanced as a result of disordered T-cell immunoregulation of B-cells. Studies in which this has been investigated provide conflicting results. In the majority of studies where peripheral blood lymphocytes from patients with alcoholic liver disease have been cultured in the presence or absence of pokeweed mitogen (a T-cell-dependent B-cell mitogen), a normal response has been reported (Dienstag *et al.* 1981; Wands *et al.* 1981; Holdstock *et al.* 1982; Rodriguez *et al.* 1984; Rong *et al.* 1984). However, a defect in helper cell function was reported in one study (Drew *et al.* 1984). Possible defects in suppressor T-cell control of B-cells have been evaluated by measuring pokeweed mitogen stimulated immunoglobulin synthesis after suppressor T-cell stimulation by concanavalin A. These experiments have shown a normal T-cell response (Wands *et al.* 1981; McKeever *et al.* 1985). One report suggesting a defect in suppressor T-cell function was possibly artifactual due to a prolonged incubation time with concanavalin A (Nouri Aria *et al.* 1986).

Evaluation of IgA production has suggested that T-cell suppressor activity is not impaired but set at a higher level (Allison and Hodgson 1989). Other reports have shown an inverse correlation between IgG synthesis and suppressor-cell activity (Rong *et al.* 1984) and numbers (Muller *et al.* 1991) in patients with alcoholic cirrhosis when compared with controls. A recent study in which a purified T-cell preparation from patients with alcoholic cirrhosis was studied showed enhanced secretion of B-cell differentiation factors for IgG and IgA but not for IgM (Giron *et al.* 1992). In the same study, greater amounts of IgG and IgA were secreted by purified B-cells from patients with alcoholic cirrhosis, both spontaneously and after activation with immunoglobulin ligands and a standard B-cell differentiation factor (Giron *et al.* 1992).

Immunoglobulin deposition on hepatocytes

IgG and IgA can be demonstrated on the cell membrane of hepatocytes in patients with alcoholic liver disease (Swerdlow *et al.* 1982; Trevison *et al.* 1983). Two patterns of monomeric IgA deposition, as determined by direct immunofluorescence, have

been described: a continuous linear or pericellular pattern and a discontinuous pattern. There is a good correlation between the proportion of subjects with IgA deposits on hepatocytes, as shown by fluorescence immunohistochemistry, and the daily alcohol consumption. About 75 percent of patients with alcoholic liver disease show deposition of IgA along hepatic sinusoids (Fig. 6.1) compared with less than 10 percent of patients with chronic non-alcoholic liver disease (Van de Wiel *et al.* 1987). This correlation is stronger than a number of other biochemical markers of alcoholic liver disease, including serum IgA levels, and has been advocated as an aid to diagnosis (Van de Wiel 1986). It has also been suggested that the pericellular pattern of deposition indicates more severe disease (Trevison *et al.* 1983). In a retrospective study, the continuous pattern of deposition appeared to be of value as a prognostic index (Vaerman and Delacroix 1984). However, IgA deposits are equally common in all histological types of alcoholic liver disease – whether fatty liver, fibrosis, hepatitis or cirrhosis – and it is difficult to reconcile this observation with the suggestion that IgA deposition is a predictive indicator of a poor prognosis (Van de Wiel *et al.* 1986). In addition, linear IgA deposition has been demonstrated in diabetic patients with fatty liver and non-alcoholic

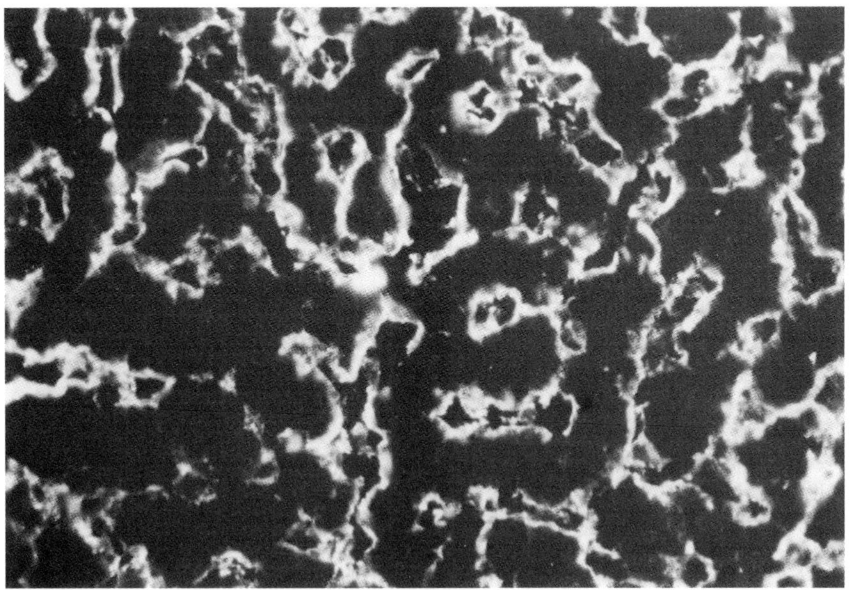

Fig. 6.1 Immunofluorescence with anti-IgA on a section of frozen liver biopsy from a patient with alcoholic liver disease. There are IgA deposits in a continuous staining pattern along sinusoids. Characteristics of serum IgA and liver IgA deposits in alcoholic liver disease. Reproduced with permission from Van de Wiel *et al.* (1987).

steatohepatitis (Nagore and Scheuer 1988). The IgA deposition in alcoholic liver disease could result from impaired clearance of IgA by the liver or could reflect the changes in the serum concentration of IgA which have already been mentioned.

Decreased IgA clearance

Several studies have provided evidence for a hepatocyte role in IgA clearance from the serum (Hopf *et al.* 1978; Kleinman *et al.* 1982; Vaerman and Delacroix 1984; Brandtzaeg 1985). In the rat there is a transport pathway for polymeric IgA across the sinusoidal membrane to the bile canalicular membrane and which is mediated by the IgA secretory component (Vaerman and Delacroix 1984). A similar mechanism has not been demonstrated in man where, however, it is biliary epithelial cells which express the secretory component (Nagura *et al.* 1981; Delacroix *et al.* 1983; Brandtzaeg 1985). Asialoglycoprotein receptors isolated from rat liver tissue bind human IgA and it has been suggested that these receptors may be involved in the endocytosis of IgA by hepatocytes and clearance of IgA from the serum (Kleinman *et al.* 1982). Changes in the structure of the asialoglycoprotein receptors by metabolites of alcohol could impair IgA binding and therefore reduce its clearance from plasma (Brown and Kloppel 1989).

IgA deposition and serum IgA levels

The question of whether IgA deposition is a reflection of raised serum levels of IgA, a non-specific effect of hepatocye damage or a specific feature of alcoholic liver disease has been examined by Van de Wiel and colleagues (1987). IgA deposition in liver biopsies of patients with alcoholic liver disease is much more common than in patients with chronic liver diseases of other aetiologies but with equally high levels of serum IgA. Measurement of the ratio of the IgA subclasses IgA_1 and IgA_2, in serum (where it is normally 4:1) and bound to hepatocytes, has shown that deposition is not simply a passive phenomenon related to serum concentration. Whereas the hepatic IgA deposits in patients with alcoholic liver disease were almost all of the IgA_1 subclass, the serum IgA subclass distribution in alcoholic patients differed from non-alcoholic patients in that there was a slight increase in IgA_2.

IgA deposition is also seen in the kidneys of 20–50 percent of patients with alcoholic liver disease and, therefore, it seems unlikely that binding of IgA to liver-specific antigens accounts entirely for the hepatic deposition (Woodroffe 1981; Berger *et al.* 1977; Montoliu *et al.* 1986). The consequences of alcoholic IgA nephropathy vary from minimal histological changes with no associated symptoms to a very active proliferative glomerulonephritis. The IgA deposition can be associated with additional deposition of IgG, IgM, C3 and fibrinogen. No glomerular antigen which binds the IgA has yet been identified (Sancho *et al.* 1981). Lomax Smith *et al.* (1983) have reported that glomerular IgA deposits have characteristics of polymerized IgA, but this has not been confirmed (Russell *et al.* 1986). As in the liver, so kidney deposits are predominantly of the IgA_1 subclass (Lomax Smith *et al.* 1983; Russell *et al.* 1986). Thus, while there are well-identified abnormalities of IgA deposition in the liver (and in the kidney) in alcoholic liver disease, it is not clear what role these have in the pathogenesis of the liver injury, or the renal injury for that matter. Recent studies have shown that, *in vitro*, polymeric and monomeric IgA stimulate monocytes to secrete tumour necrosis factor (TNF), a cytotoxic cytokine (Deviere *et al.* 1991). This could, if it operates *in vivo*, be a mechanism for tissue injury.

Non-organ-specific autoantibodies

Autoantibodies at low titre are a common feature of alcoholic liver disease, with anti-nuclear factor (ANF) and anti-smooth muscle antibodies (SMA) showing a prevalence of 12–16 percent and 12–27 percent, respectively, and with a slightly higher prevalence in woman than men (Bailey *et al.* 1976; Morgan *et al.* 1980). In one study where careful matching of controls with patients was carried out to compensate for the effect of age and sex on the prevalence of autoantibodies in normal subjects, the presence of ANF was five times more common in patients with alcoholic liver disease, and SMA eight times more common, although both antibodies were present in low titre only (McGeorge *et al.* 1984).

HLA status could have an influence on the presence of autoantibodies, as shown by the study of 69 males with alcoholic cirrhosis by Gluud *et al.* (1981a), in which ANA and SMA were more common and in higher titre in patients who were HLA B8 and/or HLA B12 than those of other haplotypes. Serum testosterone was lower in males who were ANA-positive and it was suggested that sex hormones could play a part in the increased prevalence of autoantibodies in females as compared with male patients with alcoholic liver disease. A subsequent report from the same centre evaluating 74 patients

duct epithelium (Morton *et al.* 1981). A study with a large panel of anti-cytokeratin antibodies failed to show cytoplasmic reactivity in rat or human hepatocytes in which Mallory bodies were present. It was suggested that there was a decrease, rather than an antigen change, in normal intracellular cytokeratins (as detected immunologically) of hepatocytes with Mallory bodies (Preisegger *et al.* 1991). However, there is evidence from other investigations that Mallory bodies may contain non-keratin neo-antigens which may have specific epitopes capable of provoking an immune response (Zatloukal *et al.* 1990).

Interest in the possibility that the Mallory bodies could initiate an immune response and play a role in the pathogenesis of alcoholic hepatitis was first stimulated when Mallory body antigen and antibodies to Mallory bodies were detected in the serum of patients with alcoholic hepatitis. Antibody and antigen were not detected in control groups with acute and chronic viral hepatitis, drug-induced hepatitis and other hepatic lesions (Chen *et al.* 1975; Kanagasundaram *et al.* 1977). These studies may have been flawed because of contamination of isolated Mallory body preparations by nuclear fragments (Bull 1976). Further doubt was cast on the validity of the original findings by a study using antibody to purified Mallory body raised in guinea pigs, but using the same assay systems of complement fixation and immune adherence haemagglutination; the results were consistently negative for the presence of Mallory body antigen and antibody in the sera of 32 patients with alcoholic hepatitis (Kehl *et al.* 1981).

Antibodies to acetaldehyde-modified proteins

Oxidation of ethanol to acetaldehyde is followed by covalent binding of acetaldehyde to cellular proteins (Sorrell and Tuma 1985; see also Chapter 5). This interaction has been proposed as a major underlying mechanism of tissue damage in alcoholic liver disease, both through direct toxicity and the formation of neoantigens (Tuma and Klassen 1993). Several studies have shown that acetaldehyde-modified proteins arising *in vivo* from chronic alcohol administration can result in the production of antibody directed against epitopes containing the acetaldehyde residue. In an alcohol-fed rat model, Israel *et al.* (1986) demonstrated generation of antibodies to both plasma protein–acetaldehyde and erythrocyte–

protein–acetaldehyde conjugates. The presence of antibodies against these conjugates in the serum of over 70 percent of patients with alcoholic liver disease has also been demonstrated and confirmed by others, but 39 percent of patients with chronic liver diseases of non-alcoholic aetiology also have similar antibodies (Niemela *et al.* 1986; Hoerner *et al.* 1988). In these reports, there was a positive correlation between the titre of antibody and the severity of the liver disease. The authors suggested the antibody titre could be a reflection not only of the cumulative chronic acetaldehyde load, but also the extent of hepatocyte damage, regardless of aetiology. However, there was no evidence that serum antibodies against circulating acetaldehyde adducts contributed to liver damage.

More recently, attempts by Lin *et al.* (1988) to define liver protein–acetaldehyde neo-antigen formation *in vivo* in a rat model have shown the presence of a single 37 kDa protein adduct. The appearance of this antigen was closely related to dietary intake of alcohol, and was neither an alcohol dehydrogenase nor an acetaldehyde dehydrogenase adduct. The formation of the 37 kDa adduct was increased by using cyanamide administration to block acetaldehyde oxidation, a finding strongly suggesting that the protein studied was generated after interaction with acetaldehyde. A 52 kDa acetaldehyde–protein adduct corresponding to ethanol-induced cytochrome P4502E1 has also been reported in a rat model (Behrens *et al.* 1988). Koskinas and colleagues (1992) detected a 200 kDa acetaldehyde adduct in both human and rat liver cytosol after incubation with acetaldehyde in reducing conditions. IgA class antibody specific for this adduct (Fig. 6.3) was present in 69 percent of alcoholic hepatitis patients but IgM and IgG antibodies were not detected. The prevalence of this IgA antibody was significantly lower in patients with fatty liver and inactive cirrhosis, suggesting that IgA antibody may be involved in the pathogenesis of alcoholic hepatitis (Koskinas *et al.* 1992). The 200 kDa protein awaits identification, but there is a possibility that it is a form of procollagen type I (Behrens *et al.* 1990).

The possible importance of the above findings has been highlighted by a Japanese study showing the development of hepatitis in guinea pigs immunized with acetaldehyde adducts and simultaneously given alcohol, although the histological appearance of the liver was not typical of alcohol-induced damage in the human and comprised a mononuclear infiltrate of portal tracts and perivenular areas with

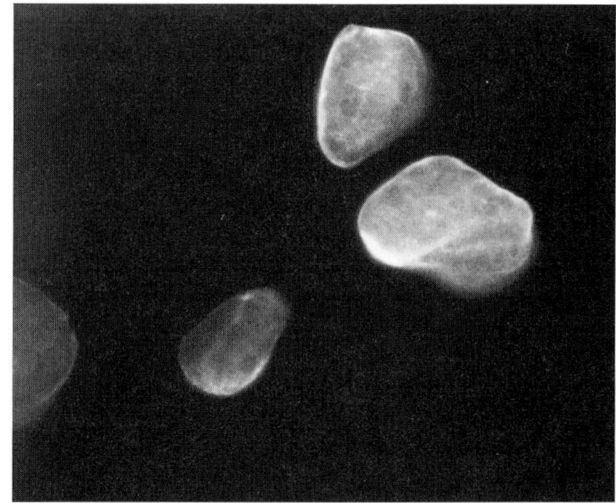

Fig. 6.3 Isolated hepatocytes from a rabbit pre-treated with alcohol, reacted with serum from a patient with alcoholic hepatitis, and then reacted with a fluorescent-conjugated anti-human IgG. There is intense immuno-staining of the hepatocytes with marginal accentuation of the positivity, indicating that the antibody reaction is with epitopes on the cell membrane.

lymphoid follicles (Yokoyama *et al.* 1993). It has been suggested that antibodies directed against acetaldehyde–protein adducts could cross-react with acetaldehyde–phospholipid adducts with the potential of damaging hepatocyte membranes (Trudell *et al.* 1990).

Circulating immune complexes

Circulating immune complexes are implicated in the pathogenesis of a number of diseases and there are several reports of their prevalence in alcoholic hepatitis and cirrhosis (Jori *et al.*1977; Andre *et al.* 1978; Penner *et al.* 1978; Thomas *et al.* 1978; Kaufman *et al.* 1979; Abrass *et al.* 1980). The nature of the antigen in the complexes is not clear. Mallory bodies can bind IgA, and IgA- and IgG-containing complexes eluted from the livers of patients with alcoholic hepatitis and active cirrhosis were reported to contain MB antigen (Kanagasundaram *et al.* 1977; Penner *et al.* 1978).

There is no general agreement as to whether the presence of circulating immune complexes in alcoholic liver disease correlates with disease activity (Penner *et al.* 1978; Abrass *et al.* 1980; Peters *et al.* 1982). Increased levels of immune complexes may

reflect an impairment of Kupffer cell function (Mannik *et al.* 1971; Lahnborg *et al.* 1981). The presence on liver cell membranes of receptors for the Fc portion of IgG and for the complement component C3 suggest a possible role for hepatocytes in immune complex clearance. Impairment of this hepatocyte function in alcohol-induced damage could promote non-specific deposition of immune complexes in the liver and also in other organs (Paronetto and Popper 1966). This possibility is of interest in that local deposition of immune complexes could produce an Arthus-like reaction, promoting the accumulation of the neutrophil infiltrate so characteristic of alcoholic hepatitis (MacSween 1978).

Cell-mediated immunity in alcoholic liver disease

Peripheral blood lymphocyte counts

Patients with alcoholic hepatitis and cirrhosis have reduced numbers of circulating lymphocytes (Fernandez *et al.* 1982), due predominantly to a reduced number of T-cells (Pelletier *et al.* 1984; Perrin *et al.* 1984), while B-cell numbers have been reported as normal (Lundy *et al.* 1975; Fernandez *et al.* 1982) or reduced (Couzigou *et al.* 1984). Abnormalities in peripheral T-cell numbers are not present in patients with alcoholic fatty liver (Pelletier *et al.* 1984) or in alcoholics without liver disease (Kawamura *et al.* 1983; Couzigou *et al.* 1984; Watson *et al.* 1985). In addition, the reduction in T-cell numbers in alcoholics with established liver disease is reported to be independent of whether they had been drinking or abstinent in the preceding 6 months, suggesting that it is the severity of liver disease and not the level of alcohol consumption which is responsible for the depletion of peripheral blood T-lymphocytes (Couzigou *et al.* 1984).

Monoclonal antibodies have enabled characterization of the relative changes in T-cell subsets and there is general agreement that the CD4/CD8 ratio is increased in patients with alcoholic hepatitis and alcoholic cirrhosis when compared with normal subjects. The increase is predominantly due to a reduction in CD8 cells (Kawamura *et al.* 1983; Pelletier *et al.* 1984; Perrin *et al.* 1984; Couzigou *et al.* 1984; Watson *et al.* 1985; Freni *et al.* 1985; Muller *et al.* 1991). Both normal (Couzigou *et al.* 1984;

Watson *et al.* 1985) and increased (Kawamura *et al.* 1983) CD4/CD8 ratios have been found in alcoholics without liver disease when compared with normal subjects. The T-cells in the peripheral blood may express the activation antigens interleukin-2 and class II HLA(DR) (Deviere *et al.* 1988; Roselle *et al.* 1988; Cook *et al.* 1991). This activation of T-cells, however, may be a direct effect of alcohol or acetaldehyde and may be found in the absence of liver disease (Cook *et al.* 1991).

Liver-associated lymphocytes

While neutrophil polymorphs are the predominant cell type in the liver in alcoholic hepatitis, lymphocytes are also part of the infiltrate and, in active cirrhosis, they are present in significant numbers. Sequestration of lymphocytes is one possible explanation for the reduced numbers of circulating lymphocytes. The majority of lymphocytes within the liver are T-cells, especially when Mallory bodies are present (Si *et al.* 1983). CD8 cells are sequestered in ascitic fluid in patients with alcoholic cirrhosis (Pirrone *et al.* 1983) and this may also contribute to low peripheral blood counts. Antigenic changes in hepatocytes could cause localized T-cell activation (Sanchez-Tapias *et al.* 1977; French *et al.* 1979). Quantitative studies of T-cell subsets in liver tissue of patients with alcoholic liver disease are consistent with the hypothesis that T-cells migrate into the liver from peripheral blood. It has been postulated that a predominantly CD8 infiltration into the hepatic parenchyma may be important in the mediation of cytotoxic hepatocyte injury (Si *et al.* 1983; Freni *et al.* 1985). The proportions of suppressor and cytotoxic T-cells in the liver have not yet been clearly defined. A recent quantitative immunohistochemical analysis showed that the number of CD8 lymphocytes in the hepatic acini in alcoholic hepatitis was similar to that found in chronic hepatitis B, and this would favour a role for cytotoxic T-cells in mediating liver injury (Sakai *et al.* 1993).

It has been suggested for some time that alcohol-induced liver disease may sometimes histologically resemble chronic active hepatitis with portal tract inflammation, piecemeal necrosis and intra-acinar lesions in which lymphocytes predominate. The topic has been a controversial one and the possibility that the chronic active hepatitis-like morphology is related to a viral infection, in particular hepatitis C, is currently under intense investigation (Takase *et al.* 1991, 1993; see also Chapters 3, 9 and 18).

Impaired cell-mediated immunity

In vivo *studies*

In vivo tests of cell-mediated immunity are impaired in alcoholic liver disease, and reduced skin reactivity to common recall antigens has been documented in all grades of alcoholic liver disease, particularly alcoholic hepatitis (Mills *et al.* 1983; Calvey *et al.* 1985). Patients with alcoholic hepatitis show improvement of skin test reactivity with clinical and histological recovery (Calvey *et al.* 1985), but it is not clear whether this is due to withdrawal of the effects of alcohol on lymphocytes or improvement in the underlying liver disease. Malnutrition is common in alcoholic hepatitis and improved nutritional status will enhance recovery of immunocompetence (O'Keefe *et al.* 1980). One study has reported an improvement in cellular immunity in patients with inactive alcoholic cirrhosis following peritoneojugular shunting for intractable ascites (Franco *et al.* 1983).

In vitro *studies*

These studies have included migration inhibition tests and lymphocyte transformation and some of the findings have shown a positive correlation with reduced skin reactivity to recall antigens (Rajkovic and Williams 1985). It has been shown that autologous liver extracts (Sorrell and Leevy 1972), Mallory body preparations (Zetterman *et al.* 1976; Triggs *et al.* 1981; Gluud *et al.* 1981b) and acetaldehyde (Actis *et al.* 1978) impair leucocyte migration in patients with alcoholic hepatitis. However, the precise nature of the antigen to which the lymphocytes were sensitized has not been established.

Lymphocyte transformation in response to non-specific mitogens such as phytohaemagglutinin is reduced in alcoholic liver disease, and there is also evidence that inhibitory factors in the serum play a role in suppression of lymphocyte function (Thestrup-Petersen *et al.* 1976; Young *et al.* 1979). Lymphocyte transformation in response to antigen has also been investigated. Mallory body preparations were reported as producing increased lymphocyte proliferation (Leevy *et al.* 1975). Exposure to Mallory bodies resulted in enhanced neutrophil polymorph chemotaxis (Peters *et al.* 1983; Samanta *et al.* 1985). However, these results have not been confirmed and convincing evidence of sensitization to Mallory bodies or Mallory body-antigens has not been produced.

One possible cause for defective lymphocyte transformation in alcoholic liver disease is an impairment in activity of the cytokines which promote lymphocyte proliferation. Production of interleukin-2 (IL-2), the major cytokine mediator of lymphocyte proliferation, is decreased in alcoholic cirrhosis, but activation markers (IL-2 receptor expression, the transferrin receptor and the Ia antigen) are increased (Deviere *et al.* 1988). The authors suggested these changes could result from prolonged exposure of T-cells to activating factors *in vivo*, although patients in whom there were histological features of alcoholic hepatitis were not studied. In contrast, Spinozzi *et al.* (1991) reported decreased IL-2 receptor expression, together with evidence of impaired intracellular signal transduction; the patients studied appeared to have only mild histological changes of alcoholic liver damage not amounting to hepatitis or cirrhosis.

Cytotoxicity

Several studies have demonstrated significant lymphocyte cytotoxicity to autologous hepatocytes from patients with alcoholic liver disease (Cochrane *et al.* 1977; Kakumu and Leevy 1977). Cytotoxicity is blocked by aggregated IgG suggesting that it is predominantly non-T-cell-mediated and antibody-dependent (Izumi *et al.* 1983). Lymphocytes harvested from patients with alcoholic hepatitis or cirrhosis demonstrate greater cytotoxicity to autologous hepatocytes than those from patients with fatty liver (Actis *et al.* 1983). Poralla *et al.* (1984) confirmed this, but in their studies there was no difference in T-cell-enriched or non-enriched lymphocyte preparations and no correlation could be shown between the presence of cytotoxicity and the degree of histological inflammation or clinical severity of liver disease. The expression of intercellular adhesion molecule-1 (ICAM-1) on hepatocytes correlates with the histological degree of hepatocellular damage and also with the expression of leucocyte function associated antigen-1 (LFA-1) on parenchymal leucocytes, suggesting this pathway may be involved in leucocyte mediated tissue damage in alcoholic hepatitis (Burra *et al.* 1992). Studies evaluating populations of natural killer (NK) cells have shown impaired activity in alcoholic liver disease (Charpentier *et al.* 1984), although, somewhat paradoxically, there was a shift in subset population to $CD56^+$ and $CD3^+$ cells, subsets associated with high NK activity (Muller *et al.* 1990). Furthermore, decreased NK activity appears to correlate more closely with the degree of malnutrition than the severity of underlying liver disease (Ledesma *et al.* 1990).

A more recent study has demonstrated a predominance of $CD4^+$ and $CD8^+$ cells in the liver parenchyma of subjects with alcoholic hepatitis and active cirrhosis, which correlated with histological features of disease severity. This adds further support to the hypothesis that a cytotoxic T-lymphocyte–hepatocyte interaction plays a role in hepatocyte damage (Chedid *et al.* 1993).

An antibody-dependent cytotoxicity assay has demonstrated the presence of antibodies directed against ethanol- or acetaldehyde-altered liver cell determinants in serum of patients with alcoholic liver disease (Neuberger *et al.* 1984). The development of antigenic determinants on the liver cell membrane probably requires metabolism of alcohol to acetaldehyde (Crossley *et al.* 1986). Consistent with this suggestion is the finding that acetaldehyde can bind to the plasma membrane of rat and human hepatocytes by the formation of an intermediate Schiff base without affecting cellular metabolism or membrane function, as assessed by alanine uptake into hepatocytes (Barry *et al.* 1983, 1984; Barry and McGiven 1985).

Role of inflammatory mediators in alcoholic liver disease

The complement system

This is a complex system of sequentially interacting, chemically and immunologically distinct plasma proteins which mediate a wide variety of responses to stimuli by the immune system. The possibility that complement activation could mediate some of the manifestations of liver disease in which an immune-mediated pathogenesis is suspected prompted several studies of serum complement levels in acute and chronic liver disease, including alcoholic liver disease. Interpretation of some of the results is hindered by the possibility that impaired hepatic synthetic capacity in patients with advanced liver disease could also cause reduced levels of complement, as the liver is the predominant source of many of the complement components in serum (Cole and Colten 1988).

Measurement of C3 in several chronic liver diseases by Fox and colleagues (1971) showed that levels in patients with alcoholic liver disease were similar to normal subjects; however, the histological type and clinical severity of the alcoholic liver disease was not recorded. Other studies in which a range of complement components including C1q, C3, C4, C5 and factor B were measured concluded that in alcoholic liver disease the level of serum complement components was normal or only slightly decreased, and that decreased levels were secondary to impaired hepatic synthesis (De Meo and Anderson 1972; Thompson *et al.* 1973; Kourilsky *et al.* 1973; Munoz *et al.* 1982). In these studies, information on the histological type of alcoholic liver disease and its clinical severity was limited, but the findings are in general agreement with reports on chronic liver disease of other aetiologies, in which no relationship between disease activity (as judged by raised transaminases or autoantibody titre) and serum complement level have been demonstrated (Finlayson *et al.* 1972).

In vitro complement activation in a laboratory model of alcoholic liver disease has been demonstrated by Barry and McGiven (1985) using liver plasma membrane vesicles incubated with acetaldehyde, which allowed covalent binding to take place without disruption to intravesicular enzyme function. Incubation of the vesicles with human serum showed activation of C3, suggesting this is a possible mechanism of hepatocyte damage.

Evidence for abnormal complement function, as opposed to serum level, has come from *in vitro* studies of neutrophil activity in serum from patients with alcoholic liver disease. De Meo and Anderson (1972) reported a disproportionate decrease in neutrophil activity in alcoholic liver disease when compared with a relatively small decrease in complement levels and suggested a serum inhibitor of complement might be present. More recent studies have demonstrated the presence of increased chemotactic factor inactivator (CFI) in patients with alcoholic hepatitis. The CFI could inhibit the chemoattractant effects of C5a, therefore impairing neutrophil chemotaxis and predisposing patients with alcoholic hepatitis to infection (Robbins *et al.* 1987; MacGregor 1990).

Eicosanoids

Interest has focused on prostaglandin E2, the predominant arachidonic acid metabolite circulating monocytes. Prostaglandin E2 has potent anti-inflammatory properties, including inhibition of T-cell aggregation, histamine release and suppression of macrophage lysosomal proteases (Goodwin and Webb 1980). In animal models it has been shown to protect the liver against galactosamine and carbon tetrachloride-induced injury (Guarner *et al.* 1985). In alcoholic liver disease, there is decreased prostaglandin E2 production by peripheral blood mononuclear cells and decreased production of the leukotriene LTB4, the major eicosanoid product of the neutrophil, which has a wide range of biological activities including aggregation and activation of neutrophils (Maxwell *et al.* 1989). The decrease in prostaglandin E2 production was most marked in patients with alcoholic hepatitis and was reversed by addition of exogenous arachidonic acid to the the culture medium.

Cytokines and the acute phase response

The acute phase response describes a group of physiological changes which include fever, granulocytosis, depressed serum levels of iron and zinc, decreased synthesis of albumin, increased synthesis of hepatic acute phase proteins and hypergammaglobulinaemia. It is induced by tissue injury secondary to infection, trauma and neoplasia as well as chronic inflammatory diseases, including rheumatoid arthritis and inflammatory bowel disease. Although the widespread presence of the acute phase response suggests it confers survival advantage, the specific functions of many acute phase proteins are not yet defined. Indeed, it has been proposed that under certain circumstances some of the effects could be harmful to the host, and this aspect has come under scrutiny as a possible mechanism in promoting hepatocyte injury, in particular in alcoholic hepatitis (Thiele 1989). The cytokines which mediate the acute phase response initiate a cascade of physiological changes which are present in a range of diseases of dissimilar aetiology. This explains how several different causes of tissue damage can give rise to the same generalized physiological features. Three cytokines central to the acute phase response are tumour necrosis factor (TNF), interleukin-1 (IL-1) and interleukin-6 (IL-6). TNF and IL-1 each comprise two structurally dissimilar proteins (designated α and β respectively) but the three cytokines have overlapping biological activities (Table 6.1). TNF, IL-1 and IL-6 are each secreted by more than one cell type and there is significant cross-induction of TNF and IL-1, both of which stimulate IL-6 production. Acute alcoholic hepatitis is accompanied by the physiological features of an acute phase response, even in the absence of infection, prompting questions as to what precipitates it and how it is related to the liver damage.

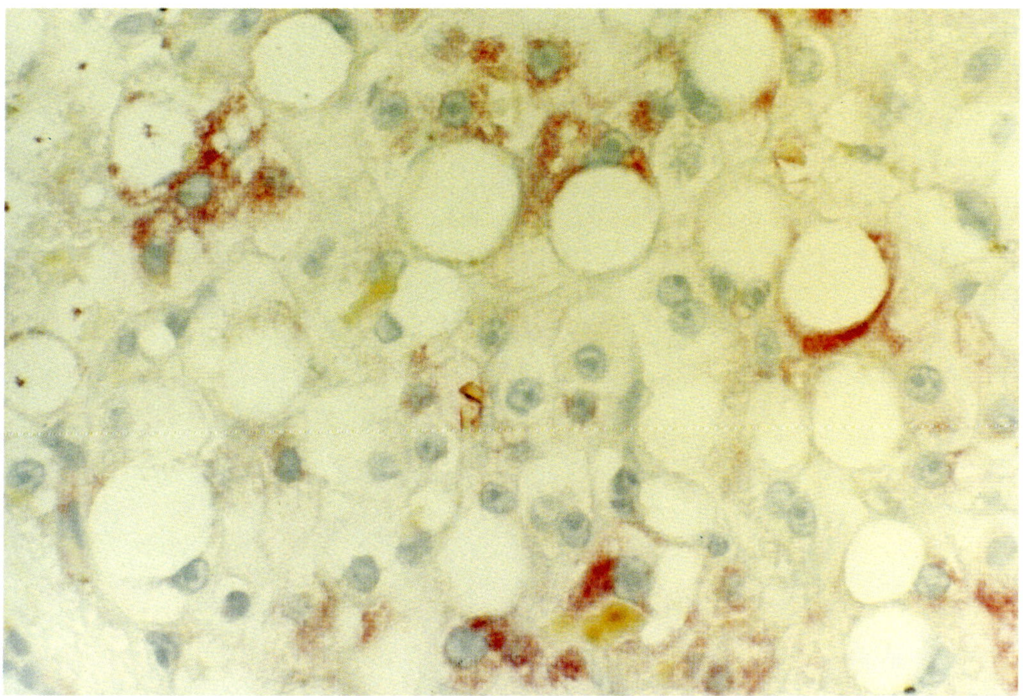

Plate 10 Immunostaining for heat shock protein (anti-HSP-60) in alcoholic hepatitis, showing pleomorphic hepatocytes with strong cytoplasmic immunoreactivity.

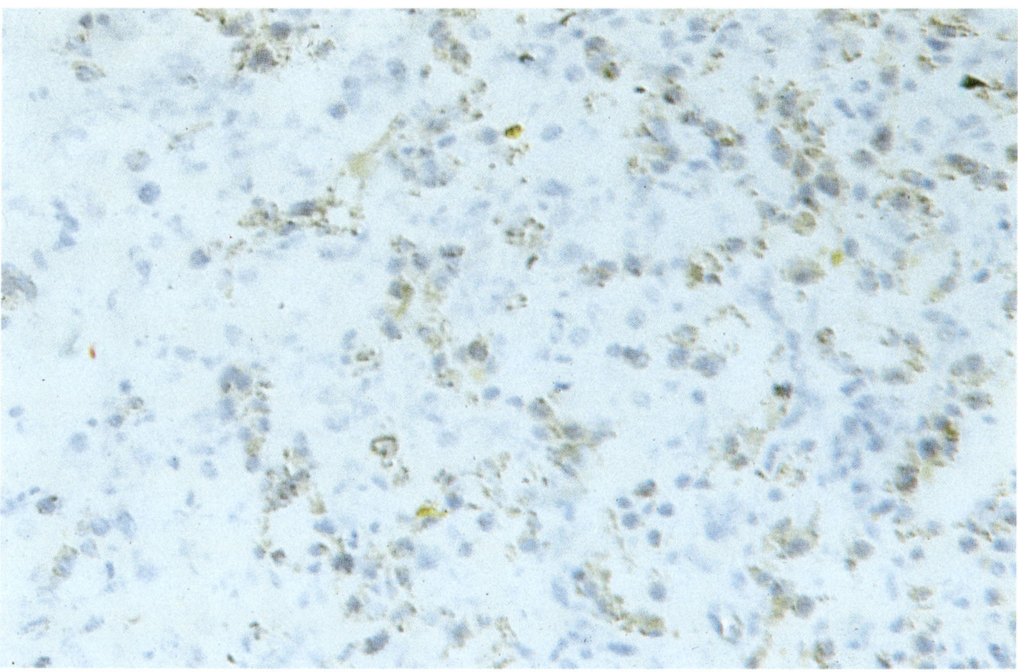

Plate 11 Immunoperoxidase staining for interleukin-8 (IL-8) in liver from a patient with severe acute alcoholic hepatitis. Elevation of local and circulating levels of the neutrophil activator IL-8 in alcoholic hepatitis.

Table 6.1   Comparison of biological characteristics of TNF, IL-1, IL-6 and IL-8

	TNF	*IL-1*	*IL-6*	*IL-8*
Stimulus for release	Infection trauma and toxins	Infection trauma and toxins	IL-1 and TNF	IL-1 and TNF
Predominant source	Monocytes, macrophages, Kupffer cells	Monocytes, macrophages, Kupffer cells	Monocytes, macrophages, Kupffer cells	Blood mononuclear cells, endothelial cells, hepatocytes
Actions				
Pyrogenic	+	+	+	−
Induction of acute phase proteins	+	+	+ +	−
Inhibiton of albumin synthesis	+	+	+ +	−
Pathogenesis of shock	+ + +	−	−	−
B-cell activation	+	+	+	−
Neutrophil activation	+	+	+	+ + +
Cytotoxic/cytostatic action on cell lines	+ +	+	−	−

Tumour necrosis factor

The clinical manifestations of acute alcoholic hepatitis, which include fever, neutrophilia and hypotension in severe cases, are similar to the biological actions of TNF. In animal models of another toxin-induced liver injury (galactosamine hepatitis), it is thought that TNF itself is a mediator of liver cell necrosis, although the mechanism of action is not clear (Lehmann *et al.* 1987). A similar mechanism has been suggested in alcoholic hepatitis, the hepatocyte injury being mediated by cytokine action (McClain and Cohen 1989).

Circulating mononuclear cells from patients with alcoholic hepatitis show higher spontaneous release of TNF in culture than do normal controls, and stimulation with lipopolysaccharide (LPS) causes a greater release of TNF (McClain and Cohen 1989). When TNF is measured directly in the plasma of patients with severe acute alcoholic hepatitis, levels are higher than in normal controls, whereas subjects with inactive alcoholic cirrhosis and alcoholics without liver disease have TNF levels which are only slightly raised or are within the normal range, respectively (Bird *et al.* 1990). Univariate analysis evaluating the relationship between plasma TNF and a number of plasma and laboratory indices of disease severity show a close correlation between TNF level and fever, peripheral blood neutrophil count, serum creatinine and serum bilirubin. In a multivariate analysis to investigate the relationship between indicators of disease severity and short-term mortality, only TNF showed a positive correlation. These findings indicate that high TNF levels correlate very closely with severity of hepatocyte injury and suggest, indirectly, that TNF could promote tissue injury (McClain 1991).

The association between increased TNF and acute alcoholic hepatitis has been confirmed by Felver and colleagues (1990), who reported a negative correlation between circulating TNF and survival over a 6 month period. The stimulus for TNF release in alcoholic hepatitis is not clear, but it is unlikely that ethanol stimulates release directly – the addition of ethanol to cell cultures decreases TNF production both in controls and in patients with alcoholic hepatitis (McClain and Cohen 1989). In a rat model, decreased serum TNF was seen in animals receiving a continuous infusion of ethanol when given a bolus dose of endotoxin compared with controls receiving no ethanol (D'Souza *et al.* 1989). However, TNF release may depend on the pattern of alcohol exposure. In another animal model, an acute alcohol bolus suppressed endotoxin-stimulated TNF release, but suppression did not occur when alcohol was administered over a prolonged period (Nelson *et al.* 1989).

Endotoxin is a potent stimulus for TNF release. Circulating levels of endotoxin are increased in alcoholic liver disease and have been positively correlated with hepatic failure, encephalopathy and death (Bigatello *et al.* 1987). However, in the studies mentioned above, there was no correlation between circulating endotoxin levels and raised plasma TNF in patients with alcoholic hepatitis, although TNF levels were higher in patients who, in addition, had some infective process (Bird *et al.* 1990).

Hepatocyte expression of type A and B receptors for TNF is upregulated in a spectrum of chronic liver diseases, including alcoholic hepatitis suggesting that hepatocytes are specific targets for TNF activity (Volpes *et al.* 1992). Chronic exposure of hepatocytes to TNF increases the expression of TNF receptors within the plasma membrane and this leads to enhanced hepatocyte responsiveness to TNF (Han *et al.* 1990). As previously noted, IgA is deposited in the liver in alcoholic liver disease and a possible role for IgA_1 in TNF release has been suggested by *in vitro* experiments in which it has been shown to increase TNF release by mononuclear cells (Deviere *et al.* 1991). There is emerging interest in the possibility that there could be a role for anti-TNF antibodies in the therapy of alcoholic liver disease and this has been stimulated by the observation that neutralizing antibodies to TNF protect animals dying of septicaemic shock (Tracey *et al.* 1987).

Interleukin-1

Interleukin-1 (IL-1) is similar to TNF in that it is released by peripheral blood mononuclear cells in response to endotoxin and gives rise to many features of the acute phase response (Table 6.1). Increased serum levels of IL-1 in alcoholic hepatitis were originally reported in six male patients by McClain and colleagues (1986) using a bioassay. Direct measurement of serum levels of IL-1 α and IL-1 β utilizing monoclonal antibodies has shown that whereas there is an increase in circulating IL-1 α in alcoholic hepatitis patients, there is not a parallel increase in IL-1 β (Bird *et al.* 1990; Khoruts *et al.* 1991). In contrast to TNF, these studies did not demonstrate a correlation between the severity of disease and increased serum levels of IL-1 .

Peripheral blood mononuclear cells from patients with acute alcoholic hepatitis do not secrete higher levels of IL-1 in the resting state when compared with normal controls, but increased IL-1 production is seen after endotoxin stimulation in patients with inactive alcoholic cirrhosis (Bird *et al.* 1989).

Interleukin-6

IL-1 and TNF induce secretion of interleukin-6 (IL-6), which itself promotes a range of physiological changes in the acute phase response and is also a likely candidate as an inflammatory mediator in acute alcoholic hepatitis (Thiele 1989). Deviere and colleagues (1989) reported an increase in IL-6 activity in abstinent patients with alcoholic cirrhosis; a positive correlation between IL-6 levels and serum IgA was also found. In a series of 58 patients with severe acute alcoholic hepatitis, Sheron *et al.* (1991) demonstrated raised IL-6 in 63.7 percent of cases. Control groups, in whom high levels were not present, included alcoholics without severe liver disease, abstinent alcoholics with established cirrhosis, patients with non-alcoholic liver disease and patients with chronic renal failure. There was a strong correlation between circulating IL-6 levels and indicators of disease severity, including serum bilirubin, prolonged prothrombin time, grade of encephalopathy, peripheral blood neutrophil count and shock. However, there was no correlation between plasma TNF and IL-6 (unlike the close correlations seen in bacterial sepsis, Waage *et al.* 1989), and no correlation between plasma endotoxin and IL-6. Whereas TNF levels in serial blood samples remained elevated, there was considerable fluctuation of IL-6 levels during the same period of observation. Khoruts *et al.* (1991) have confirmed these findings and have also reported a positive correlation between plasma IL-6 and serum transaminases as well as biochemical markers of the acute phase response over a longer term.

Exogenous administration of IL-6 even in high doses produces few toxic effects in animal models, and it therefore seems likely that it requires to act in synergy with TNF and possibly other factors in promoting hepatocyte damage in alcoholic hepatitis.

Interleukin-8

The characteristic features of acute alcoholic hepatitis include an acute inflammatory infiltrate in which neutrophils predominate, along with a high peripheral neutrophil count. Factors which govern the recruitment and activation of neutrophils are therefore potentially of prime importance in the pathogenesis of alcoholic liver disease. Interleukin-8 (IL-8), in addition to those cytokines already discussed, also has a role in neutrophil activation, as indicated by its initial identification as neutrophil-activating peptide-1. IL-8 is generated by a variety of immune and non-immune cells, including hepatocytes, and major stimuli for its release include endotoxin, IL-1 and TNF. Of these, IL-1 and TNF are capable of stimulating a prolonged and increasing IL-8 response, whereas endotoxin alone induces only a self-limiting response.

Serum IL-8 in patients with acute alcoholic hepatitis is markedly elevated when compared with normal controls and patients with inactive alcoholic cirrhosis. In contrast to TNF, IL-1 and IL-6, levels are also raised in alcoholics without overt liver disease, but are not as high as in patients with alcoholic hepatitis (Sheron *et al.* 1993; Hill *et al.* 1992). Measurement of IL-8 in liver biopsy specimens of patients with a range of acute and chronic liver diseases has confirmed IL-8 is generated locally by hepatocytes (see Plate 11 between pp. 110–111), and the highest levels occur in patients with acute alcholic hepatitis (Sheron *et al.* 1993). *In vitro* studies with rat hepatocytes have suggested ethanol can precipitate the release of IL-8 (Shiratori *et al.* 1993). However, the human Hep G2 cell line does not release IL-8 when incubated with ethanol (Sheron *et al.* 1993) and high concentrations of ethanol suppress TNF-stimulated IL-8 production (Sheron *et al.* 1992). This raises the possibility that in heavy drinkers alcohol withdrawal could precipitate a neutrophil accumulation and hepatocyte injury.

Other cytokines

The high degree of activation of the cytokines directly implicated in the acute phase response in acute alcoholic hepatitis has stimulated interest in the role of other mediators of immune activation. Interleukin-2 (IL-2) induces TNF production in cells other than monocytes and is itself induced by IL-1. However, studies of IL-2 production in alcoholic hepatitis have produced conflicting results (Bird *et al.* 1989; Vicente-Gutierrez *et al.* 1991). Gamma interferon, which upregulates IL-1 and TNF production, is not increased in alcoholic hepatitis compared with normal controls (Bird 1993) and serum levels are depressed in alcoholic cirrhosis (Vicente-Gutierrez *et al.* 1991). *In vitro* studies have suggested that ethanol may exert an inhibitory effect on the secretion of gamma interferon by peripheral blood lymphocyte (Wagner *et al.* 1992). TGF-β_1 may have a role in hepatic fibrogenesis, and fibrosis is an essential feature of alcoholic hepatitis. Significant increases in TGF-β_1 messenger RNA have been demonstrated in liver biopsies showing alcoholic

hepatitis and active cirrhosis (Milani *et al.* 1991; Annoni *et al.* 1992; Nagy *et al.* 1992).

Conclusions

A large number of reports have implicated immune mechanisms in alcoholic liver disease, and in the above review profound abnormalities have been described in both the humoral and cell-mediated immune systems. Many of the studies do not demonstrate convincingly that the patterns of abnormality have a role in the pathogenesis of liver injury, and are anything other than epiphenomena arising as a consequence of alcohol-induced liver damage. However, the studies incorporating an analysis based upon the histological type of liver damage have pointed to a striking association between the activation of the acute phase response and alcoholic hepatitis. The likelihood that activation of the cytokine cascade is central to the development of alcoholic hepatitis and the ultimate development of cirrhosis allows a number of tentative explanations to be made concerning some of the central puzzles of alcoholic liver disease. The lack of correlation between the quantity of alcohol consumed and the severity of liver damage is one such question – even with prolonged heavy intake, several years may elapse before liver cell injury arises. Although metabolic abnormalities are present in alcoholic fatty liver, these are insufficient to lead to the inflammatory features seen in alcoholic hepatitis (Lieber 1993). It seems improbable that the onset of hepatitis is due to the cumulative toxic effects of alcohol or its metabolites, and it is more feasible that triggering of the cytokine pathway in a susceptible group of individuals follows the formation of a neoantigen.

The evidence implicating HLA antigens in the predisposition of individuals to alcoholic liver disease has not yet pointed to a firm relationship between a particular haplotype and the development of alcoholic liver disease. Many of these studies have been hampered by the statistical difficulties in using relatively small numbers of patients and the importance for correcting for the large number of HLA antigens being tested (Eddleston and Davis 1982). Furthermore, ethnic differences between different study groups have not allowed any firm conclusions to be drawn (Doffoel *et al.* 1986). Studies using molecular techniques to evaluate the specific acetaldehyde dehydrogenase isoenzymes which are associated with alcoholic liver disease may well provide further information with respect to the underlying individual susceptibility to alcoholic liver disease and the formation of neoantigens incorporating acetaldehyde (Sherman *et al.* 1993.)

The characteristic IgA hypergammaglobulinaemia in alcoholic liver disease is thought to be due to a combination of enhanced IgA synthesis and impaired hepatocyte transport mechanisms. Increases in the other immunoglobulins also result in part from increased B-cell synthesis, and it is possible that the damage to the intestinal mucosa by alcohol contributes to the preponderance of IgA. Although raised circulating IgA and IgA deposition in the liver is a useful pointer in the diagnosis of alcoholic liver disease, there are as yet no indications that IgA is central to the pathogenesis of alcoholic liver disease.

The possibilty that organ-specific autoantibodies, including those to LSP, liver membrane antigen and Mallory bodies, could contribute to tissue injury in alcoholic liver disease is now thought to be unlikely, as the antibodies detected in alcoholic liver disease are seen in a wide spectrum of liver disease and are unlikely to be involved in pathogenesis. The higher incidence of autoantibodies seen in alcoholic liver disease when compared with normal subjects is probably a reflection of a generalized increase in the activation of the immune system, because of the presence of neoantigens.

It seems likely that the reaction between acetaldehyde, the major biochemically reactive metabolite of alcohol, and macromolecules is able to produce neoantigens in the form of acetaldehyde–protein adducts (see Chapter 5). Candidates for neoantigens within the liver are HSP, a 37 kDa protein and an unidentified 200 kDa protein, and there is good evidence that a vigorous humoral response to these antigens is seen in patients with alcoholic hepatitis. However, the importance of this immune reactivity in the pathogenesis of alcoholic liver disease is unknown, although it has also been suggested that extrahepatic acetaldehyde–protein adducts are responsible for alcohol-induced tissue damage elsewhere in the body (Wickramasinghe *et al.* 1987).

Some of the most compelling evidence that immune mechanisms are central to the progression of hepatic injury in alcoholic liver disease comes from recent studies showing dramatic activation of the cytokine cascade. Circulating TNF is very high in alcoholic hepatitis and levels correlate closely with indicators of hepatocyte necrosis. Interest in the role of TNF has focused on the possibility that high levels are toxic to hepatocytes and may act on specific plasma membrane receptors to cause hepa-

tocyte death. High levels of IL-6 also correlate with disease severity and IL-6 probably acts synergistically with TNF in promoting the metabolic complications of alcoholic hepatitis. Finally, it seems very likely that IL-8 has a central role in the chemotaxis and activation of neutrophils in alcoholic hepatitis: not only do high circulating levels correlate with peripheral blood neutrophilia, but increased synthesis of IL-8 in the liver, leading to high local tissue concentrations, provide a feasible explanation for the neutrophil polymorph infiltrate which is such a characteristic feature of alcoholic hepatitis.

In spite of the surfeit of information on the functioning of the immune system in the development of alcoholic liver disease, a large number of questions are still to be answered. There appears to be no single antigen which triggers the immune reaction and the exact spectrum of antigenic triggers still invites investigation. Are they predominantly acetaldehyde adducts and are they only present in the liver? What is the importance of the antigenic load arising from the gastrointestinal tract? Another area requiring further scrutiny is the factors which modulate cytokine release in alcoholic patients, and the relationship between the hepatocyte and the neutrophil in terms of cytokine release and action. Furthermore, the final pathway of hepatocyte necrosis has not been established, although there is circumstantial evidence that neutrophils and cytokines are both instrumental in cell damage.

References

Abrass, C.K., Border, W.A. and Hepner, G. (1980). Non-specificity of circulating immune complexes in patients with acute and chronic liver disease. *Clinical and Experimental Immunology* **40**, 292–298.

Actis, G., Miele-Vergani, G., Portman, B., Eddleston, A.L.W.F., Davis, M. and Williams, R. (1983). Lymphocyte toxicity to autologous human hepatocytes in alcoholic liver disease. *Liver* **3**, 8–12.

Allison, M.E.D. and Hodgson, H.J.F. (1989). Regulation of peripheral blood B-cell IgA production in alcoholic cirrhosis. *Journal of Clinical and Laboratory Immunology* **30**, 127–130.

Andre, F., Druguet, M. and Andre, C. (1978). Effect of food intake on circulating antigen–antibody complexes in patients with alcoholic cirrhosis. *Digestion* **17**, 554–559.

Annoni, G., Weiner, F.R. and Zern, M.A. (1992). Increased transforming growth factor-1 gene expression in human liver disease. *Journal of Hepatology* **14**, 259–264.

Anthony, R.S., Farquharson, M. and MacSween, R.N.M. (1983). Liver membrane antibodies in alcoholic liver diease. II. Antibodies to ethanol altered hepatocytes. *Journal of Clinical Pathology* **36**, 1302–1308.

Bailey, R.J., Krasner, N., Eddleston, A.L.W.F., Williams, R., Tee, D.E.H., Doniach, D., Kennedy, L.A. and Batchelor, J.R. (1976). Histocompatibility antigens, autoantibodies and immunoglobulins in alcoholic liver disease. *British Medical Journal* **6038**, 727–729.

Baraona, E., Pirloa, R.C. and Lieber, C.S. (1974). Small intestinal damage and changes in cell population produced by ethanol ingestion in the rat. *Gastroenterology* **66**, 226–234.

Barry, R.E., McGiven, J.D., Hayes, M. and Read, A.E. (1983). Acetaldehyde is not directly hepatotoxic in alcoholic liver disease. *Clinical Science* **65**, 23.

Barry, R.E., McGiven, J.D. and Hayes, M. (1984). Acetaldehyde binds to liver cell membranes without affecting membrane function. *Gut* **25**, 412–416.

Barry, R.E. and McGiven, J.D. (1985). Acetaldehyde alone may initiate hepatocellular damage in acute alcoholic liver disease. *Gut* **26**, 1065–1069.

Behrens, U.J., Hoerner, M., Lasker, J.M. and Lieber, C.S. (1988). Formation of acetaldehyde adducts with ethanol-inducible P450 IIE1 *in vivo*. *Biochemical and Biophysical Research Communications* **154**, 584–590.

Behrens, U.J., Ma, X.-L., Bychenok, S., Baraona, E. and Lieber, C.S. (1990). Acetaldehyde–collagen adducts in CCl$_4$-induced liver injury in rats. *Biochemical and Biophysical Research Communications* **173**, 111–119.

Berger, J., Yaneva, H. and Narra, B. (1977). Glomerular changes in patients with cirrhosis of the liver. *Advances in Nephrology* **7**, 3–14.

Bigatello, L.M., Broitman, S.A., Fattori, L., Paoli, M., Pontello, M., Bevilacqua, G. and Nespoli, A. (1987). Endotoxaemia, encephalopathy and mortality in cirrhotic patients. *American Journal of Gastroenterology* **82**, 11–15.

Bird, G.L.A. (1993). Cytokines – mediators of alcoholic hepatitis. *Advances in the Biosciences* **86**, 163–171.

Bird, G.L.A., Nouri Aria, K., Daniels, H., Alexander, G.J.N. and Williams, R. (1989). Contrasts in interleukin-1 and interleukin-2 activity in alcoholic hepatitis and cirrhosis. *Alcohol and Alcoholism* **24**, 541–546.

Bird, G.L.A., Sheron, N., Goka, A.K.J., Alexander, G.J.M. and Williams, R. (1990). Increased plasma tumor necrosis factor in severe alcoholic hepatitis. *Annals of Internal Medicine* **112**, 917–920.

Bjarnsson, I., Ward, K. and Peters, T.J. (1984). The leaky gut of alcoholism: Possible route of entry for toxic compounds. *Lancet* **i**, 179–182.

Bjorneboe, M., Prytz, H. and Orskov, F. (1972). Antibodies to intestinal microbes in serum of patients with cirrhosis of the liver. *Lancet* **i**, 58–60.

Bonanno, G., Bocchini, G., Canevari, A., Pieri, F., Ferrini, S. and Melioli, G. (1983). Immunological im-

balance in uncomplicated chronic alcoholism. *Drug and Alcohol Dependency* **12**, 189–196.

Brandtzaeg, P. (1985). Role of J chain and secretory component in receptor-mediated glandular and hepatic transport of immunoglobulins in man. *Scandinavian Journal of Immunology* **22**, 111–146.

Brown, W.R. and Kloppel, T.M. (1989). The liver and IgA: Immunological, cell biological and clinical implications. *Hepatology* **9**, 763–784.

Bull, D.M. (1974). Lymphocyte responsiveness to plant mitogens in diseases of unknown cause. *Gastroenterology* **67**, 1071–1073.

Bull, D.M. (1976). Assessment of autogenic activity of hepatic tissue components. *Gastroenterology* **71**, 164–166.

Burra, P., Hubscher, S.G., Shaw, J., Elias, E. and Adams, D.H. (1992). Is the intercellular adhesion molecule-1/leukocyte function associated antigen-1 pathway of leukocyte adhesion involved in the tissue damage of alcoholic hepatitis? *Gut* **33**, 268–271.

Burt, A.D., Anthony, R.S., Hislop, W.S., Bouchier, I.A.D. and MacSween, R.N.M. (1982). Liver membrane antibodies in alcoholic liver disease. 1. Prevalence and immunoglobulin class. *Gut* **23**, 221–225.

Calvey, H., Davis, M. and Williams, R. (1985). Controlled trial of nutritional supplementation with and without branched chain amino acid enrichment. *Journal of Hepatology* **1**, 141–151.

Cassani, F., Bianchi, F.B., Lenzi, M., Volta, U. and Pisi, E. (1985). Immunomorphological characterisation of anti-nuclear antibodies in chronic liver disease. *Journal of Clinical Pathology* **38**, 801–805.

Charpentier, B., Franco, D., Paci, L., Charra, M., Martin, B., Vuitton, D. and Fries, D. (1984). Deficient natural killer cell activity in alcoholic cirrhosis. *Clinical and Experimental Immunology* **58**, 107–111.

Chedid, A. and Mendenhall, C.L. (1990). Alcohol, immunomodulation, and AIDs: Cell-mediated immunity in alcoholic liver disease. *Progress in Clinical and Biological Research* **325**, 321–332.

Chedid, A., Mendenhall, C.L., Moritz, T.E., French, S.W., Chen, T.S., Morgan, T.R., Roselle, G.A., Nemchausky, B.A., Tamburro, C.H., Schiff, E.R., McClaim, C.J., Marsano, L.S., Allen, J.I., Samanta, A.,Weesner, R.E., Henderson, W.G. and Veterans Affairs Cooperative Study Group 275 (1993). Cell-mediated hepatic injury in alcoholic liver disease. *Gastroenterology* **105**, 254–266.

Chen, T., Kanagasarundaram, N., Kakumu, S., Luisada-Opper, A. and Leevy, C.M. (1975). Serum autoantibodies to alcoholic hyaline in alcoholic hepatitis. *Gastroenterology* **69**, 813.

Cochrane, A.M.G., Moussouros, A., Portmann, B., McFarlane, I.G., Thomson, A.D., Eddleston, A.L.W.F. and Williams, R. (1977). Lymphocyte cytotoxicity for isolated hepatocytes in alcoholic liver disease. *Gastroenterology* **72**, 918–923.

Cole, F.S. and Colten, H.R. (1988). Complement biosynthesis. In *The Complement System* (Edited by Roth, K. and Till, G.O.). Springer Verlag, Berlin.

Cook, R.T., Garvey, M.J., Booth, B.M., Golken, J.A., Stewart, B. and Noel, M. (1991). Activated CD-8 cells and HLA DR expression in alcoholics without overt liver disease. *Journal of Clinical Immunology* **11**, 246–253.

Couzigou, P., Vincendeau, P., Fleury, B., Richard-Molard, B., Pierron, A., Bergeron, J.L., Bezian, J.H., Amouretti, M. and Beraud, C. (1984). Lymphocyte subpopulations in alcoholic liver disease: Influence of alcohol, hepatocellular dysfunction and malnutrition. *Gastroenterology and Clinical Biology* **8**, 915–919.

Crossley, I.R., Neuberger, J., Davis, M., Williams, R. and Eddleston, A.L.W.F. (1986). Ethanol metabolism in the generation of new antigenic determinants on liver cells. *Gut* **27**, 186–189.

Cunningham, A.L., Mackay, I.R., Frazer, I.H., Brown, C., Pedersen, J.S., Toh, B.H., Tait, B.D. and Clark, F.M. (1985). Antibody to G-actin in different categories of alcoholic liver disease – quantification by an ELISA and significance for alcoholic cirrhosis. *Clinical Immunology and Immunopathology* **43**, 157–164.

Delacroix, D.L., Furtado-Barreira, G., De Hemptinne, B., Goudswaard, J., Dive, C. and Vaerman, J.P. (1983). The human liver and the secretory IgA immune system: Dogs, but not rats and rabbits are suitable experimental models. *Hepatology* **3**, 980–988.

De Meo, A.N. and Anderson, B.R. (1972). Defective chemotaxis associated with a serum inhibitor in cirrhotic patients. *New England Journal of Medicine* **286**, 735–740.

Deviere, J., Denys, C. and Schandene, L. (1988). Decreased proliferative activity associated with activation markers in patients with alcoholic cirrhosis. *Clinical and Experimental Immunology* **72**, 377–382.

Deviere, J., Content, J., Denys, C., Vandenbussche, P., Schandene, L. and Wybran, J. (1989). High interleukin-6 serum levels and increased production by leucocytes in alcoholic liver disease: Correlation with IgA serum levels and lymphokines production. *Clinical and Experimental Immunology* **77**, 221–225.

Deviere, J., Vaerman, J.P., Content, J., Chantal, D., Schandene, L., Vandenbussche, P., Sibille, Y. and Dupont E. (1991). IgA triggers tumor necrosis factor secretion by monocytes: A study in normal subjects and patients with alcoholic cirrhosis. *Hepatology* **13**: 670–675.

Dienstag, J.L., Weake, J.R. and Wands, J.R. (1981). Abnormalities of mononuclear cell regulation *in vitro* in primary biliary cirrhosis. *Liver* **1**, 230–243.

Doffoel, M., Tongio, M.M., Gut, J.-P., Ventre, G., Charrault, A., Vetter, D., Ledig, M., North, M.L., Mayer, S. and Bockel, R. (1986). Relationships between 34 HLA-A, HLA-B, and HLA-DR antigens and three serological markers of viral infections in alcoholic cirrhosis. *Hepatology* **6**, 457–463.

Drew, P.A., Clifton, P.M., LaBrooy, J.T. and Shear-man, D.J. (1984). Polyclonal B cell activation in alcoholic patients with no evidence of liver dysfunction. *Clinical and Experimental Immunology* **57**, 479–486.

D'Souza, N.B., Bagby, G.N., Nelson, S., Lang, C.H. and Spitzer, J.J. (1989). Acute alcohol infusion suppresses endotoxin-induced serum tumour necrosis factor. *Alcoholism: Clinical and Experimental Research* **13**, 295–298.

Eddleston, A.L.W.F. and Davis, M. (1982). Histocompatibility antigens in alcoholic liver disease. *British Medical Bulletin* **38**, 13–16.

Felver, M.E., Mezey, E., McGuire, M., Mitchell, M.C., Herlong, H.F., Veech, G.A. and Veech, R.L. (1990). Plasma tumour necrosis factor predicts decreased long term survival in severe alcoholic hepatitis. *Alcoholism: Clinical and Experimental Research* **14**, 255–259.

Fernandez, L.A., Laltoo, M. and Fox, R. (1982). A study of T cell populations in alcoholic cirrhosis and chronic alcoholism. *Clinical and Investigative Medicine* **5**, 241–245.

Finlayson, N.D.C., Krohn, K. Fauconnet, N.H. and Anderson, K.E. (1972). Significance of serum complement levels in chronic liver disease. *Gastroenterology* **63**, 653–658.

Fleming, K.A. and McGee, J.O'D. (1984). Alcohol induced liver disease. *Journal of Clinical Pathology* **37**, 721–733.

Fox, R.A., Dudley, F.J. and Sherlock, S. (1971). The serum concentration of the third component of complement B1C-B1A in liver disease. *Gut* **12**, 574–578.

Franco, D., Charra, M., Jeanbrun, P., Belghiti, J., Cortesse, A., Sossler, C. and Bismuth, M. (1983). Nutrition and immunity after peritoneovenous drainage of intractable ascites in cirrhotic patients. *American Journal of Surgery* **144**, 652–657.

Frazer, I.H., Kronborg, I.J. and Mackay, I.R. (1983). Antibodies to liver membrane antigens in chronic active hepatitis (CAH). II. Specificity for autoimmune CAH. *Clinical and Experimental Immunology* **54**, 213–218.

French, S.W. (1981). The Mallory body: Structure, composition and pathogenesis. *Hepatology* **1**, 76–83.

French, S.W., Burbige, E.J., Tarder, G., Bourke, E., Harkin, C. and Denton, T. (1979). Lymphocyte sequestration by the liver in alcoholic hepatitis. *Archives of Pathology and Laboratory Medicine* **103**, 146–152.

Freni, M.A., Ajello, A. and Resta, G. (1985). Lymphocyte subsets in liver and blood from patients with alcoholic liver disease. *Journal of Hepatology* **S1**, 54.

Giron, J.A., Alvarez-Mon, M., Menendez-Caro, J.L., Abreu, L., Albillos, A., Manzano, L. and Durantez, A. (1992). Increased spontaneous and lymphokine-conditioned IgA and IgG synthesis by B cells from alcoholic cirrhotic patients. *Hepatology* **16**, 664–670.

Gluud, C. and Tage-Jensen, U. (1981). Antigenic alterations of liver cell membrane in alcoholics. *Lancet* **ii**, 1285.

Gluud, C., Tage-Jensen, U., Bahnsen, M., Dietrichson, O. and Svejgaard, A. (1981a). Autoantibodies, HLA and testosterone in males with alcoholic liver cirrhosis. *Clinical and Experimental Immunology* **44**, 31–37.

Gluud, C., Hardt, F., Aldershvile, J., Christoffersen, P., Lyon, M. and Nielson, J. (1981b). Isolation of Mallory bodies and an attempt to demonstrate cell mediated immunity to Mallory bodies isolated in patients with alcoholic liver disease. *Journal of Clinical Pathology* **34**, 1010–1016.

Gluud, C., Tage-Jensen, U., Rubinstein, E. and Henriksen, J.H. (1984). Autoantibodies and immunoglobulins in patients with alcoholic cirrhosis – relation to measurements of hepatic function and haemodynamics. *Digestion* **30**, 1–6.

Goodwin, J.S. and Webb, D.R. (1980). Regulation of the immune response by prostaglandins. *Clinical Immunology and Immunopathology* **15**, 106–122.

Guarner, F., Fremont-Smith, M. and Prieto, J. (1985). Cytoprotective effect of prostaglandin on isolated rat liver cells. *Liver* **5**, 35–39.

Han, H.-M., Kolhatkar, A.A., Marino, M.W., de Jonge, C., Manchester, K.M. and Donner, D.B. (1990). Identification, characterisation and homologous up-regulation of latent (cryptic) receptors for tumor necrosis factor-alpha in rat liver plasma membranes. *Journal of Biological Chemistry* **265**, 18590–18594.

Hill, D.B., Marsano, L.S., Shedlofsky, S.I., Talwalkar, R., Murali, N.S. and McClain, C.J. (1992). Increased plasma interleukin-8 levels in alcoholic hepatitis. *Hepatology* **16**, 133A.

Hislop, W.S., Bouchier, I.A.D., Allan, J.G., Brunt, P.W., Eastwood, M., Finlayson, N.D., James, O., Russell, R.I. and Watkinson, G. (1983). Alcoholic liver disease in Scotland and Northeastern England: Presenting features in 510 patients. *Quarterly Journal of Medicine* **206**, 232–243.

Hoerner, M., Behrens, U.J., Worner, T.M., Blackberg, I., Braly, L.F., Schaffner, F. and Lieber, C.S. (1988). The role of alcoholism and liver disease in the appearance of serum antibodies against acetaldehyde adducts. *Hepatology* **8**, 569–574.

Holdstock, G., Ershler, W.B. and Krawitt, W.L. (1982). Demonstration of non-specific B cell stimulation in patients with cirrhosis. *Gut* **23**, 724–728.

Hopf, U., Meyer zum Buschenfelde, K.H. and Arnold, W. (1976). Detection of a liver membrane autoantibody in HBsAg negative chronic active hepatitis. *New England Journal of Medicine* **294**, 578–582.

Hopf, U., Brandtzaeg, P., Hutteroth T.H. and Meyer zum Buschenfelde, K.H. (1978). *In vivo* and *in vitro* binding of IgA to the plasma membrane of hepatocytes. *Scandinavian Journal of Immunology* **8**, 543–439.

Israel, Y., Hurwitz, B., Niemela, O. and Arnon, R. (1986). Monoclonal and polyclonal antibodies against acetaldehyde-containing epitopes in acetaldehyde–protein adducts. *Proceedings of the National Academy of Sciences, USA* **83**, 7923–7927.

Itturiaga, H., Pereda, T., Estevez, A. and Ugarte, T. (1977). Serum immunoglobulin A changes in alcoholic patients. *Annals of Clinical Research* **9**, 39–43.

Izumi, N., Hasumura, Y. and Takeuchi, J. (1983). Lymphocyte cytotoxicity for autologous human hepatocytes in alcoholic liver disease. *Clinical and Experimental Immunology* **53**, 219–224.

Izumi, N., Sato, C., Hasumura, Y. and Takeuchi, J. (1985). Serum antibodies against alcohol-treated rabbit hepatocytes in patients with alcoholic liver disease. *Clinical and Experimental Immunology* **61**, 585–592.

Izumi, N., Sakai, Y., Koyama, W. and Hasumara, Y. (1989). Clinical significance of serum antibodies against alcohol-altered hepatocyte membrane in alcoholic liver disease. *Alcoholism: Clinical and Experimental Research* **13**, 762–765.

Jori, G.D., Buonnana, G., D'Onofrio, F., Tirelli, A., Gonnella, F. and Gentile, S. (1977). Incidence and immunochemical features of serum cryoglobulin in chronic liver disease. *Gut* **18**, 245–249.

Kakumu, S. and Leevy, C.M. (1977). Lymphocyte toxicity in alcoholic hepatitis. *Gastroenterology* **72**, 594–597.

Kalsi, J., Delacroix, D.L. and Hodgson, H.J. (1983). IgA in alcoholic cirrhosis. *Clinical and Experimental Immunology* **52**, 499–504.

Kanagasundaram, N., Kakumu, S., Chen, T. and Leevy, C.M. (1977). Alcoholic hyaline antigen (AHAg) and antibody (AHAb) in alcoholic hepatitis. *Gastroenterology* **73**, 1368–1373.

Kaufman, R.L., Hoefs, J.C., Quismorio, F.C. and Tong, M. (1979). Circulating immune complexes in patients with alcoholic liver disease. *Clinical Research* **27**, 38A.

Kawamura, Y., Saito, S., Tamaki, K., Aoyagi, T. and Yamamoto, H. (1983). Observations on lymphocyte subsets defined by monoclonal antibodies in alcoholics without hepatic dysfunction. *Hepatology* **3**, 1046.

Kawanishi, H., Tavassoli, H., McDermot, R.P. and Sheagren, J.N. (1981). Impaired concanavalin A inducible suppressor T cell activity in active alcoholic liver disease. *Gastroenterology* **80**, 510–517.

Kehl, A., Schober, A., Junge, U. and Winckler, K. (1981). Solid phase radioimmunoassay for detection of alcoholic hyaline antigen (AHAg) and antibody (anti-AH). *Clinical and Experimental Immunology* **43**, 214–221.

Khoruts, A., Stahnke, L., McClain, C.J., Logan, G. and Allen, J.I. (1991). Circulating tumour necrosis factor, interleukin-1 and interleukin-6 concentrations in chronic alcoholic patients. *Hepatology* **13**, 267–276.

Kleinman, R.E., Harmatz, P.R. and Walker, W.A. (1982). The liver: An intergral part of the enteric mucosal immune system. *Hepatology* **2**, 379–384.

Koskinas, J., Kenna, J.G., Bird, G.L., Alexander, G.J.M. and Williams, R. (1992). Immunoglobulin A antibody to a 200 kilodalton cytosolic acetaldehyde adduct in alcoholic hepatitis. *Gastroenterology* **103**, 1060–1067.

Koskinas, J., Winrow, V., Bird, G., Alexander, G.J.M. and Williams, R. (1993). Hepatic 65 kDa heat shock protein in alcoholic hepatitis. *Hepatology* **17**, 1047–1051.

Kourilsky, O., Leroy, C. and Pelyier, A.P. (1973). Complement and liver cell function in 53 patients with liver disease. *American Journal of Medicine* **55**, 783–790.

Krogsgaard, K., Tage-Jensen, U. and Gluud, C. (1982). Liver membrane antibodies in alcoholic liver disease. *Lancet* **i**, 1365–1366.

Kurki, P., Miettinen, A., Salaspuro, M., Virtanen, I. and Stenman, S. (1983). Cytoskeleton antibodies in chronic active hepatitis, primary biliary cirrhosis and alcoholic liver disease. *Hepatology* **3**, 297–302.

Lahnborg, G., Friman, L. and Bergham, L. (1981). Reticuloendothelial function in patients with alcoholic liver cirrhosis. *Scandinavian Journal of Gastroenterology* **16**, 481–489.

Laskin, C.A., Vidins, E., Blendis, L.M. and Soloninka, C.A. (1990). Autoantibodies in alcoholic liver disease. *American Journal of Medicine* **89**, 129–133.

Ledesma, F., Echevarria, S., Casafont, F., Lozano, J.L. and Pons-Romero, F. (1990). Natural killer cell activity in alcoholic cirrhosis: Influence of nutrition. *European Journal of Clinical Nutrition* **44**, 733–740.

Leevy, C.M., Zetterman, R.K. and Chen, T. (1975). Alcoholic liver pathology. In *Alcoholic Liver Pathology* (Edited by Khanna, J.M., Israel, Y. and Kalant, H.), p. 157. Addiction Research Foundation of Ontario, Toronto.

Lehmann, V., Freudenberg, M.A. and Galanos, C. (1987). Lethal toxicity of lipopolysaccharide and tumor necrosis factor in normal and D-galactosamine treated mice. *Journal of Experimental Medicine* **165**, 657–663.

Lelbach, W.K. (1975). Quantitative aspects of drinking in alcoholic liver cirrhosis. In *Alcoholic Liver Pathology* (Edited by Khanna, J.M., Israel, Y. and Kalant, H.), pp. 1–18. Addiction Research Foundation of Ontario, Toronto.

Lieber, C.S. (1993). Biochemical factors in alcoholic liver disease. *Seminars in Liver Disease* **13**, 136–153.

Lin, R.C., Smith, R.C. and Lumeng, L. (1988). Detection of a protein acetaldehyde adduct in the liver of rats fed alcohol chronically. *Journal of Clinical Investigation* **31**, 615–619.

Lomax Smith, J.D., Zabrowarny, L.A., Howath, G.S., Seymour, A.E. and Woodroffe, A.J. (1983). The immunochemical characterisation of mesangial IgA deposits. *American Journal of Pathology* **113**, 359–364.

Luisada-Opper, A.V., Kanagasundaram, N. and Leevy, C.M. (1977). Chemical nature of alcoholic hyalin. *Gastroenterology* **73**, 1374–1376.

Lundy, J., Raaf, J.H. and Deakins, S. (1975). The acute and chronic effects of alcohol on the immune system. *Surgery, Gynaecology and Obstetrics* **141**, 212–218.

MacGregor, R.R. (1990). *In vivo* neutrophil delivery in men with alcoholic cirrhosis is normal despite depressed *in vitro* chemotaxis. *Alcoholism: Clinical and Experimental Research* **14**, 195–199.

MacSween, R.N.M. (1978). Alcoholic liver disease. In *Recent Advances in Histopathology* (Edited by Anthony, P.P. and Woolf, N.), pp. 193–212. Churchill Livingstone, Edinburgh.

Mallory, F.B. (1911). Cirrhosis of the liver: Five different types of disease from which it may arise. *Johns Hopkins Medical Journal* **22**, 69–75.

Mannik, M., Arend, W.P., Hall, A.P. and Filliland, B.C. (1971). Studies on antigen–antibody complexes. 1. Elimination of soluble complexes from rabbit circulation. *Journal of Experimental Medicine* **133**, 713–739.

Marbet, U.A., Bianchi, L., Meury, U. and Stalder, G.A. (1987). Long term histological evaluation of the natural history and prognostic factors of alcoholic liver disease. *Journal of Hepatology* **4**, 364–373.

Maxwell, W.J., Keating, J.J., Hogan, F.P., Kennedy, N.P. and Keeling, P.W.N. (1989). Prostaglandin E_2 and leukotriene B_4 synthesis by peripheral leucocytes in alcoholics. *Gut* **30**, 1270–1274.

McClain, C.J. (1991). Tumour necrosis factor and alcoholic hepatitis. *Hepatology* **14**, 394–396.

McClain, C.J. and Cohen, D.A. (1989). Increased tumor necrosis factor production by monocytes in alcoholic hepatitis. *Hepatology* **9**, 349–351.

McClain, C.J., Cohen, D.A., Dinarello, C.A., Cannon, J.G., Shedlofsky, S.I. and Kaplan, A.M. (1986). Serum interleukin-1 activity in alcoholic hepatitis. *Life Sciences* **39**, 1479–1485.

McFarlane, I.G. (1984). Autoimmunity in liver disease. *Clinical Science* **67**, 569–578.

McFarlane, I.G., McFarlane, B.M., Major, G.N., Tolley, P. and Williams, R. (1984). Identification of the hepatic asialoglycoprotein receptor (hepatic lectin) as a component of liver specific membrane lipoprotein (LSP). *Clinical and Experimental Immunology* **55**, 347–354.

McGeorge, J., Frazer, I.H. and Cunningham, A. (1984). Autoantibodies, sheep cell agglutinins and anti-albumin antibodies in alcoholic liver disease. *Journal of Clinical and Laboratory Immunology* **13**, 21–24.

McKeever, U., O'Mahoney, C., Whelan, C.E., Weir, D.G. and Feighery, C. (1985). Helper and suppressor T lymphocyte function in severe alcoholic liver disease. *Clinical and Experimental Immunology* **60**, 39–48.

Meliconi, R., Miglio, F., Stancari, M.V., Baraldini, M., Stefanini, G.F. and Gasbarrini, G. (1983). Hepatocyte membrane bound IgG and circulating liver-specific antibodies in chronic liver disease: Relation to hepatitis B serum markers and liver histology. *Hepatology* **3**, 155–161.

Milani, S., Herbst, H., Schuppan, D. *et al.* (1991). Transforming growth factor 1 and 2 are differentially expressed in fibrotic liver disease. *American Journal of Pathology* **139**: 1221–1229.

Millan, M.S., Morris, G.P., Beck, I.T. and Henson, J.T. (1980). Villous damage induced by suction damage and by acute ethanol intake in normal human small intestine. *Digestive Diseases and Sciences* **25**, 513–525.

Mills, P.R., Shenkin, A., Anthony, R.S., McLelland,

A.S., Main, A.N., MacSween, R.N.M. and Russell, R.I. (1983). Assessment of nutritional status and *in vitro* immune responses in alcoholic liver disease. *American Journal of Clinical Nutrition* **38**, 849–859.

Montoliu, J., Darnell, A., Torras, A. and Revert, L. (1986). Glomerular disease in cirrhosis of the liver: Low frequency of IgA deposits. *American Journal of Nephrology* **6**, 199–205.

Morgan, M.Y., Ross, M.G.R., Ng, C.R., Adams, D.M., Thomas, H.C. and Sherlock, S. (1980). HLA B8, immunoglobulins, and antibody responses in alcohol-related liver disease. *Journal of Clinical Pathology* **33**, 488–492.

Morton, J.A., Bastin, J., Fleming, K.A., McMichael, A., Burns, J. and McGee, J.O'D. (1981). Mallory bodies in alcoholic liver disease: Identification of cytoplasmic filament/cell membrane and unique antigenic determinants by monoclonal antibodies. *Gut* **22**, 1–7.

Muller, C., Wolf, H., Gottlicher, J. and Eibl, M.M. (1990). Phenotypic analysis of lymphocytes involved in major histocompatibility complex unrestricted cellular cytotoxicity in patients with alcoholic cirrhosis. *International Archives of Allergy and Applied Immunology* **91**, 329–334.

Muller, C., Wolf, H., Gottlicher, J. and Eibl, M.M. (1991). Helper inducer and suppressor inducer lymphocyte subsets in alcoholic cirrhosis. *Scandinavian Journal of Gastroenterology* **26**, 295–301.

Munoz, L.E., de Villiers, D., Markham, D., Whaley, K. and Thomas, H.C. (1982). Complement activation in chronic liver disease. *Clinical and Experimental Immunology* **47**, 548–554.

Mutchnick, M.G. and Keren, D.F. (1981). *In vitro* synthesis of antibody to specific bacterial lipopolysaccharide by peripheral blood mononuclear cells from patients with alcoholic cirrhosis. *Immunology* **43**, 177–182.

Nagore, N. and Scheuer, P.J. (1988). Does a linear pattern of sinusoidal IgA deposition distinguish between alcoholic and diabetic liver disease? *Liver* **8**, 281–286.

Nagura, H., Smith, P.D., Nakane, P.K. and Brown, W.R. (1981). IgA in human bile and liver. *Journal of Immunology* **126**, 587–595.

Nagy, P., Schaff, Z. and Lapis, K. (1992). Immunohistochemical detection of transforming growth factor-ß$_1$ in fibrotic liver diseases. *Hepatology* **14**, 269–273.

Nelson, S., Bagby, D.J., Bainton, B.G. and Summer, W.R. (1989). The effects of acute and chronic alcoholism on tumor necrosis factor and the inflammatory response. *Journal of Infectious Diseases* **160**, 422–429.

Neuberger, J., Crossley, I.R., Saunders, J.B., Davis, M., Portmann, B., Eddleston, A.L.W.F. and Williams, R. (1984). Antibodies to alcohol altered liver cell determinants in patients with alcoholic liver disease. *Gut* **25**, 300–304.

Niemela, O., Orrego, H. and Israel, Y. (1986). Antibodies against acetaldehyde-containing epitopes in human alcoholics. *Hepatology* **6**, 1105.

Nouri Aria, K.T., Alexander, G.J.M., Portmann, B.P., Hegarty, J.E., Eddleston, A.L.W.F. and Williams, R. (1986). T and B cell function in alcoholic liver disease. *Journal of Hepatology* **2**, 195–207.

O'Keefe, S.J., El-Zayadi, A.R., Carraher, T.E., Davis, M. and Williams, R. (1980). Malnutrition and immunocompetence in patients with liver disease. *Lancet* **ii**, 615–616.

Pares, A., Cabellaria, J., Bruguera, M., Torres, M. and Rodes, J. (1986). Histological course of alcoholic hepatitis: Influence of abstinence, sex and extent of hepatic damage. *Journal of Hepatology* **2**, 33–42.

Paronetto, F. and Lieber, C.S. (1976). Cytotoxicity of lymphocytes in experimental liver injury in the baboon. *Proceedings of the Society of Experimental Biology and Medicine* **153**, 495–497.

Paronetto, F. and Popper, H. (1966). Chronic liver injury induced by immunogenic reactions. Cirrhosis following immunization with heterologous sera. *American Journal of Pathology* **49**, 1087–1101.

Pelletier, G., Segond, P., Attali, P., Briantais, M.J. and Etienne, J.P. (1984). T lymphocyte populations in alcoholic liver disease. *Gastroenterology and Clinical Biology* **8**, 911–914.

Penner, E., Albini, B. and Milgrom, F. (1978). Detection of circulating immune complexes in alcoholic liver disease. *Clinical and Experimental Immunology* **34**, 28–31.

Perperas, A., Tsantoulas, D., Portmann, B., Eddleston, A.L.W.F. and Williams, R. (1981). Autoimmunity to a liver membrane lipoprotein and liver damage in alcoholic liver disease. *Gut* **22**, 149–153.

Perrin, D., Bignon, J.-D., Beaujard, E. and Cheneau, M.L. (1984). T lymphocyte populations in the peripheral blood of patients with alcoholic cirrhosis. *Gastroenterology and Clinical Biology* **8**, 907–910.

Peters, M., Tinberg, H.M. and Govindarajan, S. (1982). Immunocytochemical identity of hepatocellular hyaline in alcoholic and non-alcoholic liver disease. *Liver* **2**, 361–368.

Peters, M., Liebman, H.A., Tong, M.J. and Tinberg, M.M. (1983). Alcoholic hepatitis: Granulocyte chemotactic factor from Mallory body stimulated human peripheral blood mononuclear cells. *Clinical Immunology and Immmunopathology* **28**, 418–430.

Pirrone, S., Tosato, F., Rossi, P., Fossaluzzi, V., Torutti, E. and Sala, P.G. (1983). T cell subsets in peripheral blood and ascitic fluid of patients with alcoholic liver cirrhosis. *Lancet* **2**, 518.

Pomier-Layrargues, G., Huet, P.-M. and Richer, G. (1980). Hyperglobulinaemia in alcoholic cirrhosis: Relationship with portal hypertension and intrahepatic portal systemic shunting as assessed by Kuppfer cell uptake. *Digestive Diseases and Sciences* **25**, 489–493.

Pons Romero, F., Echevarria, S., Rodriguez de Lope, C. and San Miguel, G. (1984). Suppressor T cell activity and antibodies to alcohol altered hepatocytes. *Journal of Clinical Pathology* **37**, 598 .

Poralla, T., Hutteroth, T.H. and Meyer zum Buschenfelde, K.H. (1984). Cellular cytotoxicity against autologous hepatocytes in alcoholic liver disease. *Liver* **4**, 117–121.

Preisegger, K.-H., Zatloukal, K., Spurej, L. and Denk, H. (1991). Changes of cytokeratin filament organisation in human and murine Mallory body containing livers as revealed by a panel of monoclonal antibodies. *Liver* **11**, 300–309.

Prytz, H., Holst-Christensen, J., Korner, B. and Liehr, H. (1976). Portal venous and systemic endotoxaemia in patients without liver disease and systemic endotoxaemia in patients with cirrhosis. *Scandinavian Journal of Gastroenterology* **11**, 857–863.

Rajkovic, I.A. and Williams, R. (1985). Mechanisms of abnormalities in host defences against bacterial infection in liver disease. *Clinical Science* **68**, 247–253.

Reynolds, T.B., Benhamou, J.-P., Blake, J., Naccarato, R. and Orrego, H. (1989). Treatment of acute alcoholic hepatitis. *Gastroenterology International* **2**, 208–216.

Robbins, R.A., Zetterman, R.K., Kendall, T.J., Gossman, G.L., Mansour, H.P. and Rennard, S.I. (1987). Elevation of chemotactic factor inactivator in alcoholic liver disease. *Hepatology* **7**, 872–877.

Robinson, G.M., Orrego, H. and Israel, Y. (1981). Low molecular weight polyethylene glycol as a probe of gastrointestinal permeability after alcohol ingestion. *Digestive Diseases and Sciences* **26**, 971–977.

Rodriguez, M.A., Montano, J.D. and Williams, R.C. (1984). Immunoglobulin production by peripheral blood mononuclear cells in patients with alcoholic liver disease. *Clinical and Experimental Immunology* **55**, 369–376.

Rong, P.B., Kalsi, J. and Hodgson, H.J.F. (1984). Hyperglobulinaemia in chronic liver disease: Relationships between *in vitro* immunoglobulin synthesis, short lived suppressor cell activity and serum immunoglobulin levels. *Clinical and Experimental Immunology* **55**, 546–552.

Roselle, G.A. and Mendenhall, C.L. (1984). Ethanol induced alterations in lymphocyte function in the guinea pig. *Alcoholism: Clinical and Experimental Research* **8**, 62–67.

Roselle, G.A., Mendenhall, C.L., Grossman, C.J. and Weesner, R.E. (1988). Lymphocyte subset alterations in patients with alcoholic hepatitis. *Journal of Clinical and Laboratory Immunology* **26**, 169–173.

Russell, M.W., Mestecky, J., Julian, B.A. and Galla, J.H. (1986). IgA associated renal diseases: Antibodies to environmental antigens in sera and deposition of immunoglobulins and antigens in glomeruli. *Journal of Clinical Immunology* **6**, 74–86.

Sakai, Y., Izumi, N., Marumo, F. and Sato, C. (1993). Quantitative immunohistochemical analysis of lymphocyte subsets in alcoholic liver disease. *Journal of Gastroenterology and Hepatology* **8**, 39–43.

Samanta, A., Chen, T. and Leevy, C.M. (1985). On the mechanism of progressive liver injury: Altered DNA

and collagen synthesis induced by Mallory bodies. *Gastroenterology* **88**, 1692.

Sanchez-Tapias, J., Thomas, H.C. and Sherlock, S. (1977). Lymphocyte populations in liver biopsy specimens from patients with chronic liver disease. *Gut* **18**, 472–475.

Sancho, J., Egido, J., Sanchez-Crespo, N. and Blasco, R. (1981). Detection of monomeric and polymeric IgA containing immune complexes in serum and kidney in patients with alcoholic liver disease. *Clinical and Experimental Immunology* **47**, 327–335.

Saunders, J.B., Wodak, A.D., Haines, A., Powell-Jackson, R.R., Portmann, B., Davis, M. and Williams, R. (1982). Accelerated development of alcoholic cirrhosis in patients with HLA B8. *Lancet* **i**, 1381–1384.

Sherman, D.I.N., Ward, R.J., Williams, R. and Peters, T.J. (1994). Emerging markers of predisposition to alcoholism. In *Biological Aspects of Alcoholism* (Edited by Tabakoff, B. and Hoffman, P.). WHO Expert Series on Biological Psychiatry. WHO, Geneva (in press).

Sheron, N., Bird, G., Goka, A.K.J., Alexander, G.J.M. and Williams, R. (1991). Elevated plasma interleukin-6 and increased severity and mortality in alcoholic hepatitis. *Clinical and Experimental Immunology* **84**, 449–453.

Sheron, N., Keane, H., Bird, G.L.A., Galliati, H. and Williams, R. (1992). Soluble TNF receptors in acute alcoholic hepatitis. *Journal of Hepatology* **16**, S63.

Sheron, N., Bird, G.L.A., Koskinas, J., Ceska, M., Lindley, I., Portmann, B. and Williams, R. (1993). Circulating and tissue levels of the neutrophil chemotaxin interleukin-8 are elevated in severe acute alcoholic hepatitis and tissue levels correlate with neutrophil infiltration. *Hepatology* **18**, 41–46.

Shiratori, Y., Takada, H., Hikiba, Y., Nakata, R., Okano, K., Komatsu, Y., Niwa, Y., Matsumura, M., Shiina, S., Onata, M. and Kamii, K. (1993). Production of chemotactic factor interleukin-8 from hepatocytes exposed to ethanol. *Hepatology* **18**, 1477–1482.

Si, L., Whiteside, T.L., Schade, R.R. and Van Thiele, D. (1983). Lymphocyte subsets studied with monoclonal antibodies in liver tissue of patients with alcoholic liver disease. *Alcoholism: Clinical and Experimental Research* **7**, 431–435.

Sorensen, T.I.A., Orholm, M., Bentsen., K.D., Hoybye, G., Eghoje, K. and Christoffersen, P. (1984). Prospective evaluation of alcohol abuse and alcoholic liver injury in men as predictors of development of cirrhosis. *Lancet* **ii**, 241–244.

Sorrell, M.F. and Leevy, C.M. (1972). Lymphocyte transformation and alcoholic liver injury. *Gastroenterology* **63**, 1020–1025.

Sorrell, M.F. and Tuma, D.J. (1985). Hypothesis: Alcoholic liver injury and the covalent binding of acetaldehyde. *Alcoholism: Clinical and Experimental Research* **9**, 306–309.

Spinozzi, F., Bertotto, A., Rondoni, F., Gerli, R., Scalise, F. and Grignani, F. (1991). T lymphocyte activation pathways in alcoholic liver disease. *Immunology* **73**, 140–146.

Staun-Olsen, P., Bjorneboe, M., Prytz, H., Thomsen, A.C. and Orskov, F. (1983). *Escherichia coli* antibodies in alcoholic liver disease: Correlation to alcohol consumption, alcoholic hepatitis and serum IgA. *Scandinavian Journal of Gastroenterology* **18**, 889–896.

Swerdlow, M.A., Chowdhury, L.N. and Horn, T. (1982). Patterns of IgA deposition in liver tissues in alcoholic liver disease. *American Journal of Clinical Pathology* **77**, 259–266.

Tage-Jensen, U., Arnold, W., Dietrichson, O., Hardt, F., Hopf, U., Meyer zum Buschenfelde, K.H. and Nielsen, J.O. (1987). Liver cell membrane autoantibody specific for inflammatory liver disease. *British Medical Journal* **1**, 206–208.

Takase, S., Takada, N. and Enomoto, N. (1991). Different types of chronic hepatitis in alcoholic patients: Does chronic hepatitis induced by alcohol exist? *Hepatology* **13**, 876–881.

Takase, S., Tsutsumi, M., Kawahara, H., Takade, N. and Takada, A. (1993). The alcohol-altered liver membrane antibody and hepatitis C virus infection in the progression of alcoholic liver disease. *Hepatology* **17**, 9–13.

Thestrup-Petersen, K., Ladegoged, K. and Andersen, P. (1976). Lymphocyte transformation test with liver specific protein and phytohaemoglutinin in patients with liver disease. *Clinical and Experimental Immunology* **24**, 1–8.

Thiele, D.L. (1989). Tumor necrosis factor, the acute phase response and the pathogenesis of alcoholic liver disease. *Hepatology* **9**, 497–499.

Thomas, H.C., Freni, M., Sanchez-Tapias, J., de Villiers, D., Jain, S. and Sherlock, S. (1976). Peripheral blood lymphocyte populations in chronic liver disease. *Clinical and Experimental Immunology* **26**, 222–227.

Thomas, H.C., De Villiers, D., Potter, B., Hodgson, H., Jain, S., Jewell, D.P.P. and Sherlock, S. (1978). Immune complexes in acute and chronic liver disease. *Clinical and Experimental Immunology* **31**, 150–157.

Thompson, R.A., Carter, R., Stones, R.P., Geddes, A.M. and Goodall, J.A.D. (1973). Serum immunoglobulins, complement component levels and autoantibodies in liver disease. *Clinical and Experimental Immunology* **14**, 335–346.

Tracey, K.J., Fong, Y., Hesse, D.G., Marogue, K.R., Lee, A.T., Kuo, G.C., Lowry, S.F. and Cerami, A. (1987). Anti-cachectin/TNF monoclonal antibodies prevent septic shock during lethal bacteraemia. *Nature* **330**, 662–664.

Treichel, U., Poralla, T., Hess, G., Manns, M. and Meyer zum Buschenfelde, K.H. (1990). Autoantibodies to asialoglycoprotein receptor in autoimmune-type chronic hepatitis. *Hepatology* **11**, 606–612.

Trevison, A., Cavigli, R., Meliconi, R., Stefanini, G.F., Zotti, S., Rugge, M., Noventa, F., Betterle, C. and Realdi, G. (1983). Detection of immunoglobulin G and A on the cell membrane of hepatocyte from patients with alcoholic liver disease. *Journal of Clinical Pathology* **36**, 530–534.

Triger, D.R., Alp, M.H. and Wright, R. (1972). Bacterial and dietary antibodies in liver disease. *Lancet* **i**, 60–63.

Triger, D.R., Boyer, T.D., Redeker, A.D., Reynolds, T.B. and Waxman, A.D. (1979). Differences in intrahepatic portal-systemic shunting in alcoholic and non-alcoholic liver disease as assessed by liver scan, portal pressure and *E. coli* antibodies. *Digestive Diseases and Sciences* **24**, 509–513.

Triggs, S.M., Mills, P.R. and MacSween, R.N.M. (1981). Sensitisation to Mallory bodies (alcoholic hyaline) in alcoholic hepatitis. *Journal of Clinical Pathology* **34**, 21–24.

Trudell, J.R., Ardies, M. and Anderson, W.R. (1990). Cross-reactivity of antibodies raised against acetaldehyde adducts of protein with acetaldehyde adducts of phosphatidylethanolamine: Possible role in alcoholic cirrhosis. *Molecular Pharmacology* **38**, 587–593.

Tuma, D.J. and Klassen, L.W. (1993). Immune responses to acetaldehyde–protein adducts: Role in alcoholic liver disease. *Gastroenterology* **103**, 1969–1972.

Vaerman, J.P. and Delacroix, D.L. (1984). Role of the liver in the immunobiology of IgA in animals and humans. *Contributions to Nephrology* **40**, 17–31.

Van de Wiel, A. (1986). Immunoglobulin A and alcoholic liver disease. Thesis, University of Utrecht.

Van de Wiel, A., Schuurman, H.A. and Kater, L. (1985). Immunoglobulin A in alcoholic liver disease: Studies on serum, tissues and cells. *Plasma Therapeutics and Transfusion Technology* **6**, 733–740.

Van de Wiel, A., van Riessen, D., Haaijman, J.J., Radl, J., Delacroix, D.L., Van Hattum, J., Blok, A.P.R. and Kater, L. (1986). Characteristics of IgA deposits in liver and skin of patients with liver disease. *American Journal of Clinical Pathology* **86**, 724–730.

Van de Wiel, A., Delacroix, D.L., Van Hattum, J., Schuurman, H.J. and Kater, L. (1987). Characteristics of serum IgA and liver IgA deposits in alcoholic liver disease. *Hepatology* **7**, 95–99.

Van Epps, E., Husby, G., Williams, R.C. and Strickland, R.G. (1976). Liver disease – a prominent cause of serum IgE elevation. *Clinical and Experimental Immunology* **23**, 444–450.

Vicente-Gutierrez, M.M., Ruiz, D., Gil Extremura, B., Bermudez Garcia, J.M. and Guttierrez Gea, F. (1991). Low levels of alpha-interferon, gamma-interferon and interleukin-2 in alcoholic cirrhosis. *Digestive Diseases and Sciences* **36**, 1209–1212.

Volpes, R., Van den Oord, J.J. and De Vos, R. (1992). Hepatic expression of type A and type B receptors for tumour necrosis factor. *Journal of Hepatology* **14**, 361–369.

Waage, A., Brandtzaeg, P., Halstensen A., Kierulf, P. and Espevik, T. (1989). The complex pattern of cytokines in serum of patients with meningococcal septic shock. *Journal of Experimental Medicine* **169**, 333–337.

Wagner, F., Fink, R., Hart, R., Lersch, C., Dancygier, H. and Classen, M. (1992). Ethanol inhibits interferon-gamma secretion by human peripheral lymphocytes. *Journal of Studies on Alcohol* **53**, 277–280.

Wands, J.R., Dienstag, J.L. and Weake, J.R. (1981). *In vitro* studies of enhanced IgG synthesis in severe alcoholic liver disease. *Clinical and Experimental Immunology* **44**, 396–404.

Watson, R., Jackson, J.C. and Hartman, R. (1985). Cellular immune function, endorphins and alcohol consumption in males. *Alcoholism: Clinical and Experimental Research* **9**, 248–254.

Webb, L., Ross, M. and Markham, R.L. (1980). Immune function in patients with extrahepatic portal venous obstruction and the effects of splenectomy. *Gastroenterology* **79**, 99–103.

Wickramasinghe, S.N., Gardner, B. and Barden, G. (1987). Circulating cytotoxic protein generated after ethanol consumption: Identification and mechanism of reaction with cells. *Lancet* **ii**, 122–126.

Woodroffe, A.J. (1981). IgA, glomerulonephritis and liver disease. *Australian and New Zealand Journal of Medicine* **11**, 109–111.

Yokoyama, H., Ishii, H., Nagata, S., Kato, S., Kamegaya, K. and Tsuchiya, M. (1993). Experimental hepatitis induced by ethanol after immunisation with acetaldehyde adducts. *Hepatology* **17**, 14–19.

Young, G.P., Dudley, F.J. and Van der Weyden, M.B. (1979). Suppressive effect of alcoholic liver disease sera on lymphocyte transformation. *Gut* **20**, 833–839.

Zatloukal, K., Denk, H., Spurej, G. *et al.* (1990). High molecular weight component of Mallory bodies detected by a monoclonal antibody. *Laboratory Investigation* **62**, 427–434.

Zauli, D., Crespi, C. and Dall'Amore, P. (1985). Relationship between cytoskeleton and smooth muscle antibodies (SMA) in chronic liver disease. *Journal of Hepatology* **1**, S155.

Zetterman, R.K., Luisada-Opper, A. and Leevy, C.M. (1976). Alcoholic hepatitis. Cell-mediated immunological response to alcoholic hyaline. *Gastroenterology* **70**, 382–384.

7 Increased susceptibility of women to alcoholic liver disease: Artifactual or real?

Judith S. Gavaler and Amelia M. Arria

Introduction

The question of whether or not women are more susceptible than men to alcoholic liver disease is embedded in the larger issue of our inability to definitively identify the specific intrinsic characteristics of an individual of either gender which confer a lack of capability to resist alcohol damage to the liver. Definitive identification of susceptibility factors will require studies in which the cases of alcohol-induced liver disease have progressed to the ultimate endpoint for that individual, and in which the control group is comprised of individuals who can be defined as having been truly exposed and proven to be non-susceptible; identification of such cases and controls represents no easy task.

Although far from definitive, findings that a relatively small proportion of individuals who habitually "abuse" alcohol ultimately develop alcohol-induced cirrhosis demonstrate the extent of the conundrum. Meta-analysis of 23 biopsy series provides an estimate of the magnitude of the puzzle. Among a total of 5448 biopsied cases, approximately 25 percent had histologic findings of normal liver, 33 percent showed uncomplicated fatty liver, 20 percent showed alcoholic hepatitis alone, and only 25 percent showed cirrhosis (Lelbach 1976). Although these 23 reports analysed as a group are specific neither for dose and duration of alcohol exposure nor for gender, they do nevertheless provide a backdrop for examining the issue of susceptibility to alcoholic liver disease.

To state the obvious: susceptibility requires exposure, and identification of relative susceptibility requires reliable measurement of dose and duration of exposure. In evaluating susceptibility to alcohol-induced liver disease in general, and gender-specific susceptibility in particular, by and large we are limited to retrospective alcohol intake estimates extracted from "alcoholic" individuals who are sick and undergoing treatment for their liver disease, for their alcoholism, or for both. Further, although it has been postulated that women underestimate previous cumulative alcohol consumption to a greater degree than do men, the postulate remains unproven; indeed, in studies in which the *ranges* for reported dose and duration are available for both genders, the considerable overlap in these ranges argues against a gender differential in the self-reporting of alcoholic beverage consumption. Keeping in mind the vagaries of accurately determining alcohol exposure, let us apply them equally to both genders as we evaluate the available literature relevant to the possibility that there exist gender differences in susceptibility to alcoholic liver disease.

Approaches to evaluating the available literature

There are two ways in which to assess the available literature. The first approach would require unequivocal statistical differences between the sexes in relevant variables for alcohol dose and/or duration or in outcome variables such as prevalence of cirrhosis or cirrhosis death rates within all studies. Such an approach would demand the repeated rejection of a null hypothesis of no gender-related difference (Gavaler 1982). The second approach would allow the mosaic of patterns seen across studies to be viewed as sufficient evidence for acceptance of the alternative hypothesis that gender-related differences in alcoholic liver disease susceptibility may indeed obtain. In the absence of data from work performed using the definitive study design of following statistically adequate sample sizes of both young males and females followed for decades with precise monitoring of both alcoholic beverage consumption and status of liver histology, we must carefully evaluate the data that do exist.

If there are gender-related differences in susceptibility to alcoholic liver disease in general and to alcoholic cirrhosis in particular, then several patterns should be evident in the available literature. One piece of evidence might come from studies in which the *precipitating/perpetuating* dose of alcohol differs between female and male cirrhotics compared with controls free from liver disease. A second piece of evidence might come from reports in which alcohol exposure among females with alcoholic liver disease is lower than among males in terms of cumulative dose, regular daily dose, or duration of "excessive" alcohol intake, but the outcome is similar in terms of cirrhosis prevalence or severity of alcoholic liver disease. A third piece of evidence might come from studies in which alcohol exposure is similar but outcome is more severe in females. A fourth piece of evidence might come from studies in which the rate of progression from histologically less severe to more severe liver pathology is greater in females than in males in a setting where either the natural history runs its course or is potentially diverted by the factor of reduced or eliminated ongoing exposure to alcohol.

Precipitating/perpetuating dose of alcohol

If females are more susceptible to alcohol-induced cirrhosis than males, then risk estimates should not only be increased for females at any given level of alcohol intake, but should also be elevated at a lower *precipitating* dose than that seen in males. Table 7.1 shows the results of approximated relative risk cal-

culations using odds ratios and their 95 percent confidence intervals based on data from the available literature (Pequignot *et al.* 1974; Tuyns and Pequignot 1984; Coates *et al.* 1986). Keeping in mind that risk is statistically increased when the lower confidence interval excludes unity (the value of 1.0), several observations are evident. Within studies, although the alcohol dose level used as the risk cutoff point is two-fold lower for females (20 g of absolute ethanol per day for females, 40 g for males), the calculated risk at increasing alcohol intake levels is invariably higher among females. Across studies, this differential relationship holds, although there is variation in the absolute magnitude of the odds ratios and of the differences for these risk estimates between the genders. Finally, as depicted in Fig. 7.1, the slope for the regression equation which describes the change in risk associated with change in alcohol dose level demonstrates a statistically correlated relationship in both sexes, but a statistically steeper change in risk for females compared with males. Further confirmatory studies in females have demonstrated a statistically increased risk of alcohol-induced cirrhosis to occur at a level of 20–40 g ethanol/day (Norton *et al.* 1987). Taken together, the results of these analyses provide strong evidence that alcoholic cirrhosis is produced in females at lower regular daily alcohol exposure doses than in males.

Cumulative dose of alcohol

As enticing as the results of analyses of simple habitual alcohol dose data are, they incorporate no assessment of cumulative alcohol exposure. Specifically, they contain no information about alcohol exposure duration, a necessary component for assessing differential susceptibility. Gender-related differences in cumulative alcohol dose, or in both dose and duration of alcohol exposure, among female and male patients with the same defined degree of liver pathology would provide evidence of differential susceptibility. Five such studies are summarized in Table 7.2. Among these five reports are six independent groups of patients at stages of liver disease severity defined either by histology or by the end-stage complication of ascites.

As may be seen in Table 7.3, in three of the six groups cumulative alcohol exposure is statistically lower among females (Coates *et al.* 1986; Pares *et al.* 1986), and in a fourth group both regular daily dose and duration of alcohol exposure are statistically

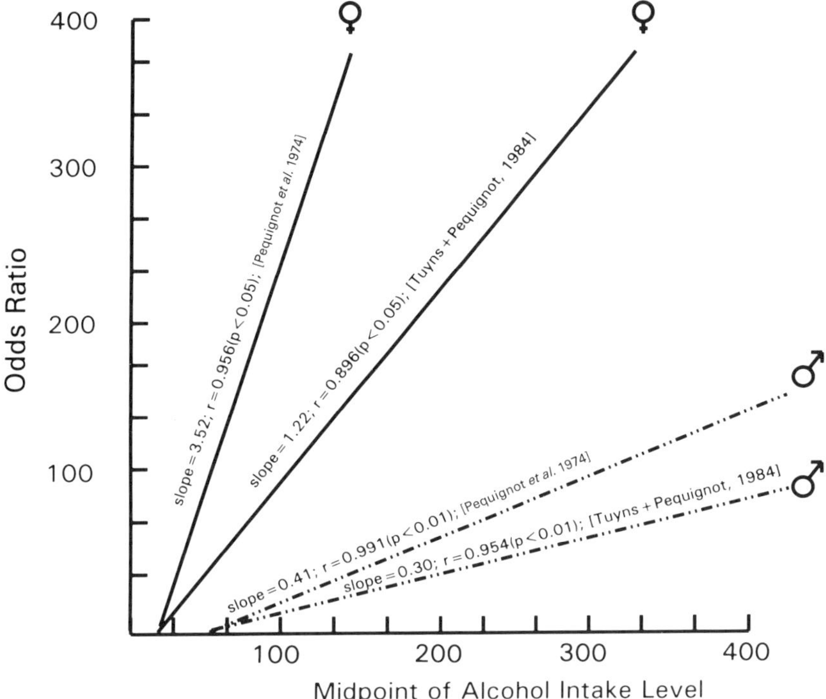

Fig. 7.1 Relationship between estimated risk of alcohol-induced cirrhosis and alcohol dose in females and males. The calculated odds ratio is plotted on the y-axis and the midpoint of each risk alcohol dose level is plotted on the x-axis. The solid (unbroken) lines are regression lines that represent the positive relationship of alcohol-induced cirrhosis risk to alcohol dosage in females. The dotted (broken) lines are regression lines that represent the positive relationship of alcohol-induced cirrhosis risk to alcohol dosage in males. The graph shows that females have a greater risk of alcohol-induced cirrhosis than males at lower midpoints of alcohol intake.

reduced in the females (Arria 1993). In the two remaining study groups, age must be used as a surrogate marker for duration under the conservative assumption that duration is proportional to age; this assumption is biased against a presumption of shorter duration in females. In one of these studies, a significantly larger proportion of females are both younger and reporting a lower habitual daily alcohol dose than males (Tuyns and Pequignot 1984), while in the second study only arithmetically lower regular daily alcohol intake is reported in gender groups of comparable age (Saunders *et al.* 1981b). Viewed together, these reports provide a strikingly consistent pattern spiced with statistical differences of reduced cumulative exposure to alcohol among females compared with males matched for stage of alcohol-induced liver disease.

Prevalence of cirrhosis

Thus far we have not approached the issue of gender-related differences in susceptibility to alcoholic liver disease from the standpoint of severity of liver disease. If we view the presence of cirrhosis as the definitive endpoint, then questions which might arise in relation to the utility of examining differences in the prevalence of less severe, potentially reversible pathology are obviated. More specifically, although denominator problems stemming from the inclusion of reliably ascertained patients at risk of having lesser stages of alcohol damage to the liver remain, numerator problems are diminished. The numerator problems related to the identification of patients with less severe histologic hepatic lesions who may not have been detected because

Table 7.1   Relative risk of cirrhosis (odds ratio with 95% confidence interval)

Authors (year)	Pequignot et al.* (1974)		Tuyns and Pequignot* (1984)		Coates et al. (1986)	
Risk dose level: cases: controls	Female 20g 83:587	Male 40g 144:542	Female 20g 149:1053	Male 40g 268:923	Female 20g 66:191	Male 40g 80:275
Dose (g ETOH/day)						
20-40 or 20-60	2.83 [$] (1.43-5.61)		4.53 [$] (2.70-7.59)		2.53 (1.0-6.4)	
40-60	11.5 [$] (2.41-15.8)	0.94 (0.42-2.11)	22.9 [$] (12.9-40.6)	2.31 [$] (1.33-3.99)		
60-80		1.98 (0.87-4.54)	40.3 [$] (18.0-90.1)	6.34 [$] (3.72-10.8)		1.83 (0.76-4.42)
80-100	109 [$] (31.2-379)	2.01 (0.95-4.02)	34.0 [$] (11.1-104)	13.5 [$] (7.87-23.2)		3.59 (0.96-13.5)
100-120		13.9 [$] (6.42-30.2)		23.6 [$] (13.0-42.9)		
120-140		17.1 [$] (7.27-40.2)		19.6 [$] (9.86-38.9)		
140-160 or 140-180		32.3 [$] (11.8-88.6)		34.6 [$] (12.9-93.1)		
>60	204 [$] (58.2-718)	8.89 [$] (5.15-15.4)	69.3 [$] (36.4-132)	14.8 [$] (9.57-22.8)	12.2 [$] (3.54-42.1)	
>80	396 [$] (42.2-3388)	6.29 [$] (3.59-11.0)	127 [$] (49.5-328)	21.8 [$] (13.8-34.3)		99.9 [$] (31.6-315)
>140		54.3 [$] (23.0-121)		54.1 [$] (27.2-108)		

* calculated using standard methods applied to data provided in the publication
$ lower confidence interval excludes unity; risk is statistically increased.

clinical symptomatology was insufficient to have brought them to the attention of treating physicians are reduced when cirrhosis is used as the endpoint. There are 12 available literature studies in which cirrhosis rates can be examined in evaluating the hypothesis that females are more susceptible than males to alcoholic cirrhosis.

The literature reports available in which cirrhosis rates, often in conjunction with alcohol dose and duration data, can be compared are summarized in Table 7.3. The first three studies report data obtained in essentially the same patient population; the study sample in the second report is an expansion of the sample of the first report, while the study sample of the third report is a selected subsample of the second report (Wilkinson et al. 1969, 1971; Bhathal et al. 1975). In the two reports from Wilkinson and colleagues (1969, 1971), cirrhosis rates among alcoholics being treated for their alcoholism are statistically higher among females than males. Further, both the duration of alcohol abuse at intake levels above 100 g of ethanol per day and habitual daily dose, and thus by extension cumulative alcohol exposure, are statistically lower among the alcoholic females. In the highly selected subgroup, dose and duration differ significantly, although cirrhosis rates do not (Bhathal et al. 1975). The findings in study samples from this large ($n = 1000$) Australian population of alcoholic individuals provide evidence of gender differences in susceptibility to alcohol-induced cirrhosis based on the parameter of a statistically lower level of alcohol exposure among females.

Rates of cirrhosis among patients with biopsy-confirmed alcoholic liver disease in nine available reports are also shown in Table 7.3. The selection criteria used in nine of the 11 studies illustrates a particularly interesting point concerning the denominator problem with which we are confronted. Specifically, risk eligibility has been defined in terms of regular alcohol consumption on a daily basis in excess of 60 g (Hislop et al. 1983), 80 g (Levi and Chalmers 1978; Bhattacharyya and Rake 1983), 88 g (Nakamura et al. 1979), 100 g (Ashley et al. 1977; Krasner et al. 1977; Morgan and Sherlock 1977) or 160 g (Alves et al. 1982). Simply looking again at Table 7.1 emphasizes the point that an index-of-suspicion or lower-limit-for-inclusion setpoint higher than 20 g for females and 40 g for males has the potential to compromise seriously con-

Table 7.2   Dose and duration of alcohol abuse among patients with alcoholic liver disease

Authors (year)	Study Population	Endpoint Lesion	Age	Dose (g ETOH/day)	Duration (years)	Cumulative dose (kg ETOH)
Saunders et al. (1981b)	Defined by >80g ETOH/day and histology. First (?) hospitalization.	cirrhosis	♀ 55 ♂ 53	♀112 ♂152		
Tuyns and Pequignot (1984)	Complete ascertainment of hospitalized cases in defined geographic area. ♀149, ♂268.	cirrhosis with ascites	age < 45 ♀24%* ♂13%	< 40 g ♀43%* ♂10%		
Coates et al. (1986)	Sequentially admitted biopsied patients; causes other than alcohol ruled out.	fatty liver alone	♀ 53 ♂ 45	♀ 22* ♂ 72		♀ 55* ♂ 476
	fatty liver alone: ♀ 47,♂ 47 cirrhosis alone: ♀ 66, ♂ 85	cirrhosis	♀ 55 ♂ 55	♀ 30* ♂ 98		♀ 163* ♂ 499
Parés et al. (1986)	Complete ascertainment of cases presenting to hospital. ♀12, ♂14.	alcoholic hepatitis without cirrhosis	♀ 49 ♂ 47	♀185 ♂215	♀10* ♂19	♀ 633* ♂1389
Arria (1993)	Cases presenting for liver transplant evaluation. ♀66, ♂189.	cirrhosis	at diagnosis ♀ 43 ♂ 45	♀153* ♂234	♀13* ♂17	

* p< at least 0.05.

clusions to be made which rely on absolute total ascertainment of cases of alcoholic liver disease.

Among the nine studies in which the prevalence of cirrhosis among patients with alcoholic liver disease can be compared between females and males, both patterns which may be considered to be indicative of gender-related differences in susceptibility are seen. In two studies, the first pattern is seen – the prevalence of cirrhosis is significantly higher among the females, although alcohol exposure estimates do not differ between the sexes (Nakamura *et al.* 1979; Alves *et al.* 1982). In five studies, the second pattern is seen – cirrhosis rates do not differ significantly between females and males, but estimates of alcohol exposure are statistically lower in the females (Ashley *et al.* 1977; Krasner *et al.* 1977; Bhattacharyya and Rake 1983; Hislop *et al.* 1983; Loft *et al.* 1987). The eighth study detects no statistical differences in the parameters of interest. The eighth study does, however, contain data which arithmetically fit smoothly into the overall mosaic of patterns of differences which provide evidence in support of the hypothesis that females may be more susceptible to alcohol-induced cirrhosis.

Thus far we have used several approaches to evaluate the available literature for evidence of differential alcohol-induced liver disease, namely the estimated relative risk *per se*, increases in relative risk with increasing alcohol dose, and duration and dose of alcohol exposure among patients with alcoholic liver disease in general and cirrhosis in particular. All of these approaches have yielded consistent findings that point to the conclusion that there do appear to be gender differences in susceptibility. An additional approach yet to be explored is an examination of severity of liver disease at time of presentation, and death rates due to cirrhosis, the ultimate marker of severity of disease. Although gender differences in severity of complications or cirrhosis death rates would not provide direct evidence relevant to differential susceptibility within the context of alcohol exposure producing liver damage *per se*, differences in severity or cirrhosis death rates could be viewed as being suggestive of qualitative differences in the course of initiated damage.

Clinical severity of alcoholic liver disease

The data in the literature in which markers of liver disease *severity* can be compared between females and males are summarized in Table 7.4 (Spain 1945; Krasner *et al.* 1977; Morgan and Sherlock 1977; Nakamura *et al.* 1979; Hislop *et al.* 1983; Pares *et al.* 1986; Loft *et al.* 1987). Notwithstanding potential confounding by factors which may result in gender differences at the stage at which patients present

Table 7.3   Prevalence of cirrhosis: Dose and duration of alcohol abuse

Authors (year)	Diagnosis Criteria	Study Population	Duration (years, or years above stated levels)	Dose (g/day)	Age
Wilkinson et al. (1969)	Alcoholism: physical or socio-economic disturbances due to heavy drinking. biopsy >91% of cirrhotics	Patients presenting with cirrhosis to alcoholism clinic. Prevalence of cirrhosis among alcoholics: ♀ 23/137(17%),♂ 54/663(8%).*	>100g/day ♀13* ♂20	♀ 140 * ♂210	♀49 ♂48
Wilkinson et al. (1971)	As above; expanded sample	As above; prevalence of cirrhosis among alcoholics: ♀29/175(17%), ♂ 69/825(8%).*	>100g/day ♀13* ♂19	♀170 * ♂265	♀48 ♂45
Bhathal et al. (1975)	As above; biopsy in 98%	Alcoholism clinic patients hospitalized for alcoholic liver disease. Prevalence of cirrhosis: ♀3/23(13%),♂10/77(13%).	>100g/day ♀13* ♂19	♀165 * ♂245	♀48 ♂44
Ashley et al. (1977)	>100g/day Hazardous drinking, liver function tests, biopsy when indicated.	Hospitalization for alcoholism. Prevalence of cirrhosis among alcoholics: ♀ 9/135(7%), ♂ 46/736(6%); among alcoholics with liver disease: ♀ 9/47(19%), ♂ 46/418(11%).	>100g/day ♀14* ♂20	♀228 * ♂316	♀ 48 ♂ 45
Krasner et al. (1977)	>100g/day regularly biopsy in 100%	Patients admitted with alcoholic liver disease. Prevalence of cirrhosis: ♀ 49/78(63%), ♂ 135/215(63%).		>150g/day ♀ 65% * ♂91%	♀ 52 ♂52
Morgan and Sherlock (1977)	>100g/day regularly biopsy in 97%	Patients admitted with alcoholic liver disease. Prevalence of cirrhosis: ♀ 16/22(73%),♂ 41/75(55%).	♀17 ♂20		♀ 48 ♂ 47
Levi and Chambers (1978)	>80g/day for >1 year biopsy in 100%	Patients admitted with alcoholic liver disease. Prevalence of cirrhosis: ♀ 15/58(26%),♂ 29/144(20%).	♀9 * ♂16	>160g/day ♀ 27%* ♂ 44%	♀ 54 ♂ 53
Nakamura et al. (1979)	>88g/day biopsy in 100%	Patients admitted with alcoholic liver disease. Prevalence of cirrhosis: ♀ 3/7(43%), ♂ 38/123(31%).*	>88g/day ♀11 ♂17	♀ 112 ♂ 117	♀ 43 ♂ 48
Alves et al. (1982)	>160g/day for > 5 years biopsy in 100%	Patients admitted with alcoholic liver disease. Prevalence of cirrhosis: ♀ 112/124(90%), ♂ 265/339(78%). *			<40 yrs ♀14% ♂13%
Bhattacharyya and Rake (1983)	>80g/day for 10-20 years biopsy in 100%	Patients admitted with alcohol abuse; prevelance of cirrhosis among alcohol abusers: ♀10/40(25%),♂ 39/121(32%).		>114g/day ♀ 52%* ♂73%	similar
Hislop et al. (1983)	>60g/day biopsy in 100%	Patients admitted for alcoholic liver disease. Prevalence of cirrhosis: ♀ 46/130(35%), ♂ 155/380(41%).		♀120 * ♂199	♀52 ♂50
Loft et al. (1987)	biopsy in 90%	Patients admitted with newly recognized alcoholic liver disease. Prevalence of cirrhosis: ♀ 8/18(44%), ♂ 15/24(62%).	lifetime total drinks ♀43000* ♂86000		♀ 54 ♂ 54

* p < at least 0.05

Table 7.4   Clinical severity of alcohol-induced liver disease

Authors (year)	Patient population	Evaluation timepoint	Jaundice	Ascites	Hepatic coma	Severity index	Peripheral neuro-pathy	Other
Spain (1945)	cirrhotics: "majority" alcoholics	autopsy	♀ 48% [*] ♂ 24%	♀ 47% [@] ♂ 37%				
Krasner et al. (1977)	alcoholic liver disease	at presentation to hospital						collateral shunting (splenic peak count rate): ♀ 55300 cpm ♂ 27350 cpm
Morgan and Sherlock (1977)	alcoholic liver disease	at presentation to hospital	liver cell failure:[#] ♀ 30% [*] ♂ 12%				♀ 57% [*] ♂ 29%	cerebellar ataxia: ♀ 13% [*] ♂ 3%
Nakamura et al. (1979)	alcoholic liver disease	at presentation to hospital	♀ 43% ♂ 31%	♀ 43% [*] ♂ 7%	♀ 29% [*] ♂ 5%			GI bleeding ♀ 29% [*] ♂ 7%
Hislop et al. (1983)	alcoholic liver disease	at presentation to hospital	♀ 42% [*] ♂ 28%	♀ 32% [*] ♂ 17%	♀ 18% [*] ♂ 10%		♀ 15% [@] ♂ 10%	
Pares et al. (1986)	alcoholic hepatitis	at diagnosis	♀ 42% ♂ 36%	♀ 58% ♂ 43%	♀ 25% ♂ 7%	grade 3: ♀ 42% ♂ 7%		
Loft et al. (1987)	alcoholic liver disease	at presentation to hospital				Pugh > 11: ♀ 33% ♂ 0%		Antipyrine clearance < 5ml/min: ♀ 28% [*] ♂ 4%

[*] p < at least 0.05.
[@] p < 0.10
[#] jaundice, ascites, and peripheral oedema.

with their alcoholic liver disease (Gavaler 1982), the pattern again is one of consistency. The prevalence of major complications and severity of impaired hepatic function is invariably higher among females than males.

To look further at severity, nine studies available in the literature in which cirrhosis death rates can be compared between females and males are summarized in Table 7.5. The first report shown is the seminal study, although it was seriously flawed in terms of case definition for alcohol aetiology. The finding of a significantly increased incidence of death due directly to liver failure and the complications of cirrhosis among presumed alcoholic females, combined with the observation that the females had died at an age a decade earlier than the males, provided the first hint that there might exist susceptibility factors related to gender (Spain 1945). A second report published 9 years later provided similar findings, but in this report the study sample was composed exclusively of chronic alcoholic individuals with biopsy-documented alcoholic cirrhosis (Phillips and Davidson 1954).

In the last two decades, several reports using a variety of types of denominator groups have been published in which gender comparisons can be made. As may be seen in Table 7.5, one study in which the denominator was composed of 200 alcoholics in a psychiatric treatment programme, over the course of 700 patient-years of follow-up, the prevalence of cirrhosis indicated on death certificates as either the primary cause or secondary finding was significantly more frequent among females (Dahlgren and Myrhed 1977). In the report in which population statistics were included, unfortunately without comparative analyses, cirrhosis/liver disease death rates were higher among females, although alcoholism rates were higher among males (Indian Health Service 1992). In this report, in which the denominator was composed of American Indians with alcohol-induced cirrhosis, case fatality rates among females were similar in one tribe and statistically higher in the second tribe (Kunitz *et al.* 1971).

Finally, in four of the studies shown in Table 7.5 the denominators were composed of patients with alcoholic liver disease (Krasner *et al.* 1977; Morgan and Sherlock 1977; Nakamura *et al.* 1979; Alves *et*

Table 7.5   Deaths due to alcohol-induced liver disease

Authors (year)	Setting	Findings
Spain (1945)	Bellevue Hospital, New York; 1936-1942; Autopsy cases; "majority alcoholics".	Age at death from cirrhosis: ♀45.7,♂ 55.1; Death due to cirrhosis: ♀51/60(85%), ♂115/190(55%)*
Phillips and Davidson (1954)	Boston City Hospital; histology in 100%; chronic alcoholics with cirrhosis. Alcohol abuse for >10 years.	Among those with severe histologic lesions: death ♀11/14(79%),♂ 7/14(50%)@ ; age at death♀ 43,♂ 47; death in entire sample ♀14/20(70%),♂9/34(26%).*
Kunitz et al. (1971)	U S Public Health Service Hospitals, Phoenix and Window Rock; complete ascertainment of alcoholic cirrhosis cases; Hopi: 1965-1967; Navaho: 1956-1967.	Case fatality rates: Hopi: ♀4/10(40%),♂6/15(40%)(♀ 5yrs younger at death). Navaho: ♀10/36(28%),♂7/55(13%)@ (ages equivalent). All:♀ 14/46(30%),♂ 13/70(19%).
Dahlgren and Myrhed (1977)	Karolinska Hospital, Stockholm; 1963-1969; early cases of alcoholism >700 patient-years follow up.	Deaths with cirrhosis as primary or secondary cause ♀13/18(72%),♂2/16(12%)*
Krasner et al. (1977)	King's College Hospital, London; 1967-1965; biopsy proven cases of alcoholic liver disease.	5 year survival rate: ♀8/28(30%),♂41/57(72%)* Among patients dying,♀9/20(45%)♂ 1/16(6%)* had stopped drinking.
Morgan and Sherlock (1977)	Royal Free Hospital, London 1975; biopsy proven cases of alcoholic liver disease.	During 1 yr period: Stopped drinking: ♀2/22(9%), ♂22/75(29%)* Deaths: ♀ 5/22(23%),♂ 10/75(13%).
Nakamura (1979)	Tohoku University Hospital, Sendai; 1972-1977; biopsy proven cases of alcoholic liver disease.	Deaths during admission: ♀ 1/7(14%),♂3/123(2%)@
Alves et al. (1982)	University Hospital Santa Maria, Lisbon; 1966-1979; first presentation; all patients with biopsy proven alcoholic liver disease.	5 year survival: ♀7/61(11%),♂ 38/116(33%).*
Indian Health Service (1992)	American Indians and Alaska Natives, U S Health Statistics for 1986-1988.	Death rate per 100,000 from chronic liver disease and cirrhosis: ♀19.7,♂12.2; age-adjusted alcoholism rates per 100,000 at least 2 fold lower in ♀ (e.g., for age 45-64: ♀54,♂ 106).

* p < at least 0.05;   @ p < 0.10

al. 1982). In these four studies, there were arithmetically or statistically increased death rates or decreased survival rates among the females compared with the males.

As a group, these reports also permit an additional aspect of gender-related differences to be explored. Specifically, if gender is indeed a factor which influences susceptibility to alcoholic liver cirrhosis, then differences in markers of susceptibility should be evident not just within relatively homogeneous groups but also across racial/ethnic groups. As in the other approaches which have been used, reproducibility is again evident, as the pattern of findings consistent with gender being a factor in alcohol-induced liver disease susceptibility is repeatedly seen in study populations drawn from Japan, Portugal, Sweden, the UK, the USA, American Indian and Alaskan Natives (the reports in Table 7.4), as well as Spain, Canada, France, Australia and Switzerland (Pares *et al.* 1986; Coates *et al.* 1986; Pequignot *et al.* 1974; Tuyns and Pequignot 1984; Wilkinson *et al.* 1969, 1971; Marbet *et al.* 1987).

We have now examined a body of available evidence gleaned from an array of studies. Support for the hypothesis that females are more susceptible than males to the development of alcohol-induced liver disease has been found using a variety of approaches to evaluate the evidence. When examining the severity of alcoholic liver disease in terms of either signs and symptoms at time of presentation or cirrhosis death rates, females consistently appear to be at increased vulnerability. When examining alcohol exposure in terms of dose and duration measures in relation to the prevalence of alcoholic liver disease in general and cirrhosis in particular, the evidence that liver pathology occurs at lower levels of exposure among females is striking. When examining odds ratios to approximate relative risk,

Table 7.6   Progression to cirrhosis

Authors (year)	Setting	Findings
Krasner et al. (1977)	King's College Hospital, London. histological follow-up 0.5-8 years in patients without cirrhosis	Among those continuing to drink, progression from alcoholic hepatitis alone to cirrhosis in ♀ 7/9(78%), ♂ 1/7(14%) (p<0.05).
Parés et al. (1986)	University of Barcelona. histological follow-up 1-3 years in patients without cirrhosis	Progression from alcoholic hepatitis to cirrhosis ♀ 7/12(58%),♂ 2/14(14%) p<0.05; progression in those who stopped or markedly reduced drinking: ♀4/8(50%), ♂ 0/9(0%) (p<0.10).
Marbet et al. (1987)	University of Basel. histological follow-up 4-8 years in patients without cirrhosis	Cumulative alcohol consumption during follow-up; 570±140 kg in ♀ ,917±80 kg in ♂ ; (p<0.10). progression to cirrhosis: ♀5/8(62%), ♂ 13/39(33%); Among those reducing intake to <40g ETOH/day, histological improvement ♀2/4(50%), ♂ 4/4(100%).

the evidence again supports the hypothesis that alcoholic cirrhosis is produced at lower habitual alcohol intake levels in females than in males.

Gender-related differences in susceptibility to alcoholic liver disease

Based on the available evidence in the literature, it is clear that females develop alcoholic liver disease at *lower levels of alcohol intake* over a *shorter period of time* compared with males. What is not clear, however, is whether or not the damage to the liver with less cumulative alcohol exposure in females represents a difference in susceptibility. The susceptibility difference to alcoholic liver disease could be a manifestation of increased sensitivity of females at a given level of ethanol exposure; the susceptibility gap could also involve gender-related differences in the mechanism(s) of disease progression once damage has been initiated or precipitated.

Gender-related differences in alcohol metabolism

Alcoholic beverages are served in unitized portions; they are not served in portions specific for body-weight, volume of distribution or gender. It is within this context that the issue of gender-related

differences in sensitivity to alcohol should be viewed. As a function of lower bodyweight, smaller blood volume, increased ratio of body fat to lean body tissue with consequent decreased volume of distribution, and decreased gastric alcohol dehydrogenase activity with consequent reduced first-pass gastric metabolism of alcohol, the bioavailability of ethanol is considered to be higher in females than in males. This increased ethanol bioavailability in females has been invoked either to explain the observed gender-related difference in susceptibility to alcoholic liver disease, or to dismiss the cumulative ethanol dose differential and thus the putative gender-related difference in susceptibility (Saunders *et al.* 1981a, 1984; Johnson and Williams 1985; Dunne 1988; Grant *et al.* 1988; Van Thiel and Gavaler 1988; Frezza *et al.* 1990; see also Chapter 2). Regardless of how one chooses to utilize the evidence of increased ethanol bioavailability in females, it is clear that females may indeed be more sensitive to a given non-gender-specific dose of ethanol.

Gender-related differences in the mechanism(s) of progression of alcoholic liver disease

Gender-related differences in the mechanism(s) of progression of alcoholic liver disease is an intriguing possibility. Although no direct evidence is available in the literature, there are data which offer indirect evidence by providing findings of gender-related differences in the histologic progression of alcohol-precipitated liver disease following cessation of exposure to ethanol (Krasner *et al.* 1977; Pares *et al.* 1986; Marbet *et al.* 1987). The data are summarized in Table 7.6. The findings of all three studies demonstrate a statistical or arithmetic increased proportion of females progressing from alcoholic hepatitis to cirrhosis with continued use of alcohol. Further, among those discontinuing or reducing exposure to ethanol, as compared with males an increased proportion of females die due to alcoholic liver disease (Krasner *et al.* 1977), an increased proportion of females progress to cirrhosis (Pares *et al.* 1986) and a decreased proportion of females show histologic improvement (Marbet *et al.* 1987). In spite of small sample sizes, the findings are not only remarkably reproducible across nationality groups, but also consistent with a hypothesis that there are gender-related differences in the mechanism(s) involved in histologically documented progression of alcohol-initiated liver damage and disease.

Conclusion

At the outset, the issue to be evaluated was that of the plausibility of gender-related differences in susceptibility to alcoholic liver disease. After extensive examination of the relevant data available in the literature, it is difficult to dismiss the reproducibility and consistency of the findings that females develop cirrhosis at a reduced cumulative ethanol dose compared with males. The findings are supported by data which point not only to gender-related differences in sensitivity to a given level of ethanol exposure due to ethanol bioavailability, but also to a gender-related differential in the mechanism(s) of the progression of initiated damage to the liver.

The larger issue remains our current inability to definitively identify the factors which are responsible for susceptibility to alcoholic liver disease in the larger population of individuals who abuse alcohol, among whom only a relatively small proportion go on to develop alcoholic liver disease. Is it possible that the factors which are involved in susceptibility are more prevalent in females than in males? Systematic evaluation of gender-related differences in thresholds of ethanol effects and susceptibility mechanisms may ultimately facilitate an answer to the question of why not all alcohol-abusing individuals of either gender develop alcoholic liver disease.

References

Alves, P., Correia, J., Borda d'Agua, C., Portugal, L., Capaz, V., Rodrigues, M. and Rodrigues, H. (1982). Alcoholic liver diseases in Portugal: Clinical and laboratory picture, mortality, and survival. *Alcoholism: Clinical and Experimental Research* **6**, 216–224.

Arria, A. (1993). Genetic and environmental influences on the age of presentation of alcoholic cirrhosis. Doctoral dissertation, University of Pittsburgh.

Ashley, M., Olin, J., le Riche, W., Kornaczewski, A., Schmidt, W. and Rankin, J. (1977). Morbidity in alcoholics. *Archives of Internal Medicine* **137**, 883–887.

Bhathal, P., Wilkinson, P., Clifton, S., Rankin, J. and Santamaria, J. (1975). The spectrum of liver disease in alcoholism. *Australian and New Zealand Journal of Medicine* **5**, 49–57.

Bhattacharyya, D. and Rake, M. (1983). Correlation of alcohol consumption with liver damage in men and women. *Alcohol and Alcoholism* **18**, 181–184.

Coates, R., Halliday, M., Rankin, J., Feinman, S. and Fisher, M. (1986). Risk of fatty infiltration or cirrhosis of the liver in relation to ethanol consumption: A case-control study. *Clinical and Investigative Medicine* **9**, 26–32.

Dahlgren, L. and Myrhed, M. (1977). Alcoholic females II. Causes of death with reference to sex differences. *Acta Psychiatrica Scandinavica* **56**, 81–91.

Dunne, F. (1988). Are women more easily damaged by alcohol than men? *British Journal of Addiction* **83**, 1135–1136.

Frezza, M., Padova, C., Pozzato, G., Terpin, M., Baraona, E. and Lieber, C.S. (1990). High blood alcohol levels in women: The role of decreased gastric alcohol dehydrogenase activity and first-pass metabolism. *New England Journal of Medicine* **322**, 1135–1136.

Gavaler, J. (1982). Sex-related differences in ethanol-induced liver disease: Artifactual or real? *Alcoholism: Clinical and Experimental Research* **6**, 186–196.

Grant, B., Dufour, M. and Harford, T. (1988). Epidemiology of alcoholic liver disease. *Seminars in Liver Disease* **8**, 12–25.

Hislop, W., Bouchier, I., Allan, J., Brunt, P., Eastwood, M., Finlayson, N., James, O., Russell, R. and Watkinson, G. (1983). Alcoholic liver disease in Scotland and northeastern England: Presenting features in 510 patients. *Quarterly Journal of Medicine* **206**, 232–243.

Indian Health Service (1992). *Trends in Indian Health – 1992*. Indian Health Service, Rockville, MD.

Johnson, R. and Williams, R. (1985). Genetic and environmental factors in the individual susceptibility to the development of alcoholic liver disease. *Alcohol and Alcoholism* **20**, 137–160.

Krasner, N., Davis, M., Portmann, B. and Williams, R. (1977). Changing pattern of alcoholic liver disease in Great Britain: Relation to sex and signs of autoimmunity. *British Medical Journal* **1**, 1497–1500.

Kunitz, S., Levy, J., Odoroff, C. and Bollinger, J. (1971). The epidemiology of alcoholic cirrhosis in two south-western Indian tribes. *Quarterly Journal of Studies on Alcoholism* **32**, 706–720.

Lelbach, W. (1976). Epidemiology of alcoholic liver disease. In *Progress in Liver Disease* (Edited by Popper, H. and Schaffner, F.), Vol. V, pp. 494–515. Grune and Stratton, New York.

Levi, A. and Chalmers, D. (1978). Recognition of alcoholic liver disease in a district general hospital. *Gut* **19**, 521–525.

Loft, S., Olesen, K. and Dossing, M. (1987). Increased susceptibility to liver disease in relation to alcohol consumption in women. *Scandinavian Journal of Gastroenterology* **22**, 1251–1256.

Marbet, U., Bianchi, L., Meury, U. and Stalder, G. (1987). Long-term histological evaluation of the natural history and prognostic factors of alcoholic liver disease. *Journal of Hepatology* **4**, 364–372.

Milman, N., Graudal, N., Strom, P. and Franzmann, M. (1988). Alcoholic hepatitis in females. *Acta Medica Scandinavica* **223**, 119–124.

Morgan, M. and Sherlock, S. (1977). Sex-related differences among 100 patients with alcoholic liver disease. *British Medical Journal* **1**, 939–941.

Nakamura, S., Takezawa, Y., Sato, T., Kera, K. and Maeda, T. (1979). Alcoholic liver disease in women. *Tohoku Journal of Experimental Medicine* **129**, 351–355.

Norton, R., Batey, R., Dwyer, T. and MacMahon, S. (1987). Alcohol consumption and the risk of alcohol-related cirrhosis in women. *British Medical Journal* **295**, 80–82.

Pares, A., Caballeria, J., Bruguera, M., Torres, M. and Rodes, J. (1986). Histological course of alcoholic hepatitis: Influence of abstinence, sex and extent of hepatic damage. *Journal of Hepatology* **2**, 33–42.

Pequignot, G., Chabert, C., Eydoux, H. and Courcoul, M. (1974). Augmentation du risque de cirrhose en fonction de la ration d'alcool. *Revue Alcoholism* **20**, 191–202.

Phillips, G. and Davidson, C. (1954). Acute hepatic insufficiency of the chronic alcoholic. *Archives of Internal Medicine* **94**, 595–603.

Saunders, J., Davis, M. and Williams, R. (1981a). Do women develop alcoholic liver disease more readily than men? *British Medical Journal* **282**, 1140–1143.

Saunders, J., Walters, J., Davies, P. and Paton, A. (1981b). A 20-year prospective study of cirrhosis. *British Medical Journal* **282**, 263–266.

Saunders, J., Wodak, A. and Williams, R. (1984). What determines susceptibility to liver damage from alcohol? *Journal of the Royal Society of Medicine* **77**, 204–216.

Spain, D. (1945). Portal cirrhosis of the liver: A review of two hundred fifty necropsies with references to sex differences. *American Journal of Clinical Pathology* **15**, 215–218.

Tuyns, A. and Pequignot, G. (1984). Greater risk of ascitic cirrhosis in females in relation to alcohol consumption. *International Journal of Epidemiology* **13**, 53–57.

Van Thiel, D. and Gavaler, J. (1988). Ethanol metabolism and hepatotoxicity: Does sex make a difference? In *Recent Developments in Alcoholism* (Edited by Galanter, M.), Vol. 6, pp. 291–303. Plenum Press, New York.

Wilkinson, P., Santamaria, J. and Rankin, J. (1969). Epidemiology of alcoholic cirrhosis. *Australian Annals of Medicine* **18**, 222–226.

Wilkinson, P., Kornaczewski, A., Rankin, J. and Santamaria, J. (1971). Physical disease in alcoholism: Initial survey of 1,000 patients. *Medical Journal of Australia* **1**, 1217–1225.

8 # The role of nutritional factors in alcoholic liver disease

Lawrence Feinman and Charles S. Lieber

Introduction

Undernutrition is common in one subset of alcoholics and is an important cause of illness for them; also animal models of liver disease due to dietary deficiencies are well known. It is not surprising that disturbances in nutrition should have been carefully considered as part of the aetiology of alcoholic liver disease. The evidence that alcohol is *per se* hepatotoxic and the way in which nutritional factors, in the setting of alcoholism, may influence the pathogenesis of liver disease, will be reviewed. The prospects for providing special nutrients to forestall the development of alcoholic cirrhosis will also be discussed.

Malnutrition as the sole cause of liver disease in the alcoholic

Malnutrition, in the absence of other aetiologic factors, has not been shown to cause cirrhosis in adult humans. Patients post-jejuno-ileal bypass for obesity may represent a partial exception in that they develop hepatic injury which resembles alcohol-associated liver disease (see Chapter 11). However, alcohol may have contributed to the liver injury in some of those cases. Starvation *per se* does not cause prominent liver injury in adult humans (Sherlock and Walshe 1948), and certainly does not cause injury that resembles that associated with alcoholism. However, experimental animals such as rodents are prone to develop fatty liver and fibrosis when placed on a choline-deficient diet. The inappropriate extrapolation of this observation to human disease was a source of confusion for a long time, as will be discussed in detail below.

Direct hepatotoxic effect of alcohol

The role of nutrition in the pathogenesis of alcoholic liver injury (fatty liver, alcoholic hepatitis and cirrhosis) has been investigated in humans from the perspectives of epidemiology and therapeutic trials, and by animal experimentation.

Our current understanding is that alcohol *per se*, given in sufficient quantities, can cause fatty liver in man (and lower animals) despite the presence of an otherwise adequate diet (see the review by Lieber and DeCarli 1991; see also Chapter 2). The lipid and protein composition of the diet have modulating effects on the amount and/or types of fat that accumulate in the liver. For example, reduction of dietary fat to 10 percent of total calories (but not lower) greatly lessens, but does not completely eliminate, hepatic fat accumulation. Fatty acids of chain length found in the diet accumulate in the liver when available from the diet; otherwise, endogenously synthesized fatty acids accumulate. Long chain fatty acids in the diet have a greater tendency than medium chain fatty acids to promote fatty liver in the presence of alcohol. Reduction of dietary protein intake to deficient levels (i.e. 4 percent of total calories) increases the fat accumulation caused by concomitant alcohol. However, provision of 25 percent of total calories as protein, which greatly exceeds the usually recommended amount of dietary protein, will not eliminate hepatic fat accumulation. The amount of fat accumulating in the alcohol-induced fatty liver is but one parameter of damage, and must be considered along with distortion of organelles such as mitochondria and the endoplasmic reticulum (Iseri *et al.* 1966), plasma membranes (Yamada *et al.* 1985) and metabolic derangements involving impaired respiration and energy production (Cederbaum *et al.* 1974, 1976), fatty acid oxidation (Cederbaum *et al.* 1975) and susceptibility to acetaldehyde toxicity (Matsuzaki and Lieber 1977), which are caused by alcohol.

The role of nutrition in the pathogenesis of alcoholic hepatitis has been studied in much less detail. Alcoholic hepatitis is considered too severe a form of injury to justify studies aimed at inducing this type of liver lesion in volunteers.

The incidence of alcoholic cirrhosis has been linked to per capita alcohol consumption. The studies of Lelbach (1967) also show the direct influence of cumulative alcohol consumption on the incidence of chronic liver disease. The beverage source of alcohol did not seem to be important, and concomitant malnutrition was not noted to be an influence. The implied direct effect of alcohol in causing hepatic fibrosis and cirrhosis has been confirmed in the baboon model of hepatic injury (Lieber *et al.* 1975).

The direct hepatotoxic effect of ethanol has been shown histologically and biochemically, in both alcoholics and non-alcoholic volunteers given alcohol, regardless of dietary variation in fat, protein, vitamins and ordinary lipotropes (Lieber *et al.* 1965; Lane and Lieber 1966; Rubin and Lieber 1967). Epidemiologic surveys, beginning with the observation that decreased cirrhosis mortality correlated with the decreased availability of alcohol during the First World War in Europe and Prohibition in the USA (Jolliffe and Jellinek 1941), went on to observe that the incidence of cirrhosis increases with the accumulated alcohol intake (g/kg/day times years) (Lelbach 1975; Pequignot *et al.* 1974, 1978; Wilkinson *et al.* 1969), females being susceptible at lower alcohol intakes than males. Processes that contribute to the pathogenesis of alcohol-related cell injury include increase of the NADH/NAD ratio (a consequence of alcohol oxidation), alterations of calcium flux and lipid peroxidation. Alcohol influences lipid peroxidation via its induction of the endoplasmic reticulum and its generation of acetaldehyde. Interactions of alcohol with selenium, iron, copper and zinc, each of which is related to cellular control of peroxidation, are under study (Lieber 1987). Dietary imbalances are not inferred from these preliminary studies.

The role of nutrition in the recovery from alcoholic liver injury was studied before its role in the pathogenesis of liver injury was understood. A normal protein, fat, and vitamin-enriched diet yielded a clinical response in cirrhosis including greater longevity. In view of our current appreciation of the direct toxicity of alcohol, and the lack of control that most alcoholics have in limiting their alcohol intake, we recommend strict abstinence from alcohol.

The significance of congeners (Feinman and Lieber 1988), moderate dosages of alcohol, genetic factors and marginal nutritional deficiencies in alcohol-related tissue injury and in the recovery phase is not yet fully elucidated.

The nutritive value of alcoholic beverages and the nutritional status of alcoholics

Nutritive value of alcoholic beverages

Alcoholic beverages contain little of nutritive value except water, variable amounts of carbohydrate, and alcohol, which can serve as an energy source, but one which requires closer analysis to appreciate its impact. The carbohydrate content of alcoholic beverages is zero for whisky, cognac and vodka, 2–10 g/l for red and dry white wine, 30 g/l for beer and dry sherry, and as much as 120 g/l for sweetened white and port wines. The amounts of protein and vitamins in these beverages is extremely low except for beer. An intake of one litre of beer daily would be required to satisfy the daily requirements of an adult male for nicotinic acid, 15–20 litres for protein and 25 litres for thiamine. Iron content may be appreciable, especially in wines. Occasionally the amounts of iron, lead or cobalt reach harmful levels. The significance of congener content is still obscure (Feinman and Lieber 1988).

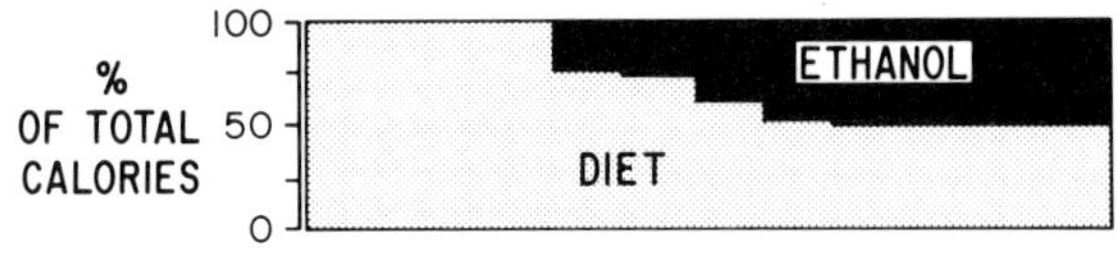

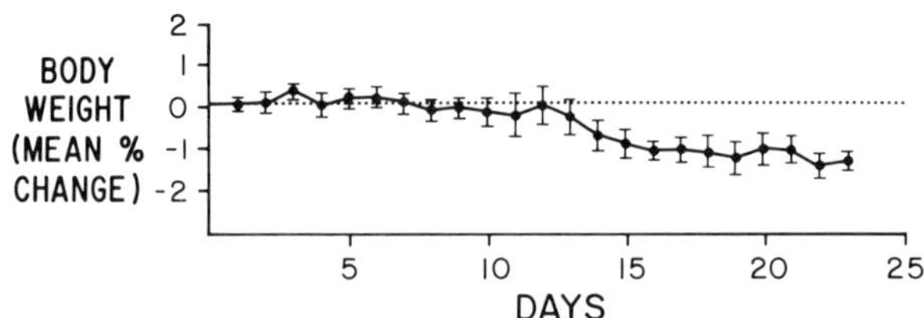

Fig. 8.1 Body weight changes after isocaloric substitution of carbohydrate by ethanol in 11 subjects (mean ± standard errors). Dotted line, mean changes in weight in control period. Reproduced with permission from Pirola and Lieber (1972).

Alcohol contributes 4.5 percent of Americans' total caloric intake (Scheig 1970), 10 percent for adult drinkers. Heavy drinkers may derive more than half their daily calories from alcohol. Although the combustion of alcohol in a bomb calorimeter indicates a value of 7.1 kcal/g, its biological value is probably less, when compared with carbohydrates. Despite higher total caloric intakes (alcohol included), drinkers are no more obese than non-drinkers (Gruchow *et al.* 1985). Subjects given additional calories as alcohol under metabolic ward conditions failed to gain weight (Lieber *et al.* 1965). Isocaloric substitution of alcohol for carbohydrate, as 50 percent of total calories in a balanced diet, resulted in a decline in body weight, and when given as additional calories, alcohol caused less weight gain than calorically equivalent carbohydrate or fat (Pirola and Lieber 1972; see Fig. 8.1). Others have reported variable responses to additional calories as alcohol (Crouse and Grundy 1984): lean individuals did not gain weight, but half of the obese individuals gained some weight. Some could detect no weight changes in healthy males over a 2 week period using moderate amounts of alcohol (Contaldo *et al.* 1989), 75 g/day substituted on a calorie basis for all foods in the diet, while others detected a drop in weight in alcoholic males after only 4 days of a substantial dose of alcohol, 40–60 percent of calories (168 g/day for a male weighing 70 kg) substituted for glucose (Reinus *et al.* 1989). Interpretation of these findings would have been made easier had the weight

changes been of sufficient magnitude to have made body composition studies feasible.

The inability of alcohol to consistently support body weight or to promote weight gain is probably due to its increase of metabolic rate. Oxygen consumption after alcohol increases in normal subjects (Tremoliere and Carre 1961; Perman, 1972), more so in alcoholics (Tremoliere and Carre 1961). Substitution of ethanol for carbohydrate increases the metabolic rate of humans and rodents (Stock *et al.* 1973; Stock and Stuart 1974; Siviy *et al.* 1987). Increase in thermogenesis occurs in humans and rats fed alcohol (Stock and Stuart 1974). A 15 percent increase in thermogenesis occurred in rats after only 10 days of alcohol intake (Stock and Stuart 1974). Although some of the energy wastage was attributable to brown fat thermogenesis in rats (Rothwell and Stock 1984) and was suppressable by sympathectomy (Larve-Achagiotis *et al.* 1989), most of it could not be so explained. Studies in "normal" males whose usual alcohol intake was less than five alcoholic beverages per day, showed a thermic effect of small doses (20 g) of alcohol (Westrate *et al.* 1990). Diet-induced thermogenesis was increased during the time of maximal alcohol oxidation, compared with the effects of an isocaloric control meal not containing alcohol, but the overall diet-induced thermogenesis for the entire 4 h post-prandial measurement period was not different. Recently, it was found that either addition of alcohol to the diet or substitution of it for other foods increased 24 h energy expenditure and decreased fat oxidation in humans (Suter *et al.* 1992). One postulated mechanism of energy wastage when alcohol is consumed is its initial oxidation without phosphorylation via the microsomal ethanol oxidizing system (MEOS). The MEOS pathway, which is engaged at higher alcohol concentrations than the alcohol dehydrogenase (ADH) pathway due to differences in their K_ms (10 *vs* 1 mm), is induced by chronic alcohol consumption, after which the wastage was noted to be aggravated (Pirola and Lieber 1975, 1976; see also Chapter 3). Other explanations have been advanced to account for energy wastage due to alcohol consumption. An uncoupling of mitochondrial NADH reoxidation, abetted by a hyperthyroid state or catecholamine release, has been proposed (Israel *et al.* 1975) and rejected (Teschke *et al.* 1983). Lands and Zakhari (1991) have postulated energy loss from "futile cycles" involving the irreversible conversion of alcohol to acetaldehyde via MEOS and back again via ADH. The inefficient utilization of metabolic intermediates, particularly relevant to dietary lipids, consequent to organelle damage (especially mitochondria) after alcohol consumption has been summarized (Lieber 1991a; see also Chapter 2).

In summary, alcoholic beverages provide little nutritive value aside from calories; as an energy source, alcohol is not as adequate as equivalent carbohydrate.

Alcohol and appetite

The intake of alcohol appears to be "unregulated" for the moderate drinker, in the context of total calories, in that alcohol intake in the range 20 g/day supplements rather than displaces macronutrient-derived calories (de Castro and Orozco 1990), thus adding 140 kcal/day. Even intakes in the range of 50 g/day generally were taken as additional calories, although at these levels alcohol began to be substituted for sucrose calories (Colditz *et al.* 1991). When individuals had been classified as restrained *vs* unrestrained eaters, it was found that alcohol consumption increased the amount of food taken by restrained eaters (Polivy and Herman 1976a, b). Patients admitted to hospital with severe liver disease are characteristically anorexic.

Alcohol and nutritional status

Patients admitted to hospital for medical complications of alcoholism often have a history of inadequate dietary protein intake (Patek *et al.* 1975) and signs of protein malnutrition (Mendenhall *et al.* 1985). In this group of hospitalized patients, anthropomorphic measurements indicate impaired nutrition: height/weight ratio is lower, muscle mass estimated by creatinine/height index is reduced, and triceps skinfolds are thinner. Continued drinking is associated with weight loss while abstinence is associated with weight gain, both in patients with and without liver disease.

Many patients who drink to excess are not clearly malnourished, or are so to a lesser extent than those hospitalized for medical problems. Patients with moderate intake of alcohol, and even those admitted for alcohol rehabilitation, hardly differ nutritionally from controls.

The broad spectrum of nutritional status that exists in alcohol drinkers prompts a closer look at what they eat. Moderate alcohol intake – that is, alcohol accounting for less than 16 percent of total calories (alcohol included) – is associated with a slightly elevated energy intake (Gruchow *et al.* 1985;

de Castro and Orozco 1990). Despite comparable levels of physical activity there is no weight gain, perhaps because of the energy considerations already discussed. Intake of alcohol above 23 percent of calories (Hillers and Massey 1985) is associated with a beginning substitution of alcohol for carbohydrate calories (Colditz *et al.* 1991) and women begin to exhibit loss of weight. When the percentage of calories as alcohol exceeds 30 percent, significant decreases in protein and fat intake occur, and the intake of vitamins A, C and thiamine may fall below the recommended dietary allowances (Hillers and Masscy 1985). Intake of calcium, iron and fibre are also appreciably lowered (Gruchow *et al.* 1985). Decreased dietary intake has been considered a major cause of malnutrition in alcoholic cirrhotics (Mezey 1978).

In summary, alcoholism is characterized by a wide spectrum of malnutrition with the vast majority of alcoholics having slight if any detectable impairment. When alcohol intake approaches about 25 percent of daily calories, deficient intake of important nutrients becomes likely. Alcoholics with medical complications requiring hospitalization generally have severe nutritional deficits.

Vitamin A

The interaction of alcoholism with vitamin A is of particular interest because it involves the intake – possibly the absorption – of the vitamin and its metabolism; there are intriguing clues that suggest that alcohol–vitamin A interactions may modulate alcohol-associated liver disease.

Vitamin A ingestion is not significantly below normal for Americans imbibing up to a mean of 400 calories of alcohol per day (or less than 20 percent of total energy) (Gruchow *et al.* 1985), since the vitamin A content of the non-alcoholic portion of the diet approximates that eaten by control populations. Americans consuming 24 percent of their energy as alcohol ingest 75 percent of the recommended daily allowance for vitamin A (Hillers and Massey 1985). Since the recommended daily allowance for vitamin A is falling (Olson 1987), these drinkers may still not have significantly subnormal intakes. We may suspect that a high alcohol intake, 50 percent or more of energy derived from alcohol, is associated with even less vitamin A intake in the USA, as has already been shown for wine drinkers in Chile, where 150 g alcohol consumption daily was associated with intake of 25 percent of the recommended daily allowance for vitamin A. Elderly American men who consume alcohol regularly have lower vitamin A intakes than their abstinent counterparts. The effect of alcohol upon vitamin A absorption in humans was shown to be inhibitory (17 percent reduction by 120 ml of wine) in a single study (Althausen *et al.* 1960). When fat malabsorption due to chronic alcoholic pancreatitis occurs, vitamin A absorption will be reduced further.

The effect of acute alcohol ingestion on blood vitamin A levels has been variously reported as unchanged in humans (Russell *et al.* 1979), increased in dogs (Lee and Lucia 1965) and increased as retinol bound to lipoproteins in rodents (Sato and Lieber 1980). However, the result of chronic alcohol consumption has been consistent and profound: hepatic vitamin A stores are decreased by alcohol consumption whether dietary vitamin A intake is low, normal or high. For example, rodents fed alcohol chronically had lower hepatic vitamin A, 5 g/kg/day yielding a 20 percent decrease in the liver. Higher alcohol intakes, 36 percent of calories or about 14 g/kg/day, decreased hepatic vitamin A by 60 percent in 4–6 weeks and 72 percent in 7–9 weeks, with no change in serum vitamin A or serum retinol binding protein and an increase in hepatic retinol binding protein (Sato and Lieber 1980). A five-fold increase in dietary vitamin A did not prevent hepatic depletion by alcohol. Once again, in the baboon model where 50 percent of caloric intake was alcohol, there was a 60 percent decrease in hepatic vitamin A after 4 months and a 95 percent decrease in 24–84 months (Sato and Lieber 1980). Finally, in humans with alcoholic liver disease, the hepatic vitamin A levels show progressive decrease as the liver injury progresses to cirrhosis (Leo and Lieber 1982; see Fig. 8.2). Recently, a positive correlation was shown between alcohol consumption and levels of plasma beta-carotene and a negative correlation between the severity of liver disease and plasma beta-carotene (Ahmed *et al.* 1992). Even when serum levels of alpha- and beta-carotene levels are normal, hepatic levels are likely to be 6–25 times lower than normals, depending on the severity of alcoholic liver disease (Leo *et al.* 1993). Alcoholism, especially when associated with chronic alcoholic liver disease, must alter the metabolism of vitamin A and related carotenes and retinoids to explain these findings. Although we have seen that vitamin A intake decreases with intensity of drinking, enhancement of hepatic vitamin A degradation due to alcohol con-

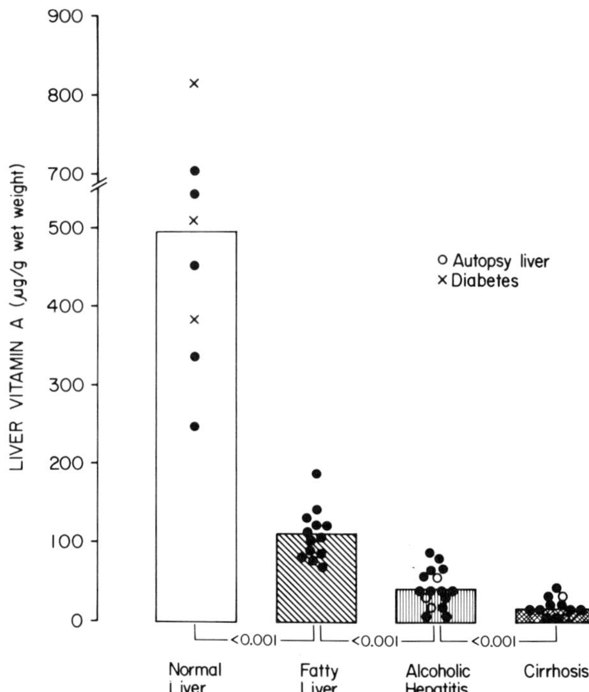

Fig. 8.2 Hepatic vitamin A levels in subjects with normal livers, and various stages of alcoholic liver injury. To convert vitamin A values to micromoles per gram, multiply by 0.003941. Figures below the graph denote *P*-values. Reproduced with permission from Leo and Lieber (1982).

sumption is the more likely explanation for vitamin A depletion. The metabolism of retinoic acid to 4-hydroxy and 4-oxoretinoic acid and other polar metabolites occurs via microsomal enzymes which are inducible by alcohol consumption (Sato and Lieber 1982), but these enzymes probably do not have sufficient activity to be largely responsible for depleting vitamin A stores. However, a newly discovered microsomal pathway for oxidation of retinol to polar metabolites (Leo and Lieber 1985), is also inducible by alcohol (Leo *et al.* 1986), and is probably the more important pathway for hepatic vitamin A depletion. In addition, alcohol promotes vitamin A mobilization from the liver.

The clinical consequences of altered vitamin A status include the increased incidence of night blindness due to lowered tissue vitamin A levels. Abnormal dark adaption occurs in 15 percent of alcoholics without cirrhosis and 50 percent of alcoholics with cirrhosis (Bonjour 1981). A serum vitamin A level of 1.4 μM or more excludes retinal dysfunction with 95 percent confidence (Carney and Russell 1980). Some claim that the relative dose response, or increase in serum retinol 5 h after a test dose of vitamin A, is necessary and helpful in predicting tissue stores of vitamin A because of the poor correlation of serum retinol, retinyl esters, retinol binding protein and albumin with tissue stores. The correlation of serum vitamin A with tissue stores is especially confounded by liver disease, protein deficiency and zinc deficiency.

Hepatotoxicity from low vitamin A intake includes the presence of multivesicular lysosomes (see Chapter 3) and is potentiated by concomitant alcohol intake (Leo *et al.* 1983). Hepatotoxicity, including fibrosis, of increased vitamin A is also potentiated by concomitant alcohol (Leo *et al.* 1982). Alcohol results in an increase in vitamin A in lungs and oesophagus (Lieber 1987). The role of alcohol in increasing vitamin A in some tissues (possibly by hepatic release of vitamin) while reducing it in others, and of speeding or altering the conversion of vitamin A to metabolites, may have important consequences for the hepatotoxicity, particularly hepatic fibrosis, associated with chronic alcohol ingestion (Leo and Lieber 1983), and may also have relevance for the association of low vitamin A or carotene levels with malignancy of various types (Lieber 1987).

Therapy is complicated by several factors: the difficulty in assessing tissue stores of vitamin A, the toxicity of high doses of vitamin A, the potential toxicity of even normal doses of vitamin A concomitant with continued intake of alcohol (or other microsome-inducing drugs), and the difficulty of monitoring vitamin A hepatotoxicity in the presence of continued alcohol intake. Therefore, vitamin A replacement should be modest for patients who cannot be assured an alcohol- and drug-free environment. Vitamin A replacement may be considered for those who can be confirmed as deficient and who can be assured abstinence from alcohol. Deficiency would be established as night blindness (or abnormal dark adaptation) with low serum vitamin A (<30 μg/dl or 1.4 μM/l) and perhaps a relative dose response $\geqslant 14$ percent (see above). Determination of hepatic vitamin A, while ideal, is not practical. Vitamin A at a dosage of 10,000 units/day for several weeks would be an adequate trial. A low serum zinc (<80 μg/dl) should prompt simultaneous replacement with $ZnSO_4$. Zinc might also be given subsequent to a failed trial of vitamin A. It must be stressed that these recommendations are not based on rigorous clinical trials.

The concept of relative nutrient deficiency

While malnutrition has been dismissed as the sole cause of liver disease in the alcoholic (*vide supra*), it is possibile that, in the setting of chronic alcohol ingestion, specific nutrients and metabolic intermediates, had they been more abundant, might have prevented hepatotoxicity. To neglect this possibility may not only diminish our appreciation of the subtleties of alcohol-induced liver injury, but may have us stumble past nutritional approaches to the prevention of that injury.

The phenomena to be considered are:

1. Alcohol metabolism, by all known pathways, with the resultant production of acetaldehyde, which has many toxic effects including its potential to promote lipid peroxidation.
2. The capacity of metabolites, dietary precursors, vitamins and trace elements such as glutathione, cysteine, methionine, *S*-adenosyl-L-methionine, vitamin E and selenium to counteract either some of the several effects of acetaldehyde and/or those of other mediators of peroxidative damage.

Approximately 90 percent of *acetaldehyde*, which is produced as the first product of alcohol metabolism and from other sources, is oxidized in the liver by cytosolic and mitochondrial aldehyde dehydrogenases (Lindros 1974). Acetaldehyde oxidation is retarded in mitochondria after chronic alcohol consumption, as first demonstrated in rats (Hasumura *et al.* 1975), and leads to elevated blood levels in humans (Korsten *et al.* 1975) and baboons (Pikkarainen *et al.* 1981). The harmful effects of acetaldehyde derive from abilities both to link covalently to proteins and to foster lipid peroxidation. Acetaldehyde also activates collagen-producing mesenchymal cells (Fig. 8.3) (see also Chapter 4), and forms protein adducts with microsomal cytochrome P4502El, tubulin, fatty acid binding protein and others, some of which form neoantigens (see Chapter 5). The mechanisms by which these events result in cell damage are discussed in detail elsewhere (Lieber and DeCarli 1991; see Chapter 2). Acetaldehyde causes lipid peroxidation in isolated perfused livers (Muller and Sies 1982), and evidence supports the occurrence of lipid peroxidation after alcohol administration in non-human primates (Shaw *et al.* 1981) and in humans (Shaw *et al.* 1983). Lipoperoxidation was long ago proposed as a mechanism of alcohol-induced hepatotoxicity (DiLuzio and

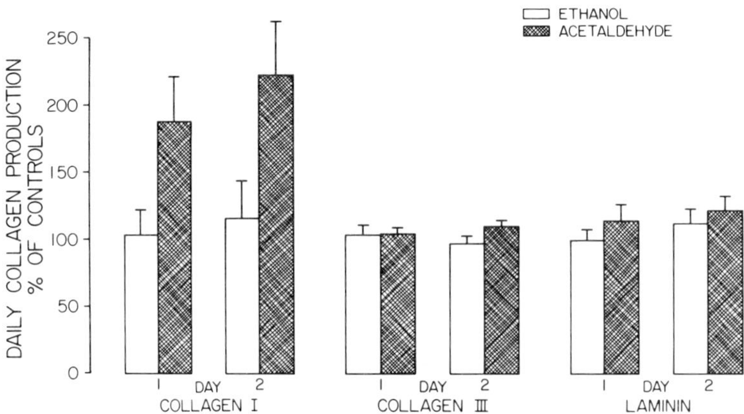

Fig. 8.3 Effects of ethanol and acetaldehyde on collagen production by fat-storing cells. Data are mean ± S.E.M. of five experiments. Data were calculated as ng/μg cellular DNA and expressed as percentage of control. The effect of acetaldehyde on type I collagen production was significant ($P < 0.01$). Days 1 and 2 refer to the first and second 24 h incubation periods of cultures with ethanol or acetaldehyde. Reproduced with permission from Moshage *et al.* (1990).

Hartman 1967; DiLuzio and Stege 1977), and, although challenged, is increasingly accepted.

Cysteine, which is a constituent of glutathione along with glutamic acid and glycine, has the capacity via its mercaptan group to react with acetaldehyde, thereby rendering it non-toxic. For example, cysteine has been shown to protect against acetaldehyde-induced death in rats and to afford protection against acetaldehyde depression of several mitochondrial functions.

Glutathione is a major cell scavenger of toxic free radicals, and also spares and potentiates the function of other of the cell's guardians against peroxidative, free radical or electrophylic attack, such as vitamin E. Hepatic glutathione is depressed by alcohol, in part due to acetaldehyde, which may selectively deplete the mitochondria of glutathione (Hirano *et al.* 1992). The liver cell is thus left vulnerable to all manner of injuries mediated by peroxidative or other (electrophylic) mechanisms. Chronic alcohol feeding in rats depresses hepatic methionine synthetase (Barak *et al.* 1987), with an eventual fall in liver S-adenosyl-L-methionine levels. It is of great interest that glutathione levels can be restored by providing *S-adenosyl-L-methionine*, thereby lessening hepatotoxicity as measured by leakage of mitochondrial glutamic dehydrogenase into the bloodstream (Lieber *et al.* 1990a). This may be a prototypical example of a nutrient in relative deficiency, by the criterion that its provision in supernormal amounts counteracts expected deleterious events.

Vitamin E and *selenium* may profitably be considered together, since they serve a protective role as antioxidants and interact physiologically. Vitamin E and selenium behave synergistically: vitamin E reduces selenium requirement, prevents its loss from the body and maintains it in an active form; selenium spares vitamin E and reduces the requirement for the vitamin.

Vitamin E deficiency was only recently recognized as a complication of alcoholism. It had been described in adults with diverse causes of severe lipid malabsorption (Bieri *et al.* 1983), including primary biliary cirrhosis (Knight *et al.* 1986). Alcoholic patients with chronic pancreatitis, especially with fat malabsorption, were reported to have low serum vitamin E levels (Kalvaria *et al.* 1986). One would anticipate that symptomatic deficiency would be delayed by large body stores in adults (Sokol 1989). Lipid peroxidation is increased in rat liver when the animals are fed alcohol chronically along with a low vitamin E diet (Kawase *et al.* 1989) and hepatic alpha-tocopherol levels are low. Alpha-tocopherol is now known to be low in advanced human alcoholic liver disease such as cirrhosis (Leo *et al.* 1993) (see Fig. 8.4). Although vitamin E seems well "positioned" metabolically, when relatively deficient, to be important in allowing alcohol to cause hepatotoxicity by the mechanisms discussed, further evidence is needed, especially at the early stages of ethanol-induced liver damage, to confirm its role in human disease. No special dietary recom-

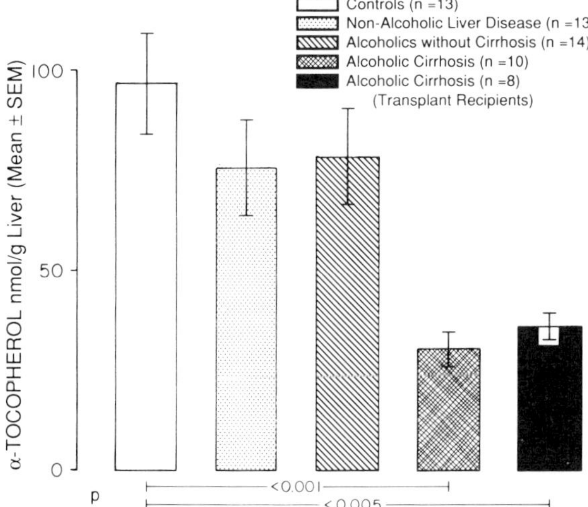

Fig. 8.4 Effect of various liver diseases on total hepatic tocopherols. Contrasting with $\alpha + \beta$ carotene and lycopene only the two cirrhotic groups had significantly lower α-tocopherol. Reproduced with permission from Leo *et al.* (1993).

mendations for vitamin E can be made for the alcoholic at this time.

Selenium metabolism is of great theoretic interest to hepatologists in view of the proposed lipoperoxidative mechanism of drug- and alcohol-induced liver injury (Lieber 1987). Serum selenium levels were noted to be low in alcoholics, especially with liver disease, but this could be a consequence of liver injury (Dworkin *et al.* 1985; Korpela *et al.* 1985a, b; Lieber 1987; Shah *et al.* 1985; Valimaki *et al.* 1983), since other, non-alcoholic patients with liver disease also have low levels. No recommendations for dietary modification of selenium intake in alcoholism are appropriate at this time.

Polyunsaturated lecithin

Choline deficiency can cause fatty liver in rats. However, there is no evidence that dietary choline deficiency causes human liver disease or is a part of alcohol-induced human liver disease. Additionally, choline therapy is not effective when alcohol intake is continued, probably reflecting low choline oxidase activity in human liver.

Alcohol-induced and choline deficiency-induced liver injury differ ultrastructurally (Iseri *et al.* 1966), in their levels of hepatic carnitine, in their response to orotic acid supplementation (Edreira *et al.* 1974)

and in their effects on lipoprotein production (Baraona and Lieber 1970; Chalvardian 1970). Even in rats, choline supplementation failed fully to prevent alcohol-induced liver injury and, at high levels, was associated with hepatotoxicity of its own. Side-effects such as nausea, vomiting, salivation, sweating and anorexia have been noted. Therefore, the current evidence shows no relevance of choline deficiency hepatotoxicity to alcohol-associated liver injury in humans or experimental animals. It is unlikely that choline supplementation could be provided safely as treatment, except in malnourished cirrhotic patients on parenteral nutrition devoid of a source of choline; these patients may be deficient in choline and may respond to choline supplementation with raised plasma choline (Chawla *et al.* 1989).

Polyunsaturated lecithin (PUL) afforded protection for baboons in the alcohol-induced model of cirrhosis in studies carried out over a 10 year span (Lieber *et al.* 1990b). Dietary polyunsaturated phosphatidylcholine is degraded by pancreatic phospholipase A2 and the products, 1-lysophosphatidylcholine and fatty acids, are absorbed in the jejunum. Isotopic labelling studies show an overall greater than 90 percent absorption of phosphatidylcholine. The polyene phosphatidylcholine is taken up by liver cells and appears in the membrane-containing fractions. It is unlikely that polyunsaturated lecithin is merely a better delivery system for choline; some of the reasons for this conclusion have already been discussed. The linoleate content of polyunsaturated lecithin is also not likely to be the beneficial component, since the control diets were already rich in that corn oil-derived fatty acid, a fatty acid which has previously been shown to be permissive rather than protective for alcoholic liver injury (Nanji and French 1989; Nanji *et al.* 1989). The mechanism by which polyunsaturated lecithin works is not fully elucidated, but several of its features are already discernible. The first feature may derive from the fact that polyene phosphatidylcholine is well positioned in the membranes to reverse the membrane alterations and related consequences of alcohol-induced injury (Thompson and Reitz 1978; Arai *et al.* 1984a, b). Feeding phosphatidylcholine has corrected the alcohol-induced decrease in hepatic phospholipids and phosphatidylcholine (Lieber *et al.* 1992), possibly related to a decreased activity of phosphatidylethanolamine-N-methyltransferase (Duce *et al.* 1988). The decrease in enzyme activity in alcohol-fed baboons precedes the development of

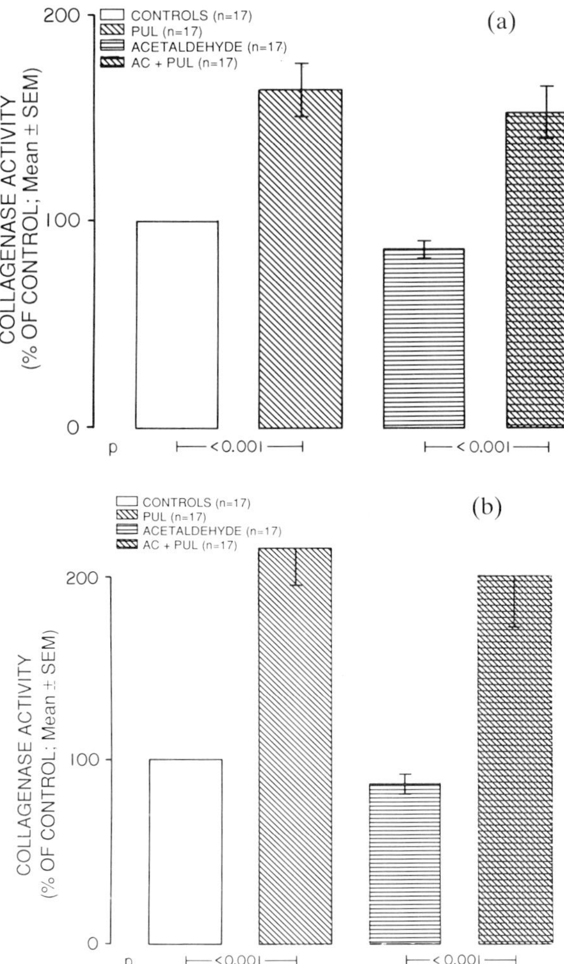

Fig. 8.5 (a) Effect of polyunsaturated lecithin (PUL) (with or without acetaldehyde) on collagenase activity of cultured lipocytes (media). (b) Effect of PUL (with or without acetaldehyde) on collagenase activity of cultured lipocytes (media + cells). PUL significantly increased collagenase activity, whereas acetaldehyde alone had no such effect. Reproduced with permission from Li *et al.* (1992).

cirrhosis (Lieber *et al.* 1994). A second feature concerns the interaction of polyunsaturated lecithin with the stimulating factors for collagen accumulation which arise from alcohol consumption. Polyunsaturated lecithin counteracts the acetaldehyde-induced increase in collagen accumulation in lipocyte cultures (Casini *et al.* 1991). Acetaldehyde stimulates collagen production, whereas polyunsaturated lecithin diminishes collagen accumulation, most likely by increasing collagenase activity (Fig. 8.5) and thereby presumably enhanc-

ing collagen degradation. Failure of collagen degradation, via collagenase, to keep pace with collagen production has been suggested as a possible factor leading to cirrhosis (Maruyama *et al.* 1982). Other phospholipids or linoleate alone, the fatty acid of polyunsaturated lecithin, do not share this property. Polyunsaturated lecithin is a mixture of lecithins containing linoleate. Since only dilinoleoylphosphatidylcholine reproduced the effect of polyunsaturated lecithin on collagenase, it must be considered to be the active component opposing collagen accumulation. Polyunsaturated lecithin can in no ordinary sense be considered lacking in the diets of alcoholics; however, should provision of dietary polyunsaturated lecithin in clinical trials prove to be effective in preventing alcoholic fibrosis, then it can be designated a "super nutrient" able to correct a relative deficiency.

Summary

We have witnessed some swings in our conception of the pathogenesis of alcoholic liver disease. In the eighteenth century, alcohol was considered a toxin. In the early part of the twentieth century, the aetiology of alcoholic liver disease was thought to be malnutrition. The failure to find cirrhosis in the adult ascribable to malnutrition *per se*, without concomitant alcoholism, has always made the malnutrition theory suspect. Experimental work since the middle of this century has established, on a firm scientific basis, that alcohol is indeed a direct hepatotoxin and causes the spectrum of liver disease despite the provision of what is acknowledged to be an adequate diet; but, in establishing the direct toxicity of alcohol, a complex interrelationship between alcohol metabolism and nutrition has been revealed. Alcoholism and the metabolism of alcohol have profound effects on the intake and metabolism of nutrients; they are responsible for many of the signs and symptoms of malnutrition typical of alcoholics with and without severe liver disease. Also, the quantitative and qualitative aspects of nutrient intake have important modulating effects on the pathogenesis of alcoholic liver disease. Recently, studies have commenced giving substances such as *S*-adenosyl-L-methionine or polyunsaturated lecithin in doses exceeding those expected in the usual diet, using them as "super-nutrients", with the exciting prospect that the development of alcoholic liver disease may thereby be thwarted.

References

Ahmed, S., Leo, M.A., Lowe, N. and Lieber, C.S. (1992). Alcohol abuse increases whereas alcoholic liver disease decreases plasma beta-carotene. *Hepatology* **16**, 78A.

Althausen, T.L., Uyeyama, K. and Loran, K. (1960). Effects of alcohol on absorption of vitamin A in normal and gastrectomized subjects. *Gastroenterology* **38**, 942.

Arai, M., Leo, M.A., Nakano, M., Gordon, E.R. and Lieber, C.S. (1984a). Biochemical and morphological alterations of baboon hepatic mitochondria after chronic ethanol consumption. *Hepatology* **4**, 165–174.

Arai, M., Gordon, E.R. and Lieber, C.S. (1984b). Decreased cytochrome oxidase activity in hepatic mitochondria after chronic ethanol consumption and the possible role of decreased cytochrome aa3 content and changes in phospholipids. *Biochimica et Biophysica Acta* **797**, 320–327.

Barak, A.J., Beckenhauer, H.C., Tuma, D.J. and Badakhsh, S. (1987). Effects of prolonged ethanol feeding on methionine metabolism in rat liver. *Biochemical Cell Biology* **65**, 230–233.

Baraona, E. and Lieber, C.S. (1970). Effects of chronic ethanol feeding on serum lipoprotein metabolism in the rat. *Journal of Clinical Investigation* **49**, 769–778.

Bieri, J.G., Corash, L. and Hubbard, V.S. (1983). Medical progress: Medical uses of vitamin E. *New England Journal of Medicine* **308**, 1063–1071.

Bonjour, J.P. (1981). Vitamin and alcoholism. *International Journal for Vitamin and Nutrition Research* **51**, 166–177.

Carney, E.A. and Russell, R.M. (1980). Correlation of dark adaptation test results with serum vitamin A levels in diseased adults. *Journal of Nutrition* **110**, 552–557.

Casini, A., Cunningham, M., Rojkind, M. and Lieber, C.S. (1991). Acetaldehyde increased procollagen type 1 and fibronectin gene transcription in cultured rat fat-storing cells through a protein synthesis-dependent mechanism. *Hepatology* **13**, 758–765.

Cederbaum, A.I., Lieber, C.S. and Rubin, E. (1974). The effect of acetaldehyde on mitochondrial function. *Archives of Biochemistry and Biophysics* **165**, 1187–1192.

Cederbaum, A.I., Lieber, C.S., Beattie, D.S. and Rubin, E. (1975). Effect of chronic ethanol ingestion on fatty acid oxidation by hepatic mitochondria. *Journal of Biological Chemistry* **250**, 5122–5129.

Cederbaum, A.I., Lieber, C.S. and Rubin, E. (1976). Effect of chronic ethanol consumption and acetaldehyde on partial reactions of oxidative phosphorylation and CO_2 production from citric acid cycle intermediates. *Archives of Biochemistry and Biophysics* **176**, 525–538.

Chalvardian, A. (1970). Mode of action of choline. V. Sequential changes in hepatic and serum lipids of choline deficient rats. *Canadian Journal of Biochemistry* **48**, 1234–1240.

Chawla, R.K., Wolf, D.C., Kutner, M.H. and Bonkovsky, H.L. (1989). Choline may be an essential nutrient in malnourished patients with cirrhosis. *Gastroenterology* **97**, 1514–1520.

Colditz, G.A., Giovannucci, E., Rimm, E.B., Stampfer, M.J., Rosner, B., Speizer, F.E., Gordis, E. and Willett, W.C. (1991). Alcohol intake in relation to diet and obesity in women and men. *American Journal of Clinical Nutrition* **54** 49–55.

Contaldo, F., D'Arrigo, E., Carandente, V., Cortese, C., Coltorti, A., Mancini, M., Taskinen, M.-R. and Nikkila, E.A. (1989). Short-term effects of moderate alcohol consumption on lipid metabolism and energy balance in normal men. *Metabolism* **38**, 166–171.

Crouse, J.R. and Grundy, S.M. (1984). Effects of alcohol on plasma lipoproteins and cholesterol and triglyceride metabolism in man. *Journal of Lipid Research* **25**, 486–496.

de Castro, J.M. and Orozco, S. (1990). Moderate alcohol intake and spontaneous eating patterns of humans: Evidence of unregulated supplementation. *American Journal of Clinical Nutrition* **52**, 246–253.

DiLuzio, N.R. and Hartman, A.D. (1967). Role of lipid peroxidation on the pathogenesis of the ethanol-induced fatty liver. *Federation Proceedings* **26**, 1436–1442.

DiLuzio, N.R. and Stege, T.E. (1977). The role of ethanol metabolites in hepatic lipid peroxidation. In *Alcohol and the Liver* (Edited by Fisher, M.M. and Rankin J.G.), pp. 45–62. Plenum Press, New York.

Duce, A.M., Ortiz, P., Cabrero, C. and Mato, J.M. (1988). *S*-adenosyl-L-methionine synthetase and phospholipid methyltransferase are inhibited in human cirrhosis. *Hepatology* **8**, 65–68.

Dworkin, B., Rosenthal, W.S. and Jankowski, R.H. (1985). Low blood selenium levels in alcoholics with and without advanced liver disease. *Digestive Diseases and Sciences* **30**, 838–844.

Edreira, J.G., Hirsch, R.L. and Kennedy, J.A. (1974). Production of fatty liver with dietary ethanol despite orotic acid supplementation. *Quarterly Journal on the Study of Alcohol* **35**, 20–25.

Feinman, L. and Lieber, C.S. (1988). Toxicity of ethanol and other components of alcoholic beverages. *Alcoholism: Clinical and Experimental Research* **12**, 2–6.

Gruchow, H.W., Sobocinski, K.A., Barboriak, J.J. and Scheller, J.G. (1985). Alcohol consumption, nutrient intake and relative body weight among US adults. *American Journal of Clinical Nutrition* **42**, 289–295.

Hasumura, Y., Teschke, R. and Lieber, C.S. (1975). Acetaldehyde oxidation by hepatic mitochondria: Its decrease after chronic ethanol consumption. *Science* **189**, 727–729.

Hillers, V.N. and Massey, L.K. (1985). Interrelationships of moderate and high alcohol consumption with diet and health status. *American Journal of Clinical Nutrition* **41**, 356–362.

Hirano, T., Kaplowitz, N., Tsukamoto, H., Kamimura,

S. and Fernandez-Checa, J.C. (1992). Hepatic mitochondrial glutathione depletion and progression of experimental alcoholic liver disease in rats. *Hepatology* **16**, 1423–1427.

Iseri, O.A., Lieber, C.S. and Gottlieb, L.S. (1966). The ultrastructure of fatty liver induced by prolonged ethanol ingestion. *American Journal of Pathology* **48**, 535–555.

Israel, Y., Videla, L. and Bernstein, L. (1975). Liver hypermetabolic state after chronic alcohol consumption: Hormonal interrelations and pathologic implications. *Federation Proceedings* **34**, 2052–2059.

Jolliffe, N. and Jellinek, E.M. (1941). Vitamin deficiencies and liver cirrhosis in alcoholism. Part Vll: Cirrhosis of the liver. *Quarterly Journal on the Study of Alcohol* **2**, 554–583.

Kalvaria, I., Labadarios, D., Shephard, G.S. *et al.* (1986). Biochemical vitamin E deficiency in chronic pancreatitis. *International Journal of Pancreatology* **1**, 119–128.

Kawase, T., Kato, S. and Lieber, C.S. (1989). Lipid peroxidation and antioxidant defense systems in rat liver after chronic ethanol feeding. *Hepatology* **10**, 815–821.

Knight, R.E., Bourne, A.J., Newton, M., Black, A., Wilson, P. and Lawson, M.J. (1986). Neurologic syndrome associated with low levels of vitamin E in primary biliary cirrhosis. *Gastroenterology* **91**, 209–211.

Korpela, H., Kumpalainen, J. and Luoma, P. (1985a) Decreased serum selenium in alcoholics as related to liver structure and function. *American Journal of Clinical Nutrition* **42**, 147–151.

Korpela, H., Kumpalainen, J. and Sotaniemi, E.A. (1985b). The role of selenium deficiency in the pathogenesis of alcoholic liver disease. *Nutrition Reviews* **40**, 424–425 (Suppl. I).

Korsten, M.A., Matszuzaki, S., Feinman, L. and Lieber. C.S. (1975). High blood acetaldehyde levels after ethanol administration in alcoholics. *New England Journal of Medicine* **292**, 386–389.

Lands, W.E.M. and Zakhari, S. (1991). The case of the missing calories. *American Journal of Clinical Nutrition* **54**, 47–48.

Lane, B.P. and Lieber, C.S. (1966). Ultrastructural alterations in human hepatocytes following ingestion of ethanol with adequate diets. *American Journal of Pathology* **49**, 593–603.

Larve-Achagiotis, C., Poussard, A.M. and Louis-Sylvestre, L. (1989). Effect of interscapular brown adipose tissue denervation on body weight and feed efficiency on alcohol drinking rats. *Physiological Behavior* **46**, 195–197.

Lee, M. and Lucia, S.P. (1965). Effect of ethanol on vitamin A mobilization in the dog and in the rat. *Journal of Studies on Alcohol* **26**, 1–8.

Lelbach, W.K. (1967). Leberschaden bei chronischen Alkoholismus. *Acta Hepatosplenology* (Stuttgart) **14**, 9–39.

Lelbach, W.K. (1975). Cirrhosis in the alcoholic and its relation to the volume of alcohol abuse. *Annals of the New York Academy of Sciences* **252**, 85–105.

Leo, M.A. and Lieber, C.S. (1982). Hepatic vitamin A depletion in alcoholic liver injury. *New England Journal of Medicine* **307**, 597–601.

Leo, M. and Lieber, C.S. (1983). Hepatic fibrosis after long term administration of ethanol and moderate vitamin A supplementation in the rat. *Hepatology* **2**, 1–11.

Leo, M.A. and Lieber, C.S. (1985). New pathway for retinol metabolism in liver microsomes. *Journal of Biological Chemistry* **260**, 5228–5231.

Leo, M.A., Arai, M., Sato, M. and Lieber, C.S. (1982). Hepatotoxicity of moderate vitamin A supplementation in the rat. *Gastroenterology* **82**, 194–205.

Leo, M.A., Sato, M. and Lieber, C.S. (1983). Effect of hepatic vitamin A depletion on the liver in humans and rats. *Gastroenterology* **84**, 562–572.

Leo, M.A., Kim, C. and Lieber, C.S. (1986). Increased vitamin A in esophagus and other extrahepatic tissues after chronic ethanol consumption in the rat. *Alcoholism: Clinical and Experimental Research* **10**, 487–492.

Leo, M.A., Rosman, A. and Lieber, C.S. (1993). Differential depletion of carotenoids and tocopherol in liver diseases. *Hepatology* **17**, 977–986.

Li, J., Kim, C.-I., Leo, M.A., Mak, K.M., Rojkind, M. and Lieber, C.S. (1992). Polyunsaturated lecithin prevents acetaldehyde accumulation by stimulating collagenase activity in cultured lipocytes. *Hepatology* **15**, 373–381.

Lieber, C.S. (1987). Alcohol and the liver. In *Liver Annual* (Edited by Arias, I.M., Frenkel, M.S. and Wilson, J.H.P.), Vol. VI, pp. 163–240. Excerpta Medica, Amsterdam.

Lieber, C.S. (1991a). Perspectives: Do alcohol calories count? *American Journal of Clinical Nutrition* **54**, 976–982.

Lieber, C.S. (1991b) Alcohol, liver, and nutrition. *Journal of the American College of Nutrition* **10**, 602–632.

Lieber, C.S. and DeCarli, L. (1991). Hepatotoxicity of ethanol. *Journal of Hepatology* **12**, 394–401.

Lieber, C.S., Jones, D.P. and DeCarli, L.M. (1965). Effects of prolonged ethanol intake: Production of fatty liver despite adequate diets. *Journal of Clinical Investigation* **4**, 1009–1021.

Lieber, C.S., DeCarli, L.M. and Rubin, E. (1975). Sequential production of fatty liver, hepatitis and cirrhosis in sub-human primates fed ethanol with adequate diets. *Proceedings of the National Academy of Sciences, USA* **72**, 437–441.

Lieber, C.S., Casini, A., DeCarli, L.M., Kim, C., Lowe, N., Sasaki, R. and Leo, M.A. (1990a). S-adenosyl-L-methionine attenuates alcohol-induced liver injury in the baboon. *Hepatology* **11**, 165–172.

Lieber, C.S., DeCarli, L.M., Mak, K.M., Kim, C.I. and Leo, M.A. (1990b). Attenuation of alcohol-induced hepatic fibrosis by polyunsaturated lecithin. *Hepatology* **12**, 1390–1398.

Lieber, C.S., Li, J.-J., Robins, S., DeCarli, L.M., Mak,

K.M. and Leo, M.A. (1992). Dietary dilinoleoylphosphatidylcholine (DLPC) is incorporated into liver phospholipids, protects against alcoholic cirrhosis, enhances collagenase activity and prevents acetaldehyde-induced collagen accumulation in cultured lipocytes. *Hepatology* **16**, 87A.

Lieber, C.S., Robins, S.J. and Leo, M.A. (1994). Hepatic phosphatidylethanolamine methyltransferase activity is decreased by ethanol and increased by phosphatidylcholine. *Alcoholism: Clinical and Experimental Research* **18** (in press).

Lindros, K.O. (1974). Acetaldehyde oxidation and its role in the overall metabolic effects of ethanol in the liver in regulation of hepatic metabolism. In *Proceedings of the Alfred Benson Symposium VI, Copenhagen 1973* (Edited by Lunquist, F. and Tygstrup, N.), pp. 417–432. Munksgaard, Copenhagen.

Maruyama, K., Feinman, L., Fainsilber, Z., Nakano, M., Okazaki, I. and Lieber, C.S. (1982). Mammalian collagenase increases in early alcoholic liver disease and decreases with cirrhosis. *Life Science* **30**, 1379–1384.

Matsuzaki, S. and Lieber, C.S. (1977). Increased susceptibility of hepatic mitochondria to the toxicity of acetaldehyde after ethanol consumption. *Biochemical and Biophysical Research Communications* **75**, 1059–1065.

Mendenhall, C., Bongiovanni, G., Goldberg, S., Miller, B., Moore, J., Rouster, S., Schneider, D., Tamburro, C., Tosch, T., Weesner, R. and the Veterans Administration Cooperative Study Group on Alcoholic Hepatitis (1985). VA cooperative study on alcoholic hepatitis III: Changes in protein-calorie malnutrition associated with 30 days of hospitalization with and without enteral nutritional therapy. *Journal of Parenteral and Enteral Nutrition* **9**, 590–596.

Mezey, E. (1978). Liver disease and nutrition. *Gastroenterology* **74**, 770–783.

Moshage, H., Casini, A. and Lieber, C.S. (1990). Acetaldehyde selectively stimulates collagen production in cultured rat liver fat-storing cells but not in hepatocytes. *Hepatology* **12**, 511–518.

Müller, A. and Sies, H. (1982). Role of alcohol dehydrogenase activity and of acetaldehyde in ethanol-induced ethane and pentane production by isolated perfused rat liver. *Biochemical Journal* **206**, 153–156.

Nanji, A.A. and French, S.W. (1989). Dietary linoleic acid is required for development of experimentally induced alcoholic liver injury. *Life Science* **44**, 223–227.

Nanji, A.A., Mendenhall, C.L. and French, S.W. (1989). Beef fat prevents alcoholic liver disease in the rat. *Alcohol: Clinical and Experimental Research* **13**, 15–19.

Olson, J.A. (1987). Recommended dietary intakes (RDI) of vitamin A in humans. *American Journal of Clinical Nutrition* **45**, 704–716.

Patek, A.J., Toth, I.G., Saunder, M.G., Castro, G.A.M. and Engel, J.J. (1975). Alcohol and dietary factors in cirrhosis. *Archives of Internal Medicine* **135**, 1053–1057.

Pequignot, G., Chabert, C., Eydoux, H. and Corcowl, M.A. (1974). Increased risk of cirrhosis with intake of alcohol. *Revue de Alcoolism* **20**, 191–202.

Pequignot, G., Tuyns, A.J. and Berta, J.L. (1978). Ascitic cirrhosis in relation to alcohol consumption. *International Journal of Epidemiology* **7**, 113–120.

Perman, E.S. (1972). Increase in oxygen uptake after small ethanol doses in man. *Acta Physiologica Scandinavica* **55**, 207–209.

Pikkarainen, P.H., Gorden, E.R., Lebsack, M.E. and Lieber, C.S. (1981). Determinants of plasma free acetaldehyde levels during the oxidation of ethanol: Effects of chronic ethanol feeding. *Biochemical Pharmacology* **30**, 799–802.

Pirola, R.C. and Lieber, C.S. (1972). The energy cost of the metabolism of drugs including alcohol. *Pharmacology* **7**, 185–196.

Pirola, R. and Lieber, C.S. (1975). Energy wastage in rats given drugs that induce microsomal enzymes. *Journal of Nutrition* **105**, 1544–1548.

Pirola, R.C. and Lieber, C.S. (1976). Hypothesis: Energy wastage in alcoholism and drug abuse. Possible role of hepatic microsomal enzymes. *American Journal of Clinical Nutrition* **29**, 90.

Polivy, J. and Herman, C.P. (1976a). Effects of alcohol on eating behavior: Disinhibition or sedation? *Addictive Behaviors* **1**, 121–125.

Polivy, J. and Herman, C.P. (1976b). Effects of alcohol on eating behavior: Influences of mood and perceived intoxication. *Journal of Abnormal Psychology* **85**, 601–606.

Reinus, J.F., Heymsfield, S.B., Wiskind, R., Casper, K. and Galambos, J.T. (1989). Ethanol: Relative fuel value and metabolic effects *in vivo*. *Metabolism* **38**, 125–135.

Rothwell, N.J. and Stock, M.J. (1984). Influence of alcohol and sucrose consumption on energy consumption and brown fat activity in the rat. *Metabolism* **33**, 768–771.

Rubin, E. and Lieber, C.S. (1967). Experimental alcoholic hepatic injury in man: Ultrastructural changes. *Federation Proceedings* **26**, 1458–1467.

Russell, R.M., Giovetti, A., Garrett, M., Thompson, J.N. and Mackey, E. (1979). Lack of direct ethanol effect on hepatic vitamin A mobilization. *Gastroenterology* **77**, 36A.

Sato, M. and Lieber, C.S. (1980). Hepatic vitamin A depletion after chronic ethanol consumption. *Gastroenterology* **79**, 1123A.

Sato, M. and Lieber, C.S. (1982). Increased metabolism of retinoic acid after chronic ethanol consumption in rat liver microsomes. *Archives of Biochemistry and Biophysics* **213**, 557–564.

Scheig, R. (1970). Effects of ethanol on the liver. *American Journal of Clinical Nutrition* **23**, 467–473.

Shah, N., Smith, A. and Picciano, M.F. (1985). Plasma selenium levels in alcoholic liver disease and primary biliary cirrhosis. *Nutrition Research* **40**, 385–387 (Suppl. I).

Shaw, S., Jayatilleke, E. and Lieber, C.S. (1981). Hepatic lipid peroxidation: Potentiation by chronic alcohol feeding and attenuation by methionine. *Journal of Laboratory and Clinical Medicine* **98**, 417–435.

Shaw, S., Rubin, K.P. and Lieber, C.S. (1983). Depressed hepatic glutathione and increased diene conjugates in alcoholic liver disease: Evidence of lipid peroxidation. *Digestive Diseases and Sciences* **28**, 585–589.

Sherlock, S. and Walshe, V. (1948). Effect of undernutrition in man on hepatic structure and function. *Nature* **161**, 604.

Siviy, S.M., Atrens, D.M., Jirasek, M. and Holmes, L.J. (1987). Effects of ethanol and tertiary-butanol on energy expenditure and substrate utilization in the rat. *Alcohol* **4**, 437–442.

Sokol, R.J. (1989). The coming of age of vitamin E. *Hepatology* **9**, 649–653.

Stock, A.L., Stock, M.J. and Stuart, J.A. (1973). The effect of alcohol (ethanol) on the oxygen consumption of fed and fasting subjects. *Proceedings of the Nutrition Society* **32**, 40A.

Stock, M.J. and Stuart, J.A. (1974). Thermic effects of ethanol in the rat and man. *Nutrition and Metabolism* **17**, 297–305.

Suter, P.M., Schutz, Y. and Jequier, E. (1992). The effect of ethanol on fat storage in healthy subjects. *New England Journal of Medicine* **326**, 983–987.

Teschke, R., Moreno, F., Heinen, E., Herrmann, J., Kruskemper, H.L. and Strohmeyer, G. (1983). Is there any evidence of a hyperthyroid hepatic state following chronic alcohol intake? *Alcohol and Alcoholism* **18**, 151–155.

Thompson, J.A. and Reitz, R.C. (1978). Effects of ethanol ingestion and dietary fat levels on mitochondrial lipids in male and female rats. *Lipids* **13**, 540–550.

Tremoliere, J. and Carre, L. (1961). Etudes sur la modalites d'oxydation de l'alcool chez l'homme normal et alcoholique. *Revue de Alcoolism* **7**, 202–227.

Valimaki, M.J., Harju, K.J. and Ylikahri, R.H. (1983). Decreased serum selenium in alcoholics – a consequence of liver dysfunction. *Clinica Chimica Acta* **30**, 291–296.

Westrate, J., Wunnink, I., Deurinberg, P. and Hautvast, J.G.A.J. (1990). Alcohol and its acute effects on resting metabolic rate and diet induced thermogenesis. *British Journal of Nutrition* **64**, 413–425.

Wilkinson, P., Santamaria, J.N. and Rankin, J.G. (1969). Epidemiology of alcoholic cirrhosis. *Australasian Annals of Medicine* **18**, 222–226.

Yamada, S., Mak, K.M. and Lieber, C.S. (1985). Chronic ethanol consumption alters rat liver plasma membranes and potentiates release of alkaline phosphatase. *Gastroenterology* **88**, 1799–1806.

9 The role of viral infections in alcoholic liver disease

Kunio Okuda and Kunihiko Ohnishi

Introduction

The suspicion that hepatitis B virus (HBV) infection aggravates alcoholic liver disease and that excess alcohol intake aggravates the disease caused by HBV has prompted numerous studies on the relationship between the two agents. While previous HBV infection in patients with alcoholic liver disease does not appear to play a major role in the rate of development or the severity of alcoholic liver disease, the co-existence of HBV infection does appear to contribute to hepatocarcinogenesis in patients with alcoholic liver disease (Brechot *et al.* 1982). Also, alcohol may expedite development of hepatocellular carcinoma in patients with liver disease due to chronic hepatitis B infection (Ohnishi *et al.* 1982) by acting as a cocarcinogen (Takada *et al.* 1986). Soon after the discovery of hepatitis C virus (HCV) and the development of an anti-HCV antibody test system (C100–3) the prevalence of anti-HCV antibodies was reported to be high in patients with alcoholic cirrhosis (Bruix *et al.* 1989) and in those with hepatocellular carcinoma (Okuda 1991; Okuda 1992). This high prevalence of HCV infection in alcoholic cirrhotics was then questioned on the grounds that hypergammaglobulinaemia, due to cirrhosis, could be causing false-positive results with the C100–3 test (Bodes *et al.* 1991). However, the early observations have been confirmed with the second-generation tests for HCV.

Estimation of relative risk of developing hepato-cellular carcinoma in a case control study showed that 25 percent of hepatocellular carcinoma cases in Italy were associated with anti-HCV positivity alone, and 20 percent with HBsAg carrier state alone (Stroffolini *et al.* 1992). It is now clear that the role of HCV infection is greater than that of HBV infection in hepatocarcinogenesis in industrialized countries such as Italy (Stroffolini *et al.* 1992), Spain (Ruiz *et al.* 1992) and Japan (Okuda 1991, 1992). Even in countries such as Taiwan, where HBV infection and HBV-associated hepatocellular carcinoma are endemic, HCV infection is prevalent among HBV-negative patients with chronic liver diseases including hepatocellular carcinoma (Chen *et al.* 1990). Currently, even more worldwide interest is focused on the relationship between alcoholic liver disease and HCV infection than on the role of HBV.

Hepatitis B virus

The role of HBV infection in alcoholic liver disease may vary with the stage of the liver injury and with the race/country of the patient. The differences in the spectrum of pathology seen in alcoholic liver disease in Japan and western countries (Ohnishi and Okuda 1986) will be discussed first, followed by a consideration of alcohol and HBV interactions.

Spectrum of alcoholic liver disease

Surveys conducted in the UK and Japan show differences in both the histological features and in the frequency of the various patterns of liver injury. For example, Japanese studies (Inoue 1977; Takada *et al.* 1982; Takeuchi 1982; Ishii *et al.* 1982; Ohnishi and Okuda 1985) have indicated that hepatic fibrosis and chronic hepatitis occur in a considerable proportion of HBsAg-negative chronic alcoholics and that the incidence of alcoholic hepatitis is very low. In these Japanese studies, the term "chronic hepatitis" has been used in accordance with the definition of the International Association for the Study of the Liver (Acapulco classification: Leevy *et al.* 1976); thus the term "chronic hepatitis" is used when portal inflammation and non-specific acinar (lobular) hepatitis, with or without piecemeal necrosis and bridging necrosis, was seen in the absence of the features of alcoholic hepatitis. Studies in the UK by Brunt *et al.* (1974), Krasner *et al.* (1977), Morgan and Sherlock (1977) and Hislop *et al.* (1983) reported the incidence of alcoholic hepatitis to range between 31 and 53 percent, while in Japan alcoholic hepatitis is seen much less frequently and Mallory bodies ("alcoholic hyaline") are rarely observed. For example, Takeuchi (1982) detected Mallory bodies in only 4 percent of patients with alcoholic hepatitis. This figure is strikingly different from the figure of 77 percent reported by French *et al.* (1977) in the USA. While no cases of chronic hepatitis were described in the four studies from the UK (Brunt *et al.* 1974; Krasner *et al.* 1977; Morgan and Sherlock 1977; Hislop *et al.* 1983), there have been occasional reports of chronic hepatitis in chronic alcoholics in other western countries, for example, Goldberg *et al.* (1977) described non-alcoholic chronic hepatitis among HBsAg-negative alcoholics, Galambos (1975) observed alcohol-induced chronic active hepatitis among alcoholics, while both Bruguera *et al.* (1977) and Levin *et al.* (1979) observed chronic active hepatitis and chronic persistent hepatitis in alcoholics. Thus, chronic hepatitis in alcoholics is not limited to the Japanese, but the incidence of this pattern of liver injury among alcoholics is considerably higher in Japan.

Another difference in the spectrum of alcoholic liver disease seen in Japan and western countries, lies in the higher incidence of hepatic fibrosis in chronic alcoholics in Japan. Pericellular fibrosis is usually present in alcoholic hepatitis and therefore is not considered a separate diagnostic category, consequently, there are no figures on the frequency of hepatic fibrosis in the studies from western countries mentioned above. Hepatocellular necrosis subsides following a short period of abstinence but pericellular fibrosis may continue to develop and certainly persists. In the Japanese studies, most of the liver biopsies were taken within the first 2 weeks of abstinence (Inoue 1977; Takada *et al.* 1982; Takeuchi 1982); thus the presence of alcoholic hepa-

titis is unlikely to have been missed. Given the rarity of alcoholic hepatitis in Japan, alcohol-associated pericellular fibrosis may be a pathological process that can occur independently of fatty liver, alcoholic hepatitis and alcoholic cirrhosis.

In any event, in Japanese patients, pericellular fibrosis and perivenular fibrosis, which are the main forms of alcohol-related hepatic fibrosis, may play an important role in the progression of the liver injury to cirrhosis. This type of progression has been demonstrated in the alcohol-fed baboon model, which develops cirrhosis without conspicuous features of alcoholic hepatitis and in which creeping fibrosis may be the main process that leads to cirrhosis (Popper and Lieber 1980).

The differences between the prevalence of Mallory bodies and other histological features seen in Japan and in western countries might be related, at least in part, to the difference in the dietary intake of fat and type of alcohol beverage consumed. Polymorphism of human liver alcohol dehydrogenase (Yin *et al.* 1984), aldehyde dehydrogenase (Harada *et al.* 1981) and the microsomal ethanol oxidizing system (Lieber and DeCarli 1970; Ohnishi and Lieber 1977, 1978) may also contribute in some way to these differences. The possibility that coexistent chronic viral infection modifies the pattern of alcohol-associated liver injury also merits consideration.

Hepatitis B virus infection in patients with alcoholic liver disease

Brechot *et al.* (1982) reported a high incidence of HBV infection in alcoholic patients in France, even in those negative for serum HBsAg. A serological study of alcoholic patients, who showed no evidence of hepatocellular carcinoma (HCC), indicated HBV exposure in 37 percent, and showed that HBV-DNA was present in liver tissue, obtained by needle biopsy, in 16 percent. However, the role of HBV infection in alcoholic liver disease with negative serum HBsAg has not been confirmed by others (Fong *et al.* 1988; Walter *et al.* 1988; Horiike *et al.* 1989). Fong *et al.* (1988) studied HBV-DNA in serum and liver from three groups of alcoholic patients: Group 1, 50 patients without liver disease; Group 2, 108 patients with alcoholic liver disease; and Group 3, five patients with alcoholic liver disease and HCCs. Serum was tested for HBsAg, anti-hepatitis B core and anti-hepatitis surface antigen by radioimmunoassay and for HBV-DNA by direct spot hybridization. Liver tissue from Groups 2 and 3 (113 patients) was examined by Southern blot analysis using ^{32}P-labelled HBV-DNA cloned from pBR 322. The controls were 21 patients with chronic hepatitis B virus (14 with chronic active hepatitis and seven with cirrhosis and HCC). Serum and tissue were analysed for HBV-DNA. Hepatitis B virus DNA was not detected in either serum or liver tissue in any of the 163 patients (Groups 1, 2 and 3). In contrast, HBV-DNA was present in the serum of 15 of the 21 controls. Tissue DNA analysis in those with chronic active hepatitis revealed free HBV-DNA in 10/14, integrated sequences in two and no viral sequences in two. All seven patients with a HCC had integrated viral DNA sequences in the tumour tissues. These results led the authors to conclude that HBV does not appear to play a role in the pathogenesis of alcoholic liver disease. Walter *et al.* (1988) investigated hepatic tumour tissue from HBsAg-negative patients with chronic alcoholic liver disease. Southern blot of DNA extracted from the tumours was negative for HBV-DNA in all 17 patients examined at a sensitivity level of less than 0.01 genome equivalent per cell. Similarly, in liver tissues from another 30 patients with alcoholic cirrhosis without HCC, no HBV-DNA was detectable. From these results, Walter *et al.* concluded that in their patients there was no molecular evidence for a contribution of HBV infection to the development of HCC in alcoholic liver disease.

Horiike *et al.* (1989) investigated HBV-DNA in the liver of 19 alcoholic patients with HCC. Hepatitis B virus-DNA was found integrated in tumour cells from five of six (83 percent) patients with HCC associated with HBsAg-positive post-hepatitic cirrhosis, but this was not related to the history of alcohol intake. HBV-DNA integration was not detected in any of the 13 patients with HBsAg-negative alcoholic liver cirrhosis and HCC. These authors concluded that HBV does not play a major role in the pathogenesis of hepatic tumours in HBsAg serum-negative alcoholics in Japan.

HBV infection and hepatocellular carcinoma in chronic alcoholics

In all parts of the world, alcohol is thought to be a risk factor for HCC, which develops in association with cirrhosis (Rogers and Conner 1986). Many reports support the association of alcoholism and HCC; for example, in alcoholic patients with hepatocellular carcinomas, 56 percent had a positive HBV serology and 100 percent had HBV-DNA in their tumours at autopsy (Brechot *et al.* 1982). These authors suggested that alcoholic patients with HBV-DNA in the liver are at high risk of developing tumours. In our study in Japan (Ohnishi *et al.* 1982), about 40–50 percent of patients with liver cirrhosis with or without HCC had a history of habitual alcohol intake of more than 69 g alcohol per day for more than 10 years. Case-control studies in the USA (Austin *et al.* 1986; Yu *et al.* 1991), Japan (Tsukuma *et al.* 1990; Tanaka *et al.* 1992), Canada (Qiao *et al.* 1988), Spain (Mayans *et al.* 1990), Taiwan (Chen *et al.* 1991) and South Africa (Mohamed *et al.* 1992) suggested a positive association of alcohol consumption with HCC, whereas a study in Greece (Trichopoulos *et al.* 1987) found no significant effect of alcohol on HCC incidence. In cohort studies, a weak or moderately positive relationship has been demonstrated between drinking and liver cancer (Hakulinen *et al.* 1974; Schmidt and Popham 1981; Trichopoulos *et al.* 1987), whereas one report in Japan indicated a considerably high risk of liver cancer among heavy drinkers of Japanese spirit (Shibata *et al.* 1986). Most of these studies support a positive relationship between drinking and HCC, but the risks estimated were far lower than those among HBV carriers. A link between HCC and alcoholic cirrhosis has also been noted. In Sakurai's (1969) series of 3000 consecutive necropsies in Japan, the prevalence of liver cirrhosis plus HCC was 20 percent in alcoholics as compared with 3 percent in non-alcoholics. In a study of 14,000 necropsies in Boston (Purtilo and Gottlieb 1973), alcohol abuse occurred in over 45 percent of the subjects who had HCC. Hepatocellular carcinoma was seen in 25 (30 percent) of 84 necropsied alcoholics with liver cirrhosis in London (Lee 1966). In the greater Copenhagen area, cirrhosis of the liver was found in 4 percent of 7763 necropsies performed in 1973, and HCC in 0.6 percent – half (56 percent) of the patients with cirrhosis and HCC were alcoholics (Norredam 1979).

However, it has become clear through the use of virus marker studies that alcoholics are often infected with HBV, making the interpretation of the data on alcoholism and HCC difficult. An aetiologic role of HBV in the development of HCC has been strongly suggested by the following (Okuda and Nakashima 1985):

(i) parallelism between the prevalence of HCC and frequency of HBsAg carriers;

(ii) high rates of positive HBV seromarkers in patients with HCC;

(iii) family clustering of HCC, liver cirrhosis and HBsAg carriers;

(iv) presence of HBsAg in the cytoplasm of non-cancerous hepatocytes in the liver of HBsAg-positive patients with HCC;

(v) production of HBsAg by several cell lines derived from human HCC;

(vi) integration of HBV genome into the cancer cell DNA;

(vii) development of HCC in certain animals infected by the indigenous hepatitis virus that is similar to human HBV;

(viii) frequent development of HCC in transgenic mice with HBV-X genome (Kim *et al.* 1991);

(ix) frequent occurrence of HCC among HBsAg carriers in comparison with non-carriers within the same population.

In Austria, where there are 47/100,000 deaths from cirrhosis per year among males, and where alcohol is the major aetiologic factor, HBsAg is detectable in the blood of 19 percent of male and 6 percent of female cirrhotics, compared with 0.5 percent of the general population (Rogers and Conner 1986). In one of our studies (Ohnishi *et al.* 1987), 25.6 percent of 156 chronic alcoholics with cirrhosis and HCC, who had a history of continuous intake of more than 69 g alcohol per day for more than 10 years, were positive for HBsAg in sera. These data not only indicate that heavy alcohol drinking *per se* may cause or promote the development of HCC, but also suggest that HBV infection plays a role in some measure in the development of HCC in chronic alcoholics. Although each factor (alcohol and chronic HBV infection) may be aetiologically related to HCC, the coexistence of both factors may cause, promote or hasten the development of HCC.

In 1983, we investigated the possibility that chronic HBV carriage expedites the development of HCC in cirrhotic patients who are drinkers (Ohnishi *et al.* 1983). In this study, 271 cirrhotic patients were divided into four groups based on the presence of HBsAg in serum and history of alcohol intake (more than 23 g alcohol/day for more than 10 years), and the frequency of development of HCC during the follow-up was compared among them. During the follow-up, 20 patients developed HCC. The frequency of development of HCC was greater in HBsAg-positive patients who were drinkers (15 percent), compared with HBsAg-negative drinking patients (7 percent), HBsAg-positive non-drinking patients (4 percent) and HBsAg-negative non-drinking patients (0 percent), although there was no significant difference in the average follow-up period from the diagnosis to the development of HCC among these groups. These results suggest that HBV carriage increases the incidence of HCC in cirrhotic patients who are drinkers.

We further attempted to determine whether HBV carriage hastens the development of liver cirrhosis and HCC in patients who are drinkers. In total, 158 patients with cirrhosis and 79 with HCC were analysed with respect to age at the time of diagnosis. They were classified into four groups based on HBsAg status and history of alcohol intake (more than 23 g alcohol/day for more than 10 years). The average age of HBsAg-positive male cirrhotics with a drinking habit (38.8 years) was less than that of HBsAg-negative male cirrhotics with the same habit (47.8 years), HBsAg-positive non-drinking male cirrhotics (49.3 years) and HBsAg-negative non-drinking male cirrhotics (58.4 years). The average age of HBsAg-positive male HCC patients with a drinking habit (48.9 years) was less that that of HBsAg-negative HCC males with the same habit (57.6 years), HBsAg-positive non-drinking HCC males (61.4 years) and HBsAg-negative non-drinking HCC males (60.6 years). These data suggest that chronic HBV carriage expedites the development of liver cirrhosis and HCC in patients who drink. However, in these studies no consideration was made for smoking, a habit frequently associated with alcoholism. In a case-control study in Greece, Trichopoulos *et al.* (1987) found an increased risk of HCC among smokers who were negative for serum HBsAg. A positive association of cigarette smoking with HCC has been demonstrated by case-control studies reported in Hong Kong (Lam *et al.* 1982), Los Angeles (Yu *et al.* 1991) and Taiwan (Chen *et al.* 1990), but has been challenged by other case-control studies in the USA (Austin *et al.* 1986), Spain (Mayans *et al.* 1990) and South Africa (Mohamed *et al.* 1992). In 1986, we investigated whether HBV carriage hastens the development of HCC in drinking patients taking smoking into consideration (Ohnishi *et al.* 1987). A total of 455 patients with HCC were analysed with respect to age at diagnosis. They were divided into eight groups based on HBsAg and anti-HBc in serum, a history of drinking more than 23 g/day for more than 10 years, and a history of smoking more than one pack of cigarettes per day for more than 10 years (Table 9.1). Among smokers with HCC, the average age of HBsAg-positive drinkers (50 years) was less

Table 9.1   Effects of HBsAg carriage and habitual alcohol intake on the ages of smoker or non-smoker HCC patients at the time of diagnosis

Group	n	Age at diagnosis (years)
HBsAg-positive, drinker and smoker	69	50 ± 10
HBsAg-negative, drinker and smoker	154	57 ± 9
HBsAg-positive, non-drinker and smoker	22	55 ± 10
HBsAg-negative, non-drinker and smoker	71	62 ± 9
HBsAg-positive, drinker and non-smoker	6	56 ± 14
HBsAg-negative, drinker and non-smoker	42	59 ± 9
HBsAg-positive, non-drinker and non-smoker	26	59 ± 8
HBsAg-negative, non-drinker and non-smoker	65	63 ± 12

Results are expressed as mean $\pm$ SD.

than that of HBsAg-negative drinkers (57 years), HBsAg-positive non-drinkers (55 years) and HBsAg-negative non-drinkers (62 years). Similarly, among non-smokers with HCC the average age of HBsAg-positive drinkers (56 years) was less than that of HBsAg-negative drinkers (59 years), HBsAg-positive non-drinkers (59 years) and HBsAg-negative non-drinkers (63 years). Furthermore, the average age of HBsAg-positive drinkers and smokers (50 years) was less than that of HBsAg-positive drinkers and non-smokers (56 years). These results suggest that both chronic HBV carriage and chronic alcohol intake hasten the development of HCC in smokers as well as non-smokers. The synergistic effect of chronic HBV carriage and chronic alcohol intake on the development of HCC may be strengthened by smoking. The following have been considered as possible mechanisms whereby alcohol abuse may promote the development of HCC:

(i) hepatocellular injury by ethanol (Ohnishi *et al.* 1982);

(ii) increase in the conversion of procarcinogen to cocarcinogen as a result of induction by alcohol of microsomal enzyme or alcohol-specific cytochrome P450 (Lieber and DeCarli 1970; Ohnishi and Lieber 1977, 1978; Capel *et al.* 1978; Ryan *et al.* 1985);

(iii) "preneoplasia" hypothesis for Mallory bodies which may be related to the genetically controlled neoplastic characteristics of the cells (Borenfreund *et al.* 1980; French 1981);

(iv) escape from the inhibitory stimulus for hepatocytic regeneration by ethanol (Bloomer *et al.* 1975), which may act as a promoter for the development of HCC. However, experiments have failed to produce evidence for the pathogenetic correlation of alcohol abuse to HCC.

Current theories of HBV-associated HCC tumorigenesis fall into two categories:

1. *Nonspecific mechanism*, in which HBV initiates a chronic inflammatory state that leads to unregulated hepatocyte proliferation, regeneration, random mutations and, ultimately, a transformed phenotype.

2. *Virally induced specific mechanism*, such as expression of viral oncogenes or transcriptional transactivating factors, inactivation of host protooncogenes, or mutations of host chromosomes such as translocations and gene rearrangements.

In the latter mechanism, integration of virus into the host DNA will be the initiating event (Brechot *et al.* 1980). Deoxyribonucleic acid integration sites may be most important in the oncogenic mechanism involved in cellular transformation and tumour formation. According to Fourel *et al.* (1990), study of woodchuck hepatomas revealed integration of the woodchuck virus, which is similar to HBV (hepadna virus) commonly occurring near the N-myc, a cell growth-related protooncogene. The "initiation" of infected hepatocytes would then be linked to cell regeneration as shown in experimental carcinogenesis. Cells with integrated sequences may escape the hepatotoxic immune effect, and interaction with chemical carcinogens and hormones could favour the clonal proliferation of these hepatocytes.

The combined role of chronic HBV infection and alcohol in the development of HCC may be due to the following:

(i) a non-specific mechanism, whereby both HBV and drinking initiate a chronic inflammatory state that leads to unregulated hepatocyte proliferation, regeneration, random mutations and, ultimately, a transformed phenotype, and/or

(ii) increased production of procarcinogens converted from their precursors by the alcohol-inducible cytochrome P450 isoenzyme (CYP2E1) or depletion of anti-tumour promoters such as retinoid as a result of drinking (Adachi *et al.* 1991), which would favour clonal proliferation of hepatocytes in which integration of the HBV genome has occurred (Ohnishi 1992).

Hepatitis C virus

It has long been known that typical alcoholic hepatitis and alcoholic cirrhosis are less common in Japan than in western countries (Table 9.2). The clinicopathological picture of alcoholic liver disease is also different (Inoue 1977; Takada *et al.* 1982, 1993a; Takeuchi 1982; Ishii *et al.* 1982; Ohnishi and Okuda 1985, 1986). In the west, alcoholic liver disease is usually classified into fatty liver, alcoholic hepatitis and cirrhosis (Hall 1985). However, in Japan, a considerable proportion of patients with alcoholic liver disease do not fall into these categories. A national study group in Japan proposed that three more histological types be added for diagnostic purposes in this country; namely, minimal or non-specific changes, alcoholic fibrosis and chronic hepatitis (Takeuchi 1982). This national Japanese study was based on 448 patients with alcoholic liver disease; fatty liver was seen in 12 percent, alcoholic hepatitis in 10 percent and cirrhosis in 33 percent of patients, leaving 45 percent not classifiable into the three basic histological types (Takeuchi 1982). In fact, fibrosis accounted for 25 percent, chronic hepatitis 10 percent and non-specific changes 11

Table 9.2 Relative frequency of alcoholic liver disease among all types of liver disease and of alcoholic cirrhosis among all types of cirrhosis in Japan, 1986–91 (National study: Chairman A. Takada)

	Liver disease		Cirrhosis	
Year	All types	Alcoholic (%)	All types	Alcoholic (%)
1986	10,445	1157 (11.1)	3858	592 (15.3)
1987	11,378	1314 (11.5)	4312	657 (15.2)
1988	12,903	1367 (1(.6)	4838	756 (15.6)
1989	13,305	1451 (10.9)	5151	786 (15.3)
1990	15,142	1463 (9.7)	5962	832 (14.0)
1991	14,839	1345 (9.1)	5812	738 (12.7)

percent. In contrast, a study in Vienna of 4060 patients with alcoholic liver disease showed fatty liver in 46 percent, 31 percent with alcoholic hepatitis, 11 percent with alcoholic fibrosis and 8 percent with alcoholic cirrhosis, but none was classified as chronic hepatitis (Thaler 1979). In a study by Rankin *et al.* (1978), of 167 patients none was described as having alcoholic fibrosis, chronic hepatitis or non-specific changes. Results of this type have led to a mounting suspicion that at least some of the Japanese patients with alcoholic liver disease had either a superimposed non-A, non-B virus infection, or that in such patients chronic non-A, non-B hepatitis was the predominant cause of liver disease with an insignificant influence from excessive alcohol intake. Some hepatologists believe that the hepatic fibrosis could have been due to a virus infection. Shortly after the discovery of HCV, the suspicion of a coexistent viral infection was shown to be correct. For example, Ishii *et al.* (1990) found that 59 percent of alcoholic patients, showing liver biopsy findings

Table 9.3 Aetiologic factors in various types of alcoholic liver disease in Japan, 1986–91 (National study: Chairman A. Takada)

Type of disease	No. of cases	Aetiologic factor		
		Alcohol alone (%)	AL + HCV (%)	AL + HBV (%)
Steatosis, others	820	84	15	1
Fibrosis	300	74	11	15
Chronis hepatitis	294	33	59	8
Alcoholic hepatitis	318	77	20	3
Cirrhosis	1141	51	44	5
Heptocellular carcinoma	981	32	59	9
All alcoholic liver disease	3854	61	33	6

AL, alcohol.

Table 9.4 Prevalence as percent of HCV-antibodies (C100-3) in patients with alcoholism and alcoholic liver disease

Authors	Country	Alcoholism with liver disease	Alcoholic Steatofibrosis	Alcoholic hepatitis	Chronic hepatitis	Cirrhosis	Hepatocellular carcinoma
Bruix et al. (1989)	Spain					38.7	76.6 (alcoholic)
Brillanti *et al.* (1989)	Italy					35.0[a]	
Pares *et al.* (1990)	Spain		20.0	21.4	25.0	42.6	
Nalpas *et al.* (1991)	France		13.0	17.5		35.9	56.2
Bodes *et al.* (1991)	Germany			6.7		38.5	
Mendenhall *et al.* (1991)	USA	4.8		27.1			
Shimizu *et al.* (1992)	Japan	5.0	3.1	0.0	73.3	46.2	83.3
Takada *et al.* (1993[b]	Japan		5.0	0.0	68.0	36.0	73.0

[a]10 of 14 had additional feature of chronic active hepatitis; [b]tests included Arima's clone #14.

compatible with chronic hepatitis, tested positive for C100–3 antibodies, while 78 percent of alcoholic patients with an hepatocellular carcinoma were also positive. Subsequent studies in Japan unanimously demonstrated that alcoholic patients with liver injury typical of western alcoholic liver disease were seldom positive for HCV, in contrast to those with chronic hepatitis and hepatocellular carcinoma who were frequently positive (Kiyosawa *et al.* 1990) (see Table 9.3). The use of the second-generation tests confirmed these findings. In the western countries where most patients show typical alcoholic liver disease, the HCV status is somewhat different, but the overall trend seems to be the same. In Spain, Pares *et al.* (1990) studied the prevalence of HCV antibodies among chronic alcoholic patients and found antibodies were present in 2.2 percent of patients without liver disease, 20 percent with steatofibrosis, 21.4 percent with alcoholic hepatitis and 42.6 percent with cirrhosis. Pares *et al.* contend that HCV infection is involved in the progression of liver damage in chronic alcoholic patients. One study in France (Nalpas *et al.* 1990) similarly showed progressive increases in HCV positivity as liver injury progressed from alcoholic steatofibrosis to alcoholic hepatitis to cirrhosis and finally to HCC, as shown in Table 9.4. It is interesting to note the difference between Japan and western countries; in Japan patients with alcoholic hepatitis, which is less common than in the west, are less frequently coinfected with HCV than patients with other patterns of alcoholic liver injury, while in western countries a considerable proportion of patients with alcoholic hepatitis do have HCV infection (Pares *et al.* 1990; Mendenhall *et al.* 1991). Figure 9.1 gives the frequency of HCV markers among Japanese patients with alcoholic liver disease and non-A, non-B liver diseases. The question asked is whether alcoholics have more frequent exposure and/or greater susceptibility to HCV. In all the four studies in which anti-HCV positivity was compared in patients with cirrhosis with and without hepatocellular carcinoma, a higher prevalence of positivity was found in the patients with tumours (Bruix *et al.* 1989; Nalpas *et al.* 1990; Shimizu *et al.* 1992; Takada *et al.* 1993a, b) (see Table 9.4). In other words, cirrhotic patients positive for anti-HCV who drink excessively develop tumours more readily than those who are negative for anti-HCV. Some studies in Europe are at variance with the these results; for example, data reported by Zarski *et al.* (1993) in France showed lower figures for HCV-antibody positivity, and HCV-RNA in serum was found to be much less

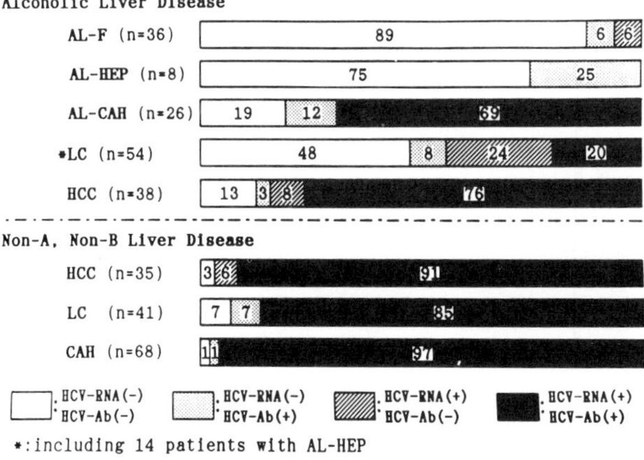

Fig. 9.1 Prevalence of HCV markers in patients with alcoholic liver disease and chronic non-A, non-B liver disease in Japan. AL, alcoholic; F, fibrosis; HEP, hepatitis; CAH, chronic active hepatitis; HCC, hepatocellular carcinoma. Courtesy of Dr A. Takada.

frequently positive. Zarski *et al.* postulated that the virus was not actively replicating and that the HCV-antibodies were anamnestic in alcoholic liver disease. However, HCV-RNA is much more frequently positive in the livers of Japanese patients with alcoholic liver disease (*vide infra*).

In liver biopsies showing chronic active hepatitis that are obtained from drinkers with chronic HCV infection, it is difficult to determine how much of the liver injury is due to virus and how much is due to alcohol. Takase *et al.* (1991) studied 27 Japanese who were heavy drinkers and showed the histological features of chronic active hepatitis: seven were positive for anti-HCV (C100–3) but negative for HCV-RNA, nine were positive for both C100–3 and HCV-RNA, seven were negative for both and four were positive for HBsAg. In the first and third groups, aspartic aminotransferase (AST) and alanine aminotransferase (ALT) quickly declined during 4 weeks of abstinence. Takase *et al.* postulated that in the first group both HCV and alcohol were contributing to the liver injury, that in the second group the chronic hepatitis was caused by HCV infection, and that in the third group the disease was caused solely by alcohol. They also studied the prognosis of alcoholic liver disease in relation to alcohol-altered liver membrane antibody (ALM-Ab) and HCV infection tested by HCV-RNA in 39 patients who were followed by repeated biopsies. They found that positivity for ALM-Ab significantly expedited development of cirrhosis, but that the presence of HCV markers did not. However, in patients with cirrhosis, the cumulative rates of development of hepatocellular carcinoma were significantly higher in HCV marker-positive patients compared with those that were negative (Takase *et al.* 1993). It is not yet clear whether HCV infection predisposes to ALM-Ab production. HCV-RNA in four heavy drinkers with chronic hepatitis became undetectable in plasma and clinical symptoms markedly improved within a few weeks after abstinence. In one patient, HCV-RNA became detectable again when he resumed drinking and the clinical status deteriorated (Takase *et al.* 1992; Takada *et al.* 1993b). These authors suggested that excess alcohol intake could enhance replication of HCV. They followed a number of patients with alcoholic liver disease: about one-third of 22 patients with alcoholic fibrosis progressed to cirrhosis within 2–7 years, and these patients were negative for HCV markers. All three patients with alcoholic hepatitis and about two-thirds of those with chronic hepatitis developed cirrhosis in 1–6 years. Thus, the development of cirrhosis was independent of HCV markers. Hepatocellular carcinoma developed in four of 14 patients with chronic hepatitis, but they were all HCV-positive. These results suggest that patients with alcoholic hepatitis and chronic hepatitis are at high risk of developing cirrhosis, and that the latter have a high risk of developing liver cancer. Based on these data, the authors postulated that, in about half of the patients with cirrhosis, the cirrhotic process developed from alcoholic hepatitis or alcoholic fibrosis, and in the other half the cirrhosis was a sequel to chronic hepatitis. In over 80 percent of patients with hepatocellular carcinoma, the tumour developed as a sequel to chronic hepatitis that had progressed to cirrhosis. Thus, heavy drinkers with chronic hepatitis C and HCV-positive alcoholic cirrhotics represent the group at greatest risk for hepatocellular carcinoma in Japan. Takada *et al.* (1993a, b) followed a total of 369 patients with cirrhosis of various aetiologies: 9.6 percent of alcoholic cirrhotics negative for HCV, 50 percent of alcoholic cirrhotics positive for HCV and 35 percent of HCV-positive patients with non-alcoholic cirrhosis developed hepatocellular carcinoma during the follow-up. The cumulative rate of tumour development was significantly higher in HCV marker-positive patients compared with those who were HCV marker-negative (Fig. 9. 2). The relative risk for the development of liver cancer in HCV carriers was estimated to be 8.3 times that in HCV-negative alcoholic cirrhotics. The probability of hepatocellular carcinoma in HCV carrier patients with alcoholic

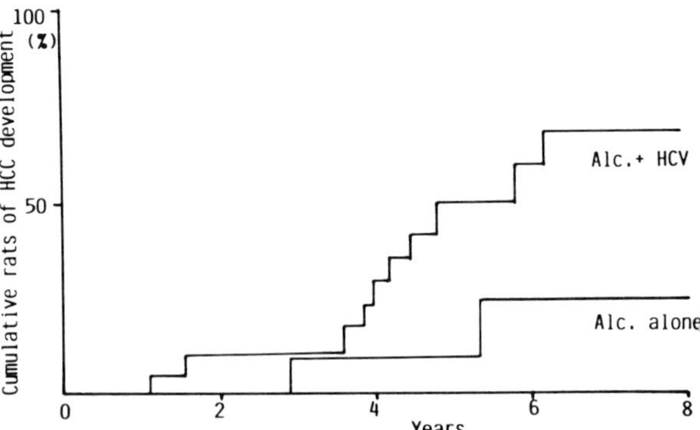

Fig. 9.2 Cumulative rate for development of hepatocellular carcinoma (HCC) in heavy drinkers with cirrhosis. HCC developed at a significantly higher rate in patients positive for HCV markers (alcohol + HCV) compared with those without HCV markers (alcohol alone). Reproduced with permission from Takada *et al.* (1993a).

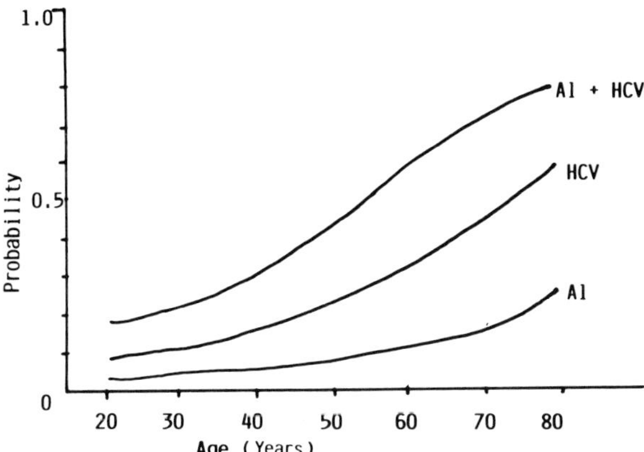

Fig. 9.3 Logistic curves illustrating the probability of HCC in patients with cirrhosis of various aetiologies. The probability of HCC in HCV-positive cirrhotics who drink excessively is significantly higher than in HCV-positive cirrhotics who do not drink. The probability of HCC is lowest among alcoholic cirrhotics who do not have HCV markers. A1, alcohol alone; HCV, HCV without alcohol; Al + HCV, alcohol and HCV. Reproduced with permission from Takada *et al.* (1993a).

cirrhosis was significantly higher (2.9 times) than that of non-alcoholic cirrhotics who carry HCV, and the probability was smallest in patients with alcoholic cirrhosis without HCV (Fig. 9.3). Takada *et al.* concluded that chronic alcoholism expedites the development of hepatocellular carcinoma in association with HCV, that alcohol and HCV are aetiopathologically dependent on one another, and that HCV infection also affects the course of alcoholic liver disease by a mechanism that is not yet well understood.

Table 9.5 gives the results of a national study in Japan on the frequency with which hepatocellular carcinoma complicates cirrhosis in alcoholics who have HBV or HCV infection. Clearly, both viruses increase the risk of liver cancer. Now that the complete nucleotide sequence of HCV is known (Okamoto *et al.* 1992), and with the development of knowledge on genotypes of HCV, questions have arisen as to whether differences in genotype make any difference in the natural history of chronic hepatitis C disease. According to Takase *et al.* (1992), 76.1 percent of Japanese patients with hepatocellular carcinoma and HCV infection had subtype K1 (type II), 17.4 percent K2a (type III) and 4.3 percent K2b (type IV). Heavy drinkers with hepatocellular carcinoma had K1 more frequently than did non-drinkers. All Chinese and Spanish patients with hepatocellular carcinomas and HCV

Table 9.5 Frequency of hepatocellular carcinoma among cirrhotic patients with different aetiologic factors in Japan, 1990–91 (National study: Chairman A. Takada)

Year	Alcohol alone	AL + HCV	AL + HBV
1990	130/495 (26.2%)	248/413 (60.0%)	38/75 (50.7%)
1991	164/536 (30.5%)	277/541 (61.4%)	46/67 (68.7%)

AL, alcohol.

Table 9.6 Relative frequency of HCV genotypes among patients with hepatocellular carcinoma

Country	No. of cases	HCV genotype (Kanazawa nomenclature)			
		PT (I)	K1 (II)	K2a (III)	K2b (IV)
Japan	46	1	35 (76.1%)	8 (17.4%)	2 (4.2%)
drinker	20	0	18 (90.0%)[a]	2 (10.0%)	0
non-drinker	26	1	17 (65.4%)[a]	6 (23.1%)	2
China	3	0	3 (100%)	0	0
Spain	7	0	7 (100%)	0	0

[a]$P < 0.05$. Reproduced with permission from Takase *et al.* (1992).

infection had subtype K1 (Table 9.6). As of writing, studies on the relationship between alcoholic liver disease and HCV infection are scarce outside Japan. The role of alcohol and HCV in other geographic areas is currently being investigated; whether the relationship between the two agents and the resultant liver disease is similar to that seen in Japan is not yet clear.

Summary

Although there is no strong evidence to suggest that alcohol intake aggravates the disease caused by hepatitis B virus, alcoholic liver disease and chronic hepatitis B virus infection may interact expediting the development of hepatocellular carcinoma. Hepatitis C virus infection is now aetiologically linked to hepatocellular carcinoma in a number of countries. Recent studies in Japan have clearly demonstrated that alcoholic cirrhotics who have chronic hepatitis C virus infection represent the highest risk group for hepatocellular carcinoma. The nature of the relationship between chronic liver disease caused by hepatitis C virus and alcoholic liver disease is as yet unresolved. It seems likely that the natural history of alcohol-related liver disease is modified by coexistent hepatitis C virus infection and that the natural history of chronic liver disease associated with the hepatitis C virus is modified by chronic alcohol ingestion.

Acknowledgement

We are indebted to Professors Akira Takase and Shujiro Takase for the provision of data and their permission to reproduce them in this chapter.

References

Adachi, S., Moriwaki, H., Muto, Y., Yamada, Y., Fukutomi, Y., Shimazaki, Y., Okuno, M. and Ninomiya, M. (1991). Reduced retinoid content in hepatocellular carcinoma with special reference to alcohol consumption. *Hepatology* **14**, 776–780 .

Austin, A., Delzelle, E., Grufferman, S., Levine, R., Morrison, A.S., Stolley, P.D. and Cole, P. (1986). A case-control study of hepatocellular carcinoma and hepatitis B virus, cigarette smoking, and alcohol consumption. *Cancer Research* **46**, 962–966.

Bloomer, J.R., Waldmann, A.T., McIntire, K.R. and Klastkin, G. (1975). Alpha-fetoprotein in non-neoplastic hepatic disorders. *Journal of the American Medical Association* **233**, 38–41.

Bodes, J.C., Biermann, J., Kohse, K.P., Walker, S. and Bode, C. (1991). High incidence of antibodies to hepatitis C virus in alcoholic cirrhosis: Fact or fiction? *Alcohol and Alcoholism* **26**, 111–114.

Borenfreund, E., Higgins, P.J. and Bendich, A. (1980). *In vivo-in vitro* rat liver carcinogenesis: Modifications in protein synthesis and ultrastructure. *Annals of the New York Academy of Science* **349**, 357–372.

Brechot, C., Pourcel, C., Louise, A., Rain, B. and Tiollais, P. (1980). Presence of integrated hepatitis B virus DNA sequence in cellular DNA of human hepatocellular carcinoma. *Nature* **286**, 533–535.

Brechot, C., Nalpas, B., Courouce, A., Duhamel, G., Callard, P., Carnot, F., Tiollais, P. and Berthelot, P. (1982). Evidence that hepatitis B virus has a role in liver-cell carcinoma in alcoholic liver disease. *New England Journal of Medicine* **306**, 1384–1387.

Brillanti, S., Barbara, K., Miglioli, M. and Bollino, F. (1989). Hepatitis C virus: A possible cause of chronic hepatitis in alcoholics. *Lancet* **ii**, 1390–1391.

Bruguera, M., Bordas, J.M. and Rodes, J. (1977). Asymptomatic liver disease in alcoholics. *Archives of Pathology and Laboratory Medicine* **101**, 644–647.

Bruix, J., Barbara, J.M., Calvet, X., Ercilla, G., Costa, J., Sanchez-Tapias, J.M., Ventura, M., Vall, M., Bruguera, M., Bru, C., Castillo, R. and Rodes, J. (1989). Prevalence of antibodies to hepatitis C virus in Spanish patients with hepatocellular carcinona and hepatic cirrhosis. *Lancet* **ii**, 1004–1006.

Brunt, P.W., Kew, M.C., Sheuer, P.J. and Sherlock, S. (1974). Studies in alcoholic liver disease in Britain. *Gut* **15**, 52–58.

Capel, I.D., Jenner, M., Pinnock, M.H. and Williams, D.C. (1978). The effect of chronic alcohol intake upon the hepatic microsomal carcinogen-activation system. *Oncology* **35**, 168–170.

Chen, C.J., Liang, K.Y., Chang, A.S., Chang, Y.C., Lu, S.N., Liaw, Y.F., Chang, W.Y., Sheen, M.C. and Lin, T.M. (1991). Effects of hepatitis B virus, alcohol drinking, cigarette smoking and familial tendency on hepatocellular carcinoma. *Hepatology* **13**, 398–406.

Chen, D.S., Kuo, G.C., Sung, J.L., Lai, M.Y., Sheu, J.C., Chen, P.J., Yang, P.M., Hsu, H.M., Chang, M.H., Chen, C.J., Hahn, L.C., Choo, Q.L., Wang, T.H. and Houghton, M. (1990). Hepatitis C virus infection in an area hyperendemic for hepatitis B and chronic liver disease: The Taiwan experience. *Journal of Infectious Diseases* **162**, 817–822.

Fong, T.L., Govindarajan, S., Valinluck, B. and Redeker, A.G. (1988). Status of hepatitis B virus DNA in alcoholic liver disease: A study of a large urban population in the United States. *Hepatology* **8**, 1602–1604.

Fourel, G., Trepo, C., Bougueleret, L., Henglein, B.,

Ponzetto, A., Tiollais, P. and Buedia, M. (1990). Frequent activation of N-myc genes by hepadnavirus insertion in woodchuck liver tumors. *Nature* **347**, 294–298.

French, S.W. (1981). The Mallory body: Structure, composition, and pathogenesis. *Hepatology* **1**, 76–83.

French, S.W., Sim, J.S., Franks, K.E., Burbige, E.J., Denton, T. and Caldwell, M.G. (1977). Alcoholic hepatitis. In *Alcohol and the Liver* (Edited by Fisher, M.M. and Rankin, J.G.), pp. 261–288. Plenum Press, New York.

Galambos, J.T. (1975). Chronic active hepatitis and ethanol – a form of drug hepatitis? *Gastroenterology* **68**, A1075.

Goldberg, S.J., Mendenhall, C.L., Connell, A.M. and Chedid A. (1977). Nonalcoholic chronic hepatitis in the alcoholic. *Gastroenterology* **72**, 598–604.

Hakulinen, T., Lehtimaki, L., Lehtonen, M. and Teppo, L. (1974). Cancer morbidity among two male cohorts with increased alcohol consumption in Finland. *Journal of the National Cancer Institute* **52**, 1711–1714.

Hall, P. (1985). Pathology and pathogenesis of alcoholic liver disease. In *Alcoholic Liver Disease: Pathobiology, Epidemiology and Clinical Aspects* (Edited by Hall, P.), pp. 41–68. Edward Arnold, London.

Harada, S., Agarwal, D.P. and Goedde, H.W. (1981). Aldehyde dehydrogenase deficiency as cause of facial flushing reaction to alcohol in Japanese. *Lancet* **ii**, 982.

Hislop, W.S., Bouchier, I.A.D. and Allan, J.G. (1983). Alcoholic liver disease in Scotland and northeastern England: Presenting features in 510 patients. *Quarterly Journal of Medicine (New Series LII)* **206**, 232–243.

Horiike, N., Michitaka, K., Onji, M., Murata, T. and Ohta, Y. (1989). HBV-DNA hybridization in hepatocellular carcinoma associated with alcohol in Japan. *Journal of Medical Virology* **28**, 189–192.

Inoue, K. (1977). The clinicopathological features of the alcoholic liver injury in Japan and its aetiological relationship to hepatitis B virus. *Gastroenterologia Japonica* **12**, 230–240.

Ishii, H., Takahashi, H., Takagi, T. and Tsuchiya, M. (1982). Alcoholic liver disease and hepatic fibrogenesis. *Journal of University of Occupational and Environmental Health* **4**, 147–156 (suppl.).

Ishii, K., Sata, M., Kumashiro, R., Ide, K., Nakano, H., Tanaka, S., Furudera, S., Tanaka, M., Majima, Y., Hirai, K., Abe, H. and Tanikawa, K. (1990). Studies on anti-HCV in hepatocellular carcinoma with alcoholic cirrhosis. *Acta Hepatologica Japonica* **31**, 1181–1185.

Kim, C.M., Koike, K., Saito, I., Miyamura, T. and Jay, G. (1991). HBx gene of hepatitis B virus induced liver cancer in transgenic mice. *Nature* **351**, 317–320.

Kiyosawa, K., Sodeyama, T., Gibo, Y., Yoshizawa, K., Nakano, Y., Furuta, S., Akahane, Y., Hishioka, K., Purcell, R. and Alter, H.J. (1990). Interrelationship of blood transfusion, non-A, non-B hepatitis and hepatocellular carcinoma: Analysis by detection of antibody to hepatitis virus. *Hepatology* **12**, 671–675.

Krasner, N., Davis, M., Portamann, B. and Williams, R. (1977). Changing pattern of alcoholic liver disease in Great Britain: Relation to sex and signs of autoimmunity. *British Medical Journal* **1**, 1497–1500.

Lam, K.C., Yu, M.C., Leung, J.W.C. and Henderson, B.E. (1982). Hepatitis B virus and cigarette smoking in risk factors for hepatocellular carcinoma in Hong Kong. *Cancer Research* **42**, 5246–5248.

Lee, F.I. (1966). Cirrhosis and hepatoma in alcoholics. *Gut* **7**, 77–85.

Leevy, C., Popper, H. and Sherlock, S. (1976). In *Diseases of the Liver and Biliary Tract: Standardization of Nomenclature, Diagnostic Criteria, and Diagnostic Methodology*, pp. 9–11. Fogarty International Center Proceedings No. 22, DHEW Publication No. (NIH) 77-725.

Levin, D.M., Baker, A.L., Riddell, R.H., Rochman, H. and Boyer, J.L. (1979). Nonalcoholic liver disease: Overlooked causes of liver inury in patient with heavy alcohol consumption. *American Journal of Medicine* **66**, 429–434.

Lieber, C.S. and DeCarli, L.M. (1970). Hepatic microsomal ethanol-oxidizing system: *In vitro* characteristics and adaptive properties *in vivo*. *Journal of Biological Chemistry* **245**, 2505–2512.

Mayans, M.Y., Calvet, X., Bruix, J., Bruguera, M., Costa, J., Esteve, J., Bosch, F.X., Bru, C. and Rodes, J. (1990). Risk factors for hepatocellular carcinoma in Catalonia, Spain. *International Journal of Cancer* **46**, 378–381 .

Mendenhall, C.L., Seeff, L., Diehl, A.M., Ghosn, S.J., French, S.W., Gartside, P.S., Rouster, S.D., Buskell-Bales, Z., Grossman, C.J., Roselle, G.A., Weesner, R.E., Garcia-Pont, P., Goldberg, S.J., Kiernan, T.W., Tamburro, C.H., Zetterman, R., Chedid, A., Chen, T., Rabin, L. and the Veterans Administration Cooperative Study Group (1991). Antibodies to hepatitis B virus and hepatitis C virus in alcoholic hepatitis and cirrhosis: Their prevalence and clinical relevance. *Hepatology* **14**, 581–589.

Mohamed, A.E., Kew, M.C. and Groeneveld, H.T. (1992). Alcohol consumption as a risk factor for hepatocellular carcinoma in urban southern African blacks. *Cancer* **51**, 537–541.

Morgan, M.Y. and Sherlock, S. (1977). Sex-related differences among 100 patients with alcoholic liver disease. *British Medical Journal* **1**, 939–941.

Nalpas, B., Driss, F., Pol, F., Hamelin, B., Housset, C., Brechot, C. and Berthelot, P. (1991). Association between HCV and HBV infection in hepatocellular carcinoma and alcoholic liver disease. *Journal of Hepatology* **12**, 70–74.

Norredam, K. (1979). Primary carcinoma of the liver: A histological study of 52 cases from Denmark. *Acta Pathologica et Microbiologica Scandinavica* **87**, 227–236.

Ohnishi, K. (1992). Alcohol and hepatocellular carcinoma. In *Alcohol and Cancer* (Edited by Watson, R.R.), pp. 179–201. CRC Press, Boca Raton, FL.

Ohnishi, K. and Lieber, C.S. (1977). Reconstitution of the microsomal ethanol-oxidizing system: Qualitative and quantitative changes of cytochrome P-450 after chronic ethanol consumption. *Journal of Biological Chemistry* **252**, 7124–7131.

Ohnishi, K. and Lieber, C.S. (1978). Respective role of superoxide and hydroxyl radical in the activity of the reconstituted microsomal ethanol oxidizing system. *Archives of Biochemistry and Biophysics* **191**, 798–803.

Ohnishi, K. and Okuda, K. (1985). The epidemiology of alcoholic liver disease in Japan. In *Alcoholic Liver Disease* (Edited by Hall, P.), pp. 167–183. Edward Arnold, London.

Ohnishi, K. and Okuda, K. (1986). Alcoholic liver disease in Japan. *Journal of Clinical Gastroenterology* **8**, 503–508.

Ohnishi, K., Iida, S., Iwama, S., Goto, N., Nomura, F., Takashi, M., Mishima, A., Kono, K., Kimura, K., Musha, H., Kotoda, K. and Okuda, K. (1982). The effect of chronic habitual alcohol intake on the development of liver cirrhosis and hepatocellular carcinoma: Relation to hepatitis B surface antigen carriage. *Cancer* **49**, 672–677.

Ohnishi, K., Iwama, S. and Nomura, F. (1983). Effects of habitual alcohol intake on the development and prognosis of chronic active hepatitis, liver cirrhosis and hepatocellular carcinoma. *Acta Hepatologica Japonica* **24**, 1341–1343.

Ohnishi, K., Terabayashi, H., Unuma, T., Takahashi, A. and Okuda, K. (1987). Effects of habitual alcohol intake and cigarette smoking on the development of HCC. *Alcoholism: Clinical and Experimental Research* **11**, 45–48.

Okamoto, H., Kurai, K., Okada, S., Yamamoto, K., Lizuka, H., Tanaka, T., Fukuda, S., Tsuda, F. and Mishiro, S. (1992). Full-length sequence of a hepatitis C virus genome having poor homology to reported isolates: Comparative study of four distinct genotypes. *Virology* **188**, 331–341.

Okuda, K. (1991). Hepatitis C virus and hepatocellular carcinoma. In *Aetiology, Pathology, and Treatment of Hepatocellular Carcinoma in North America* (Edited by Tabor, E., DiBisceglie, A.M. and Purcell, R.H.), pp. 119–126. Portofolio Publishing Co., Woodlands, TX.

Okuda, K. (1992). Hepatocellular carcinoma: Recent progress. *Hepatology* **15**, 948–963.

Okuda, K. and Nakashima, T. (1985). Primary carcinomas of the liver. In *Bockus Gastroenterology* (Edited by Berk, J.E.), 4th edn, Vol. 5, pp. 3315–3376. W.B. Saunders, Philadelphia, PA.

Pares, A., Barrera, J.M., Caballeria, J., Ercilla, G., Bruguera, M., Caballeria, L., Castillo, R. and Rodes, J. (1990). Hepatitis C virus antibodies in chronic alcoholic patients: Association with severity of liver injury. *Hepatology* **12**, 1295–1299.

Popper, H. and Lieber, C.S. (1980). Histogenesis of alcoholic fibrosis and cirrhosis in the baboon. *American Journal of Pathology* **98**, 695–716.

Purtilo, D.T. and Gottlieb, L.S. (1973). Cirrhosis and hepatoma occurring at Boston City Hospital (1917–1968). *Cancer* **32**, 458–462.

Qiao, Z.K., Halliday, M.L., Rankin, J.G. and Coates, R.A. (1988). Relationship between hepatitis B surface antigen prevalence, per capita alcohol consumption and primary liver cancer death rate in 30 countries. *Journal of Clinical Epidemiology* **41**, 787–792.

Rankin, J.G.D., Orrego-Matt, H., Deschenes, J., Medline, A., Findlay, J.E. and Armstrong, A.I. (1978). Alcoholic liver disease: The problem of diagnosis. *Alcoholism* **2**, 327–338.

Rogers, A.E. and Conner, M.W. (1986). Alcohol and cancer. *Advances in Experimental Medicine and Biology* **206**, 473–495.

Ruiz, J., Sangro, B., Cuende, J.I., Beloqui, O., Riezu-Boj, J.I., Herrero, J.I. and Prieto, J. (1992). Hepatitis B and C viral infection in patients with hepatocellular carcinoma. *Hepatology* **16**, 637–641.

Ryan, D.E., Ramanthan, L., Iida, S., Thomas, P.E., Haniu, J.E., Lieber, C.S. and Levin, W. (1985). Characterization of rat hepatic microsomal cytochrome. *Biological Chemistry* **260**, 6385–6393.

Sakurai, M. (1969). A histopathologic study on the effect of alcohol on cirrhosis and hepatoma of autopsy cases in Japan. *Acta Pathologica Japonica* **19**, 283–314.

Schmidt, W. and Popham, R.E. (1981). The role of drinking and smoking in mortality from cancer and other causes in male alcoholics. *Cancer* **47**, 1031–1041.

Shibata, A., Hirohata, T., Toshima, H. and Tashiro, H. (1986). The role of drinking and cigarette smoking in the excess deaths from liver cancer. *Japanese Journal of Cancer Research (Gann)* **77**, 287–295.

Shimizu, S., Kiyosawa, K., Sodeyama, T., Tanaka, E. and Nakano, M. (1992). High prevalence of antibody to hepatitis C virus in heavy drinkers with chronic liver diseases in Japan. *Journal of Gastroenterology and Hepatology* **7**, 30–35.

Stroffolini, T., Chiaramonte, M., Tiribelli, C., Villa, E., Simonetti, R.G., Rapicetta, M., Stazi, M.A., Bertin, T., Crece, S.L., Trande, P., Magliocco, A. and Chionne, P. (1992). Hepatitis C virus infection, HBsAg carrier state and hepatocellular carcinoma: Relative risk and population attributable risk from a case-control study in Italy. *Journal of Hepatology* **16**, 360–363.

Takada, A., Nei, J., Matsuda, Y. and Kanayama, R. (1982). Clinicopathological study of alcoholic fibrosis. *American Journal of Gastroenterology* **77**, 660–666.

Takada, A., Nei, J., Takase, S. and Matsuda, Y. (1986). Effects of ethanol on experimental hepatocarcinogenesis. *Hepatology* **6**, 65–72.

Takada, A., Takase, S. and Tsutsumi, M. (1993a). Characteristic features of alcoholic liver disease in Japan: A review. *Gastroenterologia Japonica* **28**, 181–192.

Takada, A., Takase, S. and Tsutsumi, M. (1993b). Alcohol and hepatic carcinogenesis. In: *Alcohol, Im-*

munity and Cancer (Edited by Yirmiya, R. and Taylor, A.N.), pp. 187–209. CRC Press, Boca Raton, FL.

Takase, S., Takada, N., Enomoto, N., Ysuhara, M. and Takada, A. (1991). Different types of chronic hepatitis in alcoholic patients: Does chronic hepatitis induced by alcohol exist? *Hepatology* **13**, 876–881.

Takase, S., Takada, N., Sato, I., Tsutsumi, M. and Takada, A. (1992). Relationship between alcoholic liver disease and HCV infection. In *Alcohol Metabolism and the Liver*, Vol. 12, pp. 115–120. Toyo Shoten, Tokyo. (in Japanese)

Takase, S., Tsutsumi, M., Kawahara, H., Takada, N. and Takada, A. (1993). The alcohol-altered liver membrane antibody and hepatitis C virus infection in the progression of alcoholic liver disease. *Hepatology* **17**, 9–13.

Takeuchi, J. (1982). Pathogenesis and characteristics of alcoholic liver injury in Japan. *Journal of the Japanese Society of Internal Medicine* **71**, 562–567.

Tanaka, K., Hirohata, T., Takeshita, S., Hirohata, I., Koga, S., Sugimachi, K., Kanematsu, T., Ohryohiji, F. and Ishibashi, H. (1992). Hepatitis B virus, cigarette smoking and alcohol consumption in the development of hepatocellular carcinoma: A case-control study in Fukuoka, Japan. *International Journal of Cancer (United States)* **51**, 509–514.

Thaler, H. (1979). Die Alkohol hepatitis. Ist sie die ausschleissliche Ursache einer Alkohol Zirrhose? *Internist* **20**, 179–184.

Trichopoulos, D., Day, N.E., Kaklamani, E., Tzonou, A., Munoz, N., Zavitsanos, X., Koumantaki, Y. and Trichopoulou, A. (1987). Hepatitis B virus, tobacco smoking and ethanol consumption in the aetiology of hepatocellular carcinoma. *International Journal of Cancer* **39**, 45–49.

Tsukuma, H., Hivama, T., Oshima, A., Sobue, T., Fujimoto, I., Kasugai, H., Kojima, J., Saski, Y., Imaoka, S. and Horiuchi, N. (1990). A case-control study of hepatocellular carcinoma in Osaka, Japan. *International Journal of Cancer* **45**, 231–236.

Walter, E., Blum, H.E., Meier, P., Huonker, M., Schmid, M., Maier, K.-P., Offensperger, W.-B., Offensperger, S. and Gerok, W. (1988). Hepatocellular carcinoma in alcoholic liver disease: No evidence for a pathogenetic role of hepatitis B virus infection. *Hepatology* **8**, 745–748.

Yin, S.J., Borson, W. and Li, T.K. (1984). Polymorphism of human liver alcohol dehydrogenase of ADH22–1 and ADH22–2 phenotyes in the Japanese by isoelectric focusing. *Biochemical Genetics* **22**, 169–180.

Yu, M.C., Tong, M.J., Govindarajan, S. and Henderson, B.E. (1991). Nonviral risk factors for hepatocellular carcinoma in a low-risk population, the non-Asians of Los Angeles county, California. *Journal of the National Cancer Institute (United States)* **83**, 1820–1826.

Zarski, J.P., Thelu, M.A., Moulin, C., Rachail, M. and Seigneurin, M.J. (1993). Interest of the detection of hepatitis C virus RNA in patients with alcoholic liver disease: Comparison with the HBV status. *Journal of Hepatology* **17**, 10–14.

10 Progenitor ("stem") cells in alcoholic liver disease?

Peter Van Eyken, Rita De Vos and Valeer J. Desmet

Introduction

This chapter starts with a definition of stem cells; the subsequent section briefly summarizes the currently available evidence pointing towards the existence of progenitor or stem cells in the liver. The final section reviews the data – at present very limited – on the presence and possible role of stem cells in alcoholic liver disease.

Terminology

Stem cells

Stem cells can be defined as multipotent cells that divide giving rise to two daughter cells; one cell remains a stem cell while the other daughter cell expresses a differentiated phenotype (Sell 1990). A fertilized ovum ultimately gives rise to a whole organism and as such can be considered a "totipotent stem cell" (Marceau 1990). "Pluripotent stem cells" are capable of generating several cell lineages. Progenitor cells that give rise to a single cell lineage are termed "unipotent" (Marceau 1990).

Tissue renewal

It is widely accepted that *continually renewing* cell populations such as the epidermis, the intestinal epithelium and the haematopoietic bone marrow contain a small population of stem cells (Hall 1992; Hall and Watt 1989). The identification of this population of cells has proved to be extremely difficult. Under normal circumstances, stem cells replace senescent cells. Stem cells also restore destroyed tissues in a variety of disease states (Sell 1990). In *static* cell populations, such as brain and peripheral nervous tissue, there is no cell division. *Conditional renewal* or *slowly renewing* cell populations occupy a position intermediate between static and continually renewing tissues. Normally there is little cell division, but cell proliferation can and does occur in response to certain stimuli (Hall 1992). Examples of conditional renewal tissues include the breast, pancreas and prostate gland. The liver is also usually included in this category (Hall 1992). It is claimed that conditional renewal tissues do not contain stem cells (Hall 1992).

Stem cells in the liver

It is well established that liver regeneration following a two-thirds hepatectomy in adult rats is essentially due to a rapid proliferation of the remaining hepatocytes (Marceau *et al.* 1989; Fausto and Mead 1989). Thus, in this model of liver regeneration, there is no need to invoke stem cells. The concept that the adult liver may contain a stem cell population is relatively new and derives its main support from insights gained from studies of experimental hepatocarcinogenesis, from cell culture data and from a better understanding of the normal embryonic development of the liver. In the rat, hepatocarcinogenesis caused by various chemicals is characterized at the histologic level by a proliferation of small epithelial cells termed "oval cells" because of their shape (Farber 1956; Opie 1944). The significance of oval cell proliferation and in particular the origin of these cells, their developmental fate and their relationship to the development of hepatocellular carcinoma have been debated for decades (Fausto *et al.* 1992; Farber and Sarma 1987; Sell 1990; Sell and Dunsford 1989). An exhaustive review of the currently available data on oval cells is clearly beyond the scope of this review and the reader is referred to some excellent reviews (Fausto *et al.* 1992; Sell 1990; Sell and Dunsford 1989). Detailed histologic observations, immunohistochemical analyses, radioactive labelling experiments and studies on isolated and cultured oval cells have led to the following concepts:

1. Oval cells are a *heterogeneous* population of non-parenchymal epithelial cells. A proportion of these cells express phenotypic markers of both hepatocytes and bile duct cells.
2. At least some cells in the oval cell compartment have a high *developmental plasticity*. Oval cells can differentiate into hepatocytes and can give rise to hepatocellular tumours. Other developmental options of oval cells include intestinal epithelial differentiation and formation of cholangiocarcinoma (Tatematsu *et al.* 1985; Sell and Dunsford 1989; Sell 1990).
3. The *origin* of oval cells. There is little doubt that oval cells belong to the bile duct cell lineage (Fausto 1990; Fausto *et al.* 1992; Lenzi *et al.* 1992).

Grisham (1980) deserves the credit for pointing out that normal hepatocytes in culture are non-clonogenic. Grisham suggested that the hepatic epithelial cells, isolated from normal rat livers, which retain some hepatocyte-like functions *in vitro*, derive in fact from stem cells (Grisham 1980; Tsao *et al.* 1984). Moreover, he introduced the important concept that stem cells are "facultative", that is they only proliferate in conditions of prolonged severe damage to virtually all hepatocytes coupled with inhibition of hepatocyte replication (Grisham 1980). Recent experimental data seem to confirm this hypothesis. Several groups (Lemire *et al.* 1991; Sirica and Williams 1992; Tournier *et al.* 1988) designed experimental protocols that lead simultaneously to hepatocyte damage and impaired regeneration. Treatment of rats with D-galactosamine induces the proliferation of oval cells and the appearance of both small hepatocytes and atypical duct-like structures (Lemire *et al.* 1991; Tournier *et*

al. 1988). Moreover, Lemire *et al.* (1991) were able to demonstrate that bile duct cells generated both the oval cells and the small hepatocytes. Sirica and Williams (1992) subjected rats to bile duct ligation followed by carbon tetrachloride intoxication. The (infrequent) appearance of "hepatic cell cholangioles", composed of both biliary epithelial cells and one or more ductular hepatocytes, was thought to indicate transdifferentiation of biliary epithelial cells into ductular hepatocytes.

Following studies using thymidine labelling of rat liver combined with autoradiography, Zajicek *et al.* (1985) proposed the concept of the "streaming liver". The hypothesis is that the liver is a two-compartment cell renewal system. Arber and Zajicek (1990) suggested that the ducts of Hering contain determined and uncommitted stem cells that differentiate into two committed stem cells, one a parenchymal cell and the other a biliary epithelial cell. However, the streaming liver concept – which implies that the liver stem cells are not just "facultative" – is by no means universally accepted (Tavoloni and Slott 1991).

Sigal *et al.* (1992) proposed a model in which the liver is organized in three compartments:

1. A slow cycling stem cell compartment with cells expressing a fetal phenotype and responding slowly to injury.
2. An amplification compartment with cells of intermediate phenotype rapidly proliferating in response to acute injury.
3. A terminal differentiation compartment in which cells increasingly differentiate and gradually lose their ability to divide.

With the growing evidence for the existence of stem cells in the liver, several groups became interested in normal embryonic development of the liver (Shah and Gerber 1989, 1990; Van Eyken *et al.* 1988a, b; Gall and Bhathal 1989; Shiojiri *et al.* 1991; Marceau *et al.* 1992; Marceau 1990; Germain *et al.* 1988). The early embryonic liver is composed of a population of progenitor cells that ultimately give rise to mature hepatocytes and bile duct cells (Stosiek *et al.* 1990; Desmet *et al.* 1990; Van Eyken and Desmet 1993). Immunohistochemical and cell culture studies indicate that cells forming the primitive bile duct structures or "ductal plates" during development are phenotypically equivalent to oval cells in rat liver (Shiojiri *et al.* 1991; Fausto *et al.* 1992). It is likely that a small number of progenitor cells persist in the adult liver. Unfortunately, a reliable marker for these progenitor cells is still lacking. Bisgaard and Thorgeirsson (1991) reported that cell lines established from primitive epithelial cells isolated from rat liver, comprise cells which are characterized by a unique pattern of expression of intermediate filament proteins, namely an absence of cytokeratins 18 and 19, the presence of vimentin, cytokeratins 7 and 8 and remarkably also cytokeratin 14. The observation that cytokeratin 14 was present in these cells raised the possibility that cytokeratin 14 could be used as a "marker" of progenitor cells in developing and adult liver; unfortunately, this hope has not been fulfilled (for a discussion, see Marceau *et al.* 1992).

Recent data suggest that progenitor cells in developing rat liver express the messenger RNA of a newly detected cytokeratin gene CKX and react with a monoclonal antibody BPC_5 directed against a hyperphosphorylated form of cytokeratin 8 (Marceau *et al.* 1992). It remains to be seen whether cytokeratin X and BPC_5 can be used to detect progenitor cells in adult liver. Another potentially useful marker is the 2.1 kb alpha-fetoprotein messenger RNA present in fetal livers, oval cells and hepatocellular carcinoma in the rat (Fausto *et al.* 1992).

Despite the absence of a reliable marker for liver stem cells, most authors have assumed that the stem cells reside somewhere in the biliary tree, most probably in its finest ramifications, the so-called ducts or canals of Hering which establish the continuity between the liver cell muralia and the draining bile ducts (Desmet 1987; Marceau *et al.* 1992; Sell 1990; Sell and Dunsford 1989; Lemire *et al.* 1991; Arber and Zajicek 1990). Nondescript periductular cells have also been proposed as the cells from which oval cells originate (Sell and Salman 1984; Evarts *et al.* 1990).

Although most of the available data on liver stem cells were obtained in animal models, observations implying the existence of a stem cell compartment in the human liver are beginning to appear. Immunohistochemical studies on the normal embryonic development of the liver also indicate that in humans, epithelial cells forming a partly duplicated layer of cells surrounding the portal vein branches (the "ductal plates") constitute a population of cells with phenotypic characteristics of both hepatocytes and bile duct cells (Van Eyken *et al.* 1988c; Desmet *et al.* 1990). Up to 50 percent of primary hepatocellular carcinomas express cytokeratins that are normally seen only in bile duct cells suggesting that the tumours may originate from cells with a biliary epithelial phenotype (equivalent to the oval cell in rat liver?). For a detailed discussion on the cytokeratin patterns in primary liver tumors and the implications for their histogenesis, see Van Eyken and Desmet (1993).

Regeneration following submasssive/massive hepatic necrosisis is probably partly due to a proliferation of duct-like structures, so-called "neocholangioles" (Phillips and Poucell 1981), composed of small cells often without a lumen (Gerber *et al.* 1983; Phillips and Poucell 1981). These cells express markers of hepatocytes (alpha-1-antitrypsin) and bile duct cells (carcinoembryonic antigen family of glycoproteins) and have therefore been termed "ductular hepatocytes" (Gerber *et al.* 1983). These ductular hepatocytes are thought to give rise to mature hepatocytes. Vandersteenhoven *et al.* (1990) observed that ductular hepatocytes, in a case of end-stage cirrhosis, were immunoreactive for hepatitis B surface antigen and bile duct-type cytokeratin (markers of liver parenchymal and bile duct cells, respectively). The presence of these intermediate cells was interpreted as evidence in favour of the existence of facultative stem cells. The earliest stage of regeneration following submassive/massive hepatic necrosis is characterized by the presence of small single cells with an oval nucleus, and scanty cytoplasm which is immunoreactive for the bile duct-type cytokeratin 19 and chromogranin A (Roskams *et al.* 1991). These small cells contain neuroendocrine granules, which suggests that the cells could produce substances that might play a role in the growth and/or differentiation of liver cells through an autocrine and/or paracrine pathway (Roskams *et al.* 1991). Moreover, ductular structures appearing in regenerating human liver are immunoreactive for parathyroid hormone-related peptide, a hormone which is thought to be involved in cellular growth and differentiation (Roskams *et al.* 1993). In an ultrastructural study of human livers, De Vos and Desmet (1992) described cells with an oval shape. Recently, Hsia *et al.* (1992) observed oval-type cells in non-neoplastic human liver tissue from patients with hepatocellular carcinoma.

Stem cells in alcoholic liver disease

As pointed out above, the concept of a liver stem cell is a recent one and derives its main support from animal experiments. Observations on progenitor

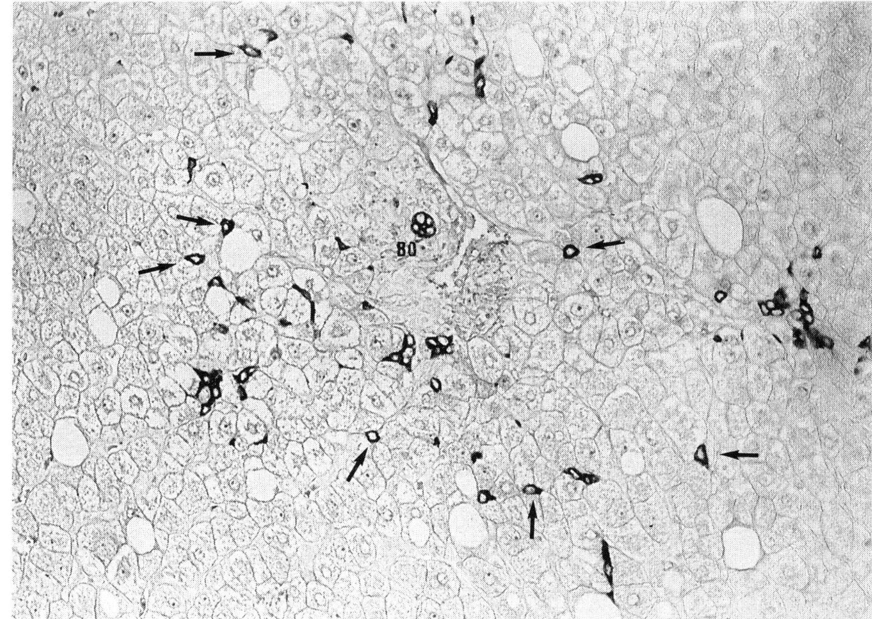

Fig. 10.1   Small epithelial cells in alcoholic steatosis. Paraffin section immunostained with a polyclonal anti-keratin antiserum. The interlobular bile duct is clearly positive. Note the presence of small, intensely positive cells with an oval shape located at some distance from the portal tract (arrows). PAP method, counterstained with Harris' haematoxylin ×300.

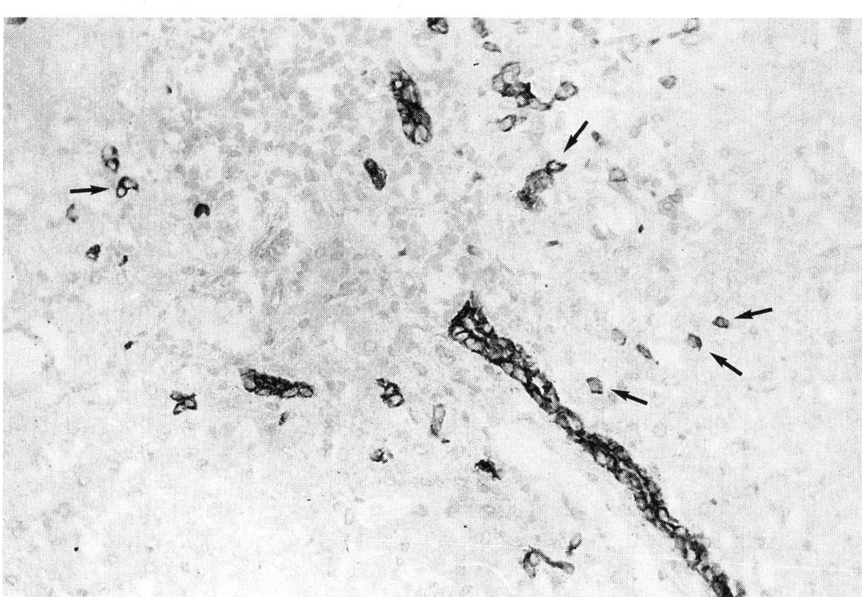

Fig. 10.2   Small epithelial cells in alcoholic steatosis. Cryostat section stained with a monoclonal antibody directed against cytokeratin 7. The interlobular bile duct and ductules are immunoreactive. A few cells with an oval shape are also positive (arrows). Indirect immunoperoxidase, counterstained with Mayer's haematoxylin ×300.

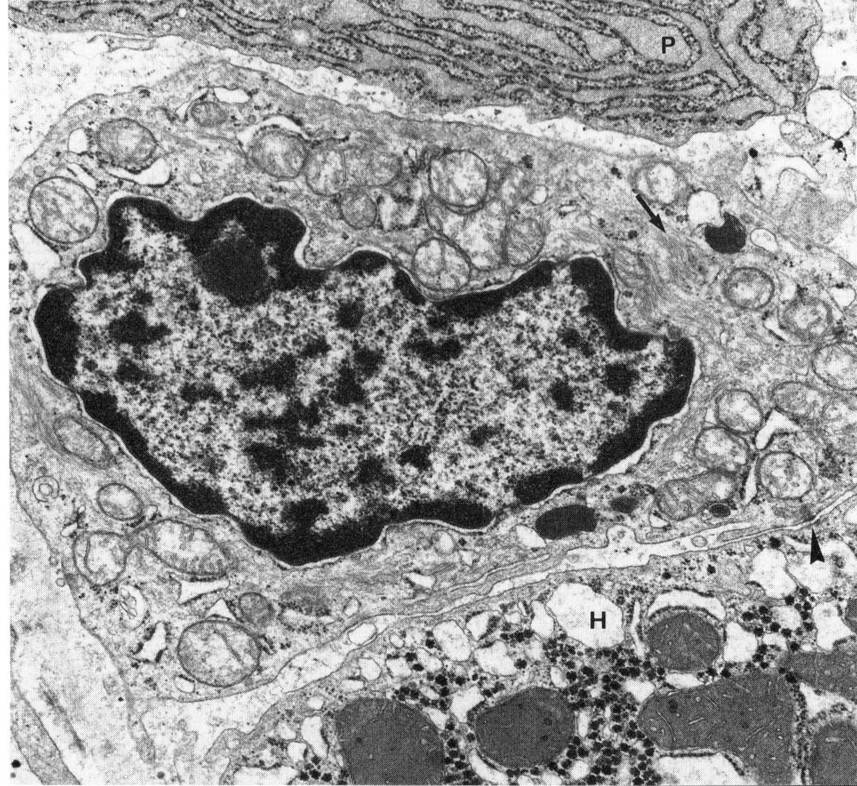

Fig. 10.3   Type I small cell in alcoholic hepatitis. The cell is situated at the sinusoidal pole of a hepatocyte (H). Note the presence of bundles of tonofilaments (arrow) and a developing desmosomal junction (arrowhead). P = plasma cell. ×16,100. Reproduced with permission from De Vos and Desmet (1992).

cells in human liver are still scarce. This section reviews the currently available data on stem cells in alcoholic liver disease and is supplemented with personal observations. In a cytokeratin-immuno-histochemical study of alcoholic liver disease, Ray (1987) noted the presence of cells which were smaller than hepatocytes, showing a central nucleus, an occasional small nucleolus, and scanty cytoplasm immunoreactive with monoclonal antibody AE1/AE3 (that in normal liver only stained the biliary epithelium). These cells, referred to by Ray (1987) as "oval" cells, were found scattered in a periportal location in non-alcoholic as well as alcoholic liver disease. Ray again stressed the morphologic similarity of these small cells in the human liver to the oval cells in experimental hepatocarcinogenesis, but he did not speculate on the significance of the finding. More recently, Ray *et al.* (1993) found small, bile duct-type cytokeratin positive "oval" cells in 98 percent of cases of alcoholic liver disease

(including cases of steatosis, fibrosis and cirrhosis). The number of "oval" cells was usually small. Lai *et al.* (1989) and Gerber and Thung (1992) also mentioned the presence of "small cells with oval nuclei" scattered as single cells or in groups between the parenchymal cell muralia; both of these studies illustrate the liver of a patient with alcoholic liver disease in which scattered "oval" cells stained positively with a polyclonal antibody to high molecular weight cytokeratins (an antibody which, in the liver, normally reacts only with bile duct cells) (Lai *et al.* 1989; Gerber and Thung 1992). "Oval" cells are not restricted to alcoholic liver disease; similar cells have been detected in "several" other types of liver disease (Ray 1987; De Vos and Desmet 1992). We have also observed small cells with an oval shape which are immunoreactive with both a polyclonal anti-cytokeratin antibody (Fig. 10.1) and with monoclonal antibodies directed against cytokeratins 7 and 19 (cytokeratins 7 and 19 are normal constituents of

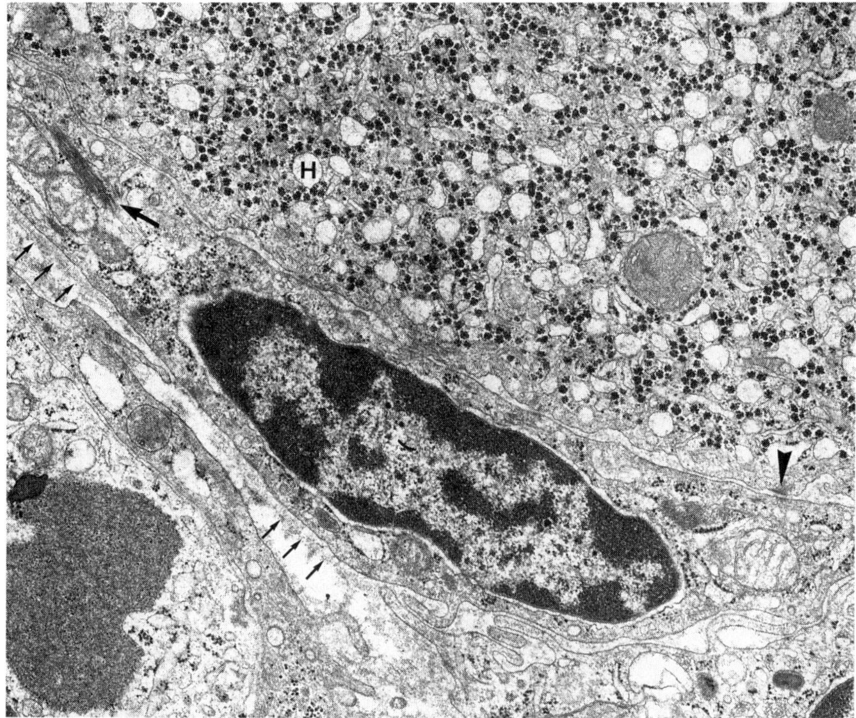

Fig. 10.4 Type I small cell in alcoholic hepatitis. The cell is situated at the sinusoidal pole of a hepatocyte (H). The cell contains bundles of tonofilaments (arrow). There is a developing desmosomal junction (arrowhead). Note a discontinuous basement membrane (small arrow). ×16,100. Reproduced with permission from De Vos and Desmet (1992).

the intermediate filament cytoskeleton of the biliary epithelium) in alcoholic liver disease (Fig. 10.2). In a detailed ultrastructural study, De Vos and Desmet (1992) analysed 13 livers, including five cases of alcoholic hepatitis and two of cirrhosis, possibly alcoholic. In all specimens, a variable number of small cells with similar epithelial characteristics were identified in the periportal area. The small epithelial cells were classified into three types:

Type I cells with a diameter of approximately 7–10 μm had an oval or oblong shape and contained an oval or oblong nucleus. A round nucleolus was often observed at the nuclear margin. The cytoplasm contained a moderate number of mitochondria, a few apparent lysosomes, slightly dilated rough endoplamic reticulum cisternae and some smooth vesicles. Several bundles of tonofilaments were always obvious. Early or well-formed junctional complexes of the desmosomal type joined these small cells with adjacent hepatocytes. Very often, a

discontinuous basement membrane surrounded the small cells (Figs 10.3, 10.4). Type I cells were typically localized at the sinusoidal pole of the hepatocytes or in the perisinusoidal recesses.

Type II cells presented the same overall characteristics as type I cells but showed in addition some features specific of biliary epithelial cells, including apical microvilli, interdigitations of the lateral membrane, basal pinocytotic vacuoles and a continuous basement membrane (Fig. 10.5). Type II small cells were preferentially localized in the vicinity of "proliferating" bile ductules, next to bile ductular cells (Fig. 10.5).

Type III cells had the characteristics of type I cells but displayed in addition features of hepatocytes. This cell type was more voluminous – approximately 10–15 μm diameter – with a more prominent nucleus. The cytoplasm contained more organelles and the cells formed a hemicanaliculus with neigh-

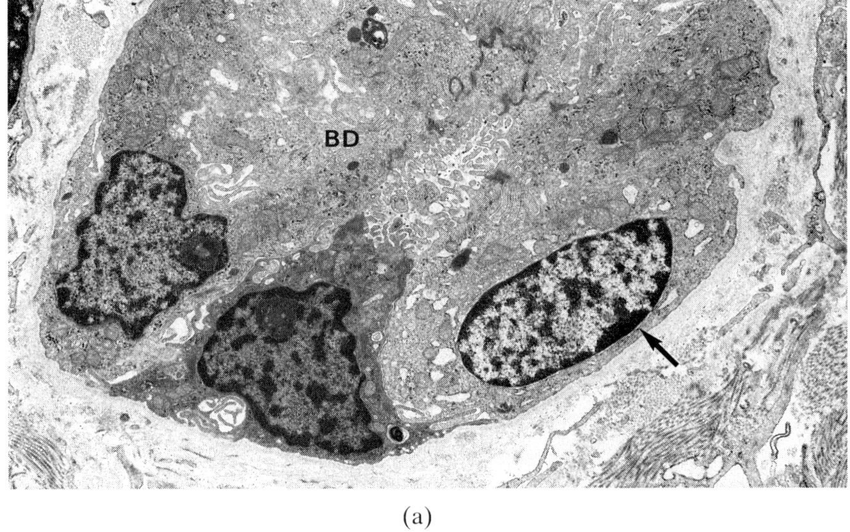

(a)

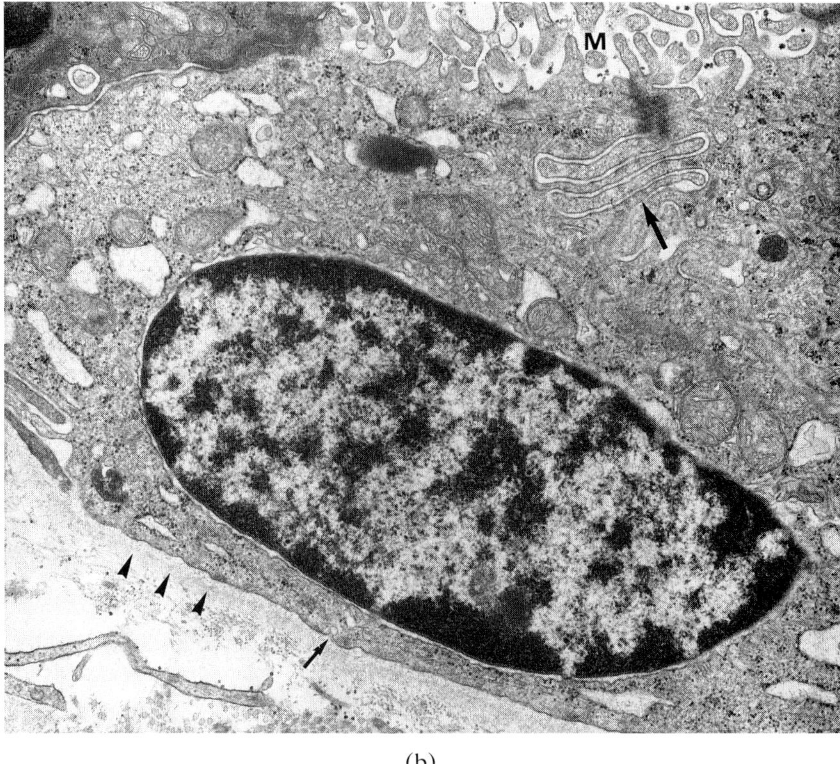

(b)

Fig. 10.5 Type II small cell in alcoholic hepatitis. (a) The cell (arrow) is located next to bile ductular cells (BD) ×5075. (b) Higher magnification of (a) showing apical microvilli (M), interdigitations of the lateral cell membrane (arrow), pinocytotic invaginations (small arrow) and a basement membrane (arrowhead). ×16,100. Reproduced with permission from De Vos and Desmet (1992).

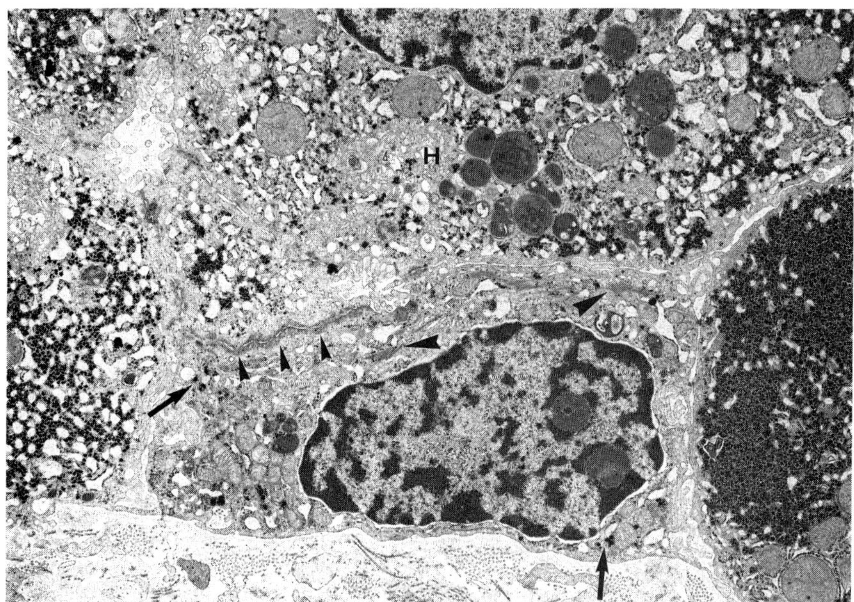

Fig. 10.6 Type III small cell in alcoholic hepatitis. The cell is situated adjacent to hepatocytes (H). Tonofilaments (arrowhead), canalicular microvilli (arrow), glycogen rosettes (small arrow) and intercellular junctions are present (small arrowhead). ×6400. Reproduced with permission from De Vos and Desmet (1992).

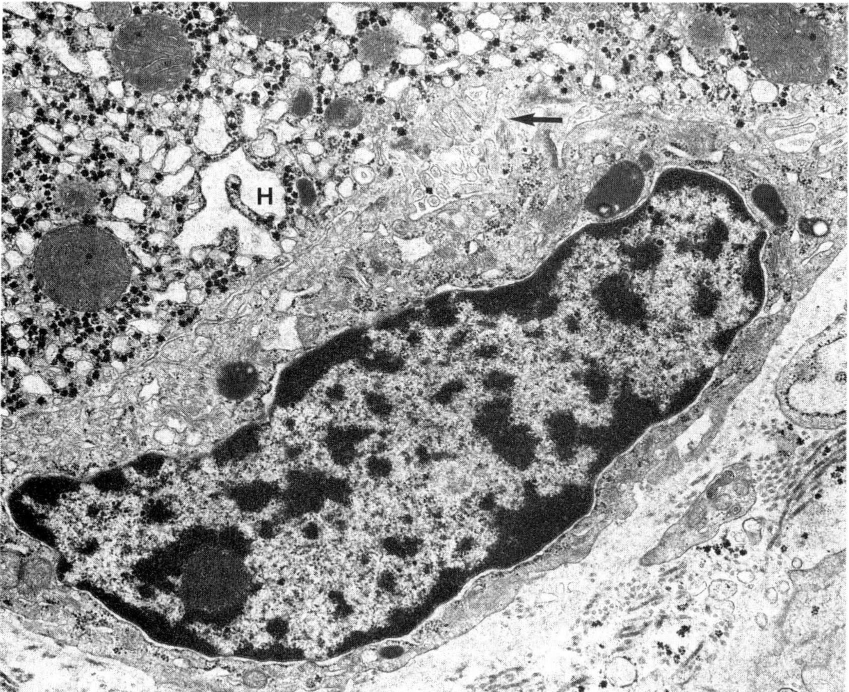

Fig. 10.7 Cell type intermediate between type I and type III in alcoholic hepatitis. The cell is situated next to a hepatocyte (H). Note the presence of canalicular microvilli (arrow). ×12,900. Reproduced with permission from De Vos and Desmet (1992).

hepatic proliferation: Antigenic expression by proliferating epithelial cells in fetal liver, massive hepatic necrosis and nodular transformation of the liver. *American Journal of Pathology* **110**, 70–74.

Germain, L., Blouin, M.J. and Marceau, N. (1988). Biliary epithelial and hepatocyte cell lineage relationships in embryonic rat liver as determined by the differential expression of cytokeratins, alphafetoprotein, albumin and cell surface-exposed components. *Cancer Research* **48**, 4909–4918.

Grisham, J.W. (1980). Cell types in long-term propagable cultures of rat liver. *Annals of the New York Academy of Sciences* **349**, 128–137.

Hall, P.A. (1992). Differentiation, stem cells and tumour histogenesis. In *Recent Advances in Histopathology* (Edited by Anthony, P.P. and MacSween, R.N.M.), Vol. 15, pp. 1–17. Churchill Livingstone, Edinburgh.

Hall, P.A. and Watt, F.M. (1989). Stem cells: The generation and maintenance of cellular diversity. *Development* **106**, 619–633.

Hsia, C.C., Evarts, R.P., Nakatsukasa, H., Marsden, E.R. and Thorgeirsson, S. (1992). Occurrence of oval-type cells in hepatitis B virus-associated human hepatocarcinogenesis. *Hepatology* **16**, 1327–1333.

Lai, Y.-S., Thung, S., Gerber, M., Chen, M.-L. and Schaffner, F. (1989) Expression of cytokeratins in normal and diseased livers and in primary liver carcinomas. *Archives of Pathology and Laboratory Medicine* **113**, 134–138.

Lemire, J.M., Shiojiri, N. and Fausto, N. (1991). Oval cell proliferation and the origin of small hepatocytes in liver injury induced by D-galactosamine. *American Journal of Pathology* **139**, 535–552.

Lenzi, R., Liu, M.H., Tarsetti, F., Slott, P.A., Alpini, G., Zhai, W.R., Paronetto, F., Lenzen, R. and Tavoloni, N. (1992). Histogenesis of bile duct-like cells proliferating during ethionine hepatocarcinogenesis: Evidence for a biliary epithelial nature of oval cells. *Laboratory Investigation* **66**, 390–402.

Marceau, N. (1990). Cell lineages and differentiation programs in epidermal, urothelial and hepatic tissues and their neoplasms. *Laboratory Investigation* **63**, 4–20.

Marceau, N., Blouin, M.J., Germain, L. and Noel, M. (1989). Role of different epithelial cell types in liver ontogenesis, regeneration and neoplasia. *In vitro Cellular and Developmental Biology* **25**, 336–341.

Marceau, N., Blouin, M.J., Noel, M., Torok, N. and Loranger, A. (1992). The role of bipotential progenitor cells in liver ontogenesis and neoplasia. In *The Role of Cell Types in Hepatocarcinogenesis* (Edited by Sirica, A.E.), pp. 121–149. CRC Press, Boca Raton, FL.

Okada, T.S. (1986). Transdifferentiation in animal cells: Fact or artifact ? *Development, Growth and Differentiation* **28**, 213–221.

Opie, E.L. (1944). The pathogenesis of tumors in the liver produced by butter yellow. *Journal of Experimental Medicine* **80**, 231–246.

Phillips, M.J. and Poucell, S. (1981). Modern aspects of the morphology of viral hepatitis. *Human Pathology* **12**, 1060–1084.

Ray, M.B. (1987). Distribution patterns of cytokeratin antigen determinants in alcoholic and nonalcoholic liver diseases. *Human Pathology* **18**, 61–66.

Ray, M.B., Mendenhall, C.L., French, S.W. and Gartside, P.S. (1993). Bile duct changes in alcoholic liver disease. *Liver* **13**, 36–45.

Roskams, T., De Vos, R., Van den Oord, J.J. and Desmet, V. (1991). Cells with neuroendocrine features in regenerating human liver. *APMIS* **23**, 32–39 (suppl.).

Roskams, T., Campos, R.V., Drucker, D.J. and Desmet, V.J. (1993). Reactive human bile ductules express parathyroid hormone-related peptide. *Histopathology* **23**, 519–525.

Scarpelli, D.G. (1985). Multipotent developmental capacity of cells in the adult animal. *Laboratory Investigation* **52**, 331–333.

Sell, S. (1990). Is there a liver stem cell? *Cancer Research* **50**, 3811–3815.

Sell, S. and Dunsford, H. A. (1989). Evidence for the stem cell origin of hepatocellular carcinoma and cholangiocarcinoma. *American Journal of Pathology* **134**, 1347–1363.

Sell, S. and Salman, J. (1984). Light- and electron-microscopic autoradiographic analysis of proliferating cells during the early stages of chemical hepatocarcinogenesis in the rat induced by feeding *N*-2-fluorenylacetamide in a choline-deficient diet. *American Journal of Pathology* **114**, 287–300.

Shah, K.D. and Gerber, M.A. (1989). Development of intrahepatic bile ducts in humans: Immunohistochemical study using monoclonal cytokeratin antibodies. *Archives of Pathology and Laboratory Medicine* **113**, 1135–1138.

Shah, K.D. and Gerber, M.A. (1990). Development of intrahepatic bile ducts in humans. *Archives of Pathology and Laboratory Medicine* **114**, 597–600.

Shiojiri, N., Lemire, J.M. and Fausto, N. (1991). Cell lineages and oval cell progenitors in rat liver development. *Cancer Research* **51**, 2611–2620.

Sigal, H., Brill, S., Fiorino, A.S. and Reid, L.M. (1992). The liver as a stem cell and lineage system. *American Journal of Physiology* **263**, G139–148.

Sirica, A.E. and Williams, T.W. (1992). Appearance of ductular hepatocytes in rat liver after bile duct ligation and subsequent zone 3 necrosis by carbon tetrachloride. *American Journal of Pathology* **140**, 129–136.

Slack, J.M.W. (1986). Epithelial metaplasia and the second anatomy. *Lancet* **ii**, 268–270.

Stosiek, P., Kasper, M. and Karsten, U. (1990). Expression of cytokeratin 19 during human liver organogenesis. *Liver* **10**, 59–63.

Tatematsu, M., Kaku, T., Medline, A. and Farber, E. (1985). Intestinal metaplasia as a common option of oval cells in relation to cholangiofibrosis in liver of rats exposed to 2-acetylaminofluorene. *Laboratory Investigation* **52**, 354–362.

Tavoloni, N. (1987). The intrahepatic biliary epithelium: An area of growing interest in hepatology. *Seminars in Liver Disease* **7**, 280–292.

Tavoloni, N. and Slott, P. A. (1991). Correspondence. *Gastroenterology* **100**, 582–583.

Thorgeirsson, S.S. and Evarts, R.P. (1992). Growth and differentiation of stem cells in adult rat liver. In *The Role of Cell Types in Hepatocarcinogenesis* (Edited by Sirica, A.E.), pp. 109–120. CRC Press, Boca Raton, FL.

Tournier, I., Legres, L., Schoevaert, D., Feldmann, G. and Bernuau, D. (1988). Cellular analysis of alpha-fetoprotein gene activation during carbon tetrachloride and D-galactosamine-induced acute liver injury in rats. *Laboratory Investigation* **59**, 657–665.

Tsao, M.-S., Smith, J.D., Nelson, K.G. and Grisham, J.W. (1984). A diploid epithelial cell line from normal adult rat liver with phenotypic properties of "oval" cells. *Experimental Cell Research* **154**, 38–52.

Uchida, T. and Peters, R.L. (1983). The nature and origin of proliferated bile ductules in alcoholic liver disease. *American Journal of Clinical Pathology* **79**, 326–333.

Vandersteenhoven, A.M., Burchette, J. and Michalopoulos, G. (1990). Characterization of ductular hepatocytes in end-stage cirrhosis. *Archives of Pathology and Laboratory Medicine* **114**, 403–406.

Van Eyken, P. and Desmet, V.J. (1993). Development of intrahepatic bile ducts, ductular metaplasia of hepatocytes and cytokeratin patterns. In *The Role of Cell Types in Hepatocarcinogenesis* (Edited by Sirca, A.E.), pp. 227–263. CRC Press, Boca Raton, FL.

Van Eyken, P., Sciot, R. and Desmet, V. (1988a). Intrahepatic bile duct development in the rat: A cytokeratin-immunohistochemical study. *Laboratory Investigation* **59**, 52–59.

Van Eyken, P., Sciot, R. and Desmet, V.J. (1988b). A cytokeratin-immunohistochemical study of alcoholic liver disease: Evidence that hepatocytes can express "bile duct-type" cytokeratins. *Histopathology* **13**, 605–617.

Van Eyken, P., Sciot, R., Callea, F., Van der Steen, K., Moerman, P. and Desmet, V.J. (1988c). The development of the intrahepatic bile ducts in man: A keratin-immunohistochemical study. *Hepatology* **8**, 1586–1595.

Van Eyken, P., Sciot, R., Paterson, A., Callea, F., Kew, M.C. and Desmet, V.J. (1988d). Cytokeratin expression in hepatocellular carcinoma: An immunohistochemical study. *Human Pathology* **12**, 562–568.

Van Eyken, P., Sciot, R. and Desmet, V.J. (1989). A cytokeratin immunohistochemical study of cholestatic liver disease: Evidence that hepatocytes can express "bile duct-type" cytokeratins. *Histopathology* **15**, 125–135.

Zajicek, G., Oren, R. and Weinreb, J.R.M. (1985). The streaming liver. *Liver* **5**, 293–300.

Part IV
Differential Diagnosis

11 Non-alcoholic steatohepatitis and other forms of pseudoalcoholic liver disease

Hyman J. Zimmerman and Kamal G. Ishak

Introduction

Non-alcoholic steatohepatitis is the term introduced by Ludwig *et al.* (1980) for an entity (or perhaps a group of entities) that is defined by histological features resembling those of alcoholic liver disease. While the name denotes simulation of alcoholic hepatitis, not all cases that have been included under this rubric resemble alcoholic hepatitis fully. Many resemble alcoholic steatosis, and those with cirrhosis resemble alcoholic cirrhosis. Indeed, the range of lesions considered to be steatohepatitis is implicit in the many other designations that have been used to refer to cases whose hepatic changes are in this category. Other terms include fatty metamorphosis of the liver in morbid obesity, diabetic hepatitis, fatty liver hepatitis, non-alcoholic fatty hepatitis, alcohol-like liver disease in non-alcoholics, fasting in obesity, liver injury with "alcoholic" hyalin, steatonecrosis and non-alcoholic Laennec's (French *et al.* 1989). Faithful resemblance to alcoholic hepatitis among the series of cases reported as non-alcoholic steatohepatitis ranges from a figure as high as 90 percent (Diehl *et al.* 1988) to one as low as 10 percent (Powell *et al.* 1990). Indeed, it is our view

that referring to the range of changes as *pseudoalcoholic liver disease* is more appropriate than the term non-alcoholic steatohepatitis.

Histological entities resembling alcoholic liver disease

There are five histological patterns that resemble those of alcoholic liver disease to a variable degree (Table 11.1). Three of them clearly warrant the designation of pseudoalcoholic liver disease in as much as they resemble phases of alcoholic liver disease. They are steatosis, steatohepatitis and cirrhosis. The fourth resembles alcoholic hepatitis because of a profusion of Mallory bodies but differs from steatohepatitis in the scantiness of steatosis. The fifth histological pattern is the presence of Mallory bodies in a histological pattern otherwise characteristic of an unrelated, specific clinical entity.

These patterns also appear to have clinical associations (Table 11.1). The patterns resembling the three phases of alcoholic liver disease, with apparent progression from steatosis to alcoholic hepatitis-like changes and cirrhosis, are seen in association with obesity (especially morbid obesity), the surgical treatment of obesity and type II diabetes mellitus. The resemblance to alcoholic hepatitis in the profusion of Mallory bodies and inflammation, but scantiness of steatosis, is seen in the lesion associated with adverse reactions to amiodarone, perhexiline maleate and Coralgil (trade name for 4-4'-diethylaminoethoxyhexestrol), as well as experimental agents including griseofulvin and environmental toxic injury (?Indian childhood cirrhosis). The fifth pattern, the finding of Mallory bodies in

Table 11.1   Histological patterns bearing resemblance to those of alcoholic liver disease

Clinical associations	Steatosis (3–4+)	Steatohepatitis Fat, inflammation ± Mallory bodies	Steato-cirrhosis	Alcoholic hepatitis Mallory bodies, inflammation ± cirrhosis	Mallory bodies in unrelated setting
Obesity/diabetes					
Obesity	3–4+	±	+		
Bypass	3–4+	3+	3+		
Diabetes mellitus (type II)	3–4+	2+	2+		
Drugs and toxins					
Amiodarone			+	2+	
Perhexiline maleate				+	
Coragil				+	
Indian childhood cirrhosis				+	−
Wilson's disease					
Miscellaneous					
Primary biliary cirrhosis					+
Chronic virus C hepatitis					+
Hepatocellular carcinoma					+

the setting of another diagnosis is exemplified by the lesion of primary biliary cirrhosis, hepatocellular carcinoma, etc. (Table 11.2). Recently, most attention has been given to the liver injury associated with obesity, particularly after surgical treatment, and diabetes mellitus, in other words the entity termed *non-alcoholic steatohepatitis* with the implicit resemblance to alcoholic hepatitis.

Alcoholic hepatitis is a characteristic form of alcohol-associated liver injury, and a classical clinicopathological entity (see Chapter 3). Alcoholic hepatitis is clearly a stage in the evolution of alcoholic liver disease, apparently preceded by steatosis and usually – perhaps always – a necessary step in the progression to *cirrhosis*. Of the three stages of alcoholic liver disease, alcoholic hepatitis has long been considered the most characteristic, since there are many other causes of steatosis and of cirrhosis. In the past, the Mallory body was thought to be pathognomonic of alcoholic liver injury and its presence essential for the diagnosis of alcoholic hepatitis.

Developments during the past quarter of a century, however, have demonstrated that the Mallory body is neither as sensitive nor as specific a marker for alcoholic hepatitis as had been believed. Alcoholic hepatitis may be diagnosed in alcoholic patients whose livers show steatosis, hepatocyte necrosis and a neutrophil polymorph infiltrate but no Mallory bodies (Harinasuta and Zimmerman 1971; Galambos 1972); on the other hand, there are a number of

disease states and drugs in the non-alcoholic patient, as well as drugs and toxins in the experimental animal that can lead to the development of Mallory bodies (French and Davies 1975; French *et al.* 1989; Hall 1987) (see Table 11.2).

Pseudoalcoholic liver disease

Hepatic injury resembling alcoholic liver disease in the non-alcoholic patient came to light in 1961 and again in 1969 with the description of hyaline degeneration "tinctorially and morphologically indistinguishable from Mallory's hyalin" in patients with Indian childhood cirrhosis (Smetana *et al.* 1961; Nayak *et al.* 1969). This curious facet of Indian childhood cirrhosis and the reports of Mallory bodies in patients with chronic cholestasis (Gerber *et al.* 1973), Wilson's disease (Sternlieb 1972), hepatocellular carcinoma (Keeley *et al.* 1972) and other conditions (Table 11.2), received relatively little attention. However, the description by Peters *et al.* (1975) of hepatic changes very similar to those of alcoholic hepatitis following intestinal bypass performed for morbid obesity, provoked much more attention. While there had been previous reports of deteriorating hepatic function after bypass surgery, the description by Peters *et al.* of steatosis, Mallory bodies, neutrophilic inflammation and cirrhosis in five morbidly obese patients was the first report of a

Table 11.2   Diseases and drugs reported to lead to Mallory bodies

Clinical conditions	*Drugs and toxins*
Alcoholism[f]	Amiodarone[d,m]
A-Beta-lipoproteinaemia[b,k]	Diethylcarboxyl 1,1-4-dihydrocollidine[3,n]
Bulimia[b,i]	Diethylstilbestrol[d,e,p]
Chronic cholestasis[g]	4,4'-Diethylaminoethoxyhexestrol[d,q]
Diabetes mellitus (type II)[f]	Glucocorticoid[d,s,o]
Focal nodular hyperplasia[b,u]	Griseofluvin[e,r]
Hepatocellular carcinoma[b]	Nifedipine[a,h]
Indian childhood cirrhosis[a,h]	Perihexiline maleate[d,t]
Intestinal bypass and related procedures[f]	
jejunocolic bypass[f]	
jejunoileal bypass[f]	
biliopancreatic diversion[j]	
gastroplasty[f]	
intestinal resection[f]	
Limb lipodystrophy[b]	
Obesity[f]	
Weber-Christian disease[b,l]	

[a]This entity has been attributed to chronic copper toxicity and, perhaps should be in column with drugs and toxins.
[b]Rare
[c]Powell *et al.* (1989).
[d]Occurs in patients.
[e]Occur in experimental animals.
[f]French and Davies (1975), French *et al.* (1989), Hall (1987), Czaja (1992).
[g]Gerber *et al.* (1973), Portmann and MacSween (1987).
[h]Smetana *et al.* (1961), Nayak *et al.* (1969).
[i]Cuellar *et al.* (1987).

[j]Grimm *et al.* (1992).
[k]Partin *et al.* (1974).
[l]Kimura *et al.* (1980).
[m]Poucell *et al.* (1984), Lewis *et al.* (1989, 1990)
[n]Yokoo *et al.* (1982).
[o]Coe *et al.* (1983), Itoh *et al.* (1977).
[p]Seki *et al.* (1983).
[q]Itoh *et al.* (1977).
[r]Denk *et al.* (1975).
[s]Babany *et al.* (1989).
[t]Poupon *et al.* (1980), Pessayre *et al.* (1979).
[u]Wetzel and Alexander (1979)

lesion fully mimicking alcoholic hepatitis developing after jejunoileal bypass. Many other reports have confirmed this observation, and it is clear that up to 50 percent of patients subjected to intestinal bypass may undergo worsening of their hepatological status with liver injury resembling alcoholic hepatitis and alcoholic cirrhosis (Snodgrass 1970; Baker *et al.* 1979, 1983; Clayman and O'Reilly 1981; Drenick *et al.* 1970, 1982; Halverson *et al.* 1978; Holzbach 1977; Kaminski *et al.* 1985; Kroyer and Talbert 1980; Peters *et al.* 1975; Peters 1977; Vyberg *et al.* 1987). The demonstration of deteriorating liver function after the various surgical procedures focused attention on the hepatic morphology in morbidly obese patients. The steatosis recorded in earlier studies of obese (Zelman 1952; Westwater and Fainer 1958) and diabetic (Zimmerman *et al.* 1950) patients had, for the most part, been considered of little consequence. The renewed attention resulting from studies of morbidly obese patients revealed that almost all had steatosis, while some had other changes as well (Table 11.3).

Only 2–12 percent of patients with morbid obesity have normal livers (Kern *et al.* 1973; Anderson and Gluud 1984; Silverman *et al.* 1990; Klain *et al.* 1989). Steatosis has been reported in 80 percent (Anderson and Gluud 1984), 94 percent (Silverman *et al.* 1990) and 97 percent (Klain *et al.* 1989) of patients, and was of moderate or severe degree in over 50 percent of patients (Fig. 11.1). Portal inflammation was found in 20–64 percent of the cases (Anderson and Gluud 1984), and lobular (acinar) inflammation has been recorded in as many as 59 percent of cases (Adler and Schaffner 1979) and as few as 9 percent (Nasrallah *et al.* 1981). Most reports have described a mononuclear inflammatory cell infiltrate, while a few reports have noted prominent neutrophilic inflammation within the lobules. The reported prevalence of fibrosis has varied widely with figures ranging from 19 to 65 percent of cases (Anderson and Gluud 1984). The fibrosis is usually portal but in up to 40 percent of obese patients it may involve zone 3 (Adler and Schaffner 1979), similar to the fibrosis of alcoholic liver disease

Table 11.3   Liver changes in obese patients

Authors	Number of patients	Fat (%)	Mallory bodies (%)	Inflammation (%)	Fibrosis (%)	Cirrhosis (%)
Anderson and Gluud (1984)	1515	80	1	335	29	3
Silverman *et al.* (1990)	100	94	1	36	65	4
Klain *et al.* (1989)	100	100	?4	19	19	6
Braillon *et al.* (1985)	50	90	0[a]	26	[a]	16[a]
Vyberg *et al.* (1987)	34	56	6	30	10	0
Marrubbio *et al.* (1976)	88	68	0	20	9	0

[a]All patients with "fatty fibrosis" or "fatty cirrhosis" and the three with Mallory bodies had moderately or severely excessive intake of alcohol.

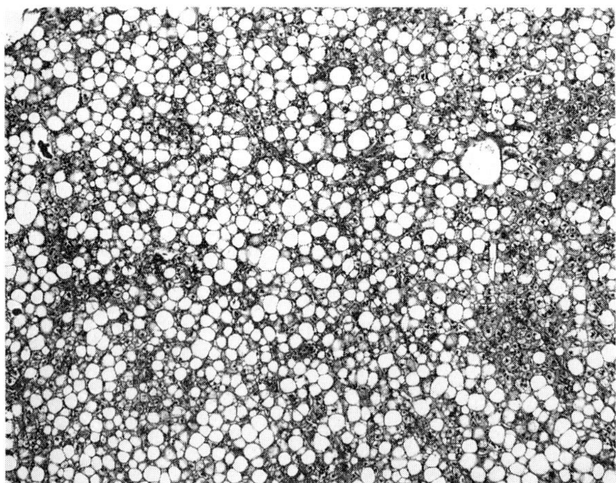

Fig. 11.1   Macrovesicular steatosis. Fatty change is seen in all acinar zones. Patient was a morbidly obese 15-year-old adolescent boy. H&E, × 50.

(Edmondson *et al.* 1967; Rabin 1989). The steatosis, with or without perivenular fibrosis, of morbidly obese patients resembles that of alcoholic liver disease. Mallory bodies have been recorded in only 1 percent of the morbidly obese patients (seven of 552 cases) summarized by Anderson and Gluud (1984), and in one of the 100 cases studied by Silverman *et al.* (1990). Klain *et al.* (1989) reported that 4 percent of their 100 morbidly obese patients showed "alcohol hepatitis-like changes", but they did not stipulate their criteria or specifically refer to Mallory bodies. Indeed, there appears to be a consensus that Mallory bodies are rarely part of the hepatic abnormalities of the morbidly obese patient (Anderson and Gluud 1984; Clain and Lefkowitch, 1987).

Progression of the steatosis of morbid obesity to cirrhosis is uncommon. While portal fibrosis has accompanied the steatosis in 25–30 percent of the patients and zone 3 fibrosis may be seen in up to 40 percent of them, cirrhosis is recorded in only 3–6 percent of patients in several large series (Kern *et al.* 1973; Anderson and Gluud 1984, Klain *et al.* 1989; Silverman *et al.* 1990). Indeed, in a study of 50 obese patients, Braillon *et al.* (1985) found "fatty fibrosis" and "fatty cirrhosis" only in the patients who were also alcoholic. Furthermore, progression of the steatosis of obesity to cirrhosis was noted in only one of 30 patients (Hilden *et al.* 1973) followed for 17–33 years and in none of 90 patients followed for 5 years (Massarat *et al.* 1979). Strikingly different, however, are the figures of Adler and Schaffner (1979), who, in a study of 29 obese patients referred for study because of mildly abnormal aminotransferase levels, found cirrhosis in 25 percent.

The hepatic disease of morbid obesity is not accompanied by clinical manifestations other than hepatomegaly. Aminotransferase levels are normal or mildly abnormal and correlate poorly with histological changes (Rozental *et al.* 1967; Galambos and Wills 1978; Klain *et al.* 1989; Silverman *et al.* 1990).

Accordingly, the liver disease of morbid obesity, can be epitomized as histological aberration with hardly any clinical reflection, with minor or no biochemical abnormality, and with little threat to well-being in most cases. Nevertheless, progression to cirrhosis, while uncommon, does occur.

Steatohepatitis, the lesion resembling alcoholic hepatitis, is uncommon in obesity with reported figures of 1–4 percent. After surgical bypass, steatohepatitis is much more common, often with Mallory bodies, and cirrhosis is distinctly more common. The presence of diabetes mellitus in the obese patient also appears to enhance the severity of the injury, leading to a higher incidence of steatohepatitis and cirrhosis (Fig. 11.2).

Obesity ——→ Steatosis - - - → Steatohepatitis - - - - → Cirrhosis

Obesity + ——→ Steatosis ——→ Steatohepatitis ——→ Cirrhosis
Diabetes

Obesity/Diabetes
+Bypass   ⟹ Steatosis ⟹ Steatohepatitis ⟹ Cirrhosis

Fig. 11.2   Relative role of obesity, diabetes and bypass in converting steatosis of obesity to steatohepatitis and cirrhosis.

Non-alcoholic steatohepatitis

Focus on the entity that has acquired the name non-alcoholic steatohepatitis (NASH) began with the reports of Miller *et al.* (1979), Adler and Schaffner (1979), Falchuk *et al.* (1980) and Ludwig *et al.* (1980), each of whom described a group of patients with liver disease which morphologically resembled alcoholic hepatitis. Ludwig *et al.* (1980) proposed the name non-alcoholic steatohepatitis and the acronym NASH was quickly acquired. However, earlier attention to non-alcoholic fatty liver that could lead to cirrhosis was contained in the report of Thaler (1962) describing *hepatitis of the fatty liver*. Miller *et al.* (1979) reported 27 non-alcoholic patients with histologic lesions "indistinguishable from alcoholic steatonecrosis": all but one had steatosis; all but two had hepatocyte degeneration and necrosis. Mallory bodies were present in 20 of the 27 cases, with neutrophilic infiltration in 16 of the 27, and varying degrees of central and portal fibrosis in all. Obesity and diabetes mellitus were present in "half of the cases". The histological features of over 200 reported cases are shown in Table 11.4.

The papers devoted to non-alcoholic steatohepatitis, under the various synonyms, have differed in their approach from those describing hepatic abnormalities in morbidly obese patients and in patients subjected to surgical treatment for the obesity. The papers on liver pathology in patients with morbid obesity or in those with bypass focused on the prevalence and character of the hepatic abnormalities, while the reports of non-alcoholic steatohepatitis have been based on groups of patients defined by having biochemical or other evidence of liver disease. Clearly, the cases of steatohepatitis are a subset of the steatosis of obesity, diabetes mellitus or of both, representing 1–4 percent of the steatosis of obesity and probably a higher proportion of those with diabetes mellitus. Only with jejunoileal bypass, gastroplasty and related procedures, or the presence of diabetes mellitus, is the proportion of cases of obesity-steatosis leading to steatohepatitis increased (Fig. 11.2).

All of the reports of steatohepatitis have in common the description of liver injury resembling those of alcoholic liver disease with all of the cases showing steatosis and variable degrees of inflammation, usually lobular. They differ, however, in the degree to which they resemble alcoholic liver disease (Table 11.4). While inflammation is included in the criteria for diagnosing steatohepatitis (French *et al.* 1989; Powell *et al.* 1990), most of the reports have described mononuclear cell prominence (Fig. 11.3) rather than the neutrophil prominence that is characteristic of alcoholic hepatitis. The prevalence of Mallory bodies ranged from 10 percent (Powell *et al.* 1990) to 90 per cent (Diehl *et al.* 1988) (Table 11.4). Nagore and Scheuer (1988), who reported hepatic changes in type II diabetes, found Mallory bodies in the livers of all nine patients studied. Significant fibrosis was present in 25 percent or more and some fibrosis is mentioned in almost all of the reports, with particular reference to the fibrosis in zone 3 in many of them (Table 11.4). Accordingly, the cases that have been grouped as steatohepatitis, with the implicit resemblance to alcoholic hepatitis, include some that resemble alcoholic steatosis, alcoholic steatofibrosis or alcoholic hepatitis.

Clinical features

Despite the differences in morphology, the clinical manifestations of the groups are similar (Table 11.5). Most patients are females and most are obese. Only in the reports of Miller *et al.* (1979) and Ludwig *et al.* (1980) did females comprise less than 75 percent of the patients; however, 70–100 percent of the reported patients were obese. However, the presence of liver injury does not depend on extreme obesity, and weights only 30–40 percent above normal are characteristic. Diabetes mellitus was present in 30–100 percent of patients. Indeed, over 90 percent of the recorded cases of steatohepatitis in one series were obese, diabetic or both (Diehl *et al.* 1988). While most patients with non-alcoholic steatohepatitis are of middle age or beyond (Czaja 1992), this type of liver injury has been reported in obese children as young as 9 years (Moran *et al.* 1983; Kinugasa *et al.* 1984).

Few of the reported patients had had clinical evidence of liver disease other than the hepatomegaly which was present in most of them (Ludwig *et al.* 1980). However, splenomegaly was recorded in

Table 11.4   Characteristics and histological features of patients described as non-alcoholic steatohepatitis

Authors	Number of patients	Females (%)	Diabetes (%)	Obesity (%)	Fat (%)	Fibrosis[a] (pericellular in zone 3) (%)	Mallory bodies (%)	Inflammation[b] M	P (%)	Cirrhosis (%)
Falchuk *et al.* (1980)	5	100	100	100	100	100	60	+	0	20
Miller *et al.* (1979)	27	56	50	50	96	100	60	+	60	0
Adler and Schaffner (1979)	29	76	61	100	100	75	33	+	40	25
Ludwig *et al.* (1980)	20	65	25	90	100	70	70	+	+	15
Itoh *et al.* (1987)	17	74	74	74	100	75	60	−	74	6
Diehl *et al.* (1988)	39	81	55	71	100	97	90	+	97	38
Lee (1989)	49	78	50	70	100	100	49	+	100	16
Powell *et al.*	42	83	36	95	100	43	10	+	±	7

[a]All reports described pericellular fibrosis. [b]M, mononuclear inflammation; P, polymorphonuclear inflammation. +, Present, 0, absent, −, no specific comment.

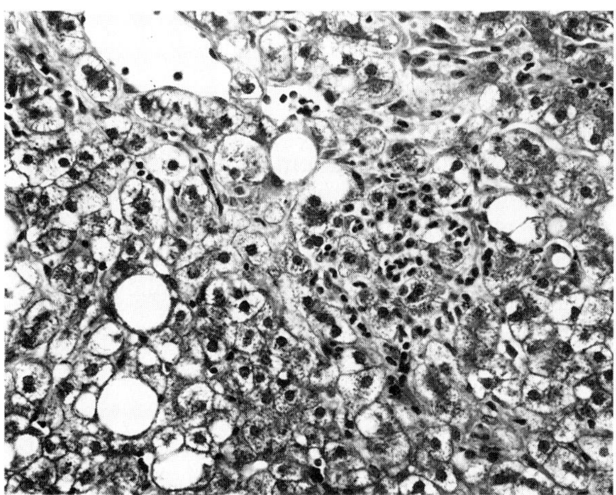

Fig. 11.3   Non-alcoholic steatohepatitis. Focal necrosis with a mononuclear cell infiltrate in zone 3. H&E, × 200.

25 percent of the cases of Ludwig *et al.* (1980) and in 33 percent of those reported by Miller *et al.* (1979). Clinical manifestations of liver disease summarized as "jaundice, ascites, oesophageal varies, encephalopathy or the hepatorenal syndrome, alone or in combination" were found in 15 percent of the cases of Diehl *et al.* (1988), a higher incidence of overt disease than any other series. However, their cases also had a higher prevalence of Mallory bodies than most other reports, presumably reflecting more severe disease. In the majority of all other cases, the liver disease was asymptomatic, and almost all of them came to medical attention because of hepatomegaly and/or minor abnormalities in serum enzyme levels.

Biochemical features

Biochemical evidence of hepatic disease is not prominent. The level of aspartate aminotransferase (AST) was elevated in 15 percent (Ludwig *et al.* 1980) to over 80 percent (Falchuk *et al.* 1980; Lee 1989) of patients; the values were only mildly elevated, ranging from 15 to 222 units. The level of alanine aminotransferase (ALT) was abnormal in 70–90 percent of patients (Lee 1989; Ludwig *et al.* 1980; Falchuk *et al.* 1980) with a range of 18–198 units recorded. Values for ALT and AST are rarely more than 10-fold the normal. While most reports do not provide the AST/ALT ratio, examination of the relative values of the two aminotransferases suggests that either the elevations of the two enzymes are approximately the same, or that the ALT values tend to exceed those of AST (Spech *et al.* 1983; Diehl *et al.* 1988). Alkaline phosphatase values are slightly elevated (two-fold or less) in most patients, although elevations as high as five-fold have been recorded (Ludwig *et al.* 1980). Serum albumin levels were almost always normal (Czaja 1992).

Special techniques for recognition

Imaging with ultrasonography, computerized tomography and magnetic resonance imaging are useful to demonstrate the presence of steatosis (French *et al.* 1989; Czaja 1992), but do not supplant liver biopsy for recognition of more specific changes. The laparoscopic appearance of the liver may suggest the presence of steatosis and cirrhosis.

Table 11.5   Clinical features of non-alcoholic steatohepatitis

	Usual	*Range*
Age	50–60	Child to senescence
Sex	Females > males	
Predisposing condition	Obesity and/or diabetes Bypass treatment	See Table 11.2
Symptoms	None	Features of cirrhosis
Signs	Hepatomegaly	
Liver enzymes AST/ALT ratio	<5 × normal ≤1	1–10 × normal <1–3 ×
Histology	Steatosis Mallory bodies Perivenular, pericellular fibrosis	None to cirrhosis

Histological features

The pattern of injury consists of macrovesicular steatosis (uncommonly microvesicular) involving mainly zone 3 or, when severe, also zone 2 and even zone 1. There may be focal hepatocyte necrosis, ballooning of hepatocytes, Mallory bodies and free acidophilic ("apoptotic") bodies, mainly in zone 3 (Figs 11.4, 11.5). Nuclear vacuolization (glycogenated nuclei) is frequently seen. Acinar inflammation is usually mononuclear and often of minor degree (Fig. 11.3). Mallory bodies, when seen, are usually small and less well-defined than those of alcoholic liver disease (Fig. 11.6), although they may be well-formed and prominent (Fig. 11.7) (Diehl *et al*. 1988). The Mallory bodies are morphologically (both by light and electron microscopy) and immunohistochemically indistinguishable from those of alcoholic liver disease (Itoh *et al*. 1982; French *et al*. 1989). Megamitochondria are seen in a frequency and prominence no different from that of alcoholic liver disease (French *et al*. 1989).

Fibrosis is present in almost all cases, usually surrounding individual cells in zone 3 and leading to a pericellular "chicken wire" pattern, similar to that of alcoholic liver disease (Fig. 11.8). Cirrhosis has been found in 7 percent (Powell *et al*. 1990), 25 percent (Adler and Schaffner 1979), 38 percent (Diehl *et al*. 1988) and even 75 percent (Miller *et al*. 1979) of patients (Figs 11.9, 11.10). The cirrhosis is rarely clinically apparent.

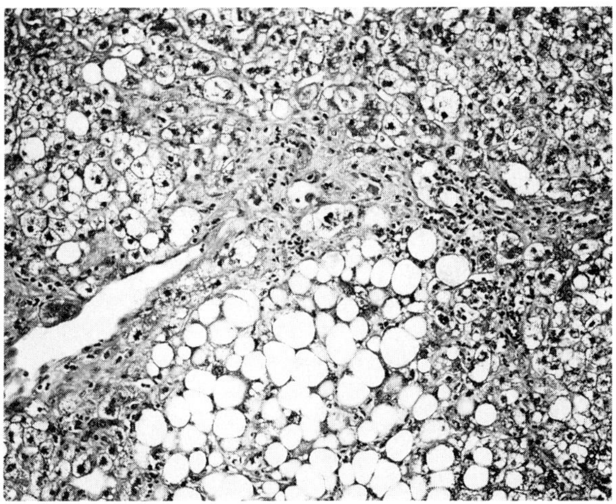

Fig. 11.4   Non-alcoholic steatohepatitis. Macrovesicular steatosis, occasional ballooned hepatocytes and focal perivenular fibrosis. H&E, × 100.

Diagnosis

The diagnosis of non-alcoholic steatohepatitis is one of exclusion. Patients come to attention as a result of finding abnormal AST and ALT levels, hepatomegaly or the abnormal appearance of the liver at laparotomy. Values of AST and ALT that are slightly to moderately elevated with the two approximately equal, in an obese or diabetic patient, should suggest the diagnosis. Under the umbrella term of steatohepatitis, there are four patterns: (1)

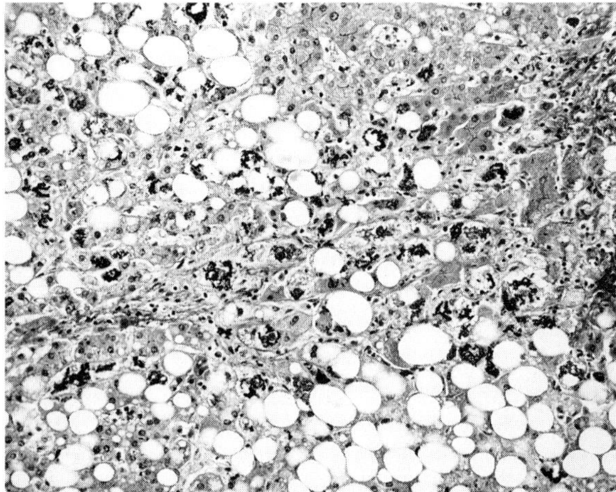

Fig. 11.5 Non-alcoholic steatohepatitis. Microvesicular steatosis and numerous darkly stained Mallory bodies in zone 3. H&E, × 110.

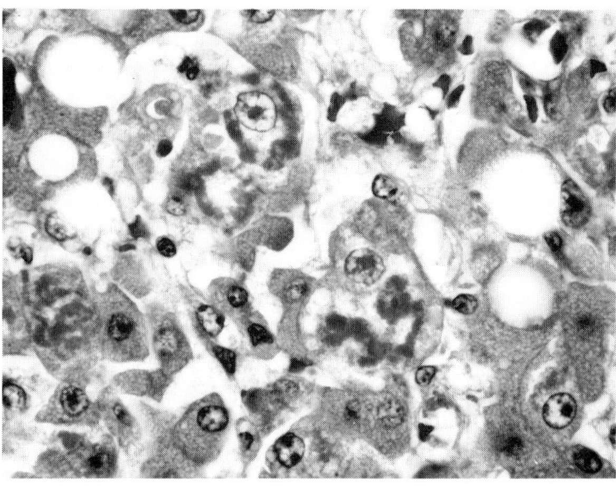

Fig. 11.7 Non-alcoholic steatohepatitis. Several zone 3 hepatocytes contain well-formed Mallory bodies. H&E, × 480

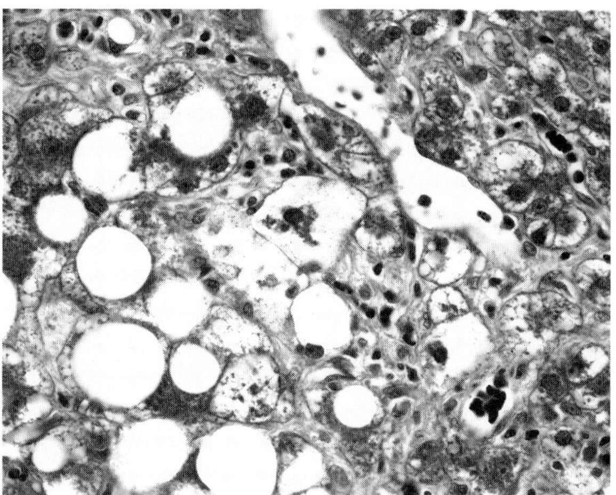

Fig. 11.6 Non-alcoholic steatohepatitis. Poorly-formed Mallory bodies in ballooned hepatocytes in zone 3. H&E, × 270.

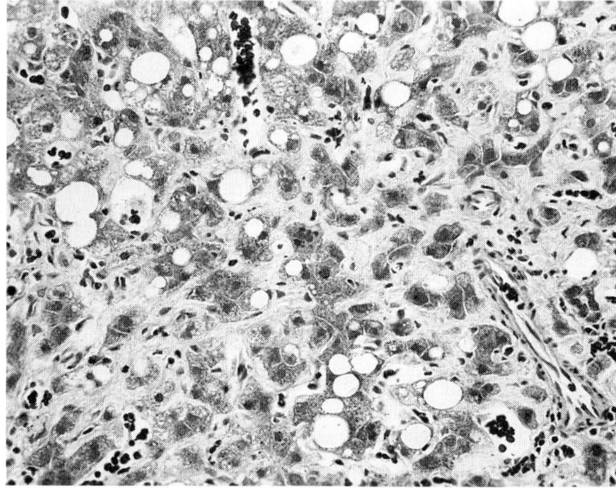

Fig. 11.8 Non-alcoholic steatohepatitis. Fibrosis in zone 3 with disruption of liver cell plates. H&E, × 110.

steatosis, with only portal inflammation, (2) fatty liver hepatitis (steatohepatitis), (3) fatty liver with portal fibrosis and (4) fatty cirrhosis (Adler and Schaffner 1979). At this juncture, it is worth noting that the terms fatty liver hepatitis and fatty cirrhosis have not gained wide acceptance. The steatohepatitis may be with or without Mallory bodies. Non-alcoholic steatosis with only portal inflammation or fibrosis needs to be distinguished from alcoholic steatosis, chronic hepatitis C and methotrexate

hepatotoxicity. Non-alcoholic steatohepatitis with Mallory bodies needs to be distinguished from alcoholic hepatitis and amiodarone toxicity. Non-alcoholic fatty cirrhosis needs to be distinguished from alcoholic cirrhosis, chronic hepatitis C and methotrexate toxicity.

The distinction of non-alcoholic steatohepatitis from alcoholic hepatitis cannot be made with confidence on histological grounds, but there are helpful clues (Table 11.6). Perivenular fibrous, pericellular

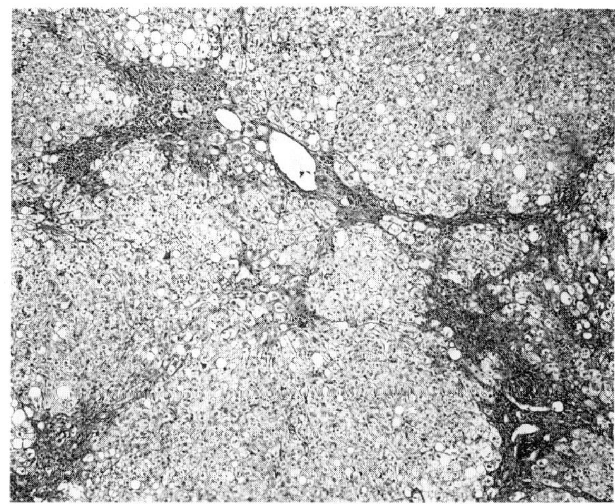

Fig. 11.9 Non-alcoholic steatohepatitis. Bridging fibrosis with incomplete cirrhosis. H&E, × 40.

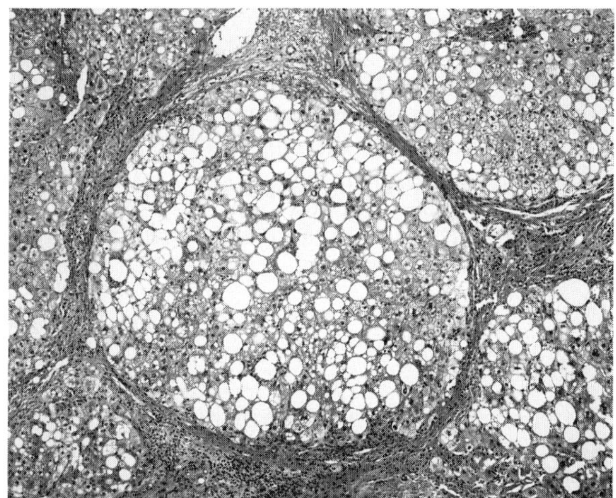

Fig. 11.10 Non-alcoholic steatohepatitis. Liver showing micronodular cirrhosis. H&E, × 170.

("chicken wire") fibrosis (Rabin 1989) and steatosis can be seen in non-alcoholic steatohepatitis and in alcoholic hepatitis. These findings, accompanied by prominent, well-formed Mallory bodies and neutrophilic infiltration of the acini suggest the diagnosis to be alcoholic hepatitis, while a mononuclear cell infiltrate and poorly formed Mallory bodies point more to non-alcoholic steatohepatitis. A striking prominence of Mallory bodies and concentration in zone 1, accompanied by little or no steatosis, would suggest a drug-associated (e.g. amiodarone) rather than obesity-related disease.

Other distinguishing features are shown in Table

11.6. Chronic hepatitis C, which is frequently accompanied by steatosis, does not show "chicken wire fibrosis", and is marked by an AST/ALT ratio of 1 or below; the diagnosis can be made serologically (Rogers *et al.* 1992). Chronic hepatitis C has been reported to have Mallory bodies (in zone 1) in a prevalence as high as 18 percent (Lefkowitch *et al.* 1993), a figure far higher than in our experience. Additionally, several other reports describing the histopathology of chronic hepatitis C fail to mention the presence of Mallory bodies (Scheuer *et al.* 1992; Bach *et al.* 1991; Gerber *et al.* 1992) Other features of chronic hepatitis C include piecemeal necrosis, lymphoplasmacytic inflammation, lymphoid aggregates, with or without lymphoid follicles with germinal centres, in the portal areas and bile duct damage (Scheuer 1992; Bach *et al.* 1992; Gerber *et al.* 1992; Lefkowitch *et al.* 1993).

Methotrexate hepatotoxicity is marked by steatosis, fibrosis and cirrhosis, and has been listed as a cause of Mallory bodies (French *et al.* 1989). While we have seen no examples of Mallory bodies attributable to methotrexate, the steatosis and fibrosis induced by methotrexate can resemble non-alcoholic steatohepatitis (French *et al.* 1989). The characteristic nuclear changes (pleomorphism and glycogenation), Ito cell prominence, minimal inflammation and the usual lack of Mallory bodies help in recognition of the methotrexate-induced lesion.

Reconciliation of the histologic features with the biochemical tests is of assistance in differential diagnosis, since an AST/ALT ratio of 1 or less is strongly against the diagnosis of alcoholic hepatitis and supportive of non-alcoholic steatohepatitis or amiodarone toxicity. Nevertheless, a ratio well above 1 may be seen in patients with non-alcoholic steatohepatitis (Falchuk *et al.* 1980), though uncommonly. However, a high AST/ALT ratio (above 3) is strongly supportive of the diagnosis of alcoholic hepatitis. Elevated levels of the mitochondrial aspartate aminotransferase are also of help in identifying alcoholism and, accordingly, alcoholic hepatitis (Nalpas *et al.* 1986); but in our view this measure serves much the same purpose as the AST/ALT ratio.

An adequate history with respect to alcohol intake, drug intake, obesity and diabetes mellitus is of considerable help in diagnosis. Serological testing is essential for the diagnosis of chronic hepatitis C, and testing for abnormal (desialylated) transferrin is of help in the diagnosis of alcoholic liver disease (Fletcher *et al.* 1991).

Table 11.6   Histological and biochemical features distinguishing non-alcoholic steatohepatitis from other conditions[a]

	Fat	*Neutrophilic inflammation*	*Zone 3 pericellular fibrosis*	*Mallory bodies*	*Piecemeal necrosis*	*AST/ALT ratio*
Non-alcoholic steatosis	3–4+	−	±	−	−	~1
Non-alcoholic steatohepatitis	4–3+	±	+	+	−	~1
Alcoholic steatosis[b]	3–4+	−	±	−	−	1–2
Alcoholic steatohepatitis[b]	1–3+	+	+	2+	−	>2
Hepatitis C	1–3+	−	−	−	+	<1
Amiodarone	±	+	+	2+	−	~1
Methotrexate	2–4+	−	+	?	−	~1

[a]1–4+, regularly present to varying degree; −, regularly absent; ±, present or absent.
[b]Elevated levels of desialylated transferase (Fletcher *et al.* 1991) or of mitochondrial isozyme of AST (Nalpas *et al.* 1986) help to identify alcoholic liver injury.

Prognosis

Steatohepatitis is a relatively non-life-threatening disease. Overt liver failure is rare. Progression to cirrhosis has been noted in one of 13 cases followed for up to 9 years by Powell *et al.* (1990) and in three of 13 cases followed by Lee (1989) for 1–7 years. As is true in alcoholic liver disease, the development of cirrhosis is accompanied by a decrease in the degree of steatosis (Powell *et al.* 1990).

Treatment

Weight reduction of modest degree achieved gradually has been successful in normalizing serum aminotransferase levels and reducing the degree of hepatomegaly and splenomegaly. Palmer and Schaffner (1990) have reported that a reduction in weight of 10 percent or more corrected the abnormal liver enzymes and reduced the hepatic enlargement of 13 of 17 patients. Watanabe *et al.* (1988) recommend that the programme of weight reduction include both diet and exercise. Rapid weight loss may have a deleterious effect. Nevertheless, controlled fasting in the obese diabetic has resulted in the disappearance of hepatic steatosis and hepatomegaly (Keeffe *et al.* 1987). The steatohepatitis that occurs in morbidly obese patients may be improved by gastroplasty or gastric bypass (Czaja 1992) in association with effective weight loss, but the improvement appears to be delayed as long as 1 year. Furthermore, rare instances of the development of steatohepatitis have been reported after gastroplasty (Hamilton *et al.* 1983).

The steatosis and steatohepatitis that develop after jejunoileal bypass have been treated by reversal of the bypass or by administration of antibiotics or metronidazole. Antimicrobial treatment is based on the hypothesis that bacterial proliferation in a blind loop of bowel leads to absorption of toxic bacterial products. However, the observation that bowel resection, leaving no blind loop, also leads to steatohepatitis suggests that the blind loop hypothesis may not be the basis for the steatohepatitis following bypass (Craig *et al.* 1980).

Pathogenesis

The pathogenesis of steatohepatitis is unclear, and a variety of factors have been considered (French *et al.* 1989; Czaja 1992). Examination of factors that enhance the severity of the steatosis of obesity and that appear to modify the progression of the steatosis to steatohepatitis and cirrhosis have a bearing on the issue. The five that warrant consideration are degree of obesity, gender, surgical treatment for obesity, rapid weight loss and diabetes mellitus.

1. *The degree of obesity* may contribute to steatosis. This seems implicit in the presence of steatosis in 80–97 percent of morbidly obese individuals. However, correlation between the degree of obesity and the severity of the steatosis or progression to cirrhosis has not been clear in most reports (Holzbach 1977). Nevertheless, the report of Wanless and Lentz (1990) showed a striking correlation between the severity of steatosis and the prevalence

of steatohepatitis, and in turn between the prevalence of steatohepatitis and that of hepatic fibrosis, suggesting that the degree of obesity has a bearing on the prevalence of steatohepatitis and fibrosis.

2. *Gender* appears to have a bearing on the incidence of the lesion. Clearly, females outnumber males among all series of patients with obesity-associated steatosis or NASH (Table 11.5). However, the studies of Kern *et al.* (1973) suggest that the severity of steatosis is correlated with the degree of obesity rather than gender *per se*. Wanless and Lentz (1990) also found that the steatosis was positively correlated with the degree of obesity and that the higher prevalence of females among patients with obesity-related hepatic disease reflected the greater proportion of females among obese patients studied.

3. *Surgical treatment* for obesity is an unequivocally identified factor leading to enhanced severity of the hepatic lesion of morbid obesity. Jejunocolic and jejunoileal bypass (Holzbach 1977), gastroplasty (Hamilton *et al.* 1983), pancreaticobiliary bypass (Grimm *et al.* 1992), as well as intestinal resection (Craig *et al.* 1980; Peura *et al.* 1980), have all been shown to enhance or produce severe hepatic injury (French *et al.* 1989). Progression to cirrhosis occurs in at least 7 percent (Halverson *et al.* 1978; Hocking *et al.* 1981) and has been reported in up to 25 percent (Haines *et al.* 1981) of cases, many resembling alcoholic liver disease. Indeed, in an analysis of 34 cases, Vyberg *et al.* (1987) found that pericellular fibrosis increased from 15 percent before bypass to 70 percent after the procedure. They also found that Mallory bodies were more than five times as frequent (32 percent) after bypass than they had been before bypass (6 percent); they also found deranged architecture, absent before bypass, in 24 percent after the procedures. Other reports have described the development of "liver failure" after jejunoileal, and less frequently, after jejunocolic bypass (DeWind and Payne 1976; Holzbach 1977). Kaminski *et al.* (1985) reported increased hepatic fibrosis in 87 percent and increased hepatic inflammation in 50 percent of a group of patients, 6 years or more after ileojejunal bypass for morbid obesity. They found that "fibrotic" liver disease, present in 10 percent of patients before bypass, had increased to 50 percent after the shunting procedures. Of particular note are the observations of Marrubbio *et al.* (1976),

who drew attention to the central lobular, pericellular fibrosis in patients with marked obesity and the enhancement after bypass. Most dramatic were the already cited observations of Peters *et al.* (1975), who described development of the full lesion of an alcohol-like hepatitis in five patients after bypass. Overall, about 5 percent of patients subjected to intestinal bypass die of liver failure and 7–10 percent develop cirrhosis (Halverson *et al.* 1978; DeWind and Payne 1976; Campbell *et al.* 1977; Schaffner and Thaler 1976). Progression of liver injury after bypass has been ascribed to protein malnutrition (Ames *et al.* 1976; Moxley *et al.* 1974; Galambos 1976; Lockwood *et al.* 1977; Ackerman 1979), the toxic effects of bacterial products or bile acids (Drenick *et al.* 1982), endogenous alcohol and acetaldehyde absorbed from the gut (Barry 1983), and rapid lipid mobilization during weight loss leading to a high concentration of free fatty acids (Mavrelis *et al.* 1983; Cairns *et al.* 1986; Wanless and Lentz 1990; French *et al.* 1989; Czaja 1992). Evidence for each of these has been inconclusive. However, a possibly injurious role of free fatty acids secondary to insulin-induced blockade of fat metabolism is contained in the hypothesis of Wanless and Lentz (1988) cited below.

4. *Rapid weight loss* has been incriminated in enhancing the hepatic injury of obesity after intestinal bypass (Capron *et al.* 1982; French *et al.* 1989; Holzbach 1977). Many of the reports have noted that progression of the hepatic injury is most apparent during periods of rapid weight loss, and that once weight has stabilized the liver injury does not progress (Haines *et al.* 1981). The possible role of rapid weight loss also seems borne out by the studies of Drenick *et al.* (1970) and Wanless and Lentz (1990), but is not supported by the studies of Rozental *et al.* (1967), who found no significant injury resulting from "crash" dietary programmes used for weight reduction in morbidly obese patients.

5. *Diabetes mellitus* appears to be an important factor in liver injury (Stone and Van Thiel 1985). In the studies of Silverman *et al.* (1990) and Wanless and Lentz (1990), the presence of diabetes mellitus appeared to enhance the likelihood of finding "steatohepatitis" and cirrhosis in the morbidly obese patient. However, other authors have not found that the presence of diabetes enhances the severity of hepatic injury in obese patients (Anderson and Gluud 1984; Adler and Schaffner 1979; Klain *et al.* 1989; Zelman 1952).

Hepatic abnormalities in the diabetic have long been of interest, but the distinction between the role of diabetes mellitus *per se*, and of the obesity that frequently accompanies type II diabetes, in provoking the hepatic abnormalities has been difficult. However, study of type II ("insulin-insensitive") diabetes reveals that virtually all have steatosis even when obesity is not marked, and that cirrhosis may be found in up to 25 percent of patients subjected to liver biopsy (Zimmerman *et al.* 1950; Nagore and Scheuer 1988). Zone 3 pericellular fibrosis is characteristic.

Balazc and Halmos (1985), in an electron microscopic study of 13 type II diabetic patients of long standing, demonstrated zone 3 perisinusoidal deposition of collagen and pericellular fibrosis accompanying "destruction of hepatic cells". These changes are to be distinguished from perisinusoidal fibrosis that occurs in both type I and type II diabetes, which is a vascular lesion related to diabetic microangiopathy (Bernuau *et al.* 1982, 1985; Latry *et al.* 1987). While steatosis, non-alcoholic steatohepatitis and cirrhosis are selectively associated with type II diabetes, obesity or both, the sinusoidal microangiopathy is a lesion of both type I and type II diabetes. Indeed, the liver disease may precede the appearance of diabetes mellitus (Batman and Scheuer 1985). Furthermore, "fatty liver hepatitis" was found in 17 of 62 (27 percent) patients with type II diabetes (Nagore and Scheuer 1988). Indeed, all of those whose liver sections were available for re-examination (nine of the 17) had Mallory bodies. The prevalence of alcoholic hepatitis-like features and cirrhosis in so high a proportion of type II diabetic patients suggests that diabetes mellitus is a risk factor separate from obesity, although the effects of the two may merge. One report (Nagore and Scheuer 1988) described the Mallory bodies of diabetes mellitus to be in zone 1 rather in the zone 3 location characteristic of alcoholic hepatitis.

The prevalence of non-alcoholic steatohepatitis in patients with type II diabetes and the observation by Wanless *et al.* (1989) that the Mallory bodies appeared in the subcapsular area of the liver in patients given intraperitoneal insulin led these authors to propose that non-alcoholic steatohepatitis results from blockade by insulin of free fatty acid oxidation leading to toxic effects of free fatty acids (Wanless *et al.* 1989; Wanless and Lentz 1990).

Pseudoalcoholic liver disease due to drugs and toxins

The observation that some drugs and other chemical agents (Table 11.2) are associated with the formation of Mallory bodies and related changes, suggests that this type of liver injury can be considered a product of toxicity. Indeed, the presence of Mallory bodies in Indian childhood cirrhosis (Smetana *et al.* 1961; Nayak *et al.* 1969) and Wilson's disease (Sternlieb 1972) may be due to chronic toxic effects of copper overload. Support for the view that Mallory bodies are a marker of toxicity came with the reports of Denk *et al.* (1975) who produced Mallory bodies in mice by the administration of griseofulvin, and of Yokoo *et al.* (1982) who produced Mallory bodies in mice by the administration of 3,5′-diethoxycarbonyl-1-4-dihydrocollidine.

Despite the association of Mallory bodies with Indian childhood cirrhosis and Wilson's disease, other toxic injury induced by copper is apparently not accompanied by Mallory body formation. Acute copper intoxication is rare and does not lead to histologic alterations likely to be confused with alcoholic or pseudoalcoholic liver disease. Copper intoxication can result from ingestion of contaminated water supplies, inhalation of metal dust, exposure to fungicides and insecticides, use of cupric sulphate as an emetic, debridement of burned skin with crystalline copper sulphate, recurrent haemodialysis, and the ingestion of copper sulphate for suicidal purposes (particularly in India) (Chuttani *et al.* 1965; Holtzman *et al.* 1966; Blomfield *et al.* 1971; Walsh *et al.* 1977). Severe liver injury, characterized by zone 3 necrosis and cholestasis, was reported by Chuttani *et al.* (1965) in five Indian patients who had committed suicide by ingesting copper sulphate.

More important are the changes associated with chronic copper overload (Table 11.7). Chronic copper toxicity can be hereditary or acquired. In humans hereditary copper overload is exemplified by Wilson's disease, and in animals by the copper toxicosis of the Bedlington terrier; both conditions have an autosomal recessive inheritance. In Wilson's disease, Mallory bodies are present typically in periportal or periseptal hepatocytes in the stages of chronic active hepatitis and cirrhosis, respectively, in contrast to their zone 3 localization in both alcoholic and pseudoalcoholic hepatitis. The hepatic morphologic changes of the Bedlington terrier also include the massive accumulation of copper (incorporated with lysosomal lipofuscin), chronic

Table 11.7   Chronic copper overload in humans

Disease or conditions	Source of copper	Pathologic effects
A. Hereditary		
Wilson's disease	Metabolic error	Acute hepatitis; steatosis, focal necrosis, glycogenated nuclei, copper storage, fibrosis. Ultrastructural changes (particularly mitochondrial). Chronic active hepatitis $\pm$ Mallory bodies. Cirrhosis with Mallory bodies and other changes. Hepatocellular carcinoma (rare)
B. Acquired		
Liver disease of vineyard sprayers	Fungicides containing $CuSo_4$	Granulomas; intra-acinar and periportal fibrosis; cirrhosis; angiosarcoma
Indian childhood cirrhosis (ICC)	Contamination of milk by copper leached from brass container	1. Pre-cirrhotic: Mallory bodies, intra-acinar and portal inflammation, ductular proliferation, copper accumulation 2. Cirrhotic: micronodular cirrhosis
ICC-like disease caused by chronic copper intoxication	High levels of copper in drinking water	Same as ICC

active hepatitis and cirrhosis (Twedt *et al.* 1979). However, steatosis and Mallory bodies have not been observed.

Acquired forms of copper overload occur in humans and animals. Sheep are particularly susceptible to copper intoxication; they can be chronically exposed to excessive copper by grazing in sprayed orchards or by eating contaminated feed. Light microscopic, ultrastructural and morphometric studies of experimentally copper-poisoned sheep have been reported by Ishmael *et al.* (1971) and Gooneratne *et al.* (1980). Light microscopic changes include steatosis, focal hepatocyte necrosis, swelling of hepatocytes and enlarged Kupffer cells; copper has been demonstrated cytochemically (incorporated in lysosomes with lipofuscin) in Kupffer cells, but Mallory bodies have not been observed.

Acquired chronic copper toxicity in humans may result from occupational or domestic exposure. An example of the former is the chronic exposure of vineyard workers to fungicide sprays containing copper sulphate. The hepatic injury is only of passing relevance to this discussion, since the lesions caused by the chronic exposure to copper are not those of steatohepatitis; they include non-caseating granulomas, intra-acinar and periportal fibrosis, cirrhosis and, rarely, angiosarcoma (Pimental and Menezes 1975, 1977). The domestic environment is the setting for Indian childhood cirrhosis and a similar disease (thus far only reported from outside the Indian subcontinent) occurring in children ingesting large quantities of copper in their drinking water.

Indian childhood cirrhosis is associated with marked hepatic copper overload. The copper storage has been demonstrated histochemically (by staining tissue sections with orcein for copper-binding protein and the rhodanine method for copper), and by quantitative techniques such as atomic absorption spectrophotometry (Portmann *et al.* 1978; Popper *et al.* 1979; Tanner *et al.* 1979; Mehrotra *et al.* 1981). It is generally accepted that the copper accumulation is directly responsible for the histopathologic lesions in Indian childhood cirrhosis. These include the presence of numerous Mallory bodies, intra-acinar and portal inflammation, copper accumulation (beginning in zone 1), periportal ductular proliferation, intra-acinar and periportal fibrosis, occlusive lesions of terminal hepatic venules and, eventually, the development of a micronodular cirrhosis (Smetana *et al.* 1961; Nayak *et al.* 1969; Bhagwat *et al.* 1983; Joshi 1987). According to Bhagwat *et al.* (1983), cases of Indian childhood cirrhosis have been reported from 17 countries. Several cases have emanated from the USA (Lefkowitch *et al.* 1982; Adamson *et al.* 1992). The non-Indian cases are also characterized by marked copper overload and histopathologic alterations indistinguishable from those of Indian childhood cirrhosis.

In 1983, Tanner *et al.* proposed that increased dietary copper (from copper contaminated milk stored in brass and copper containers) could be of aetiologic significance in Indian childhood cirrhosis. Subsequently, O'Neill and Tanner (1989) demonstrated experimentally that copper (but not zinc) is avidly taken up from brass and bound to casein from which it is completely removable by picolinate chelation. They concluded that milk is an effective carrier of copper from a brass utensil to the infant enterocyte. Lending support to a direct cytopathic effect of copper are recent reports of clinical recovery, improved survival and reversal of the hepatic histological lesion by penicillamine therapy of infants with Indian childhood cirrhosis (Tanner *et al.* 1987; Bhusnurmarth *et al.* 1991).

Of great interest are reports of several children who developed an illness, clinically and histopathogically resembling Indian childhood cirrhosis, from the chronic ingestion of well-water contaminated with high levels of copper (Walker-Smith and Blomfield 1973; Muller-Hocker *et al.* 1985, 1987; Schramel *et al.* 1988). Characteristic Mallory bodies were seen by light and electron microscopy. In all cases, the copper was leached from copper pipes into drinking water delivered to the childrens' homes. Early exposure to copper appears to be crucial, since siblings exposed after 9 months of age and the parents who drank the same water did not develop the disease (Muller-Hocker *et al.* 1988; Schramel *et al.* 1988). To date, most of the affected children have succumbed to liver failure. It is conceivable that other (and perhaps all) cases of Indian childhood cirrhosis occurring outside the Indian subcontinent are examples of chronic environmental copper toxicity.

Also of possible relevance to copper toxicity are the Mallory bodies associated with primary biliary cirrhosis, primary sclerosing cholangitis and other chronic cholestatic conditions. In primary biliary cirrhosis, the copper overload so characteristic of chronic cholestasis is in zone 1, as are the Mallory bodies (Portmann and MacSween 1987).

Of particular interest is the occurrence of Mallory bodies in a form of drug-induced liver disease (Table 11.2). Three drugs – Coralgil, perhexiline maleate and amiodarone – have been found to produce hepatic changes that resemble alcoholic hepatitis (pseudoalcoholic liver disease) accompanied by phospholipidosis (Table 11.8). Phospholipidosis is characterized by enlarged, foamy or granular hepatocytes (Fig. 11.11) and Kupffer cells (Shepherd *et al.* 1987). On electron microscopy these cells are found to contain lamellated lysosomes (Fig. 11.12), a change associated with accumulation of phospho-

Table 11.8 Drugs that produce Mallory bodies, phospholipidosis or both

	Mallory bodies	*Phospholipidosis*
Amiodarone	+	+
Coralgil[a]	+	+
Perhexiline maleate	+	+
Chlorpheniramine[b]	0	+
Thioridazine[b]	—	+
Nifedipine[c]	+	—
Diethylstilbestrol[c]	+	—
Glucocorticoids[c]	+	—
Ethanol[d] (alcoholic liver)	+	
Griseofulvin	+	—

[a]Trade name for 4,4′-diethylaminoethoxyhexestrol.
[b]Amphophilic drug, many of which can lead to phospholipidosis.
[c]Very few instances.
[d]Alcoholism leads to Mallory bodies. Alcohol *per se* does not do so in experimental animals.
+, present; 0, absent; —, no specific comment.

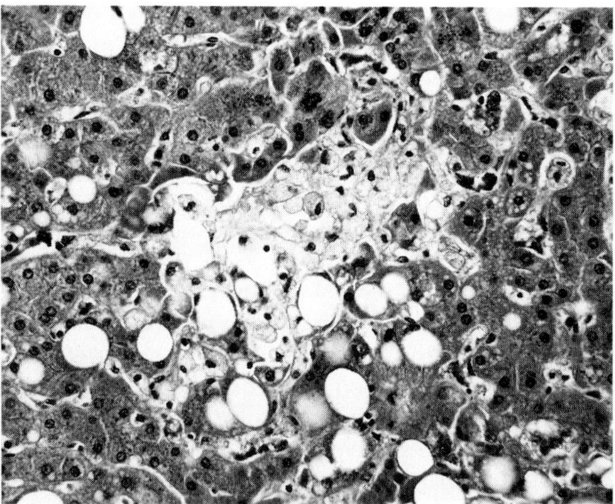

Fig. 11.11 Amiodarone-induced phospholipidosis. A cluster of foam cells is surrounded by some large lipid vacuoles. H&E, × 170.

lipids (Lullman *et al.* 1975; Lullman and Lullman-Rauch 1986; Poucell *et al.* 1984; Dake *et al.* 1985); similar changes are seen in extrahepatic sites (Lullman *et al.* 1975, Lullman and Lullman-Rauch 1986). The pseudoalcoholic liver disease lesion associated with these drugs consists of prominent Mallory bodies (Figs 11.13, 11.14), a minor degree of steatosis and neutrophil polymorph aggregates, at

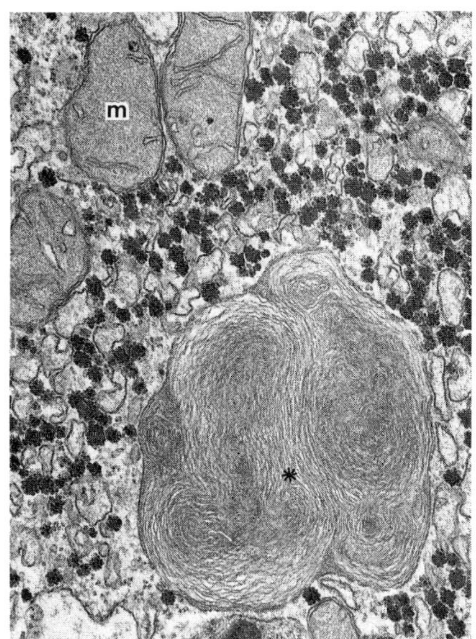

Fig. 11.12 Amiodarone-induced phospholipidosis. Large lysosomal inclusion with a fingerprint pattern (asterisk) is present in the cytoplasm of a liver cell (m = mitochondria). × 20,160.

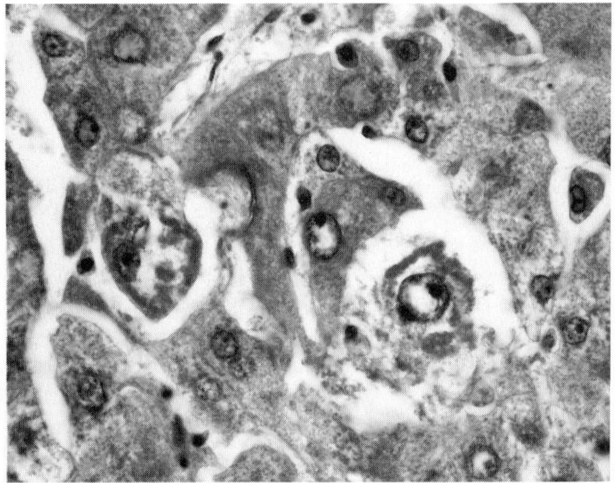

Fig. 11.13 Amiodarone-induced liver injury. Mallory bodies are seen in two hepatocytes. H&E, × 430.

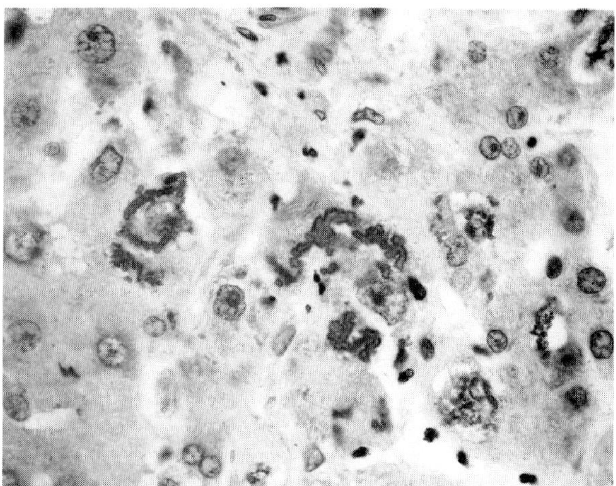

Fig. 11.14 Amiodarone-induced liver injury. Mallory bodies from case illustrated in Fig. 11.13 are well-visualized. Ubiquitin immunostain, × 410.

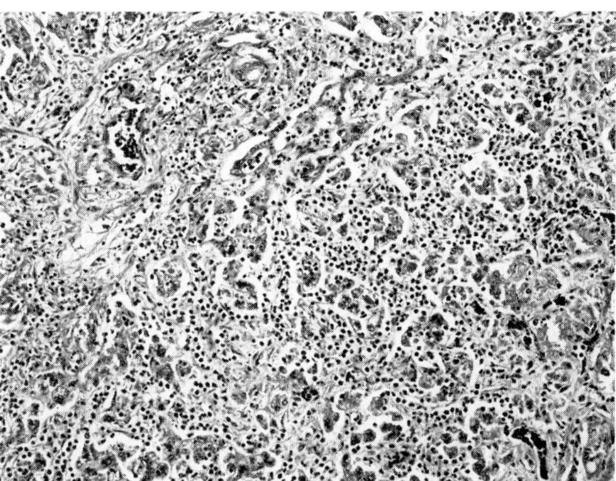

Fig. 11.15 Amiodarone-induced liver injury. Striking abscess-like outpouring of neutrophil polymorphs. Mallory bodies are present but are not well-visualized at this magnification. H&E, × 100.

times profuse (Fig. 11.15). In some cases, the Mallory bodies are predominantly located in zone 1 (Lewis *et al.* 1990). The liver injury in pseudoalcoholic liver disease may progress to cirrhosis (Simon *et al.* 1984; Poucell *et al.* 1984; Lim *et al.* 1984; Babany *et al.* 1985, 1986; Rigas *et al.* 1986; Lewis *et*

al. 1989). The combination of phospholipidosis and pseudoalcoholic liver disease was first reported in recipients of 4,4′-diethylaminoethoxyhexestrol (Coralgil) in Japan during the early 1970s (Itoh and Tsukada 1973). A similar type of liver injury was next reported in recipients of perhexiline maleate (Pessayre *et al.* 1979; Poupon *et al.* 1980) and of amiodarone (Lewis *et al.* 1989, 1990). The incidence of liver disease in recipients of these drugs (as extrapolated from amiodarone-induced disease) appears to be 1–5 percent for pseudoalcoholic liver

Table 11.9 Herpatic injury in patients taking amiodarone

Parameter	Estimated incidence (%)
Phospholipidosis	50–100
Impaired drug metabolism	~25
AST/ALT increased	~25
Mallory bodies	~1–5

disease, 25 percent for lesser parenchymal injury and, apparently, a very high incidence of phospholipidosis after prolonged administration (Table 11.9).

Despite the fact that the same drugs produce both pseudoalcoholic liver disease and phospholipidosis, the two lesions appear to be separable. Patients apparently may have either lesion or both (Lewis *et al*. 1990). However, only a small proportion of recipients of amiodarone who are found to have phospholipidosis also have pseudoalcoholic liver disease, while most patients with pseudoalcoholic liver disease also have phospholipidosis (Fig. 11.16).

There are agents that lead to only phospholipidosis and others to only pseudoalcoholic liver disease (Table 11.8). Many amphophilic compounds (Lullman and Lullman-Rauch 1986) can lead to phospholipidosis, whereas the three drugs cited above can lead both to phospholipidosis and pseudoalcoholic liver disease. Furthermore, non-amphophilic compounds (e.g. diethylstilbestrol, nifedipine) lead to only pseudoalcoholic liver disease. We infer that the two lesions in the injury produced by amiodarone and perhexiline maleate are separable effects of the agent (Fig. 11.16).

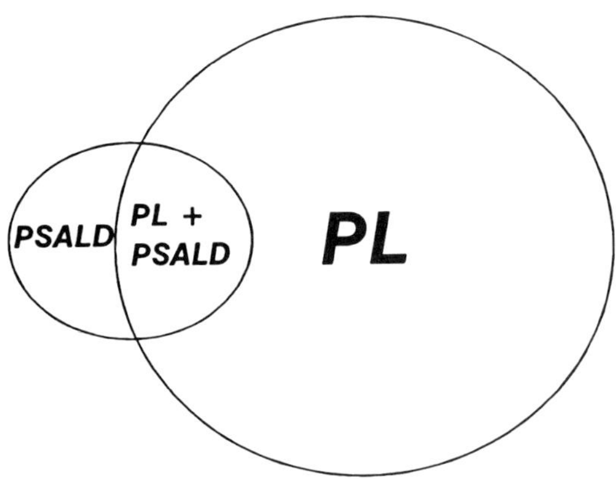

Fig. 11.16 Depiction of association of phospholipidosis (PL) with pseudoalcoholic liver disease and presence of each without the other.

Clinical features

The clinical manifestations of amiodarone-induced pseudoalcoholic liver disease/phospholipidoses may be slight, consisting only of hepatomegaly; or there may be overt liver disease including features suggesting cirrhosis, for example spider angiomas, collateral venous pattern and ascites (Lewis *et al*. 1989). Indeed, the liver disease may be fatal. However, manifestations of phospholipidosis of other organs may dominate the clinical features with prominent wasting, neuropathy, pulmonary insufficiency and thyroid dysfunction. Unfortunately, drug withdrawal may be of little benefit, since the drug remains in the body for weeks or months (Lim *et al*. 1984).

Biochemical features

Modest elevations (<five-fold) of AST and ALT are characteristic, having been reported in 14–84 percent of patients (25 percent in our experience) taking amiodarone (Lewis *et al*. 1989). The high incidence of liver enzyme abnormalities presumably reflects the phospholipidoses without Mallory bodies, inflammation or cirrhosis. However, when there is severe hepatitis or cirrhosis, hypoalbuminaemia and hypoprothrombinaemia are likely to be present.

Pathogenesis

Phospholipidosis appears attributable to binding of phospholipids within the lysosome by the amphophilic molecules (Fig. 11.17). The intralysosomal retention of phospholipids appears to be due to inhibition of phospholipase A (Kubo and Hostetler 1987) by the drug and, perhaps, to the binding of phospholipids by the drug that makes them resistant to phospholipolysis (Lullman *et al*. 1975; Lullman and Lullman-Rauch 1986). Phospholipidosis can be produced in experimental animals by a variety of amphophilic compounds and is apparently dose- and duration-dependent. Accordingly, the development of phospholipidosis appears to be a property of the drug rather than the patient. On the other hand, the development of pseudoalcoholic liver disease reflects the susceptibility of the individual patient.

Clues to the genesis of pseudoalcoholic liver disease come from studies of perhexiline toxicity. Evidence that the liver injury induced by perhexiline is due to abnormal metabolism of the drug, is provided

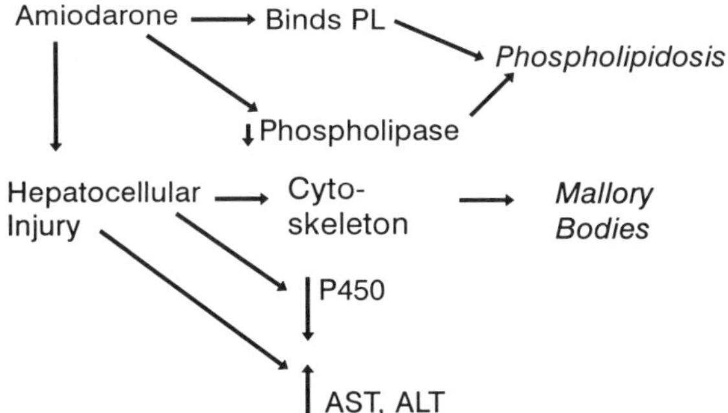

Fig. 11.17   Presumed mechanism by which amiodarone leads to hepatic injury. Phospholipidosis results from trapping of phospholipids in lysosomes due to binding by drug and inhibition of phospholipase A. Other effects of amiodarone reflect hepatocellular injury by drug or metabolite.

by the studies of Morgan *et al.* (1984). They demonstrated that patients who develop hepatic injury while taking perhexiline are far more likely to be phenotypically slow metabolizers of debrisoquine (75 percent) than those without liver injury (9 percent) (Table 11.10). Morgan *et al.* (1984) suggested that slowed metabolism of perhexiline permits the drug to exert its toxicity. There are, however, no data to indicate whether the toxicity would be due to the unchanged perhexiline molecule or to a toxic metabolite (Fig. 11.18). Similar efforts to correlate the rate of metabolism of amiodarone with hepatic injury remain to be conducted. Nevertheless, one may speculate that a metabolic defect analogous to that presumed responsible for susceptibility to per-

hexiline injury is responsible for the identical amiodarone injury (Fig. 11.18). Susceptible patients are perhaps unable or are less able than the non-susceptible to metabolize amiodarone through normal pathways. Accordingly, they would have higher levels and more prolonged retention of the drug permitting toxicity of unmetabolized drug, or of the active metabolite of the drug, produced by a normally minor pathway. Hints that the daily or total dose of the drug may have a bearing on toxicity suggest that there may be an interplay between dose-related intrinsic toxicity and genetic susceptibility. Also, the observation that quinidine and other drugs (Speirs *et al.* 1986) can inhibit debrisoquine metabolism leading to a spurious slow metabolizer phenotype, suggest a manner in which such drugs might enhance the hepatotoxic effects of perhexiline and, indeed, in which one drug might affect the toxicity of another.

In any event, while phospholipidosis is due apparently to the blockade of phospholipid escape from lysosomes, the cytologic injury that includes Mallory body production, presumably reflects impaired metabolism of amiodarone in individuals with enhanced susceptibility. The impaired metabolism could be either genetic or acquired. Whether the impaired cytochrome P450 activity and elevated blood aminotransferase levels reflect phospholipidosis or the cytologic injury associated with Mallory bodies changes, these abnormalities are a reflection of parenchymal injury (Fig. 11.17).

Table 11.10   Association of Mallory body–phospholipidosis with slow metabolizers of debrisoquine

	Metabolic phenotype[c]	
	Poor metabolizer (PM) (%)	*Extensive metabolizer (EM)* (%)
MB–PL lesion	3 (75)	1(25)[a]
Normals	9	91
Liver disease[b]	9	91

[a]Even this patient had slower than normal metabolism of the drug.
[b]Patients with other liver disease show PM and EM distribution similar to normal.
[c]From data of Morgan *et al.* (1984).

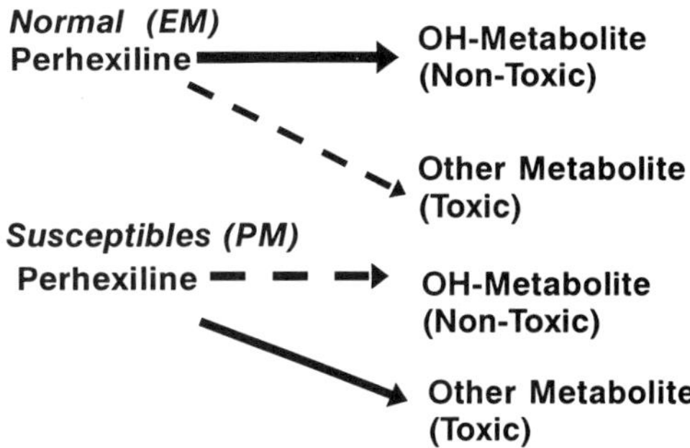

Fig. 11.18   Suggested mechanism by which perhexiline maleate leads to hepatic injury slow metabolizer converts drug to non-toxic metabolite slowly permitting greater conversion along alternative pathway to toxic metabolite.

Classification of pseudoalcoholic liver disease

Ludwig *et al.* (1980) proposed categorizing non-alcoholic steatohepatitis as primary and secondary, distinguishing between the lesion associated with obesity and diabetes mellitus as primary and other associations as secondary. We propose an alternative classification which recognizes three categories of pseudoalcoholic liver disease (Table 11.11):

1. Lesions associated with obesity and surgical treatment of it and/or diabetes mellitus.
2. Lesions associated with toxic agents and drugs.
3. A miscellaneous group of widely divergent entities.

This classification is based on the observation that the morphologic patterns of the three differ (Table 11.1).

Table 11.11   Classification of pseudoalcoholic liver disease (PSALD)

  I. PSALD associated with obesity and diabetes mellitus:
    A. Steatosis
    B. Steatohepatitis
    C. Steatofibrosis
    D. Cirrhosis

  II. PSALD associated with drugs and toxins:
    A. Copper toxicity
      1. Indian childhood cirrhosis
      2. Wilson's disease
    B. Drugs
      1. With phospholipidosis (e.g. amiodarone)
      2. Without phospholipidosis (e.g. nifedipine)

III. Miscellaneous conditions accompanied occasionally or rarely by Mallory body formation, e.g. primary biliary cirrhosis, hepatocellular carcinoma (see Table 11.2)

Concluding comments

The characteristics of steatohepatitis draw attention to several relationships (Fig. 11.19). Obesity and/or diabetes mellitus lead to liver disease resembling that caused by alcohol. Furthermore, both alcohol and obesity/diabetes mellitus can enhance the adverse effects of methotrexate on the liver, and the effects of methotrexate on the liver may sometimes resemble those of alcohol.

Of particular interest is the enhancement of the understanding of alcoholic liver disease provided by pseudoalcoholic liver disease. It has long seemed clear that the clinical manifestations of alcoholic liver disease are a composite of the effects of the hepatic injury and the extrahepatic effects of alcohol. The relatively asymptomatic nature of non-alcoholic steatohepatitis compared with the often severe clinical manifestations of alcoholic hepatitis supports the impression that the extrahepatic effects of alcohol contribute importantly to the clinical features of alcoholic liver disease.

Recognition of the liver disease associated with obesity and diabetes mellitus has helped reduce the prevalence of "cryptogenic cirrhosis". With the identification of chronic virus C hepatitis as a cause of cirrhosis and of the lesion considered in this discussion, the proportion of cases of unexplained cirrhosis is now small.

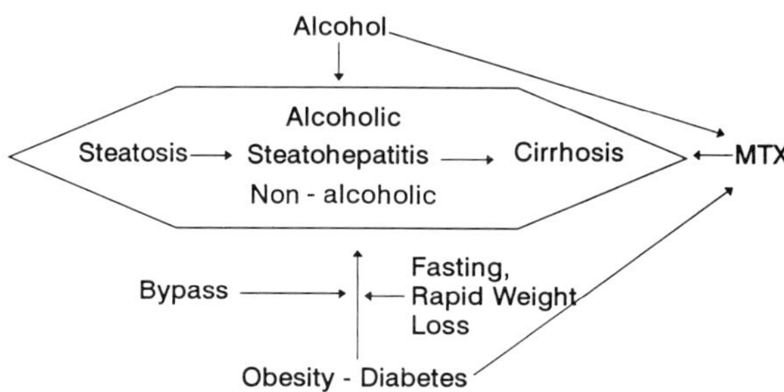

Fig. 11.19   Sequences of lesions caused by alcohol or obesity and/or diabetes. Bypass, fasting and rapid weight loss enhance the effects of obesity and diabetes. Alcohol, obesity and diabetes enhance the adverse effects of methotrexate (MTX) on the liver.

References

Ackerman, N.B. (1979). Protein supplementation in the management of degeneration of liver function after jejunoileal bypass. *Surgery, Gynecology and Obstetrics* **149**, 8–14.

Adamson, M., Reiner, B., Olson, J.L., Goodman, Z., Plotnick, L., Bermandi, I. and Gahl, W.A. (1992). Indian childhood cirrhosis in an American child. *Gastroenterology* **102**, 1771–1777.

Adler, M. and Schaffner, F. (1979). Fatty liver hepatitis and cirrhosis in obese patients. *American Journal of Medicine* **67**, 811–816.

Ames, F.C., Copeland, E.M., Leeb, D.C., Moore , D.L. and Dudrick, S.J. (1976). Liver dysfunction following small-bowel bypass for obesity: Nonoperative treatment of fatty metamorphosis with parenteral hyperalimentation. *Journal of the American Medical Association* **235**, 1249–1252.

Anderson, T. and Gluud, C. (1984). Liver morphology in morbid obesity: A literature study. *International Journal of Obesity* **8**, 97–106.

Babany, G., Saint-Marc Girardin, M.F., Zafrani, E.S., Coderci, E. and Dhumeaux, D. (1985). Deux cas de cirrhose chez des malades traites par l'amiodarone. *Gastroenterologie Clinique et Biologique* **9**, 505.

Babany, G., Mallat, A., Zafrani, E.S., Saint-Marc Giradin, M.F., Carcone, B. and Dhumeaux, D. (1986). Chronic liver disease after low daily doses of amiodarone: Report of three cases. *Journal of Hepatology* **3**, 228–232.

Babany, G., Uzzam, F., Larrey, D., Degott, C., Bourgeois, P., Rene, E., Vissuzaine, C., Erlinger, S. and Benhamou, J.-P. (1989). Alcoholic-like liver lesions induced by nifedipine. *Journal of Hepatology* **9**, 252–255.

Bach, N., Swan, N.T. and Schaffner, F. (1991). The histological features of chronic hepatitis C and autoimmune chronic hepatitis: A comparative analysis. *Hepatology* **4**, 572–577.

Baker, A.L., Elson, C.O., Jaspan, J. and Boyer, J.L. (1979). Liver failure with steatonecrosis after jejunoileal bypass: Recovery with parenteral nutrition and reanastomosis. *Archives of Internal Medicine* **139**, 289–292.

Baker, A.L., Krager, P.S., Glagov, S. and Schoeller, D.S. (1983). Aminopyrine breath test. Prospective comparison with liver histology and liver chemistry following jejunoileal bypass performed for refractory obesity. *Digestive Diseases and Sciences* **28**, 405–410.

Balazs, M. and Halmos, T. (1984). Electron microscopic study of liver fibrosis associated with diabetes mellitus. *Experimental Pathology* **27**, 153–162.

Barry, R.E. (1983). The pathogenesis of hepatitis in alcohol abuse and jejunoileal bypass. *Lancet* **1**, 489–490.

Batman, P.A. and Scheuer, P.J. (1985). Diabetic hepatitis preceding the onset of glucose intolerance. *Histopathology* **9**, 237–243.

Bernuau, D., Guillot, R., Durant, A.M., Raousc, N., Gabreau, T., Possa, P. and Feldmann, G. (1982). Ultrastructural aspects of the liver perisinusoidal space in diabetes patients with and without microangiopathy. *Diabetes* **31**, 1061–1067.

Bernuau, D., Guillot, R., Durand-Schneider, A.M., Poussier, P., Moreau, A. and Feldmann, G. (1985). Liver perisinusoidal fibrosis in BB rats with or without overt diabetes. *American Journal of Pathology* **120**, 38–45.

Bhagwat, A.G., Walia, B.N., Koshy, A. and Banerji, C.K. (1983). Will the real Indian childhood cirrhosis please stand up? *Cleveland Clinical Quarterly* **50**, 323–237.

Bhusnurmath, S.R., Walia, B.N.S., Singh, S., Parkash, D., Radotra, B.D. and Nath, R. (1991). Sequential histopathologic alterations in Indian childhood cirrhosis treated with *d*-penicillamine. *Human Pathology* **22**, 653–658.

Blomfield, J., Dixon, S.R. and McCredie, D.A. (1971). Potential hepatotoxicity of copper in recurrent hemodialysis. *Archives of Internal Medicine* **128**, 555–560.

Braillon, A., Capron, J.P., Herve, M.A., Degott, C. and Quenum, C. (1985). Liver in obesity. *Gut* **26**, 133–139.

Cairns, S.R., Kark, A.E. and Peters, T.J. (1986). Raised hepatic free fatty acids in a patient with acute fatty liver after gastric surgery for morbid obesity. *Journal of Clinical Pathology* **39**, 647–649.

Campbell, J.M., Hunt, T.K., Karam, J.H. and Forsham, P.H. (1977). Jejunoileal bypass as a treatment of morbid obesity. *Archives of Internal Medicine* **137**, 602–610.

Capron, J.-P., Delamarre, J., Dupas, J.L., Braillon, A., Degott, C. and Quenum, C. (1982). Fasting in obesity: Another cause of liver injury with alcoholic hyaline? *Digestive Disease and Sciences* **27**, 265–268.

Chuttani, H.K., Gupta, P.S., Gulati, S. and Gupta, D.N. (1965). Acute copper sulfate poisoning. *American Journal of Medicine* **39**, 849–854.

Clain, D.J. and Lefkowitch, J.H. (1987). Fatty liver disease in morbid obesity. *Gastroenterology Clinics of North America* **16**, 239–252.

Clayman, C.B. and O'Reilly, A.J. (1981). Jejunoileal bypass: Pass it by (Editorial). *Journal of the American Medical Association* **246**, 988.

Coe, J.E., Ishak, K.G. and Ross, M.J. (1983). Diethylstilbestrol-induced jaundice in the Chinese and Armenian hamster. *Hepatology* **3**, 489–496.

Craig, R.M., Neumann, T., Jeejeebhoy, K.N. and Yokoo, H. (1980). Severe hepatocellular reaction resembling alcoholic hepatitis with cirrhosis after massive small bowel resection and prolonged total parenteral nutrition. *Gastroenterology* **79**, 131–137.

Cuellar, R.E., Tarter, R., Hays, A. and Van Thiel, D.H. (1987). The possible occurrence of "alcoholic hepatitis" in a patient with bulimia in the absence of diagnosable alcoholism. *Hepatology* **7**, 878–883.

Czaja, A.J. (1992). Non-alcoholic steatohepatitis. In *Newer Aspects of Alcohol, Nutrition and Hepatic Ence-*

phalopathy (Edited by Meezy, E.), pp. 311–332. American Association for the Study of Liver Diseases.

Dake, M.D., Madison, J.M., Montgomery, C.K., Saellits, J.E., Hinchcliffe, W.A., Winkler, M.L. and Bainton, D.F. (1985). Electron microscopic demonstration of lysosomal inclusion bodies in lung, liver, lymph nodes, and blood leukocytes of patients with amiodarone pulmonary toxicity. *American Journal of Medicine* **78**, 506–512

Denk, H., Gschnaitt, F. and Wolff, K. (1975). Hepatocellular hyaline (Mallory bodies) in long term griseofulvin-treated mice: A new experimental model for the study of hyaline formation. *Laboratory Investigation* **32**, 773–776.

DeWind, L.T. and Payne, J.H. (1976). Intestinal bypass surgery for morbid obesity. Long-term results. *Journal of the American Medical Association* **236**, 2298–2301.

Diehl, A.M., Goodman, Z. and Ishak, K.G. (1988). Alcohol-like liver disease in non-alcoholics. *Gastroenterology* **95**, 1056–1062.

Drenick, E.J., Simmons, F. and Murphy, J.F. (1970). Effect on hepatic morphology of treatment of obesity by fasting, reducing diets and small bowel bypass. *New England Journal of Medicine* **282**, 829–834.

Drenick, E.J., Fisler, J. and Johnson, D. (1982). Hepatic steatosis after intestinal bypass – prevention and reversal by metronidazole, irrespective of protein-calorie malnutrition. *Gastroenterology* **82**, 535–548.

Edmondson, H.A., Peters, R.L., Frankel, H.H. and Borowsky, S. (1967). The early stage of liver injury in the alcoholic. *Medicine* **46**, 119–129.

Falchuk, K.R., Fiske, S.C., Haggitt, R.C., Federman, M. and Trey, C. (1980). Pericellular hepatic fibrosis and intracellular hyalin in diabetes mellitus. *Gastroenterology* **55**, 434–438.

Fletcher, L.M., Kwoh-Gain, I., Powell, E.E. and Halliday, J.W. (1991). Markers of chronic alcohol ingestion in patients with non-alcoholic steatohepatitis: An aid to diagnosis. *Hepatology* **13**, 455–459.

French, S.W. and Davies, P.L. (1975). The Mallory body in the pathogenesis of alcoholic liver disease. In *Alcoholic Liver Disease* (Edited by Khanna J.M., Israel Y. and Kalant H.), pp. 113–143. Addiction Research Foundation of Ontario Toronto.

French, S.W., Leslie, B.E. and Freeman, J. (1989). Nonalcoholic fatty hepatitis: An important clinical condition. *Canadian Journal of Gastroenterology* **3**, 189–197.

Galambos, J.T. (1972). Natural history of alcoholic hepatitis. III. Histological changes. *Gastroenterology* **63**, 1026–1035.

Galambos, J.T. (1976). Jejunoileal bypass and nutritional liver injury. *Archives of Pathology and Laboratory Medicine* **100**, 229–235.

Galambos, J.T. and Wills, C.E. (1978). Relationship between 505 paired liver tests and biopsies in 242 obese patients. *Gastroenterology* **74**, 1191–1195.

Gerber, M.A., Orr, W., Denk, H., Schaffner, F. and Popper, H. (1973). Hepatocellular hyalin in cholestasis and cirrhosis: Its diagnostic significance. *Gastroenterology* **65**, 89–96

Gerber, M.A., Krzysztol, K., Miriam, J., Alter, M.J., Sampliner, R.E., Margolis, H.S. and Sentinal Countries Chronic Non-A, Non-B Hepatitis Study Team (1992). Histopathology of community acquired chronic hepatitis C. *Modern Pathology* **5**, 483–486.

Gooneratne, S.R., Howell, J. and Cook, R.D. (1980). An ultrastructural and morphometric study of the liver of normal and copper-poisoned sheep. *American Journal of Pathology* **99**, 429–450.

Grimm, I.S., Schlinder, W. and Haluszka, O. (1992). Steatohepatitis and fatal hepatic failure after biliopancreatic diversion. *American Journal of Gastroenterology* **87**, 775–779.

Haines, N.W., Baker, A.L., Boyer, J.L., Glagov, S., Schnier, H., Jaspan, J. and Ferguson, D.J. (1981). Prognostic indicators of hepatic injury following jejunoileal bypass performed for refractory obesity: A prospective study. *Hepatology* **1**, 161–167.

Hall, P. de la M. (1987). Alcoholic liver disease. In *Pathology of the Liver* (Edited by MacSween, R.N.M., Anthony, P.D. and Scheuer, P.J.), 2nd edn, pp. 281–309. Churchill-Livingstone, Edinburgh.

Halverson, J.D., Wise, L., Wazna, M.F. and Ballinger, W.F. (1978). Jejunoileal bypass for morbid obesity: A critical appraisal. *American Journal of Medicine* **64**, 461–475.

Hamilton, D.L., Vest, T.K., Brown, B.S., Shah, A.N., Menguy, R.B. and Chey, W.Y. (1983). Liver injury with alcoholic like hyalin gastroplasty for morbid obesity. *Gastroenterology* **85**, 722–726.

Harinasuta, U. and Zimmerman, H.J. (1971). Alcoholic steatonecrosis: I. Relationship between severity of hepatic disease and presence of Mallory bodies in the liver. *Gastroenterology* **60**, 1036–1046.

Hilden, M., Juhl, E., Thomsen, A.C. and Christoffersen, P. (1973). Fatty liver persisting for up to 33 years. *Acta Medica Scandinavica* **194**, 485–489

Hocking, M.D., Duerson, M.L., Alexander, R.W. and Woodward, E.R. (1981). Late hepatic histopathology after jejunoileal bypass for morbid obesity: Relation of abnormalities on biopsy and clinical course. *American Journal of Surgery* **141**, 159–163.

Holtzman, N.A., Elliot, D.A. and Heller, R.H. (1986). Copper intoxication: Report of a case with observations on ceruloplasmin. *New England Journal of Medicine* **275**, 347–352.

Holzbach, R.T. (1977). Hepatic effects of jejunoileal bypass for morbid obesity. *American Journal of Clinical Nutrition* **30**, 43–52.

Ishmael, J., Gopinath, C. and Howell, J. McC. (1971). Experimental chronic copper toxicity in sheep: Histological and histochemical changes during the development of the lesions in the liver. *Research in Veterinary Science* **12**, 358–366.

Itoh, S. and Tsukada Y. (1973). Clinico-pathological and electron microscopical studies on a coronary dilating agent: 4,4′-diethylaminoethoxyhexestrol-induced liver injuries. *Acta Hepatogastroenterology (Stuttgart)* **20**, 204–215.

Itoh, S., Igarashi, M., Tsukada, Y. and Ichinoe, A. (1977). Nonalcoholic fatty liver with alcoholic hyalin after long-term glucocorticoid treatment. *Acta Hepatogastroenterology* **24**, 415–418.

Itoh, S., Matsuo, S., Ichinoe, A., Yamaba, Y. and Miyazawa, M. (1982). Nonalcoholic steatohepatitis and cirrhosis with Mallory's hyalin, with ultrastructural study of one case. *Digestive Diseases and Sciences* **27**, 341–346.

Itoh, S., Yougel, T. and Kawagoe, K. (1987). Comparison between non-alcoholic steatohepatitis and alcoholic hepatitis. *American Journal of Gastroenterology* **82**, 650–654.

Joshi, V.V. (1987). Indian childhood cirrhosis. *Perspectives in Paediatric Pathology* **11**, 175–192.

Kaminski, D.L., Hermann, V.M. and Martin S. (1985). Late effects of jejunoileal bypass operations on hepatic inflammation, fibrosis and lipid content. *Hepatogastroenterology* **32**, 159–162.

Keeffe, E.B., Adesman, P.W., Stenzel, P. and Palmer, R.M. (1987). Steatosis and cirrhosis in an obese diabetic: Resolution of fatty liver by fasting. *Digestive Diseases and Sciences* **32**, 441–445.

Keeley, A.F., Iseri, O.A. and Gottlieb, L.S. (1972). Ultrastructure of hyaline cytoplasmic inclusion in a human hepatoma: Relationship to Mallory's alcoholic hyalin. *Gastroenterology* **62**, 280–293.

Kern, W.H., Heger, A.H., Payne, J.H. and De Wind, L.T. (1973). Fatty metamorphosis of the liver in morbid obesity. *Archives of Pathology* **96**, 342–346.

Kimura, H., Kako, M., Yo, K. and Oda, T. (1980). Alcoholic hyalin (Mallory bodies) in a case of Weber-Christian disease: Electron microscopic observations of liver involvement. *Gastroenterology* **78**, 807–812.

Kinugasa, A., Tsunamoto, K., Furukawa, N., Sawada, T., Kusunoki, T. and Shimada, N. (1984). Fatty liver and its fibrous changes found in simple obesity of children. *Journal of Pediatric Gastroenterology and Nutrition* **3**, 408–413.

Klain, J., Fraser, D., Goldstein, J., Peiser, J., Avinoah, E., Ovnat, A. and Charuzi, I. (1989). Liver histology abnormalities in the morbidly obese. *Hepatology* **10**, 873–876.

Kroyer, J.M. and Talbert, W.M., Jr. (1980). Morphologic liver changes in intestinal bypass changes. *American Journal of Surgery* **139**, 855–859.

Kubo, M. and Hostetler, K.Y. (1987). Metabolic basis of diethylaminoethoxyhexesterol-induced phospholipid fatty liver. *American Journal of Physiology* **252**, E375.

Latry, P., Bioulac-Sage, P., Echinard, E., Boussarie, L., Grimaud, J.A. and Balaboud, C. (1987). Perisinusoidal fibrosis and basement membrane-like material in the livers of diabetic patients. *Human Pathology* **18**, 775–780.

Lee, R.G. (1989). Nonalcoholic steatohepatitis: A study of 49 patients. *Human Pathology* **20**, 594–598.

Lefkowitch, J.H., Honig, C.L., King, M.E. and Hagstrom, J.W.C. (1982). Hepatic copper overload and features of Indian childhood cirrhosis in an American sibship. *New England Journal of Medicine* **307**, 271–277.

Lefkowitch, J.H., Schiff, E.R., Davis, G.L., Perrillo, P., Lindsay, K., Bodenheimer, H.C., Jr., Balart, L.A., Ortego, T.J., Payne, J., Dienstag, J.L., Gibas, A., Jacobson, I.M., Tamburro, C.H., Carey, W., O'Brien, C., Sampliner, R., Van Thiel, D.H., Feit, D., Albrecht, J., Meschievitz, C., Sanghvi, B., Vaughan, R.D. and the Hepatitis Interventional Therapy Group (1993). Pathological diagnosis of chronic hepatitis C: A multicenter comparative study of chronic hepatitis C. *Gastroenterology* **104**, 595–603.

Lewis, J.H., Ranard, R.C., Caruso, A., Jackson, L.K., Mullick, F.G., Ishak, K.G., Seeff, L.B. and Zimmerman, H.J. (1989). Amiodarone hepatotoxicity: Prevalence and clinicopathologic correlations among 104 patients. *Hepatology* **9**, 679–685.

Lewis, J.H., Mullick, F.G., Ishak, K.G., Ranard, R.C., Ragsdale, B., Perse, R.M., Rusnock, E.J., Walke, A., Benjamin, S.B., Seef, L.B. and Zimmerman, H.J. (1990). Histopathologic analysis of suspected amiodarone hepatotoxicity. *Human Pathology* **21**, 59–67.

Lim, P.K., Trewby, P.N., Storey, G.C. and Holt, D.W. (1984). Neuropathy and fatal hepatitis in a patient receiving amiodarone. *British Medical Journal* **288**, 1638–1639.

Lockwood, D.H., Amatruda, J.M., Moxley, R.T., Pozefsky, T. and Boitnott, J.K. (1977). Effect of oral amino acid supplementation on liver disease after jejunoileal bypass for morbid obesity. *American Journal of Clinical Nutrition* **30**, 58–63.

Ludwig, J., Viggiano, T.R., McGill, D.B. and Ott, B.J. (1980). Nonalcoholic steatohepatitis: Mayo Clinic experience with a hitherto unnamed disease. *Mayo Clinic Proceedings* **55**, 434–438.

Lullman, H. and Lullman-Rauch, R. (1986). Drug-induced lysosomal storage diseases of the liver. In *Hepatotoxicity of Drugs* (Edited by W. Fillastre.), pp. 127–137. Universite de Rousen, Rousen.

Lullman, H., Lullman-Rauch, R. and Wassermann, O. (1975). Drug-induced phospholipidosis. *CRC Critical Reviews in Toxiciology* **4**, 185–218.

MacSween, R.N.M. (1979). Liver pathology associated with diseases of other organs. In *Pathology of the Liver* (Edited by MacSween, R.N.M., Anthony, P.P. and Scheuer, P.J.), 2nd edn, pp. 414–439. Churchill Livingstone, Edinburgh.

Marrubbio, A.T., Jr., Buchwald, H., Schwartz, M.Z. and Varco, R. (1976). Hepatic lesions of central pericellular fibrosis in morbid obesity and after jejunoileal bypass. *American Journal of Clinical Pathology* **66**, 684–691.

Massarat, S., Jordan, G., Sahrhage, G., Asholt, K., Schmitz-Moorman, P. and Bode, J.C. (1979). Follow-up studies in patients with non-alcoholic and non-diabetic fatty liver. *Acta Hepatogastroenterology* **26**, 296–301.

Mavrelis, P.G., Ammon, H.V., Gleysteen, J.J., Komorowski, R.A. and Charaf, U.K. (1983). Hepatic free fatty acids in alcoholic liver disease and morbid obesity. *Hepatology* **3**, 226–231.

Mehrotra, R., Panday, R.K. and Nath, P. (1981). Hepatic copper in Indian childhood cirrhosis. *Histopathology* **5**, 659–665.

Miller, D.J., Ishumaru, H. and Klatskin, G. (1979). Non-alcoholic liver disease mimicking alcoholic hepatitis and cirrhosis. *Gastroenterology* **77**, A27.

Moran, J.R., Ghishan, F.K. and Halter, S.A. (1983). Steatohepatitis in obese children: A cause of chronic liver dysfunction. *American Journal of Gastroenterology* **78**, 374–377.

Morgan, M.Y., Reshef, R., Shah, R.R., Oates, N.S., Idle, J.R., Sherlock, S. and Smith, R.L. (1984). Impaired oxidation of debrisoquine in patients with perhexiline liver injury. *Gut* **25**, 1057–1064.

Moxley, R.T., Pozefsky, T. and Lockwood, D.H. (1974). Protein nutrition and liver disease after jejunoileal bypass for morbid obesity. *New England Journal of Medicine* **290**, 921–926.

Muller-Hocker, J., Meyer, U., Wiebecke, B., Hubner, G., Eife, R., Kellner, M. and Schramel, P. (1985). Copper storage disease of the liver and chronic dietary copper intoxication in two further German infants mimicking Indian childhood cirrhosis. *Pathology Research and Practice* **183**, 39–45.

Muller-Hocker, J., Weiss, M., Meyer, U., Schramel, P., Wiebeck, B., Belohradsky, B.H. and Hubner, G. (1987). Fatal copper storage disease of the liver in a German infant resembling Indian childhood cirrhosis. *Virchow Archives A* **411**, 379–385.

Nagore, N. and Scheuer, P.J. (1988). The pathology of diabetic hepatitis. *Journal of Pathology* **156**, 155–160.

Nakamura, S., Takezawa, Y., Sato, T., Kera, K. and Maeda, T. (1979). Alcoholic liver disease in women. *Tohoku Journal of Experimental Medicine* **129**, 351–355.

Nalpas, B., Vassault, A., Charpin, S., Lacour, B. and Berthelot, P. (1986). Serum mitochondrial aspartate aminotransferase as a marker of chronic alcoholism: Diagnostic value and interpretation in a liver unit. *Hepatology* **6**, 608–614.

Nasrallah, S.M., Wills, C.E. and Galambos, J.T. (1981). Hepatic morphology in obesity. *Digestive Diseases and Sciences* **26**, 325–327.

Nayak, N.C., Sagreya, K. and Ramalingaswami, V. (1969). Indian childhood cirrhosis: The nature and significance of cytoplasmic hyaline of hepatocyte. *Archives of Pathology* **8**, 631–637.

Nonomura, A., Mizukami, Y., Unoura, M., Kobayashi, K., Takeda, Y. and Takeda, R. (1992). Clinicopathologic study of alcohol-like liver disease in non-alcoholics: Non-alcoholic steatohepatitis and fibrosis. *Gastroenterologica Japonica* **27**, 521–528.

Oda, T., Shikata, T., Suzuki, H., Naito, K., Kanetaka, T., Lina, S., Naito, K., Karetaka, T. and Lina, S. (1969). Pholpholipidosis der Leberzellen durch das Medikament "Coralgil". *Acta Hepatologica Japan* **10**, 530–542.

O'Leary, J.P. (1983). Hepatic complications of jejunoileal bypass. *Seminars in Liver Disease* **3**, 203–212.

O'Neill, N.C. and Tanner, M.S. (1989). Uptake of copper from brass vessels in bovine milk and its relevance to Indian childhood cirrhosis. *Journal of Pediatric Gastroenterology and Nutrition* **9**, 167–172.

Palmer, M.A. and Schaffner, F. (1990). Effect of weight reduction on hepatic abnormalities in overweight patients. *Gastroenterology* **99**, 1408–1413.

Partin, J.S., Partin, J.C., Schubert, W.K. and McAdams, J. (1974). Liver ultrastructure in abetalipoproteinemia: evaluation of micronodular cirrhosis. *Gastroenterology* **67**, 107–118.

Pessayre, D., Bichara, M., Feldmann, G., Degott, C., Potet, F. and Benhamou, J.-P. (1979). Perhexiline maleate-induced cirrhosis. *Gastroenterology* **76**, 170–177.

Peters, R.L. (1977). Patterns of hepatic morphology in jejunoileal bypass patients. *American Journal of Clinical Nutrition* **30**, 53–57.

Peters, R.L., Gay, T. and Reynolds, T.B. (1975). Post-jejunoileal-bypass hepatic disease: Its similarity to alcoholic hepatic disease. *American Journal of Clinical Pathology* **63**, 318–331.

Peura, D.A., Stromeyer, W. and Johnson, L.F. (1980). Liver injury with alcoholic hyaline after intestinal resection. *Gastroenterology* **79**, 128–130.

Pimentel, J.C. and Menezes, A.P. (1975). Liver granulomas containing copper in vineyard sprayer's lung: A new etiology of hepatic granulomatosis. *American Review of Respiratory Disease* **111**, 189–195.

Pimentel, J.C. and Menezes, A.P. (1977). Liver disease in vineyard sprayers. *Gastroenterology* **72**, 275–289.

Popper, H., Goldfischer, S., Sternlieb, I., Nayak, N.C. and Madhavan, T.U. (1979). Cytoplasmic copper and its toxic effects: Studies in Indian childhood cirrhosis. *Lancet* **i**, 1205–1208.

Portmann, B., Tanner, M.S., Mowat, A.P. and Williams R. (1978). Orcein-positive liver deposits in Indian childhood cirrhosis. *Lancet* **i**, 1338–1340.

Portmann, B. and MacSween, R.N.M. (1987). Diseases of the intrahepatic biliary tree. In *Pathology of the Liver* (Edited by MacSween, R.N.M., Anthony, P.P. and Scheuer, P.J.), 2nd edn, pp. 424–453. Churchill-Livingstone, Edinburgh.

Poucell, S., Ireton, J., Valencia-Mayoral, P., Downar, E., Larratt, L., Patterson, J., Blendis, L. and Phillips,

M.J. (1984). Amiodarone-associated phospholipidosis and fibrosis of the liver: Light, immunohistochemical, and electron microscopic studies. *Gastroenterology* **86**, 926–936.

Poupon, R., Homberg, J.C., Abauf, N., Petit, J., Bodin, F. and Darnis, F. (1980). Perhexiline maleate-associated hepatic injury: Prevalence and characteristics. *Digestion* **20**, 145–150.

Powell, E.E., Searle, J. and Mortimer, R. (1989). Steatohepatitis associated with limb lipodystrophy. *Gastroenterology* **97**, 1022–1024.

Powell, E.E., Cooksley, W.G.E., Hanson, R., Searle, J., Halliday, J.W. and Powell, L.W. (1990). The natural history of non-alcoholic steatohepatitis: A follow-up study of forty-two patients for up to 21 years. *Hepatology* **11**, 74–80.

Rabin, L. (1989). The morphological spectrum of alcoholic liver disease. In *Current Perspectives in Hepatology, Festschrift for Hyman J. Zimmerman, M.D.* (Edited by Seeff L.B. and Lewis J.H.), pp 123–139. Plenum Medical, New York.

Rigas, B., Rosenfeld, L.E., Barwick, K.W., Enriquez, R., Helzberg, J., Batsford, W.P., Josephson, M.E. and Riely, C.A. (1986). Amiodarone hepatotoxicity: A clinicopathologic study of five patients. *Annals of Internal Medicine* **104**, 348–351.

Rogers, D.W., Lee, C.H., Pound, D.C., Kumar, O.W., Cumming, S. and Lumeng, L. (1992). Hepatitis C virus does not cause non-alcoholic steatohepatitis. *Digestive Disease and Sciences* **37**, 1644–1647.

Rozental, P., Biava, C., Spencer, H. and Zimmerman, H.J. (1967). Liver morphology and function tests in obesity and during total starvation. *American Journal of Digestive Diseases* **12**, 198–208.

Rumessen, J.J. (1986). Hepatotoxicity of amiodarone. *Acta Medica Scandinavica* **219**, 235–239.

Schaffner, F. and Thaler, H. (1986). Nonalcoholic fatty liver disease. In *Progress in Liver Disease* (Edited by Popper, H. and Schaffner, F.), pp. 283–298. Grune and Stratton, New York.

Scheuer, P.J., Asbrafzadeh, P., Sherlock, S., Brown, D. and Dusheiko, G.M. (1992). The pathology of hepatitis C. *Hepatology* **15**, 567–571.

Schramel, P., Muller-Hocker, J., Meyer, U., Weiss, M. and Eife, R. (1988). Nutritional copper intoxication in three carcinoma infants with severe liver cell damage (features of Indian childhood cirrhosis). *Journal of Trace Elements and Electrocytes in Health and Disease* **2**, 85–89.

Seki, K., Minami, M., Nishwhawa, M., Kawata, S., Miyoshi, S., Imai, Y. and Tarui, S. (1983). Nonalcoholic steatohepatitis induced by massive doses of synthetic estrogen. *Gastroenterologia Japonica* **18**, 197–203.

Shepherd, N.A., Dawson, A.M., Crocker, P.R. and Levison, D.A. (1987). Granular cells a marker of early amiodarone hepatotoxicity: A pathological and analytical study. *Journal of Clinical Pathology* **40**, 418–423.

Sherr, H.P., Nair, P.P., White, J.J., Banwell, J.G. and Lockwood, D.H. (1974). Bile acid metabolism and hepatic disease following small bowel bypass for obesity. *American Journal of Clinical Nutrition* **27**, 1369–1379.

Silverman, J.F., O'Brien, K., Long, S., Leggett, N., Khazamie, P.G., Pories, W.J., Norris, H.T. and Caro, J.F. (1990). Liver pathology in morbidly obese patients with and without diabetes. *American Journal of Gastroenterology* **85**, 1349–1355.

Simon, J.B., Manley, P.N., Brien, J.F. and Armstrong, P.W. (1984). Amiodarone hepatotoxicity stimulating alcoholic liver disease. *New England Journal of Medicine* **311**, 167–172.

Smetana, H.F., Hadley, G.G. and Sirsat, S.M. (1961). Infantile cirrhosis: An analytic review of the literature and a report of 50 cases. *Pediatrics* **28**, 107–127.

Snodgrass, P.J. (1970). Obesity, small bowel bypass and liver disease. *New England Journal of Medicine* **282**, 870–871.

Spech, H.J., Liechr, H. and Mitschke, H. (1983). Nicht alkoholbedingle fettleberhepatiden und fettzirrhosen unter dem tauschenden bild alkohotloxischer lebererkrankungen. *Zeitschrift fur Gastroenterology* **21**, 651–659.

Speirs, C.J., Murray, S., Boobis, A.R., Seddon, C.E. and Dacies, D.S. (1986). Quinidine and the identification of drugs whose elimination is impaired in subjects classified as poor metabolizers of debrisoquine. *British Journal of Clinical Pharmacology* **22**, 739.

Sternlieb, I. (1972). Evolution of the hepatic lesion in Wilson's disease (hepatolenticular degeneration). *Progress in Liver Disease* (Edited by Popper, H. and Schaffner, F.), Vol. 4, pp. 511–525. Grune and Stratton, New York.

Stone, B.G. and Van Thiel, D.H. (1985). Diabetes mellitus and the liver. *Seminars in Liver Disease* **5**, 8–28.

Tanner, M.S., Portmann, B., Mowatt, A.P., Williams, R., Pandit, A.N., Mills, C.F. and Bremner, I. (1979). Increased hepatic copper concentration in Indian childhood cirrhosis. *Lancet* **i**, 1203–1205.

Tanner, M.S., Kantarjian, A.H., Bhave, S.A. and Pandit, A.N. (1983). Early introduction of copper-contaminated animal milk feed as a possible cause of Indian childhood cirrhosis. *Lancet* **ii**, 992–995.

Tanner, M.S., Bhave, S.A., Prodham, A.M. and Pandit, A.N. (1987). Clinical trails of penicillamine in Indian childhood cirrhosis. *Archives of Disease in Childhood* **62**, 1118–1124.

Thaler, H. (1962). Die Fettleber und ibre pathogenetische Beziehusg zur Leberzirrhose. *Virchows Archives A* **335**, 180–210.

Tordjman, K., Katz, I., Bursztyn, M. and Rosenthal (1985). Amiodarone and the liver. *Annals of Internal Medicine* **102**, 411.

Torosis, J.D., Barwick, K.W., Miller, D.J., Klatskin, G. and Riely, C.A. (1986). Nonalcoholic Laennec's: Clinical characteristics and long term follow-up. *Hepatology* **6**, 262A, 1170.

Trias Pulg-Sureda, Canadas, E. and Benasco, C. (1986). Toxicidad hepatica por amiodarona. Estudio necropsico de un case con afeccion multivisceral. *Gastronoenterologia Y Hepatologia* **9**, 291.

Twedt, D.C., Sternlieb, I. and Gilbertson, S.R. (1979). Clinical, morphologic and chemical studies on copper toxicosis of Bedlington terriers. *Journal of the American Veterinary Medical Association* **175**, 269–275.

Vanderhoof, J.A., Tuma, D.J., Antoson, D.L. and Sorrell, M.F. (1981). Etiology of jejunoileal bypass-induced liver dysfunction in rats. *Digestive Diseases and Sciences* **26**, 328–333.

Varma, R.R., Troup, P.J., Komorowski, R.A. and Sarna, T. (1985). Clinical and morphologic effects of amiodarone on the liver. *Gastroenterology* **88**, 1091–1092.

Vyberg, M., Ravn, V. and Andersen, B. (1987). Patterns of progression in liver injury following jejunoileal bypass for morbid obesity. *Liver* **7**, 271–276.

Walker-Smith, J. and Blomfield, J. (1973). Wilson's disease or chronic copper poisoning? *Archives of Disease in Childhood* **48**, 476–479.

Walsh, F.M., Crosson, F.J., Bayley, M., McReynolds, J. and Pearson, B.J. (1977). Acute copper intoxication: Pathophysiology and therapy with a case report. *American Journal of Diseases of Children* **131**, 149–151.

Wanless, I. and Lentz, J. (1990). Fatty liver hepatitis (steatohepatitis) and obesity: An autopsy study with analysis of risk factors. *Hepatology* **12**, 1106–1110.

Wanless, I.R., Bargman, J., Oreopoulos, D. and Vas, S.I. (1989). Subcapsular steatonecrosis of the liver in response to peritoneal insulin delivery: A clue to the pathogenesis of steatonecrosis in obesity. *Modern Pathology* **2**, 69–74.

Watanabe, A., Kobayashi, M., Morishita, N. and Nagashima, H. (1988). Multimodal treatment resulting in rapid improvement of fatty liver obese patients. *Current Therapeutic Research* **43**, 239–246.

Westwater, J.O. and Fainer, D. (1958). Liver impairment in the obese. *Gastroenterology* **34**, 688–693.

Wetzel, W.J. and Alexander, R.W. (1979). Focal nodular hyperplasia of the liver with alcoholic hyaline bodies and cytologic atypia. *Cancer* **44**, 1322–1326.

Yagupsky, P., Gazala, E., Sofer, S., Maor, E. and Abarbanel, J. (1985) Fatal hepatic failure and encephalopathy associated with amiodarone therapy. *Journal of Pediatrics* **107**, 967–970.

Yokoo, H., Harwood, T.R., Racker, D. and Arak, S. (1982). Experimental production of Mallory bodies in mice by diet containing 3,5-diethoxycarbonyl-1,4 dihydrocollidine. *Gastroenterology* **83**, 109–113.

Zelman, S. (1952). The liver in obesity. *Archives of Internal Medicine* **90**, 141–156.

Zimmerman, H.J., MacMurray, F.G., Rappoport, H. and Alpert, L.K. (1950). Studies of the liver in diabetes mellitus. I. Structural and functional abnormalities. *Journal of Laboratory and Clinical Medicine* **36**, 912–919.

12 Distinction between haemochromatosis and alcoholic siderosis

Lawrie W. Powell, Linda M. Fletcher and June W. Halliday

Introduction

Relevant historical aspects

The common association of iron overload and heavy alcohol consumption has been recognized for almost 100 years. Shortly after von Recklinghausen (1889) first suggested the terms "haemochromatosis" to describe the clinical condition of iron loading in the liver associated with tissue injury and "haemosiderin" to describe the pigment, Gilbert noted that increased hepatic iron deposits and alcohol ingestion were commonly associated. His description of "cirrhose alcoholique hypertrophique pigmentaire" (Gilbert and Grenet 1896) probably included the full spectrum of alcoholic liver disease with mild to moderate haemosiderin deposits to haemochromatosis. MacDonald (1964) concluded from an extensive study of patients and of pathological material seen at the Boston City Hospital, that "haemochromatosis" was merely the result of the combination of alcoholic cirrhosis and iron overload occurring together but not causally related. He believed that the iron loading resulted from a diet high in iron content and that some of this was derived from red wine. This led to controversy which lasted until extensive genetic and family studies by Marcel Simon and his co-workers (Simon and Bourel 1978; Simon *et al.* 1976, 1977, 1980) conclusively demonstrated that haemochromatosis is closely linked to the HLA locus on chromosome 6. These studies confirmed the earlier view of Sheldon (1935) that the disease results from an inherited defect in iron metabolism.

Nevertheless, several studies have shown that the incidence of excessive alcohol consumption is higher than expected (15–41 percent) in some groups of patients with symptomatic genetic haemochromatosis (Bomford and Williams 1976; Milder *et al.* 1980). The reason for this is unclear, but it presumably relates to the fact that alcohol and iron have a combined and possibly synergistic effect in causing liver damage and especially fibrosis (see below).

It is now firmly established that haemochromatosis is an inherited disorder closely linked to the HLA-A locus on chromosome 6 distinct from those forms of alcoholic liver disease in which some iron may be deposited in the liver. The distinction between these two conditions can now be made in most instances (see below). It is widely accepted that most, if not all, primary iron overload in Caucasoid populations (i.e. not associated with thalassaemia major or multiple blood transfusions) is due to homozygosity for HLA-linked haemochromatosis. Non-HLA-linked iron overload has been described in South African blacks (Gordeuk *et al.* 1986, 1992) and in Solomon Islanders (Eason *et al.* 1990) (see below).

It should be emphasized that the term *haemochromatosis* is used to describe an iron storage disease with excessive quantities of iron in parenchymal cells with increased total body iron content and functional impairment (present or potential) of the organs involved. The terms *haemosiderosis* or *siderosis* simply describe the presence of stainable iron in tissues. There is no implication of a progressive increase in iron content or functional impairment of the organ involved and quantitative measurement of tissue iron is necessary for accurate assessment of body iron status (see below).

The aim of this chapter is to attempt to clarify the distinction between haemochromatosis and alcoholic cirrhosis with mild to moderate haemosiderin deposits in the liver (haemosiderosis) and to discuss the role of alcoholism in the pathophysiology and symptomatology of haemochromatosis. This is preceded by a brief description of the role of the liver in iron metabolism.

The role of the liver in iron metabolism

The liver is the major iron storage organ in the body. Approximately one-third of normal body iron stores are present in the liver in the form of ferritin and haemosiderin (a breakdown product derived from ferritin). The ferritin molecule consists of a shell of 24 subunits surrounding a central hollow core which is capable of binding up to 4500 atoms of iron (Harrison *et al.* 1980). Apoferritin itself has an approximate molecular weight of 450,000 daltons and consists of subunits of two types, designated H and L, which differ in molecular weight, amino acid composition and immunological properties (Harrison *et al.* 1980). Although ferritin is predominantly intracellular, it is also present in serum (Addison *et al.* 1972) and the concentration in serum reflects body iron stores (Worwood, 1986), although concentrations have been shown to be elevated in certain conditions such as cell necrosis (Lipschitz *et al.* 1974) inflammation (Elin *et al.* 1977) and malignancy. The major iron transport protein is transferrin, which is synthesized in and secreted by the liver. Human transferrin is a glycoprotein consisting of a single polypeptide chain with two *N*-linked complex type glycan chains resulting in a molecular weight of about 80,000 daltons (de Jong *et al.* 1990). It has two iron binding sites, one in the *N*-terminal domain of the molecule and the other in the *C*-terminal domain with the iron preferentially bound in the *C*-terminal site.

Receptors for both transferrin and ferritin have been described on hepatocytes although the precise role of these proteins and their receptors in hepatic iron metabolism is yet to be elucidated. Both serum

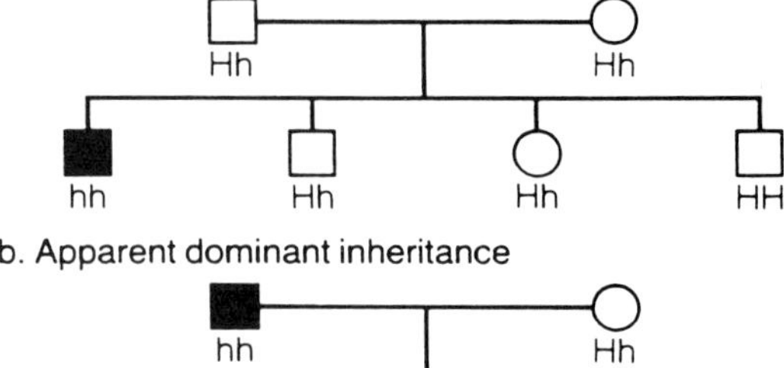

Fig. 12.1   Pattern of inheritance of haemochromatosis. (a) Mendelian autosomal recessive inheritance; (b) apparent dominant inheritance. Reproduced with permission from Halliday and Powell (1990).

ferritin and transferrin concentrations have proved useful as diagnostic tests for iron overload and alcoholism (see below).

Genetics of haemochromatosis

Although a genetic basis for haemochromatosis had been suggested earlier, it was not until the association of haemochromatosis with the HLA locus was described (Simon *et al.* 1977) that the distinction between haemochromatosis and alcoholic liver disease with iron deposition became clear. The hereditary nature of haemochromatosis was strongly suggested by these studies. An increased frequency of HLA haplotypes A3 B7, and A3 B14 was reported in patients with the disease. This was followed by the demonstration of a strong linkage between the disease gene and the HLA-A locus on chromosome 6. An apparent dominant mode of inheritance had been suggested (MacDonald 1964), but the studies of Simon and others showed that the results were best explained by an autosomal recessive mode of inheritance (Fig. 12.1a). The apparent dominance and the presence of the disease in more than one generation is then explained by a homozygous/heterozygous mating (Fig. 12.1b). Several large studies have now confirmed the strong statistical association between these HLA alleles and the development of haemochromatosis (Simon and Bourel 1978; Simon *et al.* 1976, 1977, 1980;

a Heterozygous/heterozygous mating

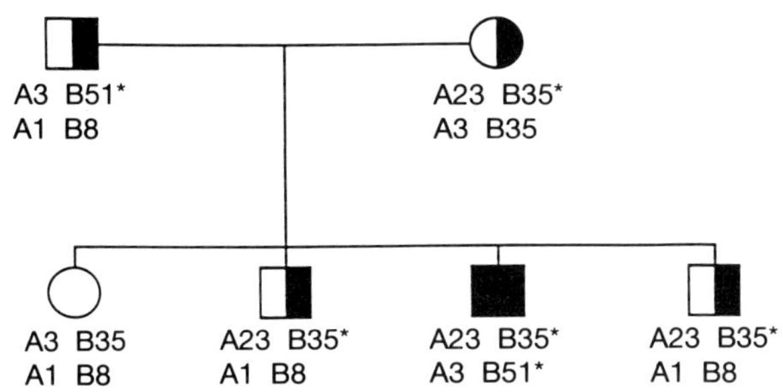

b Homozygous/heterozygous mating

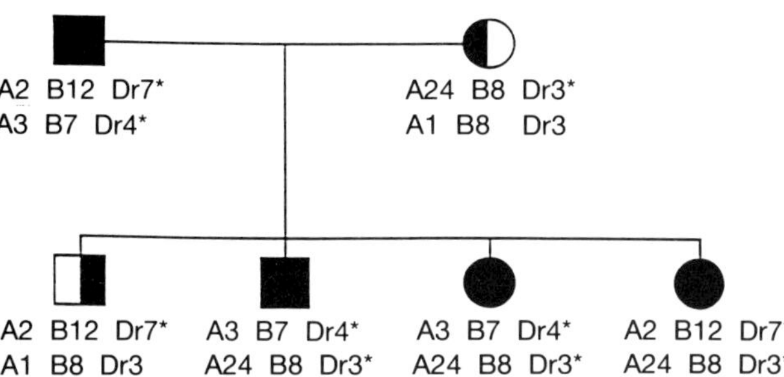

* Affected allele
◐ Heterozygous haemochromatosis
● Homozygous haemochromatosis

Fig. 12.2 Inheritance of haemochromatosis as shown by HLA haplotyping. (a) Heterozygous–heterozygous mating; (b) heterozygous–homozygous mating.

Cartwright *et al.* 1979; Doran *et al.* 1981; Bassett *et al.* 1982, 1984). HLA typing of first-degree relatives of the proband may be used to trace the pattern of inheritance of haemochromatosis. Affected siblings usually have two HLA haplotypes identical to those of the proband (putative homozygotes) whereas putative heterozygous siblings have one haplotype identical to the proband (Figs 12.2 a, b) (Simon *et al.* 1977 ; Bassett *et al.* 1979; Powell *et al.* 1990). Where sibships have resulted from a homozygous/heterozygous mating (Fig. 12.2b), affected subjects share the HLA haplotype from the heterozygous unaffected parent but may inherit either haplotype from the homozygous affected parent (Bassett *et al.* 1982). There have been a number of investigations specifically examining the relationship between heavy alcohol consumption and the development of iron overload. In studies of genetic haemochromatosis patients, an increased incidence of alcoholism has been found; however, the reason for this is

unexplained (Powell 1965, 1970; LeSage *et al.* 1983). Powell (1975) compared haemochromatosis patients who regularly drank less than 50 g alcohol per day with those who regularly ingested greater than 50 g alcohol per day. All subjects had a significant increase in iron stores i.e. greater than 5 g body iron. There were no significant differences in clinical features, pathological appearances or complications between those patients with or without heavy alcohol consumption except for those features of superimposed alcoholic liver disease in some 25 percent of the former group. Powell concluded that subjects with gross iron overload were homozygous for haemochromatosis whether or not they drank alcohol to excess. However, approximately 25 percent of the haemochromatosis subjects with heavy alcohol consumption had superimposed complications of alcoholic liver disease. These conclusions were supported and extended by a larger study from the Mayo Clinic (LeSage *et al.* 1983). There is evidence that the prognosis is worse in this group and they show no significant improvement in survival after venesection therapy (Powell 1970; Grace and Powell 1974; Grace 1978).

Population prevalence of haemochromatosis

It has become increasingly apparent that the prevalence of haemochromatosis is higher in Caucasian populations than previously thought and iron overload due to haemochromatosis constitutes a significant medical problem in developed countries of mainly Caucasian populations. Early studies based on parameters such as transferrin saturation suggested a low prevalence of the disease; however, a number of studies based on genotyping determined by HLA typing within families have confirmed the high prevalence of the disease (Table 12.1). In many Caucasian populations living in developed countries where dietary iron intake is relatively high, the prevalence of iron loading due to genetic haemochromatosis is at least 1 in 300 individuals (Leggett *et al.* 1990b) (see Table 12.1). Thus, it would now appear that haemochromatosis is the most common genetic disease inherited as an autosomal recessive trait and is also the most common inherited disease of the liver. This high prevalence of haemochromatosis in countries where alcoholism is also common, coupled with the known effects of alcohol on iron metabolism (see below) explains the frequent association of iron overload and heavy alcohol ingestion.

Table 12.1   Prevalence of haemochromatosis in Caucasian populations

Authors	Country	Prevalence	Basis of diagnosis
Beaumont *et al.* (1979)	France	0.30%	Family studies (HLA)
Olsson *et al.* (1983)	Sweden	0.50%	Male government employees – excluding blood donors
Hallberg *et al.* (1989)	Sweden	0.08%	Hospital patients
Karlsson *et al.* (1988)	Finland	0.05%	Hospital patients
Tanner *et al.* (1985)	UK	0.30%	Blood donors
Dadone *et al.* (1982)	USA	0.50%	Family studies (HLA)
Edwards *et al.* (1988)	USA	0.45%	Blood donors
Borwein *et al.* (1983)	Canada	0.30%	Family studies (HLA)
Bassett *et al.* (1982)	Australia	0.79%	Family studies (HLA)
Elliot *et al.* (1986)	Australia	1.20%	War veterans
Leggett *et al.* (1990b)	Australia	0.36%	Assymptomatic population study
Meyer *et al.* (1987)	South Africa	0.95%	Afrikaner males

Other iron-loading genes

The possible existence of other iron-loading genes has been explored, particularly in non-Caucasian populations. However, the only other primary iron overload disorder (i.e. where iron overload is present in the absence of hyperplastic refractory anaemia or blood transfusions) is Sub-Saharan African dietary iron overload. Iron overload has been known for many years to occur in Sub-Saharan Africa and it was presumed to result from increased dietary iron derived from beer brewed at home in iron drums (Bothwell and Isaacson 1962; Bothwell *et al.* 1965). In a recent survey of dietary iron overload of 505 rural Zimbabweans, iron overload was found almost exclusively among men who consumed traditional beer brewed in steel drums (Gordeuk *et al.* 1986). Approximately 21 percent of drinkers aged over 45 years had elevated serum ferritin and a transferrin saturation of greater than 70 percent. Although there is some evidence indicating that iron overload is decreasing in the urban black population in South Africa (MacPhail *et al.* 1979), Gordeuk and colleagues (1992) have recently presented evidence for a major iron-loading locus in African pedigrees that results in elevated transferrin saturation, reflecting iron loading in homozygous subjects, and which they suggest contributes to a bimodal distribution of transferrin saturation in subjects with increased dietary iron. They proposed that iron overload in Africans is due to a genetic factor in addition to the well-described dietary factor. Their analyses suggested an interaction between genotype and environment in which three genotypes responded differently to elevated levels of dietary iron. In this study, 236 members of 36 African families were chosen because they contained index subjects with iron overload. In those family members with increased dietary iron, a bimodal distribution of transferrin saturation was found, with 56 values less than 60 percent saturation and 44 higher than 60 percent. The mean serum ferritin was five times higher in the subjects with a transferrin saturation greater than 60 percent. Pedigree analysis provided evidence for both a genetic effect and an effect of increased dietary iron on transferrin saturation and unsaturated iron binding capacity, but LOD scores did not indicate linkage to the HLA loci. They concluded that the iron-loading locus in the families was not HLA-linked and different from the HLA-linked gene that is responsible for iron overload in Caucasian families.

These authors have recently extended this study to determine if this non-HLA-related iron-loading gene is present in the US African-American population (Gordeuk *et al.* 1993). They analysed data from the National Health and Nutrition Examination Survey (NHANES II) study. Their results were consistent with the presence of two populations according to transferrin saturation, approximately 70 percent having a transferrin saturation of 26 ± 6.1 percent (SD) and a second population with a transferrin saturation of 41 ± 6 percent (SD). They postulated that population one might include individuals unaffected by the iron-loading gene and that population two might include predominantly individuals with an iron-loading gene as well as some unaffected individuals with some sporadic elevations of transferrin saturation. These results, while of interest, remain to be confirmed.

Pathogenesis

The mechanisms of liver damage due to iron, alcohol and their interaction in some forms of liver damage are not clearly understood, although some theories propose similar mechanisms of tissue damage for both diseases.

Haemochromatosis

The basic biochemical defect resulting in the abnormal accumulation of hepatic iron in haemochromatosis is not understood and it is unresolved as to whether the intestine or the liver itself is the site of the defect or indeed a more generalized cellular defect may be responsible, including abnormalities in membrane iron transport proteins. There have been a number of proposed theories relating to the nature of the biochemical defect and these have been discussed recently by Halliday and Powell (1992) and by Powell *et al.* (1994). Early observations in haemochromatosis, which to date have not been fully explained, include increased iron absorption in the gut even in the presence of an increased body iron load, early deposition of iron in hepatocytes, predominantly in periportal regions, and virtually no iron in the Kupffer cells and other cells of the reticuloendothelial system.

The pathogenesis of the tissue injury in haemochromatosis also remains unresolved. Only in untreated haemochromatosis where the iron load is severe does fibrosis occur (Grace and Powell 1974). Studies by Peters *et al.* (1977) showed that hepatic lysosomes in haemochromatosis, transfusional siderosis and experimental iron overload exhibited enhanced fragility that was not detectable following removal of iron. The relationships between lysosomal fragility and hepatic fibrosis still remain unclear, although these studies are consistent with recent theories that cellular iron overload leads to lipid peroxidation of membranes by free radicals (Bacon *et al.* 1983, 1985). However, a causal link between iron-induced lipid peroxidation and liver fibrosis has yet to be established. Liver damage may indeed be initiated by moderate to severe iron overload once the capacity of the hepatocyte to maintain the iron in a non-toxic form has been exceeded (Bacon *et al.* 1983, 1985; Fletcher *et al.* 1989).

Alcoholic liver disease with siderosis

The mechanism of increase in stainable iron in some subjects with alcoholic liver disease is unknown. Despite much research on the subject, it has been considered unlikely to be related to the iron present in alcoholic beverages, or to the stimulation of iron absorption by alcohol (Celada *et al.* 1978, Chapman *et al.* 1983). It is possible that an increase in Kupffer cell iron may reflect past hepatocellular necrosis with uptake of released iron by necrotic hepatocytes or to redistribution of body iron to the liver. Of interest and relevance is the recent study by Duane *et al.* (1992). They demonstrated by *in vivo* whole-body retention studies a two-fold increase on average in intestinal iron absorption in six male chronic alcoholics and concluded that, together with previous reports of enhanced *in vitro* and *in vivo* intestinal permeability to ^{51}Cr-EDTA in chronic alcoholics, an unregulated increase in intestinal iron uptake via the non-carrier-mediated paracellular route may contribute to hepatic iron deposition in chronic alcoholics.

Although lipid peroxidation and free radicals have been proposed as mechanisms of damage in both disease conditions, it is noteworthy that inflammation is characteristic of alcoholic liver disease, particularly alcoholic hepatitis, while haemochromatosis is characterized by heavy iron deposits with little if any inflammatory infiltrate. There have been suggestions that alcohol metabolism by the liver is associated with increased rate of lipid peroxidation *in vivo* and that liver cells metabolizing alcohol generate, via a lipid peroxide intermediate, a substance that is a chemoattractant for polymorphonuclear leucocytes. Polymorphonuclear leucocytes are themselves cytotoxic to liver cells and destructive of extracellular matrix when alcoholic hepatitis is present (Roll *et al.* 1986; Roll 1991). At least half of the patients with alcoholic hepatitis who continue to drink alcohol have been reported to develop cirrhosis within 2–3 years (Pares *et al.* 1986). Stimulation of Kupffer cells leading to Ito cell activation results in an increase in collagen synthesis by these cells (Maher 1990; see also Chapter 4). Excess iron may also cause Ito cell activation resulting in collagen synthesis (Pietrangelo *et al.* 1990).

Britton *et al.* (1994) proposed two main mechanisms of hepatic injury and fibrosis resulting from the chronic iron overload, the first via a direct effect of iron on the lipocyte resulting in activation of these cells and collagen synthesis, and the second via cytokine release from activated iron-laden Kupffer cells, the cytokines in turn stimulating lipocyte to become activated collagen-producing cells.

Differentiation between haemochromatosis and alcoholic siderosis

This section will focus on those features which are useful in distinguishing between haemochromatosis and alcoholic liver disease with siderosis.

Clinical features

In 1935, Sheldon described the classic triad of hepatomegaly, diabetes and skin pigmentation in haemochromatosis. He noted that arthropathy, impotence and cardiac failure are also common complications of the disease.

The most common clinical features in symptomatic patients are weakness and lethargy (73 percent), skin pigmentation (90 percent), hepatomegaly (60 percent), unexplained arthropathy (41 percent), loss of libido (25 percent) and diabetes mellitus (20 percent) (Crawford and Halliday 1991). The diagnosis of haemochromatosis is usually suspected on the basis of clinical features and laboratory investigations consistent with excessive iron stores and then confirmed by liver biopsy (see below). It should be noted, however, that many patients are asymptomatic but may be detected on the basis of biochemical screening.

Clinical features which are more common in patients with alcoholic cirrhosis and suggest this diagnosis rather than haemochromatosis include: splenomegaly, a small liver, gonadal atrophy, gynaecosmastia, spider naevi, peripheral neuropathy and signs of alcoholism, e.g. parotomegaly (Powell *et al.* 1971). However, it should be emphasized that approximately 25 percent of patients with symptomatic haemochromatosis drink alcohol to excess and may have alcoholic liver disease superimposed on the genetic disease (Powell 1975; Powell and Kerr 1975). This is discussed later in more detail.

Special attention should be given to the skin pigmentation in attempting to differentiate between haemochromatosis and alcoholic liver disease. In the former, a characteristic "bronze pigmentation" (metallic or slate-grey hue) is often present due to the presence of increased melanin pigment (or both melanin and iron) in the dermis, together with generalized atrophy of both the epidermis and dermis. This pigmentation, while usually generalized, is frequently deeper on the face, neck, extensor aspects of the lower forearms, dorsa of the hands, lower legs, genital regions and in scars. Pigmentation of the oral mucosa, hard palate and retina has been described but is uncommon. In alcoholic liver disease, especially alcoholic cirrhosis, skin pigmentation is common due to increased melanin in the basal layers of the epidermis. It does not have the metallic slate-grey hue and is most marked on the exposed surfaces.

Thus, the distinction between alcoholic cirrhosis and haemochromatosis can be difficult for the clinician, since there may be considerable overlap in the clinical features, particularly in advanced disease. The distinction usually requires liver biopsy with estimation of the hepatic iron concentration and the hepatic iron index (see below).

Biochemical parameters

Alcohol abuse is associated with marked alterations in iron homeostasis (Potter 1991), and increased levels of serum iron, ferritin and transferrin saturation in some cases (Eichner and Hillman 1971; Krasner *et al.* 1976; Friedman *et al.* 1988; Linderbaum and Lieber 1969). Other abnormalities include changes in plasma iron turnover (Beaumier *et al.* 1984), changes in red cell iron incorporation (Beaumier *et al.* 1984; Eichner and Hillman 1971), lower levels of serum transferrin and, in approximately one-third of alcoholics, some increase in liver iron concentration (Chapman *et al.* 1982, 1983; LeSage *et al.* 1983; Bezwoda *et al.* 1985). However, these values are usually lower than those found in patients of comparable age with haemochromatosis.

Serum ferritin

In haemochromatosis, there is an increase in serum ferritin concentration which accurately reflects the degree of iron overload; however, in alcoholics, the raised serum ferritin does not necessarily correlate with hepatic iron concentration or serum iron levels (Prieto *et al.* 1975; Brissot *et al.* 1981; Kristenson *et al.* 1981; Lundin *et al.* 1981; Chapman *et al.* 1982; Valimaki *et al.* 1983; Chick *et al.* 1987) as the rise may result in part from the inflammatory process. Ferritin synthesis is stimulated by both iron and inflammation. In inflammation, the serum transaminase levels are usually raised and the serum ferritin does not reflect the iron stores. Serum ferritin is largely glycosylated, possibly resulting from an active secretory process (Worwood *et al.* 1979). Non-glycosylated serum ferritin is thought to arise from tissue damage and cell death (Chapman *et al.* 1982; Lundin *et al.* 1981; Worwood *et al.* 1982; Valimaki *et al.* 1983). Moirand *et al.* (1991) examined glycosylated and unglycosylated serum ferritin from 58 chronic hospitalized alcoholics, subdivided into three groups according to liver damage. They found that the total serum ferritin increased in alcoholics with both free and Con-A bound (glycosylated) ferritin increasing in equal amounts. In addition, both ferritins increased with severity of disease. From these studies they concluded that total serum ferritin was increased in chronic alcoholism and that at least some of this ferritin may be secreted from cells stimulated by alcohol. More studies are required to determine whether the rates of glycosylated to non-glycosylated serum ferritin is of clinical value.

The normal level of serum ferritin in adult males is 30–350 μg/l and in adult females 20–150 μg/l (Leggett *et al.* 1990a). As stated above, the serum concentration of ferritin accurately reflects the magnitude of iron stores in the body (Lipschitz *et al.* 1974) in uncomplicated haemochromatosis such that each μg/l rise in serum of ferritin is equivalent to about 10 mg of storage iron. Situations in which the serum ferritin levels are inappropriately raised include liver disease, inflammation, the leukaemias, lymphomas, cancer and infections. In alcoholic liver disease, the serum ferritin level is often elevated due to inflammation and/or cell necrosis. Several studies have shown that serum ferritin is increased in approximately 40–70 percent of alcoholics (Prieto *et al.* 1975; Kristenson *et al.* 1981; Lundin *et al.* 1981; Chapman *et al.* 1982; Valimaki *et al.* 1983; Moirand *et al.* 1991). However, the serum gammaglutamyltransferase (GGT) levels are often also raised in these subjects, suggesting that liver damage was contributing to the elevation of serum ferritin. Other studies have shown that in alcoholic subjects serum ferritin levels correlate with alcohol consumption in subjects with normal GGT levels (Meyer *et al.* 1984; Leggett *et al.* 1990a). The study of Leggett *et al.* (1990a) indicated that the serum ferritin level in asymptomatic males correlates with both the degree of meat (and presumably iron) intake and the degree of alcohol consumption.

Thus, three factors may lead to an elevation in the serum ferritin level: (1) increased body iron stores, (2) inflammation and/or necrosis and (3) excessive alcohol consumption *per se*. These factors should be considered when interpreting an elevated serum ferritin value and attention should also be directed to the transferrin saturation. Factors (2) and (3) above do not usually lead to an elevated saturation of transferrin. A serum ferritin level of less than 1000 μg/l that fluctuates in association with elevated transaminases and is associated with a normal transferrin saturation is strongly suggestive of alcoholic liver disease.

Serum iron

Serum iron levels in genetic haemochromatosis patients are usually greater than 36 μM/l (normal serum iron levels range from 10 to 30 μM/l). In iron overload conditions, such as genetic haemochromatosis, the iron-binding capacity of transferrin may be exceeded resulting in the presence of non-transferrin-bound iron (iron bound to low molecular weight iron chelates) (Batey *et al.* 1980; Brissot *et al.* 1985). There is now good evidence that hepatic uptake of this non-transferrin-bound iron is a contributing factor to excessive iron storage in the liver of haemochromatosis patients. This iron may contribute to toxicity as it may enter abnormal storage compartments. The presence of non-transferrin-bound iron in alcoholism has yet to be detected.

Transferrin saturation

Transferrin has two iron-binding sites and it is normally approximately 36 percent saturated with iron. This saturation is characteristically elevated early in the course of the disease of haemochromatosis due to both an elevated serum iron level and decreased transferrin concentration and is usually greater than 62 percent in homozygotes (Dadone *et al.* 1982). However, the specificity of the test is reduced by the relatively high number of false-positive and false-negative values, especially in relatives of patients with the disease (Bassett *et al.* 1979). Furthermore, the transferrin saturation is increased in some 25 percent of heterozygotes (Cartwright *et al.* 1979; Bassett *et al.* 1981). An increased serum iron concentration may be present in patients with alcoholic liver disease without excess iron stores. In this situation, however, the iron-binding capacity is generally not decreased and thus the percentage saturation of the transferrin is often still normal. An elevated transferrin saturation in severe alcoholic liver disease may be related to decreased transferrin synthesis by the damaged liver.

Carbohydrate-deficient transferrin (desialylated transferrin)

Excess alcohol consumption has been shown to lead to an abnormal microheterogeneity in serum transferrin resulting in an isoelectric profile different to that of normal transferrin. This form of transferrin, called carbohydrate-deficient transferrin (CDT) or desialylated transferrin (dTf), has an isoelectric point of greater than pI 5.65, whereas normal human serum transferrin has a pI between 5.2 and 5.4. This difference is due to the absence of carbohydrate groups from the glycan chains of transferrin and specifically of sialic acid, which is the only charged glycan group. Over the last decade, this form of transferrin has been increasingly used as a reliable, sensitive and specific marker of alcohol abuse (Storey *et al.* 1987; Kwoh-Gain *et al.* 1990; Stibler 1991). There are many biochemical abnormalities associated with chronic alcoholism and various laboratory markers such as gammaglutamyltransferase, mean corpuscular volume, aspartate aminotransferase (AST) and alanine aminotransferase (ALT) have been used in the diagnosis of alcoholism and ethanol-related tissue damage in suspected alcoholics. Several studies have shown that desialylated transferrin is a remarkably sensitive and specific index of chronic excessive alcohol consumption (Table 12.2), whether tissue damage is present or not (Storey *et al.* 1987; Kwoh-Gain *et al.* 1990).

Mitochondrial AST, on the other hand, has also been shown to be sensitive and more specific than the conventional markers; however, the false-positive rate is higher for this test. Carbohydrate-deficient transferrin has been shown to be most useful in the distinction between alcoholic liver disease and non-alcoholic steatohepatitis, a disease that morphologically resembles alcoholic liver disease (Fletcher *et al.* 1991) (Fig. 12.3; see also Chapter 11). Animal studies (Regoeczi *et al.* 1984) have suggested that this transferrin is more able than

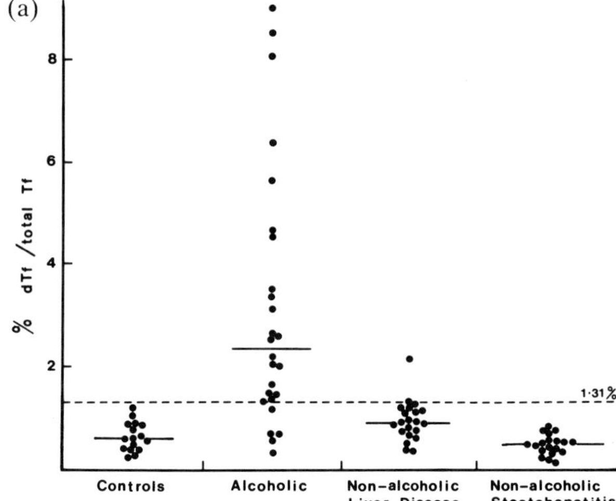

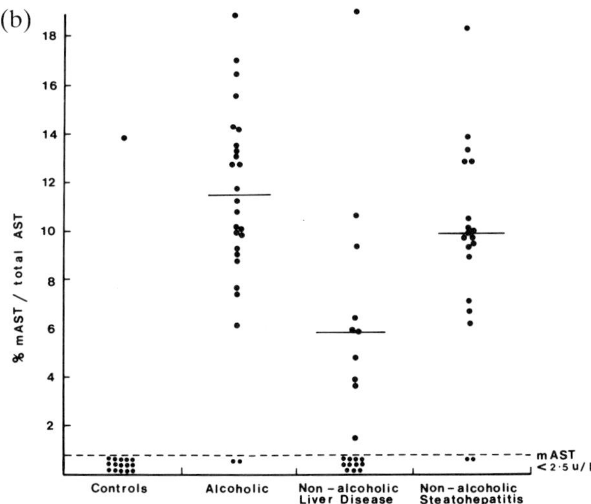

Fig. 12.3 (a) Distributions of the ratio of dTf to total Tf in controls, alcoholic subjects, patients with non-alcoholic liver disease and patients with non-alcoholic steatohepatitis. The horizontal bars represent the median values, and the dashed line the arbitrary cut-off point. (b) Distribution of the ratio of mAST/total AST expressed as a percentage in healthy controls, alcoholic subjects, patients with NALD and patients with NASH. The mAST/total AST ratio was reported only for those with elevated mAST activity (2.5 U/l). The horizontal line represents the median values, and the dashed line represents the upper limit of normal (i.e. a mAST of 2.5 U/l). Reproduced with permission from Fletcher *et al.* 1991.

Table 12.2 Sensitivity and specificity of biochemical/haematological markers

Biochemical/haematological markers	Sensitivity (%)	Specificity (%)
GGT	69	55
MCV	73	79
AST	69	66
ALT	58	50
mAST/total AST	92	50
dTf/total Tf	81	98

Reference limits: GGT > 50 IU/l; MCV > 95 fl; AST > 40 IU/l; ALT > 35 IU/l mAST > 2.5 U/l; dTf/total Tf > 1.31.
Reproduced with permission from Fletcher *et al.* (1991).

normal transferrin to deliver iron selectively to tissues and in particular to the hepatocyte. This may be one mechanism responsible for the development of alcoholic hepatic siderosis.

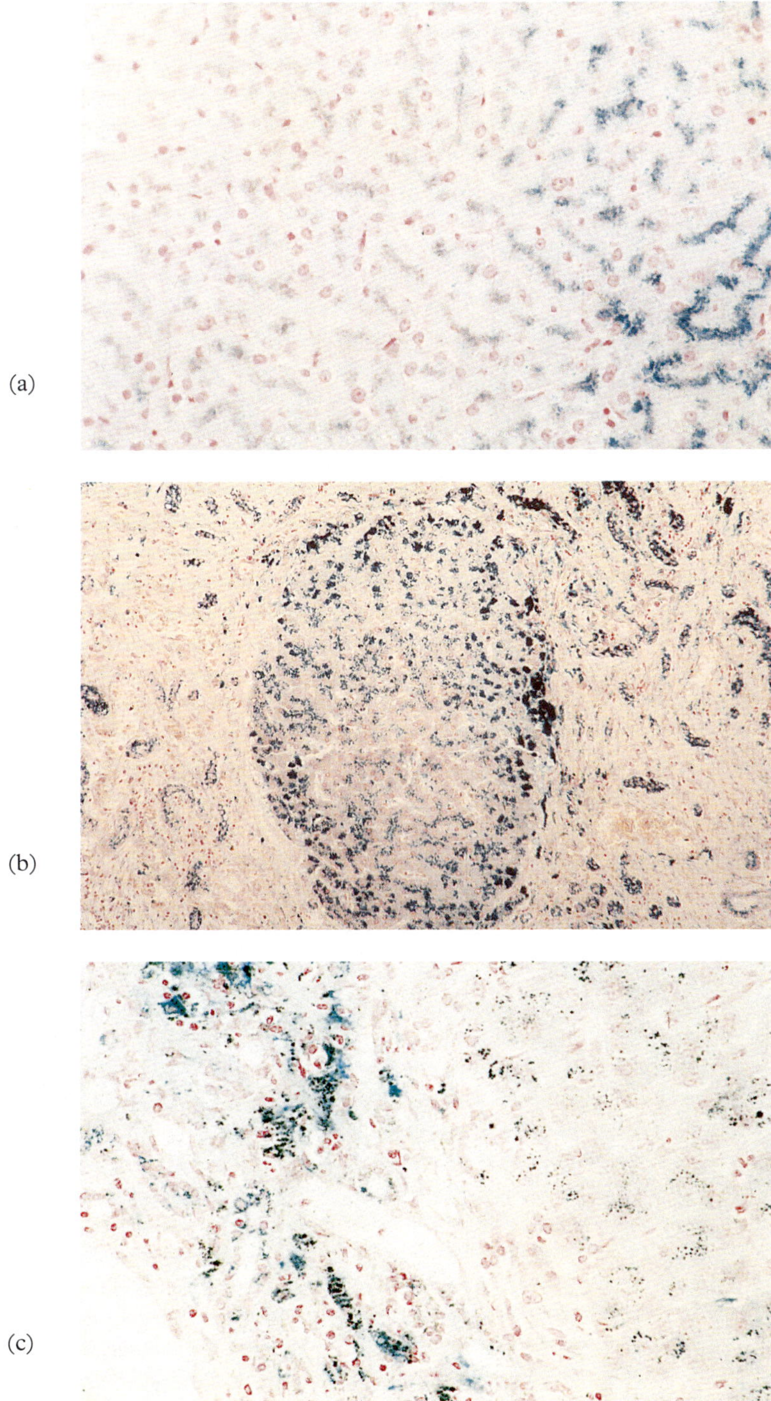

Plate 12 Liver biopsy (Perls' method for iron).
(a) Early haemochromatosis. Iron is seen in zone 1 (periportal) hepatocytes. Lipofuscin is seen in hepatocytes in zones 2 and 3.
(b) Advanced haemochromatosis. Heavy (grade 4) iron overload and cirrhosis. Heavy iron deposition is also seen in biliary epithelial cells.
(c) Alcoholic cirrhosis and mild siderosis. Cirrhotic liver showing small amounts of iron in a few hepatocytes and more pronounced iron deposition in portal tract macrophages.

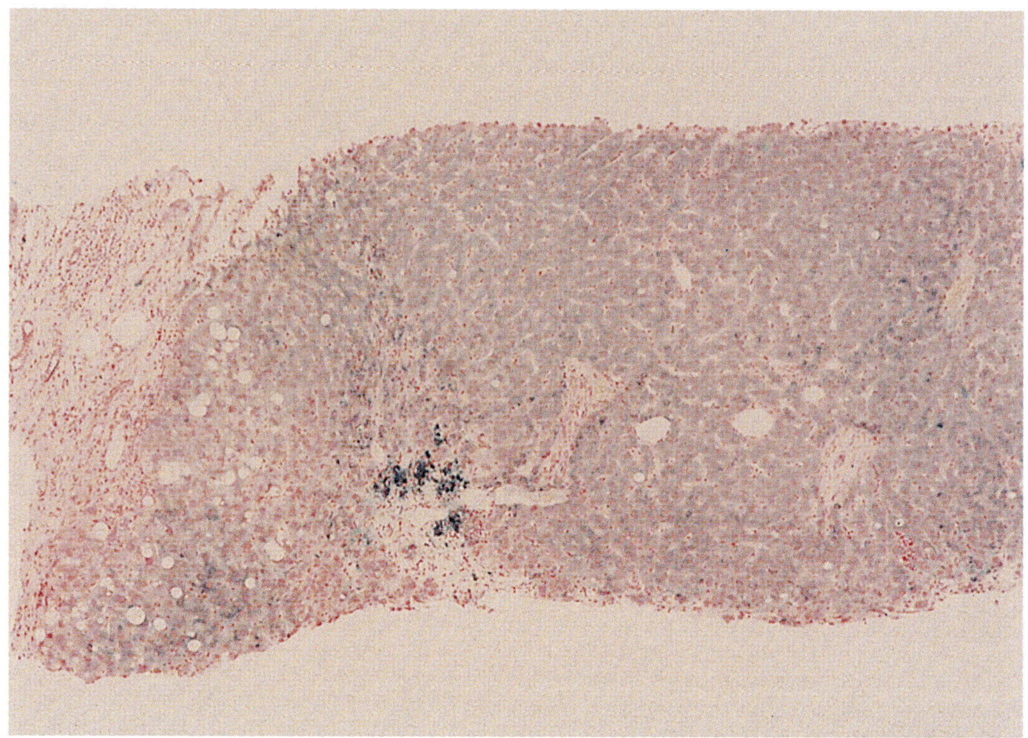

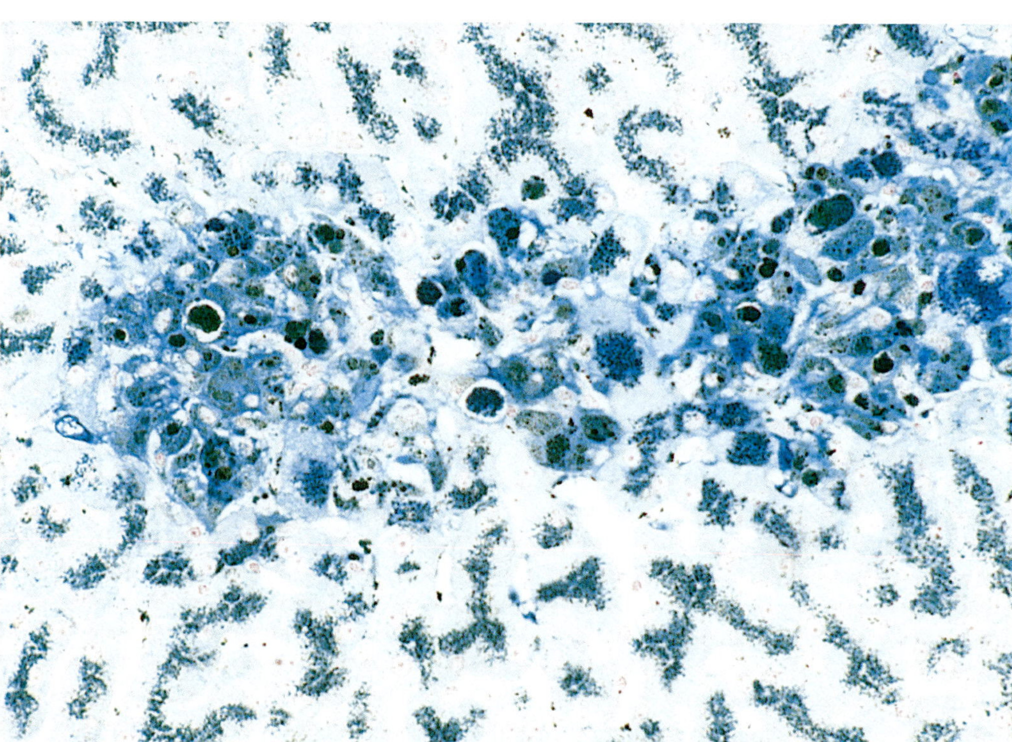

Plate 13 Haemochromatosis with heavy alcohol ingestion (Perls' method for iron).
(a) Excessive iron (grade 4) is seen in hepatocytes, Kupffer cells and portal tract macrophages. Marked portal fibrosis and focal fatty change are also seen.
(b) Marked deposition of iron in portal tract macrophages.

Pathological features

The major pathological findings in haemochromatosis relate to the deposition of massive amounts of iron in most organs, particularly the liver, pancreas, heart and endocrine glands (Sheldon 1935; Finch and Finch 1955; Powell and Kerr 1975). Iron deposition is associated with dense fibrosis in the liver and pancreas, and in the liver the fibrosis leads to cirrhosis. Cell necrosis and inflammation are usually absent and the hepatocytes usually appear normal apart from the presence of the iron (Searle *et al.* 1987, 1994). Liver biopsies from young homozygotes (Bassett *et al.* 1981) show that considerable amounts of iron have been deposited in the liver by the second decade (see Plate 12a opposite p. 206). Young males have greater amounts of iron than females of the same age. Haemosiderin is found first in hepatocytes in zone 1 of the hepatic acinus (i.e. in periportal hepatocytes). With increasing age, haemosiderin deposition progressively involves hepatocytes in all zones but the iron deposition remains most marked in acinar zone 1 (Searle *et al.* 1987, 1994). With the accumulation of more iron, increasing fibrosis develops around the portal tracts, and diffuse fibrosis occurs resulting in architectural distortion and later dissection of the acini with the formation of regenerative nodules (cirrhosis) (see Plate 12b opposite p. 206). Full clinical, biochemical and pathological expression of genetic haemochromatosis occurs only in homozygotes; however, up to 25 percent of heterozygotes may develop partial biochemical expression of the disease associated with a limited increase in hepatic iron concentration (Cartwright *et al.* 1979; Bassett *et al.* 1981).

Stainable iron has often been seen in the liver of alcoholic subjects (see Plate 12c opposite p. 206), and up to a third of patients with pre-cirrhotic alcoholic liver disease show some siderosis (Chapman *et al.* 1982, 1983; LeSage *et al.* 1983; Bezwoda *et al.* 1985). In the alcoholic siderosis seen in South African blacks, first reported by Strachan (1929), the iron overload is evident in both the reticuloendothelial system and the hepatic parenchyma (Bothwell *et al.* 1979). It has been reported, however, that changing from home-brewed beer to a commercially prepared beverage has lowered the incidence of iron overload while increasing the incidence of fatty changes or Mallory bodies in the liver in the alcoholic liver disease seen in this population. Severe iron overload to the extent seen in haemochromatosis does not normally occur in alcoholic subjects in the absence of the haemochromatosis genetic defect.

In a small proportion of patients with alcoholic cirrhosis, there is a gross deposition of iron in the liver and markedly elevated hepatic iron concentrations to the levels seen in advanced haemochromatosis, but most of these subjects are probably homozygous for haemochromatosis as well as being heavy drinkers, with the inherited disease exacerbated by alcohol (see Plates 13a and 13b opposite). The degree of parenchymal iron deposition in alcoholic cirrhosis is usually mild in comparison with the degree of fibrosis, while reticuloendothelial iron deposition is often considerable; in contrast, in genetic haemochromatosis, there is very little reticuloendothelial iron demonstrable in the early stages of the disease and the amount of parenchymal iron is out of proportion to the degree of fibrosis. These morphological features are useful in the differentiation of liver disease seen in genetic haemochromatosis from alcoholic liver disease with siderosis. Stainable hepatic iron in alcoholic liver disease is usually only minor (grade 1 or 2) and the hepatic iron concentration and hepatic iron index (see below) are either normal or marginally elevated (Bassett *et al.* 1986; Sallie *et al.* 1991). A hepatic iron index of greater than 2.0 is indicative of homozygous haemochromatosis (Fig. 12.4a, b). Often other factors contributing to the iron overload can be identified with a hepatic iron index of less than 2.0 (Bassett *et al.* 1986). These include portacaval anastomosis and haemolysis. Abnormalities of iron metabolism are not detectable with increased frequency in relatives of patients with iron overload secondary to alcoholic cirrhosis; in contrast, such abnormalities occur in over 25 percent of first-degree relatives of patients with haemochromatosis (Sabesin and Thomas 1964; Powell 1975).

Much of the confusion between haemochromatosis and alcoholic siderosis has stemmed from misinterpretation of the significance of stainable iron as a measure of tissue iron concentration and of total body iron stores. In haemochromatosis, iron is found in progressively increasing amounts in the parenchymal cells and only late in the disease is iron deposition seen in Kupffer cells, portal tract macrophages, endothelial cells lining the sinusoids and biliary epithelial cells; while alcoholic siderosis is characterized by moderate stainable iron in Kupffer cells, macrophages and sinusoidal cells in the presence of normal total body iron stores. Small amounts

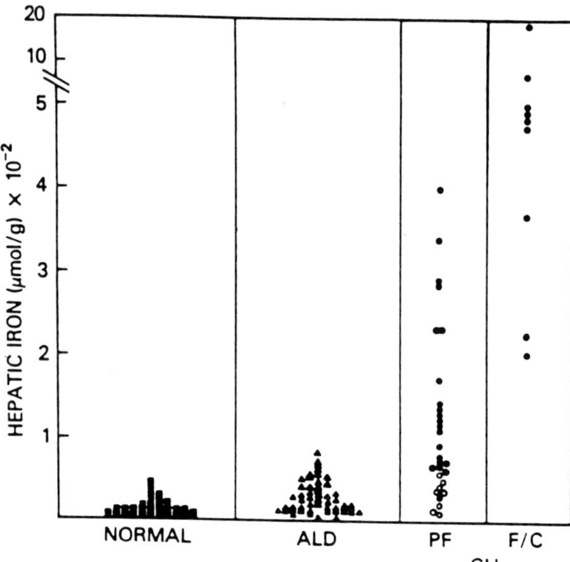

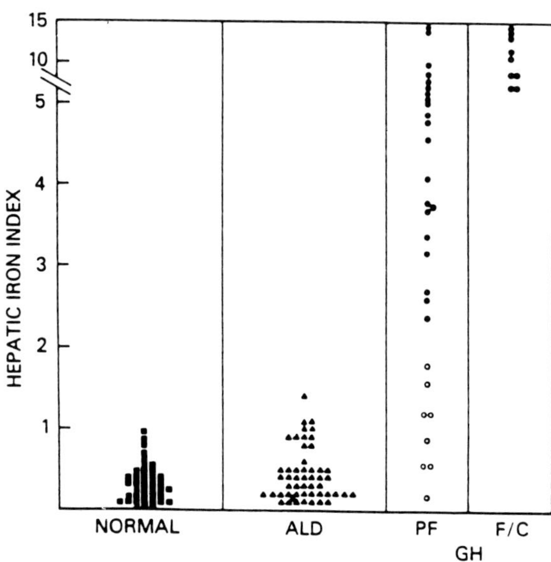

Fig. 12.4 (Top) Hepatic iron concentration; (Bottom) hepatic iron index (ratio of iron concentration to age). Normal, normal subjects; ALD, patients with alcoholic liver disease; GH, genetic haemochromatosis subjects; PF, prefibrotic; F/C, fibrotic or cirrhotic. GH heterozygotes are shown by open circles and homozygotes by closed circles. Reproduced with permission from Bassett *et al.* (1981).

of stainable iron may be present in hepatocytes. The presence of fat and other features of alcoholic liver disease may also complicate the picture of iron deposition in alcoholic subjects (Powell and Kerr 1975; see Chapter 3).

Hepatic iron concentration and hepatic iron index

Histochemical grading of hepatic iron in biopsy specimens by visual assessment of the amount of iron revealed by a Perls' stain on liver sections can rapidly provide valuable information about the level of iron stores and often about the manner by which the excessive amounts might have been acquired. The most commonly used grading system is that of Scheuer *et al.* (1962). Other studies using different criteria but with a common 0–4+ grading system have been described (Searle *et al.* 1987, 1994; Deugnier *et al.* 1993b). Patients with alcoholic liver disease often have an increase in stainable hepatic iron out of proportion to the hepatic iron concentration and this can cause difficult diagnostic problems. The reason for this disparity between stainable iron and hepatic iron concentration has never been adequately clarified. A slight to moderate increase in stainable iron is common in alcoholic cirrhosis and liver iron concentration has been shown to be higher in heavy drinkers than in a similar group of subjects with low alcohol consumption, even in the absence of liver disease (Powell 1966).

The chemical analysis of *hepatic iron concentration* in liver biopsy tissue usually distinguishes haemochromatosis from alcoholic liver disease. However, the hepatic iron concentration rises with age, minimally in normal subjects and heterozygotes for haemochromatosis, pathologically in homozygous haemochromatosis. Therefore, difficulties can arise in young homozygote haemochromatotics and also in older heterozygous subjects. It was for this reason that we suggested the use of a *hepatic iron index* based on either chemical (Bassett *et al.* 1986; Summers *et al.* 1990) or histological (Deugnier *et al.* 1993b) criteria to provide a more useful means of detection of homozygote haemochromatosis subjects and to distinguish between haemochromatosis and alcoholic siderosis (Bassett *et al.* 1986). Hepatic iron can be measured using either a colorimetric method (Torrance and Bothwell 1980) or atomic absorption spectrophotometry (Bassett *et al.* 1986) and the hepatic iron index is calculated by dividing the

Table 12.3 Studies of hepatic iron index in haemochromatosis

Authors	Normal	ALD	Hh	hh
Bassett *et al.* (1986)	<1.0	<1.4	<1.8	>2.0
Summers *et al.* (1990)	–	–	<1.5	>1.9
Olynyk *et al.* (1990)	<1.1	<1.6	–	>2.1
Bonkovsky *et al.* (1990)	<0.7	<1.1	<1.8	>2.0[a]
Saillie *et al.* (1991)	–	<1.6	–	>2.0
Deugnier *et al.* (1993b)	–	–	–	>2.0

ALD, Alcoholic liver disease; Hh, haemochromatosis, heterozygote; hh, haemochromatosis, homozygote.
[a]2/14 patients thought to have HC had HII < 2.0.

hepatic iron concentration in μmol/g dry weight by the age in years (Fig. 12.4). Computerized measurement of stainable hepatic iron in tissue sections is also now available (Olynyk *et al.* 1990); this technique also allows quantitation of stainable hepatic iron in previously obtained liver biopsy specimens. This procedure and that of Deugnier *et al.* (1993b) are particularly useful in providing an estimate of hepatic iron concentration when biochemical quantitation was not performed on the tissue obtained at the time of biopsy.

In patients with alcoholic liver disease and increased stainable iron, the liver iron rarely exceeds twice the upper limit of normal, the hepatic iron index is usually less than 2.0 and total body iron stores as determined by quantitative phlebotomy rarely exceed 3 g. Studies confirming the value of the hepatic iron index are summarized in Table 12.3.

Differentiation of genetic haemochromatosis complicated by features of alcoholic liver disease from alcoholic cirrhosis with secondary iron loading is important, since phlebotomy treatment does not prolong survival in the latter group (Grace 1978).

Thus, the distinction between haemochromatosis and alcoholic liver disease with some increase in stainable iron in the liver is usually possible on the basis of clinical, biochemical and pathological features. However, in a minority of subjects, the distinction can be quite difficult even when one includes the histological and histochemical appearances. It is in this situation that the measurement of hepatic iron concentration and hepatic iron index are most useful, since they provide a means of differentiating between the excessive iron stores of haemochromatosis and the lesser stores seen in alcoholic liver disease. A significant increase in body iron stores to an amount of 5 g or more is indicative of homozygous haemochromatosis and is rarely, if ever, seen in alcoholic liver disease without a family history of iron overload (Powell 1965; LeSage *et al.* 1983).

In summary haemochromatosis is characterized by: (1) increased serum ferritin levels, (2) an increased transferrin saturation, (3) elevated serum iron levels and (4) abnormal transaminase levels only late in the disease. Alcoholic siderosis is characterized by: (1) mildly elevated serum ferritin levels, (2) increased concentrations of carbohydrate-deficient transferrin (desialylated transferrin), (3) elevated iron levels and increased transferrin saturation, and (4) abnormal transaminase levels.

Effect of alcohol in the heterozygote for haemochromatosis

Approximately 25 percent of heterozygotes for haemochromatosis manifest some phenotypic expression of the disease, usually as an increased serum ferritin level and increased serum transferrin saturation (Bassett *et al.* 1981; Dadone *et al.* 1982). It is therefore logical to expect that alcohol abuse might accentuate these manifestations and so lead to further diagnostic confusion. However, it has now been established that significant iron loading does not occur unless there is another disorder such as hereditary spherocytosis, ß-thalassaemia minor, idiopathic refractory sideroblastic anaemia or sporadic porphyria cutanea tarda (Powell *et al.* 1994; see Chapter 13). Furthermore, heterozygous subjects do not develop significant iron overload with alcohol abuse and heavy drinkers with increased iron stores are usually homozygous for haemochromatosis (Powell 1975; Powell *et al.* 1994).

Potentiation by alcohol of the liver lesions in haemochromatosis and the interrelationships between iron, alcohol and hepatitis viruses

The studies by Irving *et al.* (1988, 1991) attempted to evaluate the possible synergistic effects of iron and ethanol with respect to hepatic damage. No synergistic effects were demonstrated with respect to amino acid uptake, protein degradation or the biosynthesis of secreted collagen; however, synergism was apparent when indices of lipid peroxidation were studied (Irving *et al.* 1988, 1991).

One of the major complications of both haemochromatosis and alcoholic liver disease is hepatic cirrhosis. The excess deposition of iron in haemochromatosis is thought to be the major contributory factor in the development of cirrhosis. Primary hepatocellular carcinoma is a common complication of haemochromatosis and is the main cause of death in about a third of cirrhotic patients (Bomford and Williams 1976; Niederau *et al.* 1985; Tiniakos and Williams 1988), but occurs only very occasionally in non-cirrhotic patients and in these cases hepatic fibrosis is usually present (Blumberg *et al.* 1988; Fellows *et al.* 1988; Kew 1990; Deugnier *et al.* 1993a). It has been estimated that the risk of the development of hepatocellular carcinoma in patients with haemochromatosis is 200 times greater than the general population (Bradbear *et al.* 1985; Niederau *et al.* 1985), but extrahepatic cancers are not increased in these subjects.

The pathogenesis of hepatocellular carcinoma is less clear because of complicating factors such as aflatoxin, alpha-1 antitrypsin deficiency, anabolic steroid use and hepatitis B infection (Anthony *et al.* 1973, Anthony 1976; Szmuness 1978). The results from many studies analysing alcohol as a risk factor for hepatocellular carcinoma in low-risk areas have highlighted the possibility of an interrelationship between hepatitis B and hepatitis C infection, iron and alcohol abuse (Naccarato and Farinati 1991; see Chapters 3 and 9). A recent study by Adami *et al.* (1992) found that alcoholism without clinically evident cirrhosis resulted in only a modest increase in primary liver cell cancer and alcoholism with cirrhosis did not increase the relative risk for liver cancer more than cirrhosis alone. They concluded that alcohol intake may be a liver carcinogen, but its role in the genesis of primary liver cancer is primarily through the development of cirrhosis. It is unclear whether the combined effect of increased tissue iron and alcoholic liver disease leads to a higher incidence of liver tumour, but the available evidence suggests that there is no increased risk.

Recent evidence suggest that chronic hepatitis C infection interferes with hepatic iron metabolism and results in increased stainable iron out of proportion to the hepatic iron stores and probably increased hepatic iron disproportionate to total body iron stores (Bacon *et al.* 1993). The precise interrelationships remain to be clarified, but in such instances accurate diagnosis of genetic haemochromatosis requires measurement of hepatic iron concentration and calculation of the hepatic iron index together with family studies.

Management

Haemochromatosis

Venesection therapy involving the removal of excess iron in genetic haemochromatosis prolongs life and may arrest tissue damage if cirrhosis is not established (Williams *et al.* 1969; Powell 1970). Many complications of the disease decrease or disappear after adequate venesection therapy, which usually involves the removal of 500 ml of blood (containing 250 mg iron) per week until the excess iron stores are removed. Treatment should be continued until the transferrin saturation falls to levels within the normal range and the haemoglobin level falls to 10.5 g/dl and fails to rise again indicating depletion of stored iron. Serum ferritin levels fall to below normal. Long-term maintenance therapy usually requires one phlebotomy every 3 months. Family screening and early detection of affected individuals is of obvious importance and it is recommended that screening studies be performed in all first-degree relatives from the age of 10 years. Transferrin saturation and serum ferritin concentrations are recommended as the best screening tests for asymptomatic pre-cirrhotic haemochromatosis. HLA typing is important in family studies where it is used to predict the genetic status of relatives.

Alcoholic siderosis

There is no evidence that removal of the iron by venesection therapy in patients with alcoholic siderosis improves liver function or prolongs life expectancy (Grace 1978).

Prognosis

In haemochromatosis, retrospective studies have shown that the 5 year survival rate with therapy increased from 33 to 89 percent (Bomford and Williams 1976). Overall cumulative survival is 76 percent at 10 years and 49 percent at 20 years (Niederau *et al.* 1985). Non-cirrhotic patients if treated early have a normal life expectancy if treatment is continued. The value of screening cirrhotic patients for early hepatocellular carcinoma is controversial, but 6 monthly ultrasound examination and determination of alpha-fetoprotein is useful although the latter may be normal in up to 50 percent of Caucasian patients with hepatocellular carcinoma. The prognosis of alcoholic siderosis is that of the underlying liver disease.

Summary

Excess alcohol consumption has profound effects on human iron metabolism and leads to increased hepatic iron deposition, apparently disproportionate to the increase in iron stores. This "siderosis" often leads to diagnostic confusion especially in differentiating the hepatic pathology from that of genetic haemochromatosis. The problem is compounded by the effects of alcohol consumption on the serum ferritin concentration, again disproportionate to any increase in body iron stores. The determination of carbohydrate-deficient transferrin (desialylated transferrin) is useful in identifying prolonged heavy alcohol consumption.

An important and consistent observation in numerous reports has been that a high proportion (approximately 20–30 percent) of patients with fully developed haemochromatosis have consumed alcohol in excess of 50 g per day. This observation was primarily responsible for the former view that haemochromatosis was not a genetic disorder, but merely a form of alcoholic or nutritional cirrhosis in subjects whose dietary intake of iron was high. However, it is now established that:

1. Caucasian subjects with heavy alcohol consumption and iron overload of the degree seen in symptomatic haemochromatosis are homozygous for haemochromatosis (Powell 1965, 1970, 1975; Powell and Kerr 1975; Le Sage *et al.* 1983).
2. Subjects heterozygous for haemochromatosis do not develop significant iron overload if they consume alcohol to excess (Powell 1975).
3. Those subjects with mild siderosis do not have an increased frequency of the HLA antigens associated with haemochromatosis (Simon *et al.* 1977).
4. In alcoholic subjects with mild hepatic haemosiderosis but without evidence of haemochromatosis, the hepatic iron concentration is not significantly elevated and the hepatic iron index is less than 2.0, in contrast to subjects homozygous for haemochromatosis (Bassett *et al.* 1986; Summers *et al.* 1990). In these alcoholic subjects, the stainable iron is found in macrophages and Kupffer cells and probably represents iron released from damaged hepatocytes.
5. For practical purposes, the only situation encountered in which heavy alcohol consumption leads to significant iron overload is in South African blacks who ingest large amounts of iron from home-made beer brewed in iron drums or pots. However, even in this situation, recent evidence suggests that the additional presence of an iron-loading gene is necessary if significant iron overload is to develop (Gordeuk *et al.* 1992).
6. Clinically, a distinction between haemochromatosis in an alcoholic subject and mild hepatic haemosiderosis associated with alcoholism can be made in most instances by hepatic biopsy and measurement of hepatic iron concentration and hepatic iron index.
7. The interrelationship between haemochromatosis and alcohol may be further compounded by the presence of hepatitic C virus (HCV) infection. Although incompletely resolved, available data suggest that HCV infection further accentuates histochemical stainable iron out of proportion to body iron stores.

Until the aberrant gene responsible for genetic haemochromatosis is cloned and DNA markers for the disease are available, the above biochemical indices together with the histological appearances and calculation of the hepatic iron index will remain the cornerstones in the differential diagnosis of haemochromatosis and alcoholic siderosis.

Acknowledgements

The authors wish to thank the National Health and Medical Research Council of Australia and the Queensland Cancer Fund for their support.

References

Adami, H.O., Hsing, A.W., McLaughlin, J.K., Trichopoulos, D., Hacker, D., Ekbom, A. and Persson, I. (1992). Alcoholism and liver cirrhosis in the etiology of primary liver cancer. *International Journal of Cancer* **51**, 898–902.

Adams, P., Speechley, M. and Kertesz, A.E. (1990). Long term survival in haemochromatosis. *Hepatology* **12**, 976.

Addison, G.M., Beamish, M.R., Hales, C.N., Hodgkins, M. and Llewellyn, P. (1972). An immunoradiometric assay for ferritin in the serum of normal subjects and patients with iron deficiency and iron overload. *Journal of Clinical Pathology* **25**, 326–329.

Anthony, P.P. (1976). Precursor lesions for liver cell cancer in humans. *Cancer Research* **36**, 2579–2583.

Anthony, P.P., Vagel, C.L. and Barker, L.F. (1973). Liver cell dysplasia: A premalignant condition. *Journal of Clinical Pathology* **26**, 217–223.

Bacon, B.R., Tavill, A.S., Brittenham, G.M., Park, C.H. and Recknagel, R.O. (1983). Hepatic lipid peroxidation *in vivo* in rats with chronic iron overload. *Journal of Clinical Investigation* **71**, 429–439.

Bacon, B.R., Tavill, A.S., Brittenham, G.M., Park, C.H. and Recknagel, R.O. (1985). Hepatotoxicity of chronic ironoverload. In *Free Radicals in Liver Injury* (Edited by Poli, G., Cheeseman, H.K., Dianzani, M.U. and Slater, T.F.), pp. 49–57. Oxford University Press, Oxford.

Bacon, B.R., Fried, M.W. and Di Bisceglie, A.M. (1993). A 39-year-old man with chronic hepatitis, elevated serum ferritin values, and a family history of hemochromatosis. *Seminars in Liver Disease* **13**, 101–105.

Bassett, M.L., Halliday, J.W. and Powell, L.W. (1979). Early detection of idiopathic haemochromatosis, relative value of serum-ferritin and HLA typing. *Lancet* **ii**, 4–7.

Bassett, M.L., Halliday, J.W. and Powell, L.W. (1981). HLA typing in idiopathic haemochromatosis: Distinction between homozygotes and heterozygotes with biochemical expression. *Hepatology* **1**, 120–126.

Bassett, M.L., Doran, T.J., Halliday, J.W., Bashir, H.V. and Powell, L.W. (1982). Idiopathic haemochromatosis: Demonstration of homozygous–heterozygous mating by HLA typing of families. *Human Genetics* **60**, 352–356.

Bassett, M.L., Halliday, J.W. and Powell, L.W. (1984). Genetic hemochromatosis. *Seminars in Liver Disease* **4**, 217–227.

Bassett, M.L., Halliday, J.W. and Powell, L.W. (1986). Value of hepatic iron measurements in early hemochromatosis and determination of the critical iron level associated with fibrosis. *Hepatology* **6**, 24–29.

Batey, R.G., Chung Fong, L., Shamir, S. and Sherlock, S. (1980). A non-transferrin-bound serum iron in idiopathic hemochromatosis. *Digestive Diseases and Sciences* **25**, 340–346.

Beaumier, D.L., Caldwell, M.A. and Holdbein, B.E. (1984). Inflammation triggers hypoferremia and ceruloplasmin in mice. *Infection and Immunity* **46**, 489–494.

Beaumont, C., Simon, M., Fauchet, R., Hespel, J.-P., Brissot, P., Genetet, B. and Bourel, M. (1979). Serum ferritin as a possible marker of the hemochromatosis allele. *New England Journal of Medicine* **301**, 169–174.

Bezwoda, W.R., Torrance, J.D., Bothwell, T.H., Macphail, A.P., Graham, B. and Mills, W. (1985). Iron absorption from red and white wines. *Scandinavian Journal of Haematology* **34**, 121–127.

Blumberg, R.S., Chopra, S., Ibrahim, R., Crawford, J., Farraye, F.A., Zeldis, J.B. and Berman. M.D. (1988). Primary hepatocellular carcinoma in idiopathic hemochromatosis after reversal of cirrhosis. *Gastroenterology* **95**, 1399–1402.

Bomford, A. and Williams, R. (1976). Long term results of venesection therapy in idiopathic hemochromatosis. *Quarterly Journal of Medicine* **180**, 611–623.

Bonkovsky, H.L., Slater, D.P., Bills, E.B. and Wolf, D.C. (1990). Usefulness and limitations of laboratory and hepatic imaging studies in iron storage disease. *Gastroenterology* **99**, 1079–1091.

Borwein, S.T., Ghent, C.N., Flanagan, P.R., Chamberlain, M.J. and Valberg, L.S. (1983). Genetic and phenotypic expression of hemochromatosis in Canadians. *Clinical and Investigative Medicine* **6**, 171–179.

Bothwell, T.H. and Isaacson, C. (1962). Siderosis in the Bantu: A comparison of the incidence in males and females. *British Medical Journal* **1**, 522–524.

Bothwell, T.H., Charlton, R.W. and Seftel, H.C. (1965). Oral iron overload. *South African Medical Journal* **39**, 892–900.

Bothwell, T.H., Charlton, R.W., Cook, J.D. and Finch, C.A. (1979). Alcohol iron and liver disease. In *Iron Metabolism in Man* (Edited by Bothwell, T.H., Charlton, R.W., Cook, J.D. and Finch, C.A.), pp. 156–174. Blackwell Scientific Publications, Oxford.

Boveris, A., Fraga, C.G., Varsavsky, A.I. and Koch, O.R. (1983). Increased chemiluminescence and superoxide production in the livers of chronically ethanol-treated rats. *Archives of Biochemistry and Biophysics* **227**, 534–541.

Bradbear, R.A., Bain, C., Siskind, V., Schofield, F.D., Webb, S., Axelsen, E.M., Halliday, J.W., Bassett, M.L. and Powell, L.W. (1985). Cohort study of internal malignancy in genetic hemochromatosis and other chronic nonalcoholic liver diseases. *Journal of the National Cancer Institute* **75**, 81–84.

Brissot, P., Bourel, M., Herry, D., Verger, J.-P., Messner, M., Beaumont, C., Regnouard, F., Ferrand, B. and Simon, M. (1981). Assessment of liver iron content in 271 patients: A reevaluation of direct and indirect methods. *Gastroenterology* **80**, 557–565.

Brissot, P., Wright, T.L., Ma, W.-L. and Weisiger, R.A. (1985). Efficient clearance of non-transferrin-bound iron by rat liver: Implications for hepatic iron loading in iron overload states. *Journal of Clinical Investigation* **76**, 1463–1470.

Britton, R.S., Tavill, A.S. and Bacon, B.R. (1994). Mechanisms of iron toxicity. In *Iron Metabolism in Health and Disease* (Edited by Brock, J., Halliday, J.W., Pippard, M. and Powell, L.W.), pp. 311–351. Balliere Tindall, London.

Cartwright, G.E., Edwards, C.Q., Kravitz, K., Skolnick, M., Amos, D.B., Johnson, A. and Buskjaer, L. (1979). Hereditary hemochromatosis: Phenotypic expression of the disease. *New England Journal of Medicine* **301**, 175–179.

Celada, A., Rudolf, H. and Donath, A. (1978). Effect of a single ingestion of alcohol on iron absorption. *American Journal of Hematology* **5**, 225–237.

Celada, A., Rudolf, H. and Donath, A. (1979). Effect of experimental chronic alcohol ingestion and folic acid deficiency on iron absorption. *Blood* **54**, 906–915.

Chapman, R.W.G., Morgan, M.Y., Laulicht, M., Hoffbrand, A.V. and Sherlock, S. (1982). Hepatic iron stores and markers of iron overload in alcoholics and patients with idiopathic haemochromatosis. *Digestive Diseases and Sciences* **27**, 909–916.

Chapman, R.W., Morgan, M.Y., Boss, A.M. and Sherlock, S. (1983). Acute and chronic effects of alcohol on iron absorption. *Digestive Diseases and Sciences* **28**, 321–327.

Chick, J., Pikkarainen, J. and Plant, M. (1987). Serum ferritin as a marker of alcohol consumption in working men. *Alcohol and Alcoholism* **22**, 75–77.

Crawford, D.H.G. and Halliday, J.W. (1991). Current concepts in rational therapy for haemochromatosis. *Drugs* **41**, 875–882.

Dadone, M.M., Kushner, J.P., Edwards, C.Q., Bishop, D.T. and Skolnick, M.H. (1982). Hereditary haemochromatosis: Analysis of the laboratory expression of the disease by genotype in 18 pedigrees. *American Journal of Clinical Pathology* **78**, 196–207.

de Jong, G., van Dijk, J.P. and van Eijk, H.G. (1990). The biology of transferrin. *Clinica Chimica Acta* **190**, 1–46.

Deugnier, Y.M., Guyader, D., Crantock, L., Lopez, J., Turlin, B., Yaouanq, J., Jouanolle, H., Campion, J., Launois, B., Halliday, J.W., Powell, L.W. and Brissot, P. (1993a). Primary liver cancer in genetic hemochromatosis: A clinical, pathological, and pathogenic study of 54 cases. *Gastroenterology* **104**, 228–234.

Deugnier, Y.M., Turlin, B., Powell, L.W., Summers, K.M., Moirand, R., Fletcher, L., Loreal, O., Brissot, P. and Halliday, J.W. (1993b). Differentiation between heterozygotes and homozygotes in genetic hemochromatosis by means of a histological hepatic iron index: A study of 192 cases. *Hepatology* **17**, 30–34.

DiLuzio, N.R. (1966). A mechanism of acute ethanol-induced fatty liver and the modification of liver injury by antioxidants. *Laboratory Investigation* **15**, 50–63.

Doran, T.J., Bashir, H.V., Trejaut, J., Bassett, M.L., Halliday, J.W. and Powell, L.W. (1981). Idiopathic haemochromatosis in the Australian population. *Human Immunology* **2**, 191–200.

Duane, P., Raja, K.B., Simpson, R.J. and Peters, T.J. (1992). Intestinal iron absorption in chronic alcoholics. *Alcohol and Alcoholism* **27**, 539–544.

Eason, R.J., Adams, P.C., Aston, C.E. and Searle, J. (1990). Familial iron overload with possible autosomal dominant inheritance. *Australian and New Zealand Journal of Medicine* **20**, 226–230.

Edwards, C.Q., Griffen, L.M., Goldgar, D., Drummond, C., Skolnick, M.H. and Kushner, J.P. (1988). Prevalence of hemochromatosis among 11,065 presumably healthy blood donors. *New England Journal of Medicine* **318**, 1355–1362.

Eichner, E.R. and Hillman, R.S. (1971). The evolution of anaemia in alcoholic patients. *American Journal of Medicine* **50**, 218–232.

Elin, R.J., Wolff, S.M. and Finch, C.A. (1977). Effect of induced fever on serum iron and ferritin concentrations in man. *Blood* **49**, 147–153.

Elliot, R., Tait, A., Lin, P.B.C., Smith, C.I. and Dent, O.F. (1986). Prevalence of haemochromatosis in a random sample of asymptomatic men. *Australian and New Zealand Journal of Medicine* **16**, 491–495.

Fellows, I.W., Steward, M., Jeffcoate, W.J., Smith, P.G. and Toghill, J. (1988). Hepatocellular carcinoma in primary haemochromatosis in the absence of cirrhosis. *Gut* **29**, 1603–1606.

Finch, S.C. and Finch, C.A. (1955). Idiopathic hemochromatosis, an iron storage disease. 1. Iron metabolism in hemochromatosis. *Medicine* **34**, 381–430.

Fletcher, L.M., Roberts, F., Powell, L.W. and Halliday, J.W. (1989). The effects of iron loading on free radical scavenging enzymes and lipid peroxidation in rat liver. *Gastroenterology* **97**, 1011–1018.

Fletcher, L.M., Kwoh-Gain, I., Powell, E.E., Powell, L.W. and Halliday, J.W. (1991). Markers of chronic alcohol ingestion in patients with nonalcoholic steatohepatitis: An aid to diagnosis. *Hepatology* **13**, 455–459.

Friedman, I.M., Kraemer, H.C., Mendoza, F.S. and Hammer, L.D. (1988). Elevated serum iron concentration in adolescent alcohol users. *American Journal of Diseases in Children* **142**, 156–158.

Gilbert, A. and Grenet, A. (1896). Cirrhose alcoholique hypertropique pigmentaire. *La Semaine Medicine* **16**, 514.

Gordeuk, V.R., Devee Boyd, R. and Brittenham, G. (1986). Dietary iron overload persists in rural Sub-Saharan Africa. *Lancet* **i**, 1310–1313.

Gordeuk, V., Mukiibi, J. and Hastedt, S.J. (1992). Iron overload in Africa. *New England Journal of Medicine* **326**, 95–100.

Gordeuk, V., McLaren, C.E., Looker, A., Brittenham, G.M. and Hasselblad, V. (1993). Evidence from NHANES II that an iron-loading gene may be present in the African-American population. *4th International Conference on Hemochromatosis and Clinical Problems in Iron Metabolism*, 29A.

Grace, N.D. (1978). Evidence for hepatic toxicity of iron: Metals and the liver. In *Health and Disease* (Edited by Powell, L.W.), pp. 131–144. Marcel Dekker, New York.

Grace, N.D. and Powell, L.W. (1974). Iron storage diseases of the liver. *Gastroenterology* **67**, 1257–1283.

Hallberg, L., Bjorn-Rasmussen, E. and Jungmer, I. (1989). Prevalence of hereditary hemochromatosis in two Swedish urban areas. *Journal of Internal Medicine* **225**, 249–255.

Halliday, J.W. and Powell, L.W. (1992). Hemochromatosis and other diseases associated with iron overload. In *Iron and Human Disease* (Edited by Lauffer, R.B.), pp. 131–160. CRC Press, Boca Raton, FL.

Harrison, P.M., Clegg, G.A. and May, K. (1980). *Iron in Biochemistry and Medicine II*. Academic Press, London.

Irving, M., Halliday, J.W. and Powell, L.W. (1988). Association between alcoholism and increased hepatic iron stores. *Alcoholism: Clinical and Experimental Research* **12**, 7–13.

Irving, M.G., Booth, C.J., Devlin, C.M., Halliday, J.W. and Powell, L.W. (1991). The effect of iron and ethanol on rat hepatocyte collagen synthesis. *Comparative Biochemistry and Physiology* (C) **100**, 583–590.

Karlsson, M., Ikkala, E., Renunanen, A., Takkunen, H., Vuori, E. and Makinen, J. (1988). Prevalence of hemochromatosis in Finland. *Acta Psychiatrica Scandinavica* **218**, 385–390.

Kew, M.D. (1990). Pathogenesis of hepatocellular carcinoma in hereditary hemochromatosis in the absence of cirrhosis. *Hepatology* **11**, 1086–1087.

Krasner, N., Cochran, K.M., Russel, R.I., Carmichael, H.A. and Thompson, G.C. (1976). Alcohol and absorption from the small intestine. 1. Impairment of absorption from the small intestine in alcoholics. *Gut* **17**, 245–248.

Kristenson, H., Fex, G. and Trell, E. (1981). Serum ferritin, gammaglutamyltransferase and alcohol consumption in healthy middle-aged men. *Drug and Alcohol Dependence* **8**, 43–50.

Kwoh-Gain, I., Fletcher, L.M., Price, J., Powell, L.W. and Halliday, J.W. (1990). Desialylated transferrin and mitochondrial aspartate aminotransferase compared as laboratory markers of excessive alcohol consumption. *Clinical Chemistry* **36**, 841–845.

Leggett, B.A., Brown, N.N., Bryant, S.J., Duplock, L., Powell, L.W. and Halliday, J.W. (1990a). Factors affecting the concentrations of ferritin in serum in a healthy Australian population. *Clinical Chemistry* **36**, 1350–1355.

Leggett, B.A., Halliday, J.W., Brown, N.N., Bryant, S. and Powell, L.W. (1990b). Prevalence of haemochromatosis amongst asymptomatic Australians. *British Journal of Haematology* **74**, 525–530.

LeSage, G.D., Baldus, W.P., Fairbanks, V.F., Baggenstoss, A.H., McCall, J.T., Breanndan Moore, S., Taswell, H.F. and Gordon, H. (1983). Hemochromatosis: Genetic or alcohol induced? *Gastroenterology* **84**, 1471–1477.

Lieber, C.S. (1980). Alcohol, protein metabolism, and liver injury. *Gastroenterology* **79**, 373–390.

Linderbaum, J. and Lieber, C.S. (1969). Hematologic effects of alcohol in man in the absence of nutritional deficiency. *New England Journal of Medicine* **281**, 333–338.

Lipschitz, D.A., Cook, J.D. and Finch, C.A. (1974). A clinical evaluation of serum ferritin as an index of iron stores. *New England Journal of Medicine* **290**, 1213–1216.

Lundin, L., Hallgren, R., Birgegard, G. and Wide, L. (1981). Serum ferritin in alcoholics and the relation to liver damage, iron status and erythropoietic activity. *Acta Psychiatrica Scandinavica* **209**, 327–331.

MacDonald, R.A. (1964). *Hemochromatosis and Hemosiderosis*. C.C. Thomas, Springfield, IL.

MacPhail, A.P., Simon, M.O., Torrance, J.D., Charlton, R.W., Bothwell, T.H. and Isaacson, C. (1979). Changing patterns of dietary iron overload in black South Africans. *American Journal of Clinical Nutrition* **32**, 1272–1278.

Maher, J.J. (1990). Hepatic fibrosis caused by alcohol. *Seminars in Liver Disease* **10**, 66–74.

Meyer, T.E., Kassianides, C., Bothwell, T.H. and Green, A. (1984). Effects of heavy alcohol consumption on serum ferritin concentrations. *South African Medical Journal* **66**, 573–575.

Meyer, T.E., Ballot, D., Bothwell, T.H., Green, A., Derman, D.P., Baynes, R.D., Jenkins, T., Jooste, P.L., du Toit, E.D. and Jacobs, P. (1987). The HLA linked iron loading gene in an Afrikaner population. *Journal of Medical Genetics* **24**, 348–356.

Milder, M.S., Cook, J.D., Stray, S. and Finch, C.A. (1980). Idiopathic haemochromatosis, an interim report. *Medicine (Baltimore)* **59**, 34–49.

Moirand, R., Lescoat, G., Delamaire, D., Lauvin, L., Campion, J.P., Deugnier, Y. and Brissot, P. (1991). Increase in glycosylated and nonglycosylated serum ferritin in chronic alcoholism and their evolution during alcohol withdrawal. *Alcoholism: Clinical and Experimental Research* **15**, 963–969.

Morgan, M.Y. (1991). Alcoholic liver disease: Natural history, diagnosis, clinical features, evaluation, management, prognosis, and prevention. In *Oxford Textbook of Clinical Hepatology* (Edited by McIntyre, N., Benhamou, J.-P., Bircher, J., Rizzetto, M. and Rodes, J.), pp. 815–855. Oxford University Press, Oxford.

Mufti, S.I. (1991). Cancer: Role of alcohol and other factors. In *Drug and Alcohol Abuse Reviews Vol. 2: Liver Pathology and Alcohol* (Edited by Watson, R.R.), pp. 195–219. Humana Press, Totowa.

Naccarato, R. and Farinati, F. (1991). Hepatocellular carcinoma, alcohol, and cirrhosis: Facts and hypotheses. *Digestive Diseases and Sciences* **36**, 1137–1142.

Niederau, C., Fischer, R., Sonnenberg, A., Stremmel, W., Trampish, H.J. and Strohmeyer, G. (1985). Survival and causes of death in cirrhotic and in noncirrhotic patients with primary haemochromatosis. *New England Journal of Medicine* **313**, 1256–1262.

Olsson, K.S., Ritter, B., Rosen, V., Heedman, P.A. and Staugard, F. (1983). Prevalence of iron overload in central Sweden. *Acta Psychiatrica Scandinavica* **213**, 105–112.

Olynyk, J., Hall, P., Sallie, R., Reed, W., Shilkin, K. and Mackinnon, M. (1990). Computerised measurement of iron in liver biopsies: A comparison with biochemical and iron measurement. *Hepatology* **12**, 26–30.

Pares, J., Caballeria, M., Bruguera, M., Torres, M. and Rodes, J. (1986). Histological course of alcoholic hepatitis: Influence of abstinence, sex and extent of hepatic damage. *Journal of Hepatology* **2**, 33–42.

Peters, T.J., Selden, C. and Seymour, C.A. (1977). Lysosomal disruption in the pathogenesis of hepatic damage in primary and secondary haemochromatosis.

In *CIBA Foundation Symposium 51*, pp. 317–329. Elsevier, Amsterdam.

Pietrangelo, A., Rocchi, E., Schiaffonati, L., Ventura, E. and Cairo, G. (1990). Liver gene expression during chronic dietary iron in rats. *Hepatology* **11**, 798–804.

Potter, B.J. (1991). Alcohol and hepatic iron homeostasis. In *Drug and Alcohol Abuse Reviews Vol. 2: Liver Pathology and Alcohol* (Edited by Watson, R.R.), pp. 1–60. Humana Press, Totowa.

Powell, L.W. (1965). Iron storage disease in relatives of patients with alcoholic cirrhosis and hemosiderosis: A comparative study of 27 families. *Quarterly Journal of Medicine* **34**, 427.

Powell, L. (1966). Normal human iron storage and its relationship to ethanol consumption. *Australian Annals of Medicine* **15**, 110.

Powell, L.W. (1970). Changing concepts in haemochromatosis. *Postgraduate Medicine Journal* **46**, 200–209.

Powell, L.W. (1975). The role of alcoholism in hepatic iron storage disease. *Annals of the New York Academy of Science* **252**, 124–134.

Powell, L.W. and Kerr, J.F.R. (1975). The pathology of the liver in haemochromatosis. In *Pathobiology Biology Annual* (Edited by Joachim, H.), pp. 71–81. Appleton-Century Crofts, New York.

Powell, L.W., Mortimer, S. and Harris, I. (1971). Cirrhosis of the liver – a comparative study of the 4 major aetiological groups. *Medical Journal of Australia* **1**, 940–950.

Powell, L.W., Summers, K.M., Board, P.G., Axelsen, E., Webb, S. and Halliday, J.W. (1990). Expression of hemochromatosis in homozygous subjects: Implications of early diagnosis and prevention. *Gastroenterology* **98**, 1625–1632.

Powell, L.W., Jazwinska, E. and Halliday, J.W. (1994). Primary iron overload. In *Iron Metabolism in Health and Disease* (Edited by Brock J., Halliday, H.W., Pippard, M. and Powell, L.W.), pp. 227–240. Bailliere Tindall, London.

Prieto, J., Barry, M. and Sherlock, S. (1975). Serum ferritin in patients with iron overload and with acute and chronic liver diseases. *Gastroenterology* **68**, 525–533.

Regoeczi, E., Chindemi, P.A. and Debanne, M.T. (1984). Transferrin glycans: A possible link between alcoholism and hepatic siderosis. *Alcoholism: Clinical and Experimental Research* **8**, 287–292.

Reitz, R.C. (1975). A possible mechanism for the peroxidation of lipids due to chronic ethanol consumption. *Biochimica et Biophysica Acta* **380**, 145–154.

Roll, F.J. (1991). The pathogenesis of inflammation in alcoholic liver disease. In *Liver Pathology and Alcohol* (Edited by Watson, R.R.), pp. 61–89. Humana Press, Totowa.

Roll, F.J., Bissell, D.M. and Perez, H.D. (1986). Human hepatocytes metabolizing ethanol generate a non-polar chemotactic factor for human neutrophils. *Biochemical and Biophysical Research Communications* **137**, 688–694.

Sabesin, S.M. and Thomas, C.B. (1964). Parenchymal siderosis in preexisting portal cirrhosis: A pathologic entity stimulating idiopathic and transfusional hemochromatosis. *Gastroenterology* **46**, 477–485.

Sallie, R.W., Reed, W.D. and Shilkin, K.B. (1991). Confirmation of the efficacy of hepatic tissue iron index in differentiating genetic haemochromatosis from alcoholic liver disease complicated by alcoholic haemosiderosis. *Gut* **32**, 207–210.

Scheuer, P.J., Williams, R. and Muir, A.R. (1962). Hepatic pathology in relatives of patients with haemochromatosis. *Journal of Pathology and Bacteriology* **84**, 53–64.

Searle, J.W., Kerr, J.F.R., Halliday, J.W. and Powell, L.W. (1987). Iron storage disease. In *Pathology of the Liver* (Edited by MacSween, R.N.M., Anthony, P.P. and Scheuer, P.J.), pp. 181–201. Churchill Livingstone, Edinburgh.

Searle, J.W., Kerr, J.F.R., Halliday, J.W. and Powell, L.W. (1994). Iron storage disease. In *Pathology of the Liver* (Edited by MacSween, R.N.M., Anthony, P.P., Scheuer, P.J., Portmann, B.C. and Burt, A.D.), 3rd edn. Churchill Livingstone, Edinburgh (in press).

Seumatsu, T., Matsumura, T., Sato, N., Miyamoto, T., Ooko, T., Kamada, T. and Abe, H. (1981). Lipid peroxidation in alcoholic liver disease in humans. *Alcoholism: Clinical and Experimental Research* **5**, 427–430.

Sheldon, J.H. (1935). *Haemachromatosis*, p. 382. Oxford University Press, Oxford.

Simon, M. and Bourel, M. (1978). Heredite de l'hemochromatose idiopathique demonstration de la transmission recessive et mise en evidene du gene responsable porte par le chromosome 6. *Gastroenterologie Clinique et Biologique* **2**, 573–577.

Simon, M., Bourel, M., Fauchet, R. and Genetet, B. (1976). Association of HLA-A3 and HLA-B14 antigens with idiopathic haemochromatosis. *Gut* **17**, 332–334.

Simon, M., Bourel, M., Genetet, B. and Fauchet, R. (1977). Idiopathic haemochromatosis: Demonstration of recessive transmisssion and early detection by family HLA typing. *New England Journal of Medicine* **297**, 1017–1021.

Simon, M., Fauchet, R., Hespel, J.P., Beaumont, C., Brissot, P., Hery, B., Hita De Nercy, Y., Genetet, B. and Bourel, M. (1980). Idiopathic haemochromatosis: A study of biochemical expression in 247 heterozygous members of 63 families. Evidence for a single major HLA-linked gene. *Gastroenterology* **78**, 703–708.

Sorensen, T.I.A., Orholm, M., Bentsen, K.D., Hoybye, G., Eghoje, K. and Christoffersen, P. (1984). Prospective evaluation of alcohol abuse and alcoholic liver injury in men as predictors of development of cirrhosis. *Lancet* **ii**, 241–244.

Stibler, H. (1991). Carbohydrate-deficient transferrin in serum: a new marker of potentially harmful alcohol consumption reviewed. *Clinical Chemistry* **37**, 2029–2037.

Storey, E.L., Anderson, G., Mack, U., Powell, L.W. and Halliday, J.W. (1987). Desialylated transferrin as a serological marker of chronic excessive alcohol consumption. *Lancet* **i**, 1292–1293.

Strachan, A.S. (1929). Haemochromatosis and haemosiderosis in South African natives. MD thesis, University of Glasgow.

Summers, K.M., Halliday, J.W. and Powell, L.W. (1990). Identification of homozygous hemochromatosis subjects by measurement of hepatic iron index. *Hepatology* **12**, 20–25.

Szmuness, W. (1978). Hepatocellular carcinoma and the hepatitis B virus. *Progress in Medical Virology* **24**, 40–69.

Tanner, A.R., Desai, S., Lu, W. and Wright, R. (1985). Screening for haemochromatosis in the UK: Preliminary results. *Gut* **26**, A1139.

Tiniakos, G. and Williams, R. (1988). Cirrhotic process, liver cell carcinoma, and extrahepatic malignant tumors in idiopathic haemochromatosis: Study of 71 patients treated with venesection therapy. *Applied Pathology* **6**, 128–138.

Torrance, J.D., and Bothwell, T.H. (1980). Iron. In *Methods in Haematology* (Edited by Cook, J.D.), pp. 116–133. Churchill Livingstone, Edinburgh.

Valimaki, M., Harkonen, M. and Ylikahri, R. (1983). Serum ferritin and iron levels in chronic male alcoholics before and after ethanol withdrawal. *Alcohol and Alcoholism* **18**, 255–260.

von Recklinghausen, F.D. (1889). Uber Hamochromatose. *Tagebl Versamml Natur Arzte Heidelberg* **62**, 324–325.

Williams, R., Smith, P.M., Spicer, E.J.F., Barry, M. and Sherlock, S. (1969). Venesection therapy in idiopathic haemochromatosis. *Quarterly Journal of Medicine* **38**, 1–16.

Worwood, M. (1986). Serum ferritin. *Clinical Science* **70**, 215–220.

Worwood, M., Cragg, S.J., Wagstaff, M. and Jacobs, A. (1979). Binding of human serum ferritin to concanavalin A. *Clinical Science* **56**, 83–87.

Worwood, M., Cragg, S.J., Williams, A.M., Wagstaff, M. and Jacobs, A. (1982). The clearance of ^{131}I-human plasma ferritin in man. *Blood* **60**, 827–833.

Part V
Alcohol and Porphyria

13 Porphyria cutanea tarda

Richard Hift and Ralph E. Kirsch

Introduction

Porphyria cutanea tarda illustrates many of the issues facing those seeking to understand the pathogenesis of alcohol-induced liver disease in general. Porphyria cutanea tarda, a syndrome due to decreased activity of a single enzyme, uroporphyrinogen decarboxylase, is strongly associated with excessive alcohol ingestion, but appears to require an underlying genetic predisposition as well as co-existent iron overload for its clinical expression. A biochemical defect resembling porphyria cutanea tarda may be induced in animals by polyhalogenated hydrocarbons, but the mechanism by which the defect is produced remains unclear. Significantly, the defect in these animal models is enhanced by iron overload but not by the short-term administration of alcohol. Although iron appears to play an important role, the rarity of porphyria cutanea tarda in patients with genetic haemochromatosis, as opposed to its relative frequency in iron overload conditions associated with alcohol excess, suggests that iron overload and alcohol act synergistically in the pathogenesis of this syndrome. This chapter will concentrate on current knowledge of the mechanisms by which alcohol may induce porphyria cutanea tarda, and which may provide insights into the pathogenesis of alcohol-induced liver disease in general. The clinical features and therapy of porphyria cutanea tarda are described for background purposes only, and the reader is referred to other sources for more detailed clinical information (Moore *et al.* 1987).

Pathogenesis of porphyria cutanea tarda

Haem synthesis

The porphyrias are a group of diseases arising from disturbances of haem synthesis (Fig. 13.1). The first porphyrin precursor, 5-aminolaevulinic acid (ALA), is formed by the reaction of glycine and succinyl CoA. Two molecules of ALA condense to form the monopyrrole, porphobilinogen (PBG). Four molecules of porphobilinogen combine to form the linear tetrapyrrole hydroxymethylbilane, which is cyclized in a specific fashion to produce a tetrapyrrolic macrocycle, uroporphyrinogen. This octacarboxylic molecule undergoes four successive decarboxylations to produce the tetracarboxylic coproporphyrinogen, which is further converted via the dicarboxylic protoporphyrinogen to protoporphyrin and to haem. The successive decarboxylations from uroporphyrinogen to coproporphyrinogen are catalysed by a single enzyme, uroporphyrinogen decarboxylase (UROD). Defective activity of UROD has been shown repeatedly to be responsible for the clinical and biochemical effects of porphyria cutanea tarda (Kushner *et al.* 1976; Elder and Evans 1978; Doss *et al.* 1980; Felsher *et al.* 1982; Kushner 1982).

Haem synthesis in the organism occurs at two principal sites; in erythroid precursor cells for incorporation into haemoglobin, and in non-erythroid cells where it is required for myoglobin and haemoproteins such as the cytochromes. The liver is an important haem-requiring organ and is responsible for much of the non-erythroid haem synthesis. Con-

disease tended to have the lowest specific activity. Equally exciting was the finding that in remission induced by venesection, both enzyme activity and concentration returned to normal levels.

Since the sporadic disease is characterized by deficiency of the hepatic form of UROD only, investigators have looked for liver-specific isoenzymes of UROD which might be particularly vulnerable to inhibition. Since hepatic and erythroid UROD have been shown to originate from mRNA of the same size and to have similar chemical, immunological and physical properties, and the complementary DNAs for mRNAs from different cell lines are very similar (Elder *et al.* 1989), it seems that human UROD must be encoded by a single autosomal gene which is transcribed and translated identically in all tissues. This strongly suggests that the sporadic condition results from a potentially reversible, liver-specific inactivation of UROD triggered directly or indirectly by an exogenous agent or agents.

There is clear evidence for the concept that genetic factors, though not of the same importance as they are in the familial form, may influence susceptibility to sporadic porphyria cutanea tarda. Family studies (Elder *et al.* 1989; Nordmann and Deybach 1990; Roberts *et al.* 1988) have demonstrated siblings with classical sporadic disease, that is normal erythroid UROD activity and reduced hepatic UROD activity which improves after venesection. Since erythrocyte UROD activity was normal, the defect cannot be the classic inherited mutant UROD shown in the familial disease, yet the occurrence of this condition in several family members suggests that a mutation at some locus other than the UROD locus itself may predispose individuals to develop porphyria cutanea tarda when exposed to factors such as alcohol and oestrogen (Elder *et al.* 1989).

Although Beaumont *et al.* (1987) claimed that the long history of alcohol intake classically associated with sporadic porphyria cutanea tarda is not found in patients with the familial form, others have commented on the frequency with which a history of exposure to alcohol is present in patients with expressed familial disease (Elder *et al.* 1980; de Verneuil *et al.* 1984b; Doss *et al.* 1980). In most kindreds, a large number of asymptomatic family members with no more than decreased UROD activity are encountered, which suggests that the presence of an inherited defect in the UROD gene alone may be insufficient for clinical expression of the disease. It seems that in these cases, a pathogenic process specific to the liver may additionally be responsible to a greater or lesser extent for converting a potentially rate-limiting step in haem synthesis to a block in the pathway sufficient to allow porphyrin accumulation. This is supported by the observation that the decrease in specific activity of UROD in clinically active familial porphyria cutanea tarda is greater than that observed in clinically quiescent familial disease (Elder *et al.* 1985a), and, in both forms of the disease, venesection is followed by an improvement in the specific activity of enzyme. These observations suggest that both familial and sporadic porphyria cutanea tarda may require a blend of genetic and environmental influences for their clinical expression. What remains to be shown is how these environmental factors, of which the most important is alcohol, interact with an underlying genetic predisposition to precipitate disease.

The role of alcohol

Alcohol is the factor most commonly associated with the development of porphyria cutanea tarda in humans. More than 80 percent of our patients had a history of excessive alcohol ingestion. The amount of alcohol required may be modest, especially when associated with a high iron content, and porphyria cutanea tarda will often arise in people with minimal evidence of chronic alcohol-induced liver damage.

The strong association of alcohol with porphyria cutanea tarda has led to a search for a causal mechanism. Alcohol affects the activities of several haem synthetic enzymes in both humans and rodents. Thus alcohol increases the activity of ALA synthase and porphobilinogen deaminase and decreases the activity of ALA dehydratase (ALA-D), coproporphyrinogen oxidase, ferrochelatase and UROD in normal subjects (McColl *et al.* 1980). This effect has been particularly well studied for ALA-D, where the acute ingestion of alcohol has a marked and direct effect on its activity (Moore *et al.* 1984). Sieg *et al.* (1991) have shown differences in the response of this enzyme to acute alcohol exposure in normal subjects and to chronic exposure in alcoholics. Following the administration of alcohol to a group of six normal subjects, ALA-D activity was diminished by 44 percent. The activity could be largely restored towards normal in the presence of dithiothreitol and zinc. ALA-D activity in a group of alcoholic subjects was found to be even more strongly inhibited, by a factor of 57 percent on average. Whereas an increase in ALA, porphobilinogen deaminase and coproporphyrin excretion, implying an induction of ALA synthase and of porphyrin synthesis, was noted in the normal subjects, the alcoholics showed little tendency to an enhanced urinary ALA excretion. It seems, therefore, that chronic alcohol use leads to an adaptive response with a reduction in ALA synthase activity adapting this to the level appropriate for haem production in the face of a reduction in catalytic activity of ALA-D. Since others have described increased ALA synthase activity in alcoholics (Bonkovsky and Pomeroy 1977; McColl *et al.* 1981), the nature of the adaptive response must be considered conjectural.

ALA-D contains sulph-hydryl groups and zinc which are essential for full activity (Shemin 1976; Anderson and Desnick 1979; Tsukamoto *et al.* 1979). It is possible that alcohol influences ALA-D activity by the oxidation of sulph-hydryl groups and reducing the hepatic concentration of sulph-hydryl donors like cystein or glutathione which are thought to bind to acetyldehyde (Moore *et al.* 1971) This may explain the effects of dithiothreitol and zinc in restoring ALA-D activity following exposure to alcohol.

Unfortunately, in animal studies, the short-term administration of iron and alcohol shows no synergistic effect and does not produce uroporphyria, the animal equivalent of porphyria cutanea tarda. Similarly, no additional effect has been shown when hexachlorobenzene-exposed rats are treated acutely with alcohol or oestrogens (Kondo and Shimuzu 1986). There is thus no animal model for the direct induction of porphyria cutanea tarda by the short-term administration of alcohol, even in the presence of an excess of iron. In contrast, the disease may easily be induced, in both humans and animals, by aromatic hydrocarbons such as hexachlorobenzene. This has led to the suggestion that, although alcohol may play some role in inducing ALA synthase and inhibiting UROD, its contribution to the development of porphyria cutanea tarda may be indirect, perhaps by potentiating iron absorption and by depleting hepatic glutathione stores (Moore *et al.* 1987). Alternatively, the effect of alcohol may be time-related; whereas hydrocarbons will induce porphyria cutanea tarda in humans in months, alcohol may require years.

The role of iron overload

Evidence of hepatic iron overload is almost invariable in porphyria cutanea tarda. In our series, 90 percent of patients had evidence of excessive iron stores, either on serum ferritin estimation, liver biopsy or both. Despite the importance of iron in this condition, it is noteworthy that iron overload is rarely accompanied by porphyria cutanea tarda in the absence of an additional trigger which is usually alcohol. However, the fundamental importance of the association between porphyria cutanea tarda and iron overload is shown by the predictable clinical and biochemical response to iron-reducing measures, such as phlebotomy and desferrioxamine infusion.

The strength of the association of iron overload with porphyria cutanea tarda must indicate a pathogenic role for iron in this disorder. However, the influence of iron is disproportionate to the modest elevation in iron stores encountered. The total body iron is usually increased by only 1–2 g, which represents a 20 percent increase over the usual body store of 5 g. In contrast, genetic haemochromatosis is characterized by the accumulation of much larger amounts of iron, as much as 15–50 g or a 1000 percent expansion in iron stores (Powell 1992). This difference in the degree of iron overload is reflected by the response to therapy. In porphyria cutanea tarda normal iron stores are achievable after modest courses of venesection, while genetic haemochromatosis may require several years of venesection to mobilize the excess iron.

Some authors have suggested that porphyria cutanea tarda arises in people heterozygous for the haemochromatosis allele. This claim is largely based on the occasional finding of the two diseases in the same family (Seymour *et al.* 1990). Thus, Kushner *et al.* (1985) described a single pedigree in which the proband carried one HLA-A3 allele (a surrogate marker of the haemochromatosis gene) and had sporadic porphyria cutanea tarda, while several family members had evidence of minor iron overload also associated with HLA-A3. They subsequently described 14 patients with sporadic porphyria cutanea tarda and hepatic siderosis, and reported that HLA-A3 was present in 57 percent of these patients, which would indeed suggest an association between the HLA-A3 allele and porphyria cutanea tarda. However, in a much larger study, Beaumont *et al.* (1987) found that HLA-A3 was no more prevalent in sporadic or in familial porphyria cutanea tarda than in a control population and concluded that the two diseases are not associated. In a review of more than 250 families with haemochromatosis, Adams and Powell (1987) could find no patients with coexistent overt porphyria cutanea tarda. Certainly, in our experience, porphyria cutanea tarda is common in the black South African population where genetic haemochromatosis of the classical HLA-3-associated type described in Europe and North America is extremely rare. Thus, though heterozygosity for genetic haemochromatosis may contribute to the iron overload associated with porphyria cutanea tarda in isolated cases, it is not an an important factor in most cases of this disease.

Mukerji and Pimstone (1986) suggested that ferrous iron might damage UROD directly. They reported that ferrous iron could competitively inhibit partially purified UROD, and postulated an interaction of ferrous iron with cysteinyl residues at the active site of UROD. They had previously found that UROD in two patients with familial porphyria cutanea tarda appeared to be more susceptible to inhibition by ferrous iron than that from a normal subject (Mukerji *et al.* 1985). Certainly, work from the Netherlands (Siersema *et al.* 1991) suggests an "intimacy" between iron loading and aberrant porphyrin synthesis. They induced uroporphyria in C57BL/10 mice by the administration of iron-dextran with or without coincidental treatment with hexachlorobenzene and found, on histological and ultrastructural examination, that uroporphyrin crystals and ferritin coexisted in close proximity within the hepatocyte. However, despite these studies, the bulk of available evidence suggests that a direct interaction of iron and UROD is unlikely to be the major mechanism by which iron operates in porphyria cutanea tarda.

Deam and Elder (1991) induced severe uroporphyria in iron-overloaded C57BL/6 mice when ALA was added to the drinking water. This was accompanied by an 80 percent decrease in hepatic UROD activity. A second group of DBA/2 mice did not develop porphyria under the same conditions. In neither strain could porphyria be induced by the addition of ALA alone. The significance of this is three-fold:

1. This observation suggests the importance of a genetic predisposition in determining the inducibility of porphyria.
2. Iron overload appears to be essential for the defect to be manifest.
3. Uroporphyria can be induced without the mediation of aromatic hydrocarbons, but in response to ALA.

These observations raise the possibility that inactivation of UROD in iron-loaded mice may require interaction between iron and ALA or a subsequent haem biosynthetic intermediate.

Furthermore, the same interaction may play a role in producing uroporphyria following the administration of aromatic hydrocarbons, since the porphyrinogenic effect of the aromatic hydrocarbons is potentiated by ALA (Urquhart *et al.* 1988; Sinclair *et al.* 1989) as indeed it is by iron (Taljaard *et al.* 1972; Blekkenhorst *et al.* 1980). Even some non-halogenated chemicals and drugs will cause uroporphyria in iron-loaded mice of susceptible strains (Francis and Smith 1987; Urquhart *et al.* 1988; Sinclair *et al.* 1989). Many of these recent studies show that in susceptible strains of mice – particularly the C57BL group – uroporphyria will occur under the influence of iron overload alone or together with the administration of ALA, suggesting that uroporphyria is the outcome of an endogenous malfunction of iron and haem metabolism, and that drugs and chemicals such as acetone and hexachlorobenzene (and by analogy, alcohol in humans) might function merely to exacerbate this intrinsic malfunction (Smith *et al.* 1990).

Whereas Elder (1976) proposed the formation of an iron chelate which binds to the active centre of UROD, catalysing the formation of free radicals which thereafter damage UROD, others have suggested that this theory does not explain sufficiently the involvement of cytochrome P450, which has repeatedly been implicated in this process (Sinclair *et al.* 1984, 1986, 1987). Sinclair and others (Francis and Smith 1987) have suggested that the 3-methylcholanthrene type cytochrome P448 may be induced under those circumstances which give rise to porphyria cutanea tarda resulting in the generation of reactive oxygen radicals. Iron, as a ready electron donor, may be implicated in the formation of free radicals (Aust and Svingen 1982); as illustrated by the following Haber-Weiss reaction:

$$\frac{\begin{array}{l} Fe^{3+} + O_2^- \rightarrow Fe^{2+} + O_2 \\ Fe^{2+} + H_2O_2 \rightarrow Fe^{3+} + OH^- + OH \cdot \end{array}}{O_2^- + H_2O_2 \rightarrow O_2 + OH^- + OH \cdot}$$

Such a reaction generates the highly reactive hydroxyl radical which is able to effect subcellular molecular damage (Visser *et al.* 1989). In the context of porphyria cutanea tarda, such radicals may well damage the active site of UROD itself or, more probably, might catalyse the conversion of an endogenous substrate to an inhibitor of UROD activity.

In addition to their effect on UROD, there is evidence that iron and hydrocarbons act synergistically on the function of the mitochondrial respiratory chain (Feldman and Bacon 1989). Hexachlorobenzene alone was shown to produce uncoupling which could be reversed by albumin. The latter was postulated to act as a scavenger of pentachlorophenyl, a product of hexachlorobenzene metabolism, which probably functions as the uncoupler. However, where both iron loading and hexachlorobenzene were used, the inhibitory effect produced was only partially reversed. This was interpreted as suggesting both a reversible uncoupling and an irreversible inhibition of mitochondrial electron transport. Thus iron and hydrocarbon may be acting on different sites within the respiratory chain, rather than merely potentiating a single effect. Others have shown that where higher iron levels are achieved, evidence of mitochondrial dysfunction – in the form of uncoupling of oxidative metabolism – may indeed be obtained in the absence of hexachlorobenzene (Hanstein *et al.* 1975, 1981).

In summary, it appears that iron may exert its permissive effect in porphyria cutanea tarda by facilitating the formation of free radicals in a process which requires the participation of exogenous precipitants such as alcohol or aromatic hydrocarbons, or possibly endogenous substances which include intermediates of haem synthesis.

Hexachlorobenzene-induced uroporphyria

Though toxins such as hexachlorobenzene and tetrachloro-*p*-dioxin are now uncommon causes of porphyria cutanea tarda, they reliably induce uroporphyria which biochemically closely resembles human porphyria cutanea tarda. Hexachlorobenzene-induced uroporphyria in animals and in cell culture systems may offer important insights into the pathogenesis of porphyria cutanea tarda and are thus discussed in some detail.

Uroporphyria induced by aromatic hydrocarbons is clearly associated with a diminution in activity of hepatic UROD without alteration in the amount of enzyme protein present (Elder and Sheppard 1982). This suggests that, in contrast to alcohol-related porphyria cutanea tarda, aromatic hydrocarbons reduce the activity of the enzyme without affecting its synthesis or degradation. This is not due to covalent binding of the hydrocarbon or its metabolites to UROD (Smith and Francis 1987), suggesting that the aromatic hydrocarbons have an indirect effect on the enzyme, probably mediated by the production of a UROD inhibitor.

Several studies suggest the importance of the generation of reactive oxygen species and free radicals in this process. Hexachlorobenzene has been shown to increase the production of reactive oxygen species by the microsomal mixed function oxidase system (Elder *et al.* 1985b). These reactive oxygen species may convert uroporphyrinogen to uroporphyrin. The conversion may be mediated in the presence of NADPH by a specific isozyme of cytochrome P450, induced by polyhalogenated aromatic hydrocarbons (Sinclair *et al.* 1987). Uroporphyrin is not a substrate for the UROD reaction, which may explain the massive accumulation of uroporphyrin seen in uroporphyria and porphyria cutanea tarda in the presence of a rather modest inhibition of UROD activity, and in addition, uroporphyrin may itself function as an inhibitor of UROD (Elder *et al.* 1983). It is possible that hydrocarbons may effect the transformation of endogenous substances other than uroporphyrinogen to inhibitors of UROD. Several investigators have suggested the presence of an inhibitor of UROD in murine liver following the administration of hydrocarbons (Smith *et al.* 1987; Cantoni *et al.* 1984; Billi *et al.* 1986). Uroporphyrin is only one candidate inhibitor for UROD, and porphyrin-free fractions of liver cytosol from porphyric mice have been found to inhibit UROD (Cantoni *et al.* 1984).

Visser *et al.* (1989) determined the time sequence of the development of hexachlorobenzene-induced uroporphyria in rats and related this to the production of malondialdehyde, a marker of lipid peroxidation and indirectly of free radical activity. Uroporphyria was induced in the rats with a combination of hexachlorobenzene and intramuscular iron. Their results showed that uroporphyria developed in two distinct phases. In the first phase, there was a moderate but significant increase in liver porphyrins and in markers of fatty acid metabolism. During this phase, however, hepatic UROD activity remained normal and there was no increase in the urinary excretion of porphyrins. This is evidence that in the initial stages of uroporphyria, UROD activity is not decreased, no UROD inhibitor can yet have been formed and an explanation must be sought for the accumulation of uroporphyrin in the absence of diminished UROD activity. The direct oxidation of uroporphyrinogen to uroporphyrin, which cannot itself be further metabolized, would seem reasonable. The simultaneous accumulation of malondialdehyde suggests that free radicals may play a role in this phase. Indeed, it has been shown, *in vitro*, that uroporphyrinogen may be oxidized to uroporphyrin in the presence of free radicals

(Sinclair *et al.* 1987; de Matteis *et al.* 1988). In contrast, in the second phase, there is a marked inhibition of UROD activity; porphyrins rise to higher levels, are excreted in the urine, and malondialdehyde accumulates to an even greater extent. Support for such a two-stage model of uroporphyrin accumulation has also been put forward by Lambrecht *et al.* (1988), who found that, in cultured chick-embryo hepatocytes, polyhalogenated hydrocarbons cause accumulation of uroporphyrin without affecting UROD activity.

There is increasing evidence that cytochromes are involved in the induction of uroporphyria. The 3-methylcholanthrene type of the cytochrome P450 family (cytochrome P448) in particular appears to be important (Sinclair *et al.* 1984). Rodent susceptibility to polyhalogenated aromatic hydrocarbon-induced uroporphyria is very dependent on species and strain. This porphyria appears to depend to a large degree on induction of an arylhydrocarbon-inducible microsomal cytochrome of the P4501A subfamily (Sinclair *et al.* 1986; Hahn *et al.* 1988) and susceptibility has been shown to correlate partially with the responsiveness of this cytochrome (Greig *et al.* 1984). Thus, hexachlorobenzene produces porphyria much more easily in iron-loaded mice of the C57BL strain, which are arlhydrocarbon-responsive than in the non-responsive DBA/2 strain.

Francis and Smith (1987) were able to show that even non-halogenated polycyclic aromatic hydrocarbons, when fed to iron-loaded mice, could induce uroporphyria and UROD inhibition. Like the polyhalogenated hydrocarbons, these are inducers of cytochrome P450 1 but are themselves poor substrates for this isozyme. They suggested that the cytochrome P450 1 system was uncoupled, releasing activated oxygen, which would react with iron leading to an oxidative process and the conversion of some endogenous substrate to a UROD inhibitor. Taking this further, Marks has suggested that the propensity of a chemical compound to induce uroporphyria depends on its ability to induce specific isozymes of cytochrome P450, releasing activated oxygen which mediates the formation of a stable UROD inhibitor (Marks *et al.* 1989). Unfortunately, there is evidence that this proposal may not be entirely correct. Sinclair has demonstrated that a severe uroporphyria may be induced by the administration of acetone, iron dextran and ALA (Sinclair *et al.* 1989). Although acetone appeared to play a major role in the induction of this form of uroporphyria, it did not induce those isozymes induced by hexachlorobenzene or 3-methylcholanthrene (cyto-

chrome P448). Indeed, cytochrome P450 2E1, which is induced in rodents by acetone, does not appear to oxidize uroporphyrinogen to uroporphyrin. Thus, if any specific form of cytochrome P450 is involved in the uroporphyria caused by acetone, it is not the same form that is inducible by other substances such as hexachlorobenzene.

Smith *et al.* (1990) induced uroporphyria in C57BL/10ScSn mice following the administration of a single dose of iron dextran in the absence of aromatic hydrocarbons. Co-administration of nafenopin completely abrogated the development of uroporphyria, even though UROD activities were moderately decreased. Thus nafenopin (which is an inducer of a novel isozyme of cytochrome P450 named 1VA1), protects the iron-loaded animal against uroporphyria. The authors speculate that whereas induction of cytochrome P450 1A may lead to the presence of uroporphyria, induction of cytochrome P450 1VA1 appears to be protective. The mechanism of this protection is not understood. Nafenopin may prevent oxidation of uroporphyrinogen or may induce protective systems possibly associated with its known ability to cause peroxisome proliferation. Unfortunately, there is no therapeutic role for nafenopin as it was ineffective in reducing uroporphyria once established.

Despite much interest, the pathogenesis of aromatic hydrocarbon-induced uroporphyria remains unclear. It is disappointing that alcohol does not exert the same effects as the aromatic hydrocarbons on UROD in the experimental model. However, the synergism shown between the aromatic hydrocarbon and iron, and the importance of genetic factors in determining the inducibility of uroporphyria, may assist in the understanding of its human counterpart porphyria cutanea tarda. In view of the central position of the cytochrome P450 system in the metabolism of both ethanol and other hydrocarbons and their implication in the genesis of uroporphyria, it seems probable that variability in this enzyme, whether genetic or acquired, may prove important in determining the susceptibility of the human subject to alcohol-induced porphyria cutanea tarda. To what extent the aromatic hydrocarbon in the animal model and alcohol in the human disorder play analogous roles is curently unknown.

Clinical features

In the early stages, porphyria cutanea tarda may be clinically silent though biochemically expressed. In our experience, dark-skinned people may present with nothing more than an increase in pigmentation. However, the classical presentation is with a typical vesicular-erosive photodermatitis characterized by blistering, fragility of the skin, sores and scabs in sun-exposed areas, particularly the face and the backs of the hands and forearms. This may be followed by chronic pigmentary changes including hyperpigmentation, hirsutism and occasionally pseudosclerodermatous appearances with marked skin atrophy and resorption of the terminal phalanges. These changes are thought to result from photoactivation of porphyrins deposited in the skin and may be mediated via the generation of free radicals (Poh-Fitzpatrick 1985; Athar *et al.* 1988) and the activation of complement (Baart de la Faille-Kuiper *et al.* 1968; Baart de la Faille *et al.* 1978; Lim and Gigli 1981; Lim *et al.* 1981; Pigatto *et al.* 1986).

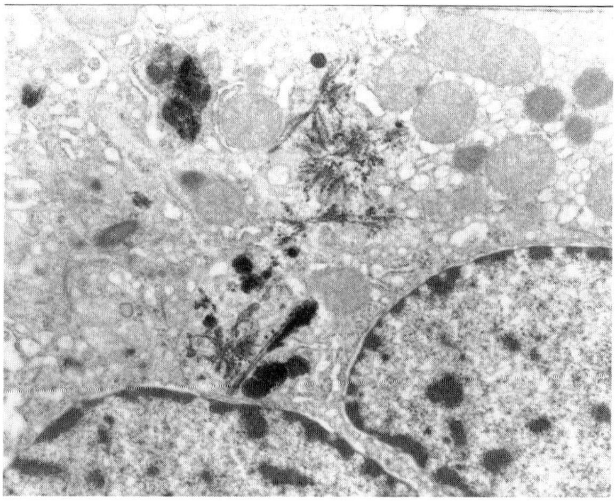

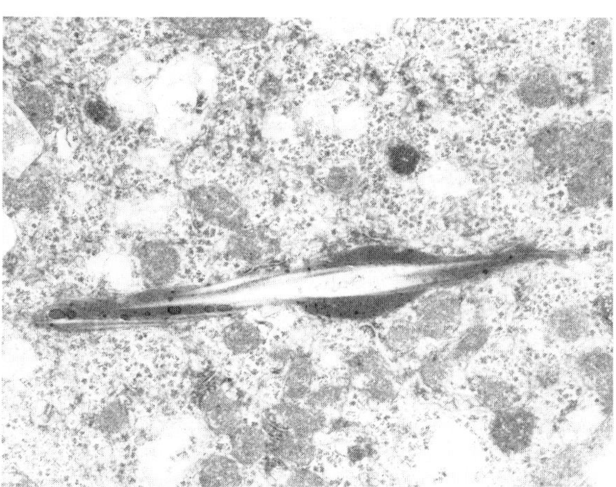

Fig. 13.2 Uroporphyrin crystals. Liver from a patient with porphyria cutanea tarda showing both needle-shaped and stellate uroporphyrin crystals. ×7680.

Pathology

Liver function is usually abnormal. In 40 patients investigated by us, moderately elevated transaminases were noted in 38. Most patients showed a raised serum ferritin as well. Only 13 patients, however, had clinical evidence of liver disease and this was usually limited to hepatomegaly.

Liver histology is almost invariably abnormal in porphyria cutanea tarda. In our patients, as well as those reported by others (Grossman *et al.* 1979; Campo *et al.* 1990), abnormalities were detected in all on liver biopsy. The predominant abnormalities are steatosis and perisinusoidal and perivenular fibrosis. Periportal inflammation and cellular necrosis are less commonly observed and frank cirrhosis is rare. These changes are indistinguishable from those seen in alcohol abuse *per se* and may indeed be secondary to it. Indeed, it is unclear whether porphyria cutanea tarda independently contributes to the hepatic damage seen histologically or is itself a consequence of that damage.

Characteristic, however, of porphyria cutanea tarda is the accumulation of iron within the liver which is usually readily apparent on light microscopy, particularly if sections are selectively stained for iron. In contrast to genetic haemochromatosis, iron accumulation is seldom massive, and is commonly found in both the Kupffer cells and periportal hepatocytes. The association of portal inflammation, haemosiderosis and steatosis appears to be characteristic of porphyria cutanea tarda and

Fig. 13.3 Uroporphyrin crystals. Needle-shaped crystals in the cytoplasm of an hepatocyte. ×38,400.

occurs in over 50 percent of cases, but is very much less common in the absence of porphyria cutanea tarda (Campo *et al.* 1990).

A distinctive but not invariable finding in porphyria cutanea tarda is the demonstration of needle-shaped inclusions in hepatocytes representing aggregated uroporphyrin crystals. These are occasionally seen under light microscopy but are more readily visualized by their brilliant fluorescence under ultraviolet light and are also well shown on electron microscopy (Figs 13.2, 13.3).

Diagnosis

Though the diagnosis of porphyria cutanea tarda may be suspected on clinical grounds, the disorder must be differentiated from other causes of pigmentation or of bullous or vesiculo-erosive skin disease, including other forms of porphyria, pseudoporphyria and pellagra. A tentative diagnosis may be made where grossly elevated urinary porphyrins are demonstrated. It must in all cases be confirmed by demonstrating, by high-performance liquid chromatography or thin-layer chromatography, the characteristic accumulation of porphyrins in urine, with high levels of uroporphyrin and decreasing amounts of hepta-, hexa-, pentacarboxylic and coproporphyrin. A similar pattern is seen in plasma and a characteristic abnormal porphyrin, isocoproporphyrin, is shown in the faeces. This pattern of accumulation is easily explicable since the defective enzyme, UROD, is responsible for the intermediate decarboxylations.

Determination of UROD activity is rarely necessary, but will help to distinguish the familial form from the sporadic form. In the latter, erythrocyte UROD activity is normal, whereas in the former it is reduced by approximately 50 percent. Following confirmation of the diagnosis, biochemical tests of liver function, estimation of iron stores such as ferritin and transferrin saturation and liver biopsy are indicated to delineate the extent of associated alcohol-related liver damage and iron overload.

Conclusion

In this chapter, we have attempted to highlight some of the issues facing those seeking to understand the role of alcohol in the pathogenesis of porphyria cutanea tarda. The apparent synergism of the major causal factors, alcohol and iron, has been stressed and the possibility that an underlying genetic predisposition may be required before the syndrome can be expressed has been raised. The nature of these genetic factors remains to be precisely identified. In familial porphyria cutanea tarda, an inherited defect in UROD is obviously important; in sporadic porphyria cutanea tarda, inherited variations in the propensity to iron accumulation, in expression of cytochrome P450 enzymes and in their inducibility, in the inducibility of ALA synthase and conceivably in the hepatic metabolism of ethanol itself, may determine susceptibility to porphyria

cutanea tarda. The nature of the biochemical defect – decreased activity of uroporphyrinogen decarboxylase – has been explored, as have the many animal experiments which have provided valuable insight into the potential mechanisms by which this enzyme and the haem synthetic pathway may be affected. The gap between the almost invariable finding that patients with porphyria cutanea tarda consume relatively large amounts of alcohol and the tenuous link between alcohol and disturbed porphyrin metabolism remains an exciting challenge for those interested in understanding how alcohol affects the liver.

References

Adams, P.C. and Powell, L.W. (1987). Porphyria cutanea tarda and HLA-linked hemochromatosis – all in the family? *Gastroenterology* **92**, 2033–2035.

Anderson, P.M. and Desnick, R.J. (1979). Purification and properties of δ-aminolevulinate dehydratase from human erythrocytes. *Journal of Biological Chemistry* **254**, 6924–6930.

Andrew, T.L., Riley, P.G. and Dailey, H.A. (1990). Regulation of heme biosynthesis in higher animals. In *Biosynthesis of Heme and Chlorophyll* (Edited by Dailey, H. A.), pp. 163–200. McGraw-Hill, New York.

Athar, M., Mukhtar, H., Elmets, C.A., Zaim, M.T., Lloyd J.R and Bickers, D.R. (1988). *In situ* evidence for the involvement of superoxide anions in cutaneous porphyrin photosensitization. *Biochemical and Biophysical Research Communications* **151**, 1054–1059.

Aust, S.D. and Svingen, B.A. (1982). The role of iron in enzymatic lipid peroxidation. In: *Free Radicals in Biology* (Edited by Pryor, W. A.), Vol. V, pp. 1–28. Academic Press, New York.

Baart de la Faille, H., Beerens, E.G.J., van Weelden, H. *et al.* (1978). Complement components in blood serum and suction blister fluid in erythropoietic protoporphyria. *British Journal of Dermatology* **99**, 401–404.

Baart de la Faille-Kuyper, E.H. and Cormane, R.H. (1968). The occurrence of certain serum factors in the dermo-epidermal junction and vessel walls of the skin in lupus erythematosus and other (skin) diseases. *Acta Dermatologica et Venereologica* **48**, 578–588.

Barnard, G.F. and Akhtar, M. (1979). Stereochemical and mechanistic studies on the decarboxylation of uroporphyrinogen III in haem biosynthesis. *Journal of the Chemical Society, Perkin Transactions* 1, 2354–2359.

Beaumont, C., Fauchet, R., Phung, L.N., de Verneuil, H., Gueguen, M. and Nordmann, Y. (1987). Porphyria cutanea tarda and HLA-linked hemochromatosis: Evidence against a systematic association. *Gastroenterology* **92**, 1833–1838.

Billi, S.C., Wainstock de Calimanovici, R. and San Martin de Viale, S.C. (1986). Rat liver porphyrinogen carboxylase inhibition as a function of the degree of hexachlorobenzene-induced porphyria. In *Hexachlorobenzene: Proceedings of an International Symposium* (Edited by Morris, C.R. and Cabral, J.R.P.), pp. 487–491. IARC Scientific Publication No. 77, Lyon.

Blekkenhorst, G.H., Day, R.S. and Eales, L. (1980). The effect of bleeding and iron administration on the development of hexachlorobenzene-induced rat porphyria. *International Journal of Biochemistry* **12**, 1013–1017.

Bonkovsky, H.L. and Pomeroy, J.S. (1977). Human hepatic delta-aminolaevulinic acid synthase: Requirement of an exogenous system for succinyl-coA generation to demonstrate increased activity in cirrhotic liver. *Clinical Science and Molecular Medicine* **52**, 509–521.

Campo, E., Bruguera, M. and Rodes, J. (1990). Are there diagnostic histologic features of porphyria cutanea tarda in liver biopsy specimens? *Liver* **10**, 185–190.

Cantoni, L., dal Fiume, D., Rizzardini, M. and Ruggieri R. (1984). *In vitro* inhibitory effect on porphyrinogen carboxylase of liver extracts from TCDD treated mice. *Toxicology Letters* **20**, 211–217.

de Matteis, F., Harvey, C., Reed, C. and Hempenious R. (1988). Increased oxidation of uroporphyrinogen by an inducible liver microsomal system. *Biochemical Journal* **250**, 161–169.

de Verneuil, H., Sassa, S. and Kappas, A. (1983). Purification and properties of uroporphyrinogen decarboxylase from human erythrocytes: A single enzyme catalysing the four sequential decarboxylations of uroporphyrinogens I and III. *Journal of Biological Chemistry* **258**, 2454–2460.

de Verneuil, H., Beaumont, C., Deybach, J.C., Nordmann, Y., Sfar, Z. and Kastally, R. (1984a). Enzymatic and immunological studies of uroporphyrinogen decarboxylase in familial porphyria cutanea tarda and hepato-erythropoietic porphyria. *American Journal of Human Genetics* **36**, 613–622.

de Verneuil, H.B., Grandchamp, B., Foubert, C., Weil, D., N'Guyen, V.C., Gross, M.S., Sassa, S. and Nordmann, Y. (1984b). Assignment of the gene for uroporphyrinogen decarboxylase to human chromosome 1 by somatic cell hybridization and specific enzyme immunoassay. *Human Genetics* **66**, 202–205.

de Verneuil, H.B., Grandchamp, C., Beaumont, C., Picat, C. and Nordmann Y. (1986). Uroporphyrinogen decarboxylase structural mutant (gly^{281glu}) in a case of porphyria. *Science (Washington, DC)* **234**, 732–734.

Deam, S. and Elder, G.H. (1991). Uroporphyria produced in mice by iron and 5 aminolaevulinic acid. *Biochemical Pharmacology* **41**, 2019–2022.

Doss, M., von Tiepermann, R., Look, D., Menning, M., Nikolowski, J., Rickmans, F. and Braun Falco, O. (1980). Hereditary and non-hereditary form of chronic hepatic porphyria: Different behaviour of uroporphyrinogen decarboxylase in liver and erythrocytes. *Klinische Wochenschrift* **58**, 1347–1356.

Dubart, A., Mattei, M.G., Raich, N., Beaupain, D., Romeo, P.H., Mattei, J.F. and Goossens, M. (1986). Assignment of human uroporphyrinogen decarboxylase (Uro-D) to the P34 band of chromosome 1. *Human Genetics* **73**, 277–280.

Elder, G.H. (1976). Acquired disorders of haem synthesis. *Essays in Medical Biochemistry* **2**, 75–114.

Elder, G.H. and Evans, J.O. (1978). Evidence that the coproporphyrinogen oxidase activity of rat liver is situated in the intermembrane space of mictochondria. *Biochemical Journal* **172**, 345–352.

Elder, G.H. and Sheppard, D.M. (1982). Immunoreactive uroporphyrinogen decarboxylase is unchanged in porphyria caused by TCDD and hexachlorobenzene. *Biochemical and Biophysical Research Communications* **109**, 113–120.

Elder, G.H., Sheppard, D.M., Enriques de Salamanca, R. and Olmos A. (1980). Identification of two types of porphyria cutanea tarda by measurement of erythrocyte uroporphyrinogen decarboxylase. *Clinical Science* **58**, 477–484.

Elder, G.H., Tovey, J.A. and Sheppard, D.M. (1983). Purification of uroporphyrinogen decarboxylase from human erythrocytes. *Biochemical Journal* **214**, 45–55.

Elder, G.H., de Salamanca, R.E., Urqhart, A.J., Munoz, J.J. and Bonkovsky, H.L. (1985a). Immunoreactive uroporphyrinogen decarboxylase in the liver in porphyria cutanea tarda. *Lancet.* **ii**, 229–233.

Elder, G.H., Roberts, A.G. and Urquhart A.J. (1985b). Acquired uroporphyrinogen decarboxylase defects: Molecular mechanisms. In *Porphyrins and Porphyrias* (Edited by Nordmann, Y.), pp. 147–152. Colloque. INSERM/John Libbey Eurotext Ltd., Paris.

Elder, G.H., Roberts, A.G. and Enriques de Salamanca, R. (1989). Genetics and pathogenesis of human uroporphyrinogen decarboxylase defects. *Clinical Biochemistry* **22**, 163–168.

Feldman, E.S. and Bacon, B.R. (1989). Hepatic mitochondrial oxidative metabolism and lipid peroxidation in experimental hexachlorobenzene-induced porphyria with dietary carbonyl iron overload. *Hepatology* **9**, 686–692.

Felsher, B.F., Carpio, N.M., Engleking, D.W. and Nunn, A.T. (1982). Decreased hepatic uroporphyrinogen decarboxylase activity in porphyria cutanea tarda. *New England Journal of Medicine* **306**, 766–769.

Francis, J.E. and Smith, A.G. (1987). Polycyclic aromatic hydrocarbons cause hepatic porphyria in iron-loaded C57BL/10 mice: Comparison of uroporphyrinogen decarboxylase inhibition with induction of alkoxyphenoxazone dealkylations. *Biochemical and Biophysical Research Communications* **146**, 13–20.

Garey, J.R., Hansen, J.L., Harrison, L.M., Kennedy, J.B. and Kushner J.P. (1989). A point mutation in the coding region of uroporphyrinogen decarboxylase associated with familial porphyria cutanea tarda. *Blood* **73**, 892–895.

Garey, J.R., Harrison, L.M., Franklin, K.F., Metcalf, K.M., Radisky, E.S. and Kushner J.P. (1990). Uroporphyrinogen decarboxylase: A splice site mutation causes the deletion of exon 6 in multiple families with porphyria cutanea tarda. *Journal of Clinical Investigation* **86**, 1416–1422.

Greig, J.B., Francis, J.E., Kay, S.J.E., Lovell, D.P. and Smith A.G. (1984). Incomplete corelation of 2,3,7,8-tetrachlorodibenzo-p-dioxin hepatotoxicity with Ah phenotype in mice. *Toxicology and Applied Pharmacology* **74**, 17–25.

Grossman, M.E., Bickers, D.R., Poh-Fitzpatrick, M.B., Deleo, V.A. and Harber, L.C. (1979). Porphyria cutanea tarda: Clinical and laboratory findings in 40 patients. *American Journal of Medicine* **67**, 277–286.

Hahn, M.E., Gasiewicz, T.A., Linko, P. and Goldstein J.A. (1988). The role of the Ah locus in hexachlorobenzene-induced porphyria: Studies in congenic C57BL/6J mice. *Biochemical Journal* **254**, 245–254.

Hanstein, W.G., Sacks, P.V. and Muller-Eberhard, U. (1975). Properties of liver mitochondria from iron-loaded rats. *Biochemical and Biophysical Research Communications* **67**, 1175–1184.

Hanstein, W.G., Heitmann, T.D., Sandy, A., Biesterfeldt, H.L., Liem, H.M. and Muller-Eberhard, U. (1981). Effects of hexachlorobenzene and iron loading on rat liver mitochondria. *Biochimica et Biophysica Acta* **678**, 293–299.

Jackson, A.H., Sancovich, H.A. and Ferramola, A.M. (1980). Synthetic and biosynthetic studies of porphyrins. III. Structures of the intermediates between uroporphyrinogen III and coproporphyrinogen III: Synthesis of fourteen heptacarboxylic, hexacarboxylic, and pentacarboxylic porphyrins related to uroporphyrin III. *Bioorganic Chemistry* **9**, 71–120.

Jordan, P.M. (1990). Biosynthesis of 5-aminolevulinic acid and its transformation into coproporphyrinogen in animals and bacteria. In *Biosynthesis of Heme and Chlorophylls* (Edited by Dailey, H.A.), pp. 55–121. McGraw-Hill, New York.

Kondo, M. and Shimuzu, Y. (1986). The effects of ethanol, estrogen and hexachlorobenzene on the activities of hepatic delta-aminolevulinate synthase, delta-aminolevulinate dehydratase, and uroporphyrinogen decarboxylase in male rats. *Archives of Toxicology* **59**, 141–145.

Kushner, J.P. (1982). The enzymatic defect in porphyria cutanea tarda. *New England Journal of Medicine* **306**, 799–800.

Kushner, J.P., Barbuto, A.J. and Lee, G.R. (1976). An inherited enzymatic defect in porphyria cutanea tarda: Decreased uroporphyrinogen decarboxylase activity. *Journal of Clinical Investigation* **58**, 1089–1097.

Kushner, J.P., Edwards, C.Q., Dadone, M.M. and Skolnick, M.H. (1985). Heterozygosity for HLA-linked hemochromatosis as a likely cause of the hepatic siderosis associated with sporadic porphyria cutanea tarda. *Gastroenterology* **88**, 1232–1238.

Lambrecht, R., Sinclair, P., Bement, W., Sinclair, J., Carpenter, H., Buhler, D., Urquhart, A. and Elder, G. (1988). Hepatic uroporphyrinogen decarboxylase activity in cultured chick-embryo hepatocytes and in Japanese quail and mice treated with polyhalogenated aromatic compounds. *Biochemical Journal* **253**, 131–138.

Lim, H.W. and Gigli, I. (1981). Role of complement in porphyrin-induced photosensitivity. *Journal of Investigative Dermatology* **76**, 4–9.

Lim, H.W., Perez, H.D., Goldstein, I.M. and Gigli, I. (1981). Complement-derived chemotactic activity is generated in human serum containing uroporphyrin after irradiation with 405 nm light. *Journal of Clinical Investigation* **67**, 1072–1077.

Marks, G.S., McCluskey, S.A., Mackie, J.E., Riddick, D.S. and James, C.A. (1989). Interaction of chemicals with cytochrome P-450: Implications for the porphyrinogenicity of drugs. *Clinical Biochemistry* **22**, 169–175.

Mauzerall, D. and Granick, S. (1958). Porphyrin biosynthesis of erythrocytes. III. Uroporphyrinogen and its decarboxylase. *Journal of Biological Chemistry* **232**, 1141–1162.

McColl, K.E.L., Thompson, G.G., Moore, M.R. and Goldberg, A. (1980). Acute ethanol ingestion and haem biosynthesis in healthy subjects. *European Journal of Clinical Investigation* **10**, 107–112.

McColl, K.E.L., Moore, M.R., Thompson, G.G. and Goldberg, A. (1981). Abnormal haem biosynthesis in chronic alcoholics. *European Journal of Clinical Investigation* **11**, 461–468.

McLellan, T., Pryor, M.A., Kushner, J.P., Eddy, R.L. and Shows, T.B. (1985). Assignment of uroporphyrinogen decarboxylase (UROD) to the pter-p21 region of human chromosome 1. *Cytogenetics and Cell Genetics* **39**, 224–227.

Moore, M.R., Beattie, A.D., Thompson, G.G. and Goldberg, A. (1971). Depression of δ-aminolevulinic acid dehydratase activity by ethanol in man and rat. *Clinical Science* **40**, 81–88.

Moore, M.R., McColl, K.E.L. and Goldberg, A. (1984). The effects of alcohol on porphyrin biosynthesis and metabolism. In *Clinical Biochemistry of Alcoholism* (Edited by Rosalki, S.B.), pp. 161–187. Churchill Livingstone, Edinburgh.

Moore, M.R., McColl, K.E.L., Rimington, C. and Goldberg, A. (1987). *Disorders of Porphyrin Metabolism.* Plenum Press, New York.

Mukerji, S.K. and Pimstone, N.R. (1986). *In vitro* studies of the mechanism of inhibition of rat liver uroporphyrinogen decarboxylase activity by ferrous iron under anaerobic conditions. *Archives of Biochemistry and Biophysics* **244**, 619–629.

Mukerji, S.K., Pimstone, N.R. and Tan, K.T. (1985). A potential biochemical explanation for the genesis of porphyria cutanea tarda. *FEBS Letters* **189**, 217–220.

Nordmann, Y. and Deybach, J.-C. (1990). Human hereditary porphyrias. In *Biosynthesis of Heme and Chlorophylls* (Edited by Dailey, H.A.), pp. 491–542. McGraw-Hill, New York.

Pigatto, P.D., Polenghi, M.M., Altomare, G.F., Giacchetti, A., Cirillo, R. and Finzi, A.F. (1986). Complement cleavage products in the phototoxic reaction of porphyria cutanea tarda. *British Journal of Dermatology* **114**, 567–573.

Poh-Fitzpatrick, M.B. (1985). Porphyrin sensitised cutaneous photosensitivity – Pathogenesis and treatment. In *Porphyria: Clinics in Dermatology* (Edited by Disler P.B. and Moore M.R.), pp. 41–82. Lippincott, Philadelphia.

Powell, L.W. (1992). Haemochromatosis and related iron storage diseases. In *Wright's Liver and Biliary Disease* (Edited by Millward-Sadler, G.H., Wright, R. and Arthur, M.J.P.), pp. 976–994. W.B. Saunders, London.

Roberts, A.G., Elder, G.H., Newcombe, R.G., De Salamanca, R.E. and Munoz, J.J. (1988). Heterogeneity of familial porphyria cutanea tarda. *Journal of Medical Genetics* **10**, 669–676.

Romana, M., Dubart, A., Beaupain, D., Chabret, C., Goossens, M. and Romeo, P.-H. (1987). Structure of the gene for human uroporphyrinogen decarboxylase. *Nucleic Acid Research* **15**, 7343–7353.

Romeo, P.H., Raich, N., Dubart, A., Beaupain, D., Pryor, M., Kushner, J., Cohen-Solal, M. and Goossens, M. (1986). Molecular cloning and nucleotide sequence of a complete human uroporphyrinogen decarboxylase cDNA. *Journal of Biological Chemistry* **261**, 9825–9831.

Seymour, D.G., Elder, G.H., Fryer, A., Jacobs, A. and Williams, G.T. (1990). Porphyria cutanea tarda and haemochromatosis: a family study. *Gut* **31**, 719–721.

Shemin, D. (1976). 5-Aminolevulinic acid dehydratase: Structure, function and mechanism. *Philosophical Transactions of the Royal Society of London B***273**, 109–115.

Sieg, I., Doss, M.O., Kandels, H. and Schneider, J. (1991). Effect of alcohol on δ-aminolevulinic acid dehydratase and porphyrin metabolism in man. *Clinica Chemica Acta* **202**, 211–218.

Siersema, P.D., van Helvoirt, P., Ketelaars, D.A.M. *et al.* (1991). Iron and uroporphyrin in hepatocytes of inbred mice in experimental porphyria: A biochemical and morphological study. *Hepatology* **14**, 1179–1188.

Sinclair, P.R., Bement, W.J., Bonkovsky, H.L. and Sinclair, J.F. (1984). Inhibition of uroporphyrinogen decarboxylase by halogenated biphenyls in chick hepatocyte cultures. *Biochemical Journal* **222**, 737–748.

Sinclair, P.R., Bement, W., Bonkovsky, H.L., Lambrecht, R.W., Frezze, J.E., Sinclair, J.F., Urquhart, A.J. and Elder, G.H. (1986). Uroporphyrin accumulation produced by halogenated biphenyls in chick embryo hepatocytes: Reversal of the accumulation by piperonyl butoxide. *Biochemical Journal* **237**, 61–73.

Sinclair, P., Lambrecht, R. and Sinclair, J. (1987). Evidence for cytochrome P-450 mediated oxidation of uroporphyrinogen by cell-free liver extracts from chick embryos treated with 3-methylcholanthrene. *Biochemical and Biophysical Research Communications* **146**, 1324–1329.

Sinclair, P.R., Bement, W.J., Lambrecht, R.W., Jacobs, J.M. and Sinclair, J.F. (1989). Uroporphyria caused by acetone and 5-aminolevulinic acid in iron-loaded mice. *Biochemical Pharmacology* **38**, 4341–4344.

Smith, A.G. and Francis, J.E. (1981). Investigations of rat liver uroporphyrinogen decarboxylase. *Biochemical Journal* **195**, 241–250.

Smith, A.G. and Francis, J.E. (1987). Chemically induced formation of an inhibitor of hepatic uroporphyrinogen decarboxylase in inbred mice with iron overload. *Biochemical Journal* **246**, 221–226.

Smith, A.G., Francis, J.E., Walters, D.G. and Lake, B.G. (1990). Protection against iron-induced uroporphyria in C57BL/10ScSn mice by the peroxisome proliferator nafenopin. *Biochemical Pharmacology* **40**, 2564–2568.

Taljaard, J.J.F., Shanley, B.C., Deppe, W.M. and Joubert, S.M. (1972). Porphyrin metabolism in experimental hepatic siderosis in the rat. II. Combined effect of iron overload and hexachlorobenzene. *British Journal of Haematology* **23**, 513–519.

Tsukamoto, I., Yoshinaga, T. and Sano, S. (1979). The role of zinc with special reference to the essential thiol groups in δ-aminolevulinic acid dehydratase of bovine liver. *Biochimica et Biophysica Acta* **570**, 167–178.

Urquhart, A.J., Elder, G.H., Roberts, A.G., Lambrecht, R.W., Sinclair, P.R., Bement, W.J., Gorman, N. and Sinclair, J.A. (1988). Uroporphyria produced in mice by 20-methylcholanthrene and 5-aminolaevulinic acid. *Biochemical Journal* **253**, 357–362.

Visser, O., Van den Berg, J.W.O., Edixhoven-Bosdijk, A., Koole-Lesuis, R., Rietveld, T. and Wilson, J.H.P. (1989). Development of hexachlorobenzene porphyria in rats: Time sequence and relationship with lipid peroxidation. *Food and Chemical Toxicology* **27**, 317–321.

Part VI
Experimental Studies on Alcohol and the Liver

14 Effect of alcohol on hepatic blood flow and the microvasculature of the liver

Robert S. McCuskey

Introduction

Alcohol ingestion produces increased hepatic oxygen consumption, fatty liver, hepatomegaly, hepatocellular damage and, with prolonged consumption, liver injury may progress to alcoholic hepatitis, fibrosis and cirrhosis. In recent years, an important role has been demonstrated for perisinusoidal cells, cytokines, free radicals and eicosanoids in the pathophysiology of liver injury resulting from alcohol, eithor alone or in combination with gut-derived endotoxin, other hepatotoxins or infection. Alterations in hepatic blood flow, particularly in the microcirculation, accompany these responses. The purpose of this chapter is to summarize the current knowledge of the pathophysiology of alcohol on the circulation of blood through the liver; this will be preceded by an overview of the hepatic circulation and microvasculature in health.

Hepatic circulation and microvascular system

The mammalian liver has a dual blood supply. Approximately 80 percent of the blood entering the liver is poorly oxygenated venous blood supplied by the portal vein, whereas the remainder is well oxyge-

nated and supplied by the hepatic artery. These blood vessels enter at the hilum (porta hepatis), where efferent bile ducts as well as lymphatics also exit the organ. The venous drainage of the liver courses independent of the above structures to drain into the inferior vena cava near the diaphragm.

Within the liver, distributing branches of the portal vein and hepatic artery course in parallel and, after repeated branching, terminal branches of these vessels (portal venules and hepatic arterioles) supply blood to the hepatic sinusoids. The sinusoids are the principal vessels involved in transvascular exchange between the blood and the parenchymal cells. Branches of hepatic arterioles also supply the peribiliary plexus which, in turn, drains into the sinusoids. Because all these vessels are independently contractile, the sinusoids receive a varying mixture of portal venous and hepatic arterial blood (Knisely *et al.* 1948; Irwin and MacDonald 1953; McCuskey 1966, 1986; Bloch 1970). Portal and arterial blood flowing through the sinusoids is collected in small branches of hepatic veins termed central venules or terminal hepatic venules (see below), through which the blood is returned through larger hepatic veins to the inferior vena cava. Lymphatic vessels originate as blind-ending capillaries in the connective tissue spaces (portal tracts) associated with the portal veins and hepatic arteries. The fluid contained in these lymphatics flows towards the hepatic hilus and eventually into the cisternae chyli.

The hepatic microvascular system comprises all of the intrahepatic vessels having internal diameters less than 300 μm. It thus includes all blood and lymphatic vessels immediately involved in the delivery and removal of fluids to and from the hepatic parenchyma, namely portal venules, hepatic arterioles, sinusoids, central venules and lymphatics. The organization of these vessels into structural or functional units related to liver function and disease has been the subject of considerable debate during the past century, however, none of the following proposed concepts are mutually exclusive.

The classic hepatic lobule (Kiernan 1883) is a polygonal structure bounded at its periphery by terminal branches of the hepatic artery and portal vein, plus accompanying bile ducts, lymphatics, and nerves coursing in the portal tract. The axis of the lobule is the central venule, which is the origin of hepatic venous drainage. The peripheral boundaries of these lobules are poorly defined in most species, including man. As a result, considerable sinusoidal anastomoses occur between adjacent lobules, and thus the blood collected by each central venule is supplied by several portal venules. For these reasons and because of intralobular regional differences in oxygenation, metabolic functions, and responses to some diseases, an acinar concept was proposed (Rappaport *et al.* 1954; Rappaport 1973) to define the hepatic functional unit.

The hepatic acinus is a unit having no distinct morphologic boundaries. Its axis is a portal tract containing a terminal portal venule and hepatic arteriole. The peripheral boundary is circumscribed by an imaginary line connecting the neighbouring terminal hepatic venules (central venules of the classic lobule), which collect blood from sinusoids supplied by a portal venule and hepatic arteriole forming the stem or axis of the acinus. Contained within the acinus are three zones, each having different levels of oxygenation and metabolic function. Although the acinar concept has been widely accepted, it fails to account for those mammalian species (e.g. pig, seal) that have connective tissue boundaries circumscribing classic lobules. Additional inconsistencies increasingly have been identified in three-dimensional studies of metabolic heterogeneity and microvascular structure (Sasse 1986; Teutsch 1986, 1988; McCuskey 1987; Lamers *et al.* 1989a, b; Quistorff and Romert 1989; Quistorff 1990; Ekataksin and Wake 1991; Ekataksin *et al.* 1992; Teutsch *et al.* 1992).

Currently, the concept of subunits of the classic lobule forming functional units is the most consistent with existing evidence (Matsumoto and Kawakami 1982; Ekataksin and Wake 1991; Ekataksin *et al.* 1992, 1993a, b, c). The original concept (Matsumoto and Kawakami 1982) demonstrated that each "classic" lobule consists of several "primary" lobules. Each primary lobule is cone-shaped, having its convex surface at the periphery of the classic lobule supplied by terminal branches of

portal venules and hepatic arterioles and its apex at the centre of the classic lobule drained by a central (terminal hepatic) venule. Recently, these "primary lobules" were renamed hepatic microvascular subunits (HMS), which were demonstrated to consist of a group of sinusoids supplied by a single inlet venule and its associated termination of a branch of the hepatic arteriole from the adjacent portal space (Ekataksin and Wake 1991; Ekataksin *et al.* 1992, 1993c). Further confirmation of this HMS concept was very recently obtained by studying their development in neonatal livers (Ekataksin *et al.* 1993a, b).

Terminal portal venules contribute·to a "vascular septum" formed by themselves and the sinusoids that intervene between parallel terminal portal venules originating from the same distributing portal venule (Matusumoto and Kawakami 1982). A nodal point or mid-septal point in the vascular septum also exists between the approximated tips of terminal portal venules originating from neighbouring, parallel distributing portal venules coursing on opposing sides of the lobule. That this vascular septum functions as a "watershed" to supply sinusoids of adjacent lobules (Matsumoto and Kawakami 1982) has been confirmed by *in vivo* microscopy (McCuskey 1987; Ekataksin *et al.* 1992, 1993c), as has the mid-septal or nodal point being an area of marginal or limited blood flow. Hepatocellular metabolic gradients also have demonstrated to conform to this proposed functional-unit concept (Teutsch 1986, 1988; Teutsch *et al.* 1992).

Sinusoids

The principal site for regulating blood flow and solute exchange occurs in the sinusoid network, which exhibits structural and functional heterogeneity. The structure of the hepatic sinusoid is unique; in all mammalian livers studied to date, it is composed of endothelial cells, Kupffer cells and perisinusoidal cells (Wisse 1977; Fahimi 1982; Jones 1982; Wisse *et al.* 1983). Additional cells may be present, most notably mast cells (McCuskey 1989) and "pit" cells which are thought to be natural killer cells (Kaneda *et al.* 1983).

The endothelial cells have an attenuated cytoplasm that is highly fenestrated. Most of the fenestrae are 100–150 nm in diameter and tend to be clustered together to form sieve plates; none of the fenestrae are bridged by diaphragms. The endothelial fenestrae are dynamic structures whose diameters are affected by luminal blood pressure, vasoactive substances, drugs and toxins, including alcohol (Boler and Bibighaus 1967; Napanitaya *et al.* 1976; Frenzel *et al.* 1977; Fraser *et al.* 1980a, b; McCuskey *et al.* 1983; Wisse *et al.* 1985; Oda *et al.* 1987a, b, 1990; see also Chapter 15). Phagocytic Kupffer cells are attached to the luminal surface of the endothelium. These cells are also a source of a variety of vasoactive substances that may influence sinusoidal blood flow and exchange processes through their action on sinusoid lining cells. Beneficial and toxic mediators are also produced by Kupffer cells; these substances participate in non-specific host defence mechanisms, as well as liver injury (McCuskey *et al.* 1982, 1987; Decker 1989, 1990). Phagocytosis and the release of these various substances are thought to be modulated in part by gut-derived endotoxins; Kupffer cells are the principal cells responsible for clearance of these bacterial products (Morrison and Ulevitch 1978; Mathison and Ulevitch 1979; Rosenstreich and Vogel 1980; Ruiter *et al.* 1981; McCuskey *et al.* 1982, 1987; Decker 1989, 1990) that are normally present in portal blood. As a result, Kupffer cell dysfunction and endotoxin have been implicated in the pathophysiology of a variety of liver diseases, including those elicited by alcohol (Nolan and Camara 1982; McCuskey *et al.* 1987; Nolan 1989; see also Chapter 6).

External to the endothelium, perisinusoidal cells (fat-storing cells or Ito cells) are located in the perisinusoidal space of Disse. The thin, multiple cytoplasmic processes of the Ito cells course though the perisinusoidal space and embrace the abluminal surfaces of the endothelium. In health, little or no basal lamina and collagen are associated with the sinusoidal endothelium. As a result, the sinusoid wall is a highly permeable structure that permits continuity of plasma between the blood and the hepatocyte. As alcoholic liver disease progresses basement membrane-like material and collagen fibrils accumulate in the perisinusoidal space, resulting in "capillarization" of the sinusoid and impaired transvascular exchange (LeBail *et al.* 1990; see Chapters 3 and 4). The perisinusoidal cells are thought to be the cells responsible for the synthesis of this material.

The perisinusoidal space is thought by some to function as a lymphatic space that channels plasma to the true lymphatics coursing in the portal tract. Although this hypothesis would help to explain the large efflux of lymph from the liver, it may not be valid. Anatomic connections between the space of Disse and the portal tract have not been identified (Niiro and O'Morchoe 1986). Furthermore, plasma

flow in the space of Disse would have to occur against a pressure gradient if one assumes equalization of pressure between the sinusoid and the space of Disse caused by the porosity of the sinusoid wall. However, such retrograde flow might occur through the influence of leucocytes massaging the endothelium to create a roller-pump effect (Wisse *et al.* 1985; Wisse and McCuskey 1986).

Microvascular heterogeneity

Near their origins from portal venules and hepatic arterioles, sinusoids are slightly narrower as well as being tortuous and anastomotic forming interconnecting polygonal networks; farther away from the portal venules the sinusoids become organized as parallel vessels that terminate in central venules (terminal hepatic venules) (Hase and Brim 1966; Miller *et al.* 1979; Kardon and Kessel 1980; Matsumoto and Kawakami 1982; Wisse *et al.* 1983, 1985). Short intersinusoidal sinusoids connect adjacent parallel sinusoids (McCuskey 1966). The periportal tortuous, anastomotic network of sinusoids becomes almost non-existent at the point in the vascular septum formed by sinusoids that intervene between terminal portal venules. As a result, a "sickle-shaped" zone of tortuous, anastomotic sinusoids is formed, which is thought to provide a haemodynamically equipotential line at its edge where the parallel sinusoids begin (Matsumoto and Kawakami 1982). The latter converge in a radial fashion to terminate in the central venule. That a sickle-shaped flow front exists has also been demonstrated by *in vivo* microscopy by monitoring the inflow of dye injected into the portal vein (McCuskey 1987; Ekataksin *et al.* 1992, 1993c).

In the periportal area, the volume of liver occupied by sinusoids is greater than that surrounding central venules (Miller *et al.* 1979; Conway *et al.* 1985). However, because of the smaller size and anastomotic nature of the periportal sinusoids, the surface available for exchange in this area (surface/volume ratio) is greater than in centrilobular sinusoids (Miller *et al.* 1979; Conway *et al.* 1985). Kupffer cells are also more numerous in the periportal region (Dimlich *et al.* 1982; Sleyster and Knook 1982; McCuskey *et al.* 1984). The size and pattern of distribution of endothelial fenestrae differs along the length of the sinusoid (Wisse *et al.* 1983, 1985). At the portal end, the fenestrae are larger but comprise less of the endothelial surface area than they do in the pericentral region (Wisse *et al.* 1983,

1985). The functional significance of these regional differences is unclear, but it is tempting to relate them to the functional metabolic heterogeneity that has been demonstrated for hepatocytes in different regions of the lobule (Gumucio and Miller 1982; Jungermann and Katz 1982; Sleyster and Knook 1982; Teutsch 1986, 1988). This, in turn, may depend on the recognized portal-to-central intra-lobular oxygen gradient (Lemasters *et al*. 1981).

Intrahepatic regulation of blood flow

Portal venules and central venules contain limited amounts of smooth muscle in their walls relative to their luminal size, but nevertheless are contractile and respond to pharmacologic agents (reviewed in McCuskey and Reilly 1993). Hepatic arterioles are more responsive because of a complete investment of smooth muscle and relatively small lumens. However, the principal intrahepatic site for the regulation of blood flow resides in the sinusoid where the major blood pressure drop occurs in the liver (Nakata *et al*. 1961; McCuskey 1966, 1971; Nakata 1967; Rappaport 1977). Blood pressures in portal and central venules have been measured to be about 6–7 cm H_2O and 1.5–3.0 cm H_2O, respectively (Nakata 1967), while arterial blood intermittently enters the sinusoid at pressures ranging from 12–25 cm H_2O (Rappaport 1977).

In the sinusoids, the endothelial cells and Kupffer cells are responsive to a wide variety of pharmacody-namic substances. By contracting (or swelling), they may selectively reduce the patency of the sinusoid lumen, thereby altering the rate and distribution of blood flow (McCuskey 1966, 1971). The partici-pation of perisinusoidal cells in regulating sinusoidal diameter has yet to be established, although studies *in vitro* have demonstrated contractile responses (Sakamoto 1991; Pinznai *et al*. 1992), while one *in vivo* microscopic report is strongly suggestive (Zhang *et al*. 1994). It should be noted, however, that all three sinusoidal cell types contain filaments, tubules and contractile proteins suggestive of con-tractile activity (Oda *et al*. 1987b).

Because of these structures, blood flow through individual sinusoids is variable. The average veloc-ity of erythrocyte flow in sinusoids of the rat has been measured to range between 25 and 300 μm/sec, with the volumetric rate of flow averaging 6.0 μl/sec (Koo *et al*. 1976; Koo and Liang 1979; Cilento *et al*. 1981; Koo 1987; Sherman and Fisher 1987). The wide variations in flow are due to the structural features previously described for sinusoids and also are due to intermittent arterial inflow into the sinus-oids (Bloch 1955; McCuskey 1966; Rappaport 1977). In addition, at sites where the lumen is narrowed by the bulging, nuclear regions of sinus-oidal lining cells, flow may be impeded by leuco-cytes that transiently plug the vessel and obstruct flow (Wisse *et al*. 1985, 1986). Transient leucocyte plugging is more frequent in the narrower and more tortuous periportal sinusoids than in the wider, more parallel sinusoids of the centrilobular region. The more plastic erythrocytes usually flow easily through such sites unless the lumen is reduced to near zero.

Effect of alcohol on hepatic blood flow and the microvasculature

Acutely administered alcohol generally increases hepatic blood flow (Castenfors *et al*. 1960; Shaw *et al*. 1977; Orrego and Carmichael 1992). The acute vasodilator effect of alcohol is not thought to be a result of vascular actions of metabolites of alcohol, acetaldehyde or acetate (Altura and Gebrewold 1981; Altura and Altura 1982; Carmichael *et al*. 1988; Orrego *et al*. 1988), but is suggested to be due to adenosine and an increase in splanchnic blood flow (Carmichael *et al*. 1988). Very recently, how-ever, high doses of alcohol in the perfused liver have been shown to have a vasoconstrictive effect on the intrahepatic vasculature followed by a slow "escape" phase thought to be due initially to the release of endothelin, a potent vasoconstrictor, and the sub-sequent release of the vasodilator, nitric oxide (Oshita *et al*. 1992a, b, 1993). Chronic ingestion of alcohol results in reduced flow and portal hyper-tension (Mezey 1982), which has been attributed to hepatocellular swelling since it was seen in the absence of perisinusoidal and perivenular collagen formation (Blendis *et al*. 1982; Vidins *et al*. 1985). More recently, it has been suggested that the portal hypertension may also be due to a dominant action of endothelin over nitric oxide (Oshita *et al*. 1992b, 1993).

At the microcirculatory level, acute, oral adminis-tration of alcohol to rats increases both portal and hepatic arterial blood flow resulting in an average net increase in the velocity of erythrocyte flow through the sinusoids (Sato *et al*. 1987a; Sherman *et al*. 1987). The increased flow in the sinusoids, however, was heterogeneous, with some sinusoids exhibiting dramatic increases in cellular velocity while others had little or no increase and some a decrease (Sherman and Fisher 1987). As a result, some perivenular areas became hypoxic while others exhibited an increase in oxygenation (Sato *et al.* 1987a, b). The reasons for this heterogeneity are not clear but the appearance of "fast" sinusoids suggests "arterialized" vessels due to the dilation of "arterio-sinus twigs", which supply scattered sinusoids at the periphery of the lobule (Sherman *et al.* 1987). Reduced flow in other sinusoids may have been due to hepatocellular swelling and/or plugging of some sinusoids by formed blood elements. In addition, alcohol may have elicited constriction of some sinusoids through the local release of vasoactive substances (e.g. from Kupffer cells – see below) or the modification of the action of such substances. Such alterations in vascular responsiveness to agonists in the presence of alcohol have been demonstrated in other microvascular beds (Altura and Altura 1982, 1983), where alcohol interacts with prostaglandins in bizarre ways and which is dose-dependent. At low doses of alcohol, vascular responses to agonists can be either potentiated or attenuated while high doses usually are depressive. Similar dose-dependent interactions with adrenergic, cholinergic and aminergic substances have also been reported (reviewed by Altura and Altura 1982).

Acutely administered alcohol also results in a dose-dependent increase in leucocyte adhesion and endothelial cell swelling in the sinusoids (Eguchi *et al.* 1991a; McCuskey 1991a, b; McCuskey *et al.* 1991b, 1993b). Activation of Kupffer cells is elicited at low doses of alcohol while depression occurs at high alcohol doses and with chronic exposure (Abril *et al.* 1991; Jolley *et al.* 1991, 1993; Nishida *et al.* 1992a; McCuskey *et al.* 1993b). The acute responses to alcohol are exacerbated in the presence of endotoxaemia and abolished or minimized with anti-TNFα, suggesting that TNFα is a primary mediator initiating these events either directly or through an intermediary substance, e.g. IL-1 (Eguchi *et al.* 1991a, b). Subsequently, free radicals, such as superoxide derived from activated leucocytes plugging the sinusoids, may play a role in exacerbating liver injury (Bautista and Spitzer 1992). None of the above responses were seen in alcohol-treated endotoxin-resistant mice (C$_3$H/HeJ). Taken together, these data suggest a role for endotoxin in alcohol-induced hepatic injury (McCuskey *et al.* 1990; Eguchi *et al.* 1991a; McCuskey 1991b). Further support is provided by the demonstration that alcohol exacerbates the progression of sepsis by

accelerating the elevation of plasma endotoxin levels, the time to achieve lethality, as well as the hepatic microvascular inflammatory response as evidenced by increased leucocyte adhesion and plugging of sinusoids, perhaps due to increased TNFα release from the initially activated Kupffer cells (McCuskey *et al.* 1993b; Nishida *et al.* 1994a). Alcohol also enhances the hepatotoxic effects of cocaine both in mice (see Chapter 17) and, to a lesser extent, in rats, with a loss of Kupffer cells in both species and assumption of phagocytic function by sinusoidal endothelial cells (McCuskey *et al.* 1991a, b; Earnest *et al.* 1993). The latter response, as well as leucocyte adhesion, may be due to IL-1, since this cytokine induces similar changes within 1 h after administration (McCuskey *et al.* 1991b; Nishida *et al.* 1993).

The effects of long-term exposure to alcohol on the hepatic microcirculation also has been studied, but to a lesser extent (McCuskey *et al.* 1991a, 1993a, b; Nishida *et al.* 1992; Earnest *et al.* 1993). The phagocytic activity of Kupffer cells and changes in the hepatic microcirculation were examined up to 24 weeks after mice and rats had been maintained on ethanol-containing liquid diets. The phagocytic activity of Kupffer cells showed a significant decrease in the alcohol-treated animals, but the blood flow of the sinusoids was relatively normal in both groups with little or no leucocyte plugging or sticking in the sinusoids or central venules. These results suggest that long-term alcohol suppresses the release and/or production of mediators (e.g. TNF and IL-1) that alter the hepatic microcirculation following acutely administered alcohol. It should be noted, however, that while these animals had fatty livers, there was no significant increase in collagen deposition along the sinusoids or infiltration of leucocytes into the parenchyma.

Unfortunately, attempts to provide a small animal model of alcoholic fibrosis and cirrhosis have had only limited success. As a result, most microcirculatory studies of the fibrotic and/or cirrhotic liver have been in chemically induced models. During fibrosis induced by a choline-deficient diet and cirrhosis produced by administering carbon tetrachloride (CCl$_4$), there is a dilation of central venules (Koo *et al.* 1976; Koo and Liang 1976; Sherman and Fisher 1987). While the average velocity of cellular flow in sinusoids did not increase significantly in livers with moderate fibrosis, there was a marked increase in the average flow velocities in sinusoids and central venules of cirrhotic livers (Koo *et al.* 1976; Koo and Liang 1976; Sherman and Fisher 1987). In large part, this was due to the appearance of "fast" sinusoids which dramatically increased in proportion in cirrhotic livers compared with controls. As with acute alcohol treatment, these "fast" sinusoids may function as intrahepatic shunts (Sherman and Fisher 1987), since these appeared to represent "arterialized" vessels; further support for this interpretation is that ligation of the hepatic artery abolished the presence of such "fast" sinusoids (Koo *et al.* 1976). The dilation of central venules is probably a reflection of increased flow and not the result of downstream distortion or stenosis of hepatic veins, since pressures in central venules do not rise significantly under these conditions and the pressure gradient between cenral venules and the vena cava remains unchanged (Shibayama and Nakata 1985). This supports the view that alterations in the sinusoids are responsible for a major component of the portal hypertension. However, pressures in terminal portal venules also rise significantly under these conditions, so that attributing increased flow to a hyperdynamic splanchnic circulation can not be completely discounted.

Alcohol, Kupffer cell function and hepatic injury

Following the ingestion of alcohol, significant alterations occur in host defence mechanisms, including depressed reticuloendothelial function as well as altered lymphocyte, granulocyte and platelet functions, all of which increase the host's susceptibility to infection (Louria 1963; Nolan 1965; Adams and Jordan 1984; see also Chapter 6). Kupffer cells are the largest cell population within the reticuloendothelial system. Several studies have demonstrated that Kupffer cell function is affected by alcohol in both experimental animals and man. Clearance of micro-aggregated albumin and endotoxin is depressed in rats following both acute and chronic administration of alcohol (Ali and Nolan 1967; Nolan *et al.* 1980; Nolan and Camara 1982). Acute human alcoholics with no evidence of liver disease have also demonstrated a depressed reticuloendothelial system which returns to normal several days following alcohol withdrawal (Liu 1979). Furthermore, reticuloendothelial system depression has been demonstrated by reduced clearance of micro-aggregated albumin (Cooksley *et al.* 1973), and the lack of a concentration gradient of immune complexes between portal and hepatic veins (Kaufman *et al.* 1982). Finally, elevated levels of systemic, circu-

lating endotoxin have also been reported in humans intoxicated with alcohol (Bode *et al.* 1987) as well as during alcoholic liver disease (Liu 1979; Nolan and Camara 1982; Bhagwandeen *et al.* 1987), suggesting spill-over of gut-derived endotoxin due to alcohol-depressed clearance by hepatic Kupffer cells. As a result, Kupffer cell dysfunction and endotoxin have been implicated in the aetiology of alcoholic liver disease (Ali and Nolan 1967; Cooksley *et al.* 1973; Liu 1979; Nolan *et al.* 1980; Nolan and Camara 1982). This concept is further supported by animal studies, which demonstrated that, in the presence of alcohol, normally innocuous doses of endotoxin become toxic and result in severe liver damage (Cooksley *et al.* 1973; Bhagwandeen *et al.* 1987; Shibayama *et al.* 1991; see also Chapters 4 and 6). Hypoxia, such as reported for centrilobular hepatocytes in rats acutely dosed with alcohol (Sato *et al.* 1987a; see also Chapters 3 and 19), also potentiates the hepatotoxicity of endotoxin (Shibayama 1987).

Kupffer cells are the principal site for the removal of circulating endotoxins from the blood (Mathison and Ulevitch 1979; Mairer and Ulevitch 1981; Ruiter *et al.* 1981). Following the endocytosis of endotoxin, a variety of toxic and beneficial mediators are released from Kupffer cells, e.g. TNFα, IL-1, eicosanoids and reactive free radicals (for a more detailed discussion, see Chapter 6). These cytokines are thought to participate in the host response to endotoxin (reviewed in McCuskey 1987; Decker 1989, 1990; Wake *et al.* 1989), and has led to the concept of macrophages playing a central role in the host response to endotoxin (reviewed in McCuskey *et al.* 1987, 1991b, 1993b; Decker 1989, 1990; Wake *et al.* 1989). As indicated above, a variety of evidence also implicates Kupffer cells and endotoxin in the aetiology of alcoholic liver disease (Nolan *et al.* 1980; Nolan and Camara 1982; Liehr 1983; Bhagwandeen *et al.* 1987), as well as hepatic microvascular and parenchymal dysfunction during sepsis and shock (Cooksley *et al.* 1973; Munford 1978; Kaufman *et al.* 1982; Bode *et al.* 1987; McCuskey *et al.* 1993b; Nishida *et al.* 1994a). Since the liver receives 25 percent of the cardiac output in mammals, mechanisms which limit or modify hepatic blood flow may have profound effects on venous return to the heart as well as in influencing blood flow and parenchymal function in the liver and in extrahepatic splanchnic viscera.

Kupffer cell function is impaired in liver disease. Studies of experimental alcoholic liver disease in rats showed that the lysozyme content of Kupffer cells is decreased (Kelly *et al.* 1989). Human monocytes also showed both a decrease in lysozyme content and secretion when they were treated *in vitro* with alcohol (McCarthy *et al.* 1990). Kupffer cells from chronic alcohol-fed rats demonstrated markedly depressed phagocytic capacity (Shiratori *et al.* 1989).

Nitric oxide is a potent pharmacodynamic substance produced in the liver by both Kupffer cells (Billiar *et al.* 1989) and hepatocytes (Curran *et al.* 1989) and perhaps by sinusoidal endothelial cells (Salvemini *et al.* 1990). Nitric oxide synthetase exists in both constitutive (endothelial) and inducible (macrophage) forms (Moncada *et al.* 1991; Nathan 1992). Nitric oxide's myriad functions include inhibition of vascular smooth muscle contraction, platelet aggregation and adherence, protein synthesis in macrophages and hepatocytes, as well as stimulating chemotaxis by neutrophils and signalling by neurotransmitters (Moncada *et al.* 1991; Nathan 1992). Recent evidence suggests that the synthesis of nitric oxide in the liver has a protective function preventing hepatic injury during the inflammatory response (Billiar *et al.* 1990) and following ethanol administration (Oshita *et al.* 1992a, c, 1993). Inhibition of nitric oxide synthesis during endotoxaemia promotes intrahepatic thrombosis and an oxygen radical-mediated hepatic injury (Hambrecht *et al.* 1992). High levels of nitric oxide have also been associated with endotoxaemia in septic patients (Ochoa *et al.* 1991), and both protective and pathological roles for nitric oxide have been reported in endotoxin shock (Wright *et al.* 1992) as well as in ischaemia/reperfusion injury (Carey *et al.* 1992). In other microvascular beds, nitric oxide has been shown to be an endogenous modulator of leucocyte adhesion (Kubes *et al.* 1991). Nitric oxide is released from bovine aortic endothelial cells stimulated with endotoxin (Salvemini *et al.* 1990) and appears to play a role in maintaining vascular integrity in endotoxin-induced acute intestinal damage (Hutcheson *et al.* 1992). Nitric oxide has been implicated in the regulation of intrahepatic vascular tone following infusion of alcohol (Hutcheson *et al.* 1992; Oshita *et al.* 1992a, b; 1993); very recently, nitric oxide has been demonstrated to affect hepatic sinusoid diameter, blood flow and leucocyte adherence. Inhibition of nitric oxide expression leads to increased microvascular dysfunction during endotoxaemia (Nishida *et al.* 1994b) and increased liver injury following alcohol (Oshita *et al.* 1992a, c, 1993). All of the above suggests that nitric oxide may play an important role in coordinating the time course for the expression of the inflammatory response and hepatic microvascular dysfunction during infection and that this may be modified by alcohol.

Conclusion

Alcohol affects Kupffer cell function which in turn alters the host defence functions of these cells, including phagocytosis of particulates, endocytosis of endotoxin and the production of cytokines as well as other inflammatory or vasoactive mediators. The resulting hepatic injury is exacerbated when alcohol is present in combination with other toxic substances (e.g. endotoxin, cocaine) or infection. It is anticipated that studies currently in progress in various laboratories around the world will provide new knowledge which should be beneficial in understanding alcohol-induced perturbations in the hepatic microcirculation, as well as the role of cytokines and nitric oxide in host defence and in modulating microvascular function and blood flow in the liver.

References

Abril, E.R., Jolly, C.S., Krasovich, M.A., McCuskey, R.S. and Earnest, D.L. (1991). Divergent effects of chronic ethanol ingestion on Kupffer cell function: Implications for alcoholic liver disease. *Hepatology* **14**, 139A.

Adams, H.G. and Jordan, C. (1984). Infections in the alcoholic. *Medical Clinics of North America* **68**, 179–200.

Ali, M.V. and Nolan, J.P. (1967). Alcohol induced depression in reticuloendothelial function in the rat. *Journal of Laboratory and Clinical Medicine* **70**, 295–301.

Altura, B.M. and Altura, B.T. (1982). Microvascular and vascular smooth muscle actions of ethanol, acetaldehyde, and acetate. *Federation Proceedings* **41**, 2447–2451.

Altura, B.M. and Altura, B.T. (1983). Peripheral vascular actions of ethanol and its interaction with neurohumoral substances. *Neurobehavior, Toxicology and Teratology* **5**, 211–220.

Altura, B.M. and Gebrewold, A. (1981). Failure of acetaldehyde or acetate to mimic the splanchnic arteriolar or venular dilator actions of ethanol: Direct *in situ* studies on the microcirculation. *British Journal of Pharmacology* **73**, 580–582.

Annoni, G., Weiner, F.R. and Zern, M.A. (1992). Increased TGF-β1 gene expression in human liver disease. *Journal of Hepatology* **14**, 259–264.

Bautista, A.P. and Spitzer, J.J. (1992). Acute ethanol

intoxication stimulates superoxide anion production by *in situ* perfused rat liver. *Journal of Hepatology* **15**, 892–898.

Bhagwandeen, B.S., Apte, M., Manwarring, L. and Dickenson, J. (1987). Endotoxin induced hepatic necrosis in rats on an alcohol diet. *Journal of Pathology* **152**, 47–53.

Billiar, T.R., Curran, R.D., Stuehr, D.J., West, M.A., Bentz, B.G. and Simmons, R.L. (1989). An L-arginine dependent mechanism mediates Kupffer cell inhibition of hepatocyte protein synthesis *in vitro*. *Journal of Experimental Medicine* **169**, 1467–1472.

Billiar, T.R., Curran, R.D., Harbrecht, B.G., Stuehr, D.J., Demetris, A.J. and Simmons, R.L. (1990). Modulation of nitric oxide synthesis *in vivo*: N^G-momomethyl-L-arginine inhibits endotoxin-induced nitrite/nitrate biosynthesis while promoting hepatic damage. *Journal of Leukocyte Biology* **48**, 565–569.

Blendis, L.M., Orrego, H., Crossley, I.R., Blake, J.E., Medline, A. and Israel, Y. (1982). The role of hepatocyte enlargement in hepatic pressure in cirrhotic and noncirrhotic alcoholic liver disease. *Hepatology* **2**, 539–546.

Bloch, E.H. (1955). The *in vivo* microscopic vascular anatomy and physiology of the liver as determined with the quartz-rod method of transillumination. *Angiology* **6**, 340–349.

Bloch, E.H. (1970). The termination of hepatic arterioles and the functional unit of the liver as determined by microscopy of the living organ. *Annals of the New York Academy of Science* **170**, 78–87.

Bode, C., Kugler, V. and Bode, J.C. (1987). Endotoxemia in patients with alcoholic and non-alcoholic cirrhosis and in subjects with no evidence of chronic liver disease following acute alcohol excess. *Journal of Hepatology* **4**, 8–14.

Boler, R.K. and Bibighaus, A.J. (1967). Ultrastructural alterations of dog livers during endotoxin shock. *Laboratory Investigation* **17**, 537–561.

Carey, C., Siegfried, M.R., Ma, X., Weyrich, A.S. and Lefer, A.M. (1992). Antishock and endothelial protective actions of NO donor in mesenteric ischemia and reperfusion. *Circulatory Shock* **38**, 209–216.

Carmichael, F.J., Saldivia, V., Varghese, G.A., Israel, Y. and Orrego, H. (1988). Ethanol-induced increase in portal blood flow: Role of acetate and A_1- and A_2-adenosine receptors. *American Journal of Physiology* **255**, G417–423.

Castenfors, H., Hultman, E. and Josephson, B. (1960). Effect of intravenous infusions of ethyl alcohol on estimated hepatic blood flow in man. *Journal of Clinical Investigation* **39**, 776–781.

Cilento, E.V., Reilly, F.D. and McCuskey, R.S. (1981). Quantification of volumetric flow within segments of the hepatic microvasculature following norepinephrine administration. *Microvascular Research* **21**, 239.

Conway, J.G., Popp, J.A. and Thurman, R.G. (1985).

Microcirculation in periportal and pericentral regions of lobule in perfused rat liver. *American Journal of Physiology* **249**, G449–456.

Cooksley, W.G.E., Powell, L.W. and Halliday, J.W. (1973). Reticuloendothelial phagocytic function in human liver disease and its relationship to haemolysis. *British Journal of Haematology* **25**, 147–152.

Curran, R.D., Billiar, T.R., Stuehr, D.J., Hofmann, K. and Simmons, R.L. (1989). Hepatocytes produce nitrogen oxides from L-arginine in response to inflammatory products of Kupffer cells. *Journal of Experimental Medicine* **170**, 1769–1774.

Decker, K. (1989). Hepatic mediators of inflammation in cells of the hepatic sinusoids. In *Cells of the Hepatic Sinusoid* (Edited by Wisse, E., Knook, D.L. and Decker, K.), pp. 171–175. Kupffer Cell Foundation, Leiden.

Decker, K. (1990). Biologically active products of stimulated liver macrophages. *European Journal of Biochemistry* **192**, 245–361.

Dimlich, R.V.W., Reilly, F.D. and McCuskey, R.S. (1982). Alterations in Kupffer cells following administration of compound 48/80. In *Sinusoidal Liver Cells* (Edited by Knook, D.L. and Wisse, E.), pp. 463–466. Elsevier/North-Holland, Amsterdam.

Earnest, D.L., Abril, E.R., Jolley, C.S., Nishida, J., Krasovich, M.A., McDonnell, D., Watson, R.R. and McCuskey, R.S. (1993). Ethanol feeding significantly potentiates cocaine-induced Kupffer cell dysfunction. In *Cells of the Hepatic Sinusoid* (Edited by Wisse, E. and Knook, D.L.), Vol. IV, pp. 400–402. Kupffer Cell Foundation, Leiden.

Eguchi, H., McCuskey, P.A. and McCuskey, R.S. (1991a). Kupffer cell activity and hepatic microvascular events after acute ethanol ingesion in mice. *Hepatology* **13**, 751–757.

Eguchi, H., McCuskey, P.A., Scuderi, P. and McCuskey, R.S. (1991b). $TNF\alpha$ plays a role in hepatic microvascular events following acute ethanol ingestion in $C_{57}Bl/6$ mice. In *Cells of the Hepatic Sinusoid* (Edited by Wisse, E., Knook, D.L. and McCuskey, R.S.), Vol. III, pp. 465–468. Kupffer Cell Foundation, Leiden.

Ekataksin, W. and Wake, K. (1991). Liver units in three dimensions: 1. Organization of argyrophilic connective tissue skeleton in porcine liver with particular reference to the "compound hepatic lobule". *American Journal of Anatomy* **191**, 113–153.

Ekataksin, W., Wake, K. and McCuskey, R.S. (1992). Liver units in three dimensions: *In vivo* microscopy and computer-aided reconstruction of microvascular zonation in mammalian livers. *Hepatology* **16**, 135A.

Ekataksin, W., Nishida, J., McDonnell, D., Krasovich, M. and McCuskey, R.S. (1993a). Postnatal development of the hepatic microvasculature and microcirculation in rats. *Hepatology* **18**, 157A.

Ekataksin, W., Wake, K., Nishida, J., Krasovich, M. and McCuskey, R. (1993b). HMS, hepatic microcirculatory subunit: Three dimensional observations on development and spacial distribution in mammalian livers. *Hepatology* **18**, 153A.

Ekataksin, W., Wake, K., Nishida, J. and McCuskey, R. (1993c). Mammalian liver units as revealed by temporal and spacial reconstructions: Recognition of the hepatic microcirculatory subunits. *Anatomical Record* **1**, 48 (suppl.).

Fahimi, H.D. (1982). Sinusoidal endothelial cells and perisinusoidal fat-storing cells: Structure and function. In *The Liver: Biology and Pathobiology* (Edited by Arias, I., Popper, H. and Schacter, D.), pp. 507–523. Raven Press, New York.

Fraser, R., Bolen, L.M. and Day, W.A. (1980a). Damage of rat liver sinusoidal endothelium by ethanol. *Pathology* **12**, 371–376.

Fraser, R., Boler, L.M., Day, W.A., Bobbs, B., Johnson, H.D. and Lee, D. (1980b). High pressure perfusion damages the sieving ability of sinusoidal endothelium in rat livers. *British Journal of Experimental Pathology* **61**, 222–228.

Fraser, R., Day, W.A. and Fernando, N.S. (1986). Review: The liver sinusoidal cells. Their role in disorders of the liver, lipoprotein metabolism and atherogenesis. *Pathology* **18**, 5–11.

Frenzel, H., Kremer, B. and Hucker, H. (1977). The liver sinusoids under various pathological conditions: A TEM and SEM study of rat liver after respiratory hypoxia, telecobalt-irridation and endotoxin application. In *Kupffer Cells and Other Sinusoidal Cells* (Edited by Wisse, E. and Knook, D.L.), pp. 213–222. Elsevier/North-Holland, Amsterdam.

Gumucio, J.J. and Miller, D.L. (1982). Liver cell heterogeneity. In *The Liver: Biology and Pathobiology* (Edited by Arias, I., Popper, H. and Schacter, D.), pp. 647–661. Raven Press, New York.

Hambrecht, B.G., Billiar, T.R., Demetris, A.J., Stadler, J., Ochoa, J., Curran, R.D. and Simmons, R.L. (1992). Inhibition of nitric oxide synthesis during endotoxemia promotes intrahepatic thrombosis and an oxygen radical mediated hepatic injury. *Journal of Leukocyte Biology* **52**, 390–394.

Hase, T. and Brim, J. (1966). Observation of the microcirculatory architechture of the rat liver. *Anatomical Record* **156**, 157–174.

Hutcheson, I.R., Wittle, B.J.R. and Boughton-Smith, N.K. (1992). Role of nitric oxide in maintaining vascular integrity of endotoxin-induced acute intestinal damage in the rat. *British Journal of Pharmacology* **101**, 815–820.

Irwin, J.W. and MacDonald, J. (1953). Microscopic observations of the intrahepatic circulation of living guinea pigs. *Anatomical Record* **117**, 1–15.

Jolley, C., Zhu, W., Abril, E., Eguchi, H., McCuskey, P., McCuskey, R. and Earnest, D. (1991). High resolution *in vivo* microscopy (HRM) detects subtle changes in Kupffer cell phagocytic function weeks before standard intravenous particle clearance tests. *Gastroenterology* **100**, A757.

Jolley, C.S., Abril, E.R., Olson, G.B., Earnest, D.L., McDonnell, D., Nishida, J. and McCuskey, R.S. (1993). Effects of ethanol on *in vivo* and *in vitro* Kupffer cell function, DNA profile and cytoskeletal staining. In *Cells of the Hepatic Sinusoid* (Edited by Wisse, E. and Knook, D.L.), Vol. IV, pp. 417–420. Kupffer Cell Foundation, Leiden.

Jones, E.A. (1982). Kupffer cells. In *The Liver: Biology and Pathobiology* (Edited by Arias, I., Popper, H. and Schacter, D.), pp. 507–523. Raven Press, New York.

Jungermann, K. and Katz, N. (1982). Functional hepatocellular heterogeneity. *Hepatology* **2**, 385–395.

Kaneda, K., Dan, C. and Wake, K. (1983). Pit cells as natural killer cells. *Biomedical Research* **4**, 567–576.

Kardon, R.H. and Kessel, R.G. (1980). Three-dimensional organization of the hepatic microcirculation in the rodent as observed by scanning electron microscopy of corrosion casts. *Gastroenterology* **79**, 72–81.

Kaufman, R.L., Hoefs, J.C. and Quismorio, F.P., Jr. (1982). Immune complexes in the portal and systemic circulation of patients with alcoholic liver disease. *Clinical Immunology and Immunopathology* **22**, 44–54.

Kelly, P.M., Heryet, A.R. and McGee, J.O. (1989). Kupffer cell number is normal, but their lysozyme content is reduced in alcoholic liver disease. *Journal of Hepatology* **8**, 173–180.

Kiernan, F. (1883). The anatomy and physiology of the liver. *Transactions of the Royal Society of London* **123**, 711–770.

Knisely, M.H., Bloch, E.H. and Warner, L. (1948). Selective phagocytosis I. Microscopic observations concerning the regulation of the blood flow through the liver and other organs and the mechanism and rate of phagocytic removal of particles from the blood. *Det Kongelige Danske Videnskabernes Selskab, Biologiske Skrifter* **4**, 1–93.

Koo, A. (1987). Nervous control of the hepatic microcirculation. In *Microcirculation: An Update* (Edited by Tsuchiya, M., Asano, M. and Oda, M.), pp. 335–338. Excerpta Medica, Amsterdam.

Koo, A. and Liang, L.Y.S. (1976). Intrahepatic microvascular changes in carbon tetrachloride-induced cirrhotic livers in the rat. *Australian Journal of Experimental Biology and Medical Science* **54**, 277–286.

Koo, A. and Liang, I.Y.S. (1979). Microvascular filling pattern in liver sinusoids during vagal stimulation. *Journal of Physiology* **295**, 191–199.

Koo, A., Liang, I.Y.S. and Cheng, K. (1976). Effect of the ligation of the hepatic artery on the microcirculation in the cirrhotic liver in the rat. *Australian Journal of Experimental Biology and Medical Science* **54**, 287–295.

Kubes, P., Suzuki, M. and Granger, D.N. (1991). Nitric oxide: An endogenous mediator of leukocyte adhesion. *Proceedings of the National Academy of Science* **88**, 4651–4655.

Lamers, W.H., Moorman, A.F.M. and Charles, R.

(1989a). The metabolic lobulus, a key to the architecture of the liver. *Cell Biology Review* **19**, 5–26.

Lamers, W.H., Hilberts, A., Furt, E., Smith, J., Jonges, G.N., van Noorden, C.J.F., Janzen, J.W.G., Charles, R. and Moorman, A.F.M. (1989b). Hepatic enzyme zonation: A reevaluation of the concept of the liver acinus. *Hepatology* **10**, 72–76.

LeBail, B., Bioulac-Sage, P., Senuita, R., Quinton, A., Saric, J. and Ballabaud, C. (1990). Fine structure of hepatic sinusoids and sinusoidal cells in disease. *Journal of Electron Microscopic Techniques* **14**, 257–282.

Lemasters, J.J., Ji, S. and Thurman, R.G. (1981). Centrilobular injury following hypoxia in isolated, perfused rat liver. *Science* **213**, 661–663.

Liehr, H. (1983). Endotoxins and alcoholic hepatitis. In *Clinical Hepatology* (Edited by Cosmos, G. and Thaler, T.), pp. 336–339. Berlin.

Liu, Y.K. (1979). Phagocytic capacity of reticuloendothelial system in alcoholics. *Journal of the Reticuloendothelial Society* **25**, 605–613.

Louria, D.B. (1963). Susceptibility to infection during experimental alcohol intoxication. *Transactions of the Association of American Physicians* **76**, 102–112.

Mairer, R.V. and Ulevitch, R. (1981). The response of isolated rabbit hepatic macrophages (h-MO) to lipopolysaccharide (LPS). *Circulatory Shock* **8**, 165–181.

Mathison, J.C. and Ulevitch, R. (1979). The clearance, tissue distribution and cellular localization of intravenously injected lipopolysaccharide in rabbits. *Journal of Immunology* **123**, 2133–2143.

Matsumoto, T. and Kawakami, M. (1982). The unit-concept of hepatic parenchyma – a reexamination based on angio architectural studies. *Acta Pathologica Japonica* **32**, 285–314.

McCarthy, S.P., Lewis, C.E. and McGee, J.O. (1990). Effects of ethanol on human monocyte/macrophage lysozyme storage and disease: Implications for the pathobiology of alcoholic liver disease. *Journal of Hepatology* **10**, 90–98.

McCuskey, R.S. (1966). A dynamic and static study of hepatic arterioles and hepatic sphincters. *American Journal of Anatomy* **119**, 455–487.

McCuskey, R.S. (1971). Sphincters in the microvascular system. *Microvascular Research* **2**, 428–433.

McCuskey, R.S. (1986). Microscopic methods for studying the microvasculature of internal organs. In *Physical Techniques in Biology and Medicine: Microvascular Technology* (Edited by Baker, C.H. and Nastuk, W.H.), pp. 247–264. Academic Press, New York.

McCuskey, R.S. (1987). Hepatic microvascular heterogeneity and functional units: current concepts and unresolved problems. In *Microcirculation: An update* (Edited by Tsuchiya, M., Asano, M., Mishima, Y. and Oda, M.), pp. 313–316. Excerpta Medica, Amsterdam.

McCuskey, P.A. (1989). Electron and fluorescence microscopic study of mast cells and adrenergic innervation in Beagle dog liver. In *Cells of the Hepatic Sinusoids*

(Edited by Wisse, E., Knook, D.L. and Decker, K.), Vol. II, pp. 260–265. Kupffer Cell Foundation, Leiden.

McCuskey, R.S. (1991a). *In vivo* microscopy of the effects of ethanol on the liver. In *Alcohol and Drug Abuse Reviews: Liver Pathology and Alcohol* (Edited by Watson, R.R. and Clifton, N.J.), pp. 563–574. Humana Press, Totowa.

McCuskey, R.S. (1991b). Responses of the hepatic sinusoid lining and microcirculation to combinations of endotoxin, cytokines and ethanol. In *Cells of the Hepatic Sinusoid* (Edited by Wisse, E., Knook, D.L. and McCuskey, R.S.), Vol. III, pp. 1–5. Kupffer Cell Foundation, Leiden.

McCuskey, R.S. and Reilly, F.D. (1993). Hepatic microvasculature: Dynamic structure and its regulation. *Seminars in Liver Disease* **13**, 1–12.

McCuskey, R.S., Urbaschek, R., McCuskey, P.A., Sacco, N., Stauber, W., Pinkstaff, C.A. and Urbaschek, B. (1982). Studies of Kupffer cells in mice sensitized or tolerant to endotoxin. In *Sinusoidal Liver Cells* (Edited by Knook, K.L. and Wisse, E.), pp. 387–392. Elsevier/North-Holland, Amsterdam.

McCuskey, R.S., Vonnahme, F.J. and Grun, M. (1983). *In vivo* microscopic and electron microscopic observations of the heaptic microvascular system following portacaval anastomosis. *Hepatology* **3**, 96–104.

McCuskey, R.S., McCuskey, P.A., Urbaschek, R. and Urbaschek, B. (1984). Species differences in Kupffer cells and endotoxin sensitivity. *Infection and Immunity* **45**, 278–280.

McCuskey, R.S., McCuskey, P.A., Urbaschek, R. and Urbaschek, B. (1987). Kupffer cell function in host defense. *Reviews of Infectious Disease* **5**, S616-S619.

McCuskey, R.S., McCuskey, P.A., Eguchi, H., Crichton, E.G., Urbaschek, R. and Urbaschek, B. (1990). *In vivo* microscopy of the liver following acute administration of ethanol. In *Alcohol, Immunosuppression and AIDS* (Edited by Pawlowski, A., Seminara, D. and Watson, R.), pp. 341–350. Alan R. Liss, New York.

McCuskey, R.S., Eguchi, H., McCuskey, P.A., Krasovich, M.A., Watzl, B. and Watson, R.R. (1991a). Long-term exposure to cocaine in combination with ethanol elicits fibrosis, necrosis and microvascular dysfunction in murine liver. *Gastroenterology* **100**, 773A.

McCuskey, R.S., Eguchi, H., McCuskey, P.A., Urbaschek, R. and Urbaschek, B. (1991b). Some effects of ethanol in Kupffer cell function and host defense mechanisms in the liver. In *Frontiers of Mucosal Immunology* (Edited by Tsuchiya, M., Nagura, H., Hibi, T. and Mono, I.), pp. 187–192. Excerpta Medica, Amsterdam.

McCuskey, R.S., Eguchi, H., Nishida, J., Krasovich, M.A., McDonnell, D., Watzl, B., Jolley, C.S., Abril, E.R., Earnest, D.L. and Watson, R.R. (1993a). Effects of ethanol and cocaine alone or in combination on hepatic sinusoids of mice and rats. In *Cells of the Hepatic*

Sinusoid (Edited by Wisse, E. and Knook, D.L.), Vol. IV, pp. 376–380. Kupffer Cell Foundation, Leiden.

McCuskey, R.S., Eguchi, H., Nishida, J., Urbaschek, R. and Urbaschek, B. (1993b). Effects of ethanol alone or in combination with infection, toxins or drugs of abuse on the hepatic microcirculation. *Advances in Biological Science* **86**, 227–234.

Mezey, E. (1982). Alcoholic liver disease. In *Progress in Liver Disease* (Edited by Popper, H. and Schaffner, F.), Vol. VII, pp. 555–572. Grune and Stratton, New York.

Miller, D.L., Zanolli, C.S. and Gumucio, J.J. (1979). Quantitative morphology of the sinusoids of the hepatic acinus. *Gastroenterology* **76**, 965–969.

Moncada, S., Palmer, R.M.J. and Higgs, E.A. (1991). Nitric oxide: Physiology, pathophysiology and pharmacology. *Pharmacological Reviews* **43**, 103–142.

Morrison, D.C. and Ulevitch, R.J. (1978). The effects of bacterial endotoxins on host mediation systems. *American Journal of Pathology* **93**, 525–618.

Munford, R.S. (1978). Endotoxins and the liver. *Gastroenterology* **75**, 532–535.

Nakata, K. (1967). Microcirculation and hemodynamical analysis of the blood circulation in the liver. *Acta Pathologica Japonica* **17**, 361–376.

Nakata, K., Leong, G.F. and Brauer, R.W. (1961). Direct measurement of blood pressures in minute vessels of the liver. *American Journal of Physiology* **199**, 1181–1188.

Napanitaya, W., Lamb, J.C., Grisham, J.W. and Carson, J.L. (1976). Effect of venous outflow obstruction on pores and fenestrations in sinusoidal endothelium. *British Journal of Experimental Pathology* **57**, 604–609.

Nathan, C. (1992). Nitric oxide as a secretory product of mammalian cells. *FASEB Journal* **6**, 3051–3064.

Niiro, G.K. and O'Morchoe, C.C.C. (1986). Pattern and distribution of intrahepatic lymph vessels in the rat. *Anatomical Record* **215**, 351–360.

Nishida, J., Abril, E.R., McDonnell, D., Jolley, C.S., Krasovich, M.A., McCuskey, R.S., Earnest, D.L. and Watson, R.R. (1992). Effects of the combination of ethanol and cocaine on hepatic sinusoids in rats. *Hepatology* **16**, 235A.

Nishida, J., McDonnell, D., Krasovich, M.A. and McCuskey, R.S. (1993). Effects of IL-1 on Kupffer cells and the hepatic sinusoidal microcirculation. In *Cells of the Hepatic Sinusoid* (Edited by Wisse, E. and Knook, D.L.), Vol. IV, pp. 148–151. Kupffer Cell Foundation, Leiden.

Nishida, J., Ekataksin, W., McDonnell, D., Unbaschek, R., Unbaschek, B. and McCuskey, R.S. (1994a). Ethanol exacerbates hepatic microvascular dysfunction, endotoxemia and lethality in septic mice. *Shock* **1**, 413–418.

Nishida, J., McCuskey, R.S., McDonnell, D. and Fox, E.S. (1994b). Protective role of nitric oxide in hepatic microcirculatory dysfunction during endotoxemia. *American Journal of Physiology* (in press).

Nolan, J.P. (1965). Alcohol as a factor in the illness of university service patients. *American Journal of Medical Science* **249**, 135–142.

Nolan, J.P. (1989). Intestinal endotoxins as mediators of hepatic injury – an idea whose time has come again. *Hepatology* **10**, 887–891.

Nolan, J.P. and Camara, D.S. (1982). Endotoxin, sinusoidal cells, and liver injury. In *Progress in Liver Disease* (Edited by Poppen, H. and Schaffner, F.), Vol. 7, pp. 361–376. Grune and Stratton, New York.

Nolan, J.P., Leibowitz, A. and Vladutiu, A.L. (1980). Influence of alcohol on Kupffer cell function and possible significance in liver injury. In *The Reticuloendothelial System and the Pathogenesis of Liver Disease* (Edited by Liehr, H. and Grun, M.), pp. 125–136. Elsevier/North-Holland, Amsterdam.

Ochoa, J.B., Ukekwu, A.O., Billiar, T.R., Curran, R.D., Cerra, F.B., Simmons, R.L. and Peitzman, A.B. (1991). Nitrogen oxide levels in patients after trauma and during sepsis. *Annals of Surgery* **214**, 621–626.

Oda, M., Nakamura, M., Watanabe, N., Ohiya, Y., Sekizuka, E., Tsuckoda, N., Yonei, Y., Komatsu, H., Nagata, H. and Tsuchiya, M. (1987a). Some dynamic aspects of the hepatic microcirculation – demonstration of sinusoidal endothelial fenestrae as a possible regulatory factor. In *Intravital Observation of Organ Microcirculation* (Edited by Tsuchiya, M., Wayland, H., Oda, M. and Okazaki, I.), pp. 105–138. Excerpta Medica, Amsterdam.

Oda, M., Tsukado, N., Honda, K., Komatsu, H., Kaneko, K., Azuma, T., Nishizaki, N., Watanabe, N. and Tsuchiya, M. (1987b). Hepatic sinusoidal endothelium – its functional implications in the regulation of sinusoidal blood flow. In *Microcirculation: An Update* (Edited by Tsuchiya, M., Asano, M., Mishima, Y. and Oda, M.), pp. 317–320. Excerpta Medica, Amsterdam.

Oda, M., Azuma, T., Watanabe, N., Nishizaki, Y., Nishida, J., Ishii, K., Suzki, H., Kaneko, H., Komatsu, H., Tsukada, N. and Tsuchiya, M. (1990). Regulatory mechanism of hepatic microcirculation: Involvement of contraction and dilatation of sinusoids and sinusoidal endothelial fenestrae. *Progress in Applied Microcirculation* **17**, 103–128.

Orrego, H. and Carmichael, F.J. (1992). Review article: Effects of alcohol on liver haemodynamics in the presence and absence of liver disease. *Journal of Gastroenterology and Hepatology* **7**, 70–89.

Orrego, H., Carmichael, F.J., Saldivia, V., Giles, H.G., Sandrin, S. and Israel, Y. (1988). Ethanol-induced increase in portal blood flow: Role of adenosine. *American Journal of Physiology* **254**, G495–501.

Oshita, M., Sato, N., Yoshihara, H., Takei, Y., Hijioka, T., Fukui, H., Goto, M., Matsunaga, T., Kashiwagi, T., Kawano, S., Fusamoto, H. and Kamada, T. (1992a). Ethanol-induced vasoconstriction causes focal hepatocellular injury in the isolated perfused rat liver. *Hepatology* **16**, 1007–1013.

Oshita, M., Takei, Y., Hijioka, T., Goto, M., Fukui, H., Nishimura, Y., Kawano, S., Fusamoto, H., Kamada,

T. and Sato, N. (1992b). Ethanol induced vasoconstriction in perfused rat liver. *Microcirculation Annals* **8**, 19–22.

Oshita, M., Takei, Y., Kawano, S., Hijioka, T., Fukui, H., Nishimura, Y., Fusamoto, H. and Kamada, T. (1992c). Nitric oxide attenuates ethanol induced hepatic injury. *Hepatology* **16**, 109A.

Oshita, M., Takei, Y., Kawano, S., Yoshihara, H., Hijioka, T., Fukui, H., Goto, M., Masuda, E., Nishimura, Y., Fusamoto, H. and Kamada, T. (1993). Roles of endothelin-1 and nitric oxide in the mechanism for ethanol-induced vasoconstriction in the rat liver. *Journal of Clinical Investigation* **91**, 1337–1342.

Pinznai, M., Faili, P., Ruocco, C., Casini, A., Milani, S., Baldi, E., Giotti, A. and Gentilini, P. (1992). Fat-storing cells as liver-specific pericytes: Spatial dynamics of agonist-stimulated intracellular calcium transients. *Journal of Clinical Investigation* **90**, 642–646.

Quistorff, B. (1990). Metabolic heterogeneity of liver parenchymal cells. *Essays in Biochemistry* **25**, 83–136.

Quistorff, B. and Romert, P. (1989). High zone-selectivity of cell permeabilization following digitonin-pulse perfusion of rat liver: A reinterpretation of the microcirculatory zones. *Histochemistry* **92**, 487–498.

Rappaport, A.M. (1973). The microcirculatory hepatic unit. *Microvascular Research* **6**, 212–228.

Rappaport, A.M. (1977). Microcirculatory units in the mammalian liver. *Bibliotheca Anatomica* **16**, 116–120.

Rappaport, A.M., Borowy, Z.J., Lougheed, W.M. and Lotto, W.N. (1954). Subdivision of the hexagonal liver lobules into a structural and functional unit. *Anatomical Record* **119**, 11–34.

Rosenstreich, D.L. and Vogel, S.N. (1980). The central role of macrophages in endotoxin reactions. In: *Microbiology – 1980* (Edited by Schlessinger, D.), pp. 11–38. American Society of Microbiology, Washington, DC.

Ruiter, D.J., van der Meulen, J., Brouwer, A., Hummel, M.J., Mauw, B.J., van der Ploeg, J.C. and Wisse, E. (1981). Uptake by liver cells of endotoxin following its intravenous injection. *Laboratory Investigation* **45**, 38–45.

Sakamoto, M. (1991). Effects of endothelin-1 on the contraction of Ito cells (fat-storing cells). *Acta Hepatologica Japonica* **32**, 1027–1033.

Salvemini, D., Korbut, R., Anggard, E. and Vane, J. (1990). Immediate release of a nitric oxide-like factor from bovine aortic endothelial cells by *E. coli* LPS. *Proceedings of the National Academy of Sciences (USA)* **87**, 2593–2597.

Sasse, E. (1986). Liver structure and innervation. In *Regulation of Hepatic Metabolism: Intra- and Intercellular Compartmentation* (Edited by Thurman, R.G., Kauffman, K.C., and Jungermann, K.), pp. 3–25. Plenum Press, New York.

Sato, N., Eguchi, H., Takei, Y., Hijioka, T., Tsuji, S., Matsumura, T., Hayashi, N., Kawano, S. and Kamada, T. (1987a). Microcirculatory aspects of the mechanism of alcoholic liver disease – sinusoidal blood flow and oxygenation at periportal regions of hepatic lobules in rats. In *Microcirculation Vol. 2: An Update* (Edited by Tsuchiya, M., Asano, M., Michima, Y. and Oda, M.), pp. 357–360. Excerpta Medica, Amsterdam.

Sato, N., Matsumura, T., Kawano, S. and Kamada, T. (1987b). Hepatic microcirculation and hepatic cellular metabolism. In *Microcirculation Vol. 2: An update* (Edited by Tsuchiya, M., Asano, M., Mishima Y. and Oda, M.), pp. 309–312. Excerpta Medica, Amsterdam.

Shaw, S., Heller, E.A. and Friedman, H.S. (1977). Increased hepatic oxygenation following ethanol administration in the baboon. *Proceedings of the Society for Experimental Biology and Medicine* **156**, 509–513.

Sherman, I.A. and Fisher, M.M. (1987). Hepatic microvascular patterns in normal and diseased liver. In *Microcirculation Vol. 2: An Update* (Edited by Tsuchiya, M., Asano, M., Mishima, Y. and M. Oda, M.), pp. 345–348. Excerpta Medica, Amsterdam.

Shibayama, Y. (1987). Enhanced hepatotoxicity of endotoxin by hypoxia. *Pathology Research and Practice* **182**, 390–395.

Shibayama, Y. and Nakata, K. (1985). Localization of increased hepatic vascular resistance in liver cirrhosis. *Hepatology* **5**, 643–648.

Shibayama, Y., Asaka, S. and Nakata, N. (1991). Endotoxin hepatotoxicity augmented by ethanol. *Experimental Molecular Pathology* **55**, 196–202.

Shiratori, Y., Teraoka, H., Matano, S., Matsumoto, K., Kamii, K. and Tanaka, M. (1989). Kupffer cell function in chronic ethanol fed rats. *Liver* **9**, 351–359.

Sleyster, E.C.H. and Knook, D.L. (1982). Relation between localization and function of rat liver Kupffer cells. *Laboratory Investigation* **47**, 484–490.

Teutsch, H.F. (1986). A new sample isolation procedure for microchemical analysis of functional liver cell heterogeneity. *Journal of Histochemistry and Cytochemistry* **34**, 263–267.

Teutsch, H.F. (1988). Regionality of glucose-6-phosphate hydrolysis in the liver lobule of the rat: Metabolic heterogeneity of "portal" and "septal" sinusoids. *Hepatology* **8**, 311–317.

Teutsch, H.F., Altemus, J., Gerlach-Arbeiter, S. and Kyander-Teutsch, T.L. (1992). Distribution of 3-hydroxybutyrate dehydrogenase in primary lobules of the rat liver. *Journal of Histochemistry and Cytochemistry* **40**, 213–219.

Vidins, E.I., Britton, R.S., Medline, A., Blandis, L.J., Israel, Y. and Orrego, H. (1985). Sinusoidal caliber in alcoholic and nonalcoholic liver disease: Diagnostic and pathologic implications. *Hepatology* **5**, 408–414.

Wake, K., Decker, K., Kirn, A., Knook, D.K., McCuskey, R.S. and Wisse, E. (1989). Cell biology and kinetics of Kupffer cells in the liver. *International Review of Cytology* **118**, 173–229.

Wisse, E. (1977). Ultrastructure and function of Kupffer cells and other sinusoidal lining cells. In *Kupffer Cells and Other Sinusoidal Lining Cells* (Edited by Wisse, E.

and Knook, D.L.), pp. 33–60. Elsevier/North-Holland, Amsterdam.

Wisse, E. and McCuskey, R.S. (1986). On the interactions of blood cells with the sinusoidal wall as observed by *in vivo* microscopy of rat liver. In *Cells of the Hepatic Sinusoids* (Edited by Kirn, A., Knook, D.L. and Wisse, E.), pp. 477–482. Kupffer Cell Foundation, Leiden.

Wisse, E., De Zanger, R.B., Jacobs, R. and McCuskey, R.S. (1983). Scanning electron microscopic observations on the structure of portal veins, sinusoids and central veins. *Scanning Electron Microscopy* **III**, 1441–1452.

Wisse, E., De Zanger, R.B., Jacobs, R., Charels, K., Van Der Smissen, P. and McCuskey, R.S. (1985). The liver sieve: Consideration concerning the structure and function of endothelial fenestrae, the sinusoid wall and the space of Disse. *Hepatology* 5, 683–692.

Wright, C.E., Rees, D.D. and Moncada, S. (1992). Protective and pathological roles of nitric oxide in endotoxin shock. *Cardiovascular Research* **26**, 48–57.

Zhang, J., Pegoli, W. and Clemens, M.G. (1994). Endothelin-1 induces direct constriction of hepatic sinusoids. *American Journal of Physiology* **29**, G624–G632.

15 Alcohol and the "liver sieve"

Robin Fraser, George W.T. Rogers and Bruce R. Dobbs

Introduction

Disorder of the "liver sieve" (the fenestrated hepatic
sinusoidal endothelium) induced by alcohol abuse is
an important event in the pathogenesis of alcoholic
cirrhosis. Sited strategically between the blood and
the hepatocytes, the "liver sieve" functions as a
dynamic bio-filter of blood-borne macromolecules.
Interference with this structure will hinder both
sieving and the free diffusion of nutrients to and
from the hepatocytes. This may arise either directly
by alterations to the degree of fenestration, or porosity of the endothelium, or indirectly following
perisinusoidal fibrosis and the formation of a basement membrane.

In this chapter, we focus our attention not only on
the effects of alcohol on the "liver sieve", but also
examine the role of the other sinusoidal (non-
parenchymal) cells in the pathogenesis of alcoholic
liver disease, since these cells are intimately related
in location and function.

The "liver sieve"

It was known that gaps occurred in the hepatic
sinusoidal wall, but it was not appreciated how small
these fenestrae were until the advent of electron
microscopy and whole organ perfusion fixation
(Yamagishi 1959; Laschi and Casanova 1969; Wisse
1970; Orci *et al.* 1971; Motta and Porter 1974).
These fenestrae, with diameters of about 100 nm,
occur within an endothelium lacking a basement
membrane or a distinct matrix in the underlying
space of Disse. Fraser and colleagues (1968) showed
that chylomicrons, the lipoproteins which transport
dietary lipid from the intestines, are normally larger
than 100 nm diameter, depending on dietary fat
intake. Shortly after, Wisse (1970) postulated that
the fenestrated sinusoidal endothelium might act as
a filter for chylomicrons.

This structure, termed the "liver sieve" (Fig.
15.1), has been demonstrated in humans, other
mammals, birds and fish (Fraser *et al.* 1986a;
McCuskey *et al.* 1986). Many factors influence the
"liver sieve" to have profound effects on hepatic
function generally and lipid metabolism specifically
(Wisse *et al.* 1985; Fraser *et al.* 1986a).

Hepatic sinusoidal cells

Four different types of sinusoidal cells are known:
Kupffer cells, Ito cells, endothelial cells and "pit
cells". Kupffer, an early investigator, described the
first two types of sinusoidal cells, probably without
recognizing their differences. In 1876, Kupffer described the *Sternzellen*, dendritic or star-shaped cells
seen in livers stained with gold chloride. These
Sternzellen are now known as the fat-storing, perisinusoidal stellate cells of Ito (Wake 1982). In 1898,
with the then current interest in phagocytosis,
Kupffer described the phagocytic intrasinusoidal
cells which presently carry his name (Aterman
1979).

Meticulous ultrastructural studies have cemented
the concept of the four distinct families of sinusoidal
cells. The fenestrated endothelial cells lining the
sinusoids were shown to be quite distinct from the

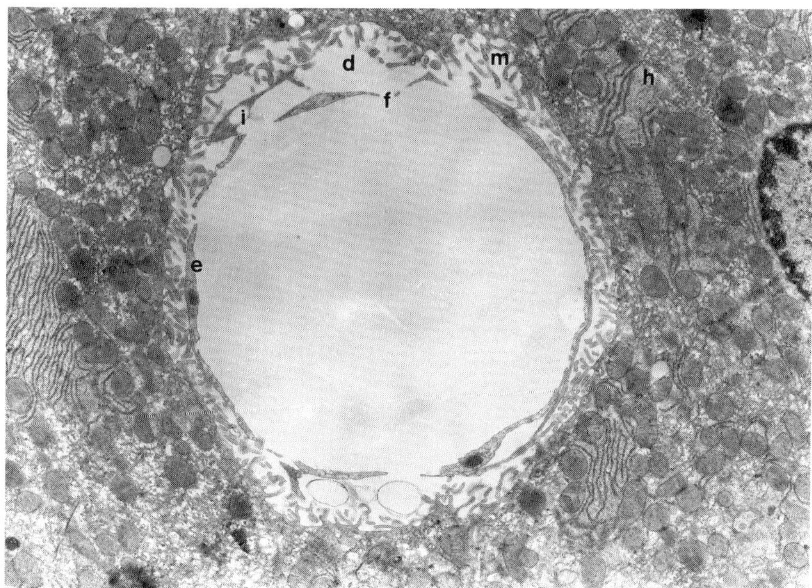

Fig. 15.1   Transmission electron micrograph of a hepatic sinusoid showing: (e) endothelial lining; (f) fenestrae; (m) microvilli; (d) space of Disse; (h) hepatocyte; (i) Ito cell process. ×2170.

intrasinusoidal Kupffer cell (Wisse 1972). The perisinusoidal stellate cell was rediscovered by Ito in 1951 (Ito 1973) and further differentiated from the Kupffer cell by Wake (1971). The fourth cell, the intrasinusoidal "pit cell", was so named because of its distinctive granules or pits (Dutch for pips) (Wisse *et al.* 1976). These cells are now recognized as the large granular lymphocytes or natural killer cells resident in the liver (Bouwens and Wisse 1988).

While the role or function of hepatic sinusoidal cells had been addressed since von Kupffer studied hepatic phagocytosis, the relationship of structure and function has taken enormous strides over the last 20 years. The interested reader is referred to the biennial series, *Cells of the Hepatic Sinusoid*, which are the proceedings of the International Symposia on "Cells of the Hepatic Sinusoids", 1986–1993 .

Although alcohol may affect all the sinusoidal cells, at present its major action seems to be related to the Kupffer, Ito and endothelial cells. The function of, and communication between, these three cell types will be discussed, albeit briefly, before examining the role of alcohol on the "liver sieve".

Kupffer cells

The phagocytic Kupffer cells lie within the sinusoids (Fig. 15.2). They originate both from the bone

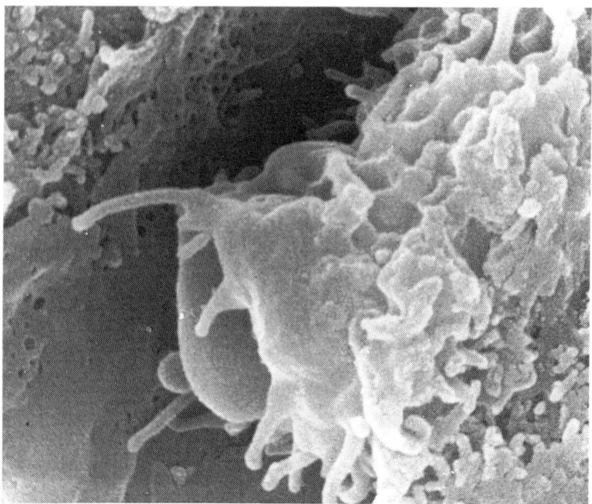

Fig. 15.2   Scanning electron micrograph of a Kupffer cell within the lumen of a fenestrated hepatic sinusoid. ×7000.

marrow monocytic phagocytic system, as well as from division within the liver, to become resident hepatic histiocytes (Bouwens *et al.* 1984). Kupffer cells are well situated to guard against viruses, bacteria and bacterial endotoxins derived from the gastrointestinal tract. Kupffer cells release many mediators including tumour necrosis factor alpha (TNFα), transforming growth factor beta (TGFβ), prostaglandins and free radicals which influence other sinusoidal cells in their vicinity (Fraser *et al.* 1986a; Wake *et al.* 1989; Fukui *et al.* 1991; McCuskey 1991; see also Chapters 4, 6 and 14).

Exposure of rats to alcohol or carbon tetrachloride alters the number and the phagocytic activity of Kupffer cells (Lautenschlager *et al.* 1982). In contrast, acute alcohol ingestion by mice has been shown to activate the phagocytic activity of Kupffer cells (Eguchi *et al.* 1991). The release by Kupffer cells of cytokines that stimulate Ito cells is one of the more important events in the pathogenesis of hepatic fibrosis (Tsukamoto *et al.* 1990; see also Chapter 4).

Ito cells

The fat storing stellate cells of Ito lie in a perisinusoidal position within the space of Disse; the cells are surrounded by hepatocyte microvilli, and often reside between hepatocytes (Fig. 15.3). As well as containing retinol (vitamin A) rich fat droplets the Ito cells have morphological characteristics in common with fibroblasts and are often found in close proximity to collagen bundles in the space of Disse (McGee and Patrick 1972; Kent *et al.* 1977; Nakano and Lieber 1982). Their stellate processes have intimate contact with the sleeve-like fenestrated endothelium, and function as a supporting scaffold

(Wake 1988). The Ito cells also have contractile properties, and appear to be innervated in some species including humans (Lafon *et al.* 1989; Lee *et al.* 1992). For a detailed description of the structure and function of Ito cells see Chapter 4.

Endothelial cells

Endothelial cells may be able to function in a similar manner to Kupffer cells, producing cytokines, such as TNFα after administration of a bacterial endotoxin (Nagano *et al.* 1992). These workers also showed that the endothelium became damaged or "leaky" after exposure to endotoxin as indicated by the presence of lymphocytes within the space of Disse.

Endothelial cells appear to play a subsidiary role in phagocytosis and may support the Kupffer cells in this regard in the ethanol-fed rat (Shiratori *et al.* 1989). Receptors for glycoproteins are expressed by endothelial cells and have different specificity from those on Kupffer cells, suggesting that the two cell types have independent roles in glycoprotein catabolism (Sano *et al.* 1990).

Maintenance of the integrity of the endothelium appears to be important in the preservation of the liver for transplantation. Although parenchymal cell function was preserved after 24–48 h cold storage of rat livers, severe damage was noted to the non-parenchymal cells, including denudation of the sinusoidal lining (Caldwell-Kenkel *et al.* 1989).

Communication between sinusoidal cells

Intersinusoidal cell communication is important in the pathogenesis of alcoholic fibrosis and cirrhosis (Gressner 1991). Endothelial cells, *in vitro*, release an inhibitor of Ito cell growth or multiplication which may regulate fibrogenesis (Rosenbaum *et al.* 1989). They also have a scavenger function in the homeostatic control of the extracellular matrix (Smedsrod *et al.* 1990). Damaged membranes of hepatocytes release the cytokine "hepitoin" (*hepa*tocellular *I*to cell *in*itiator), which stimulates the multiplication of Ito cells (Gressner *et al.* 1992). (For a detailed discussion, see Chapter 4.)

Defenestration of endothelial cells, which has been shown to precede fibrosis, may elevate the concentration of cytokines in the space of Disse, and

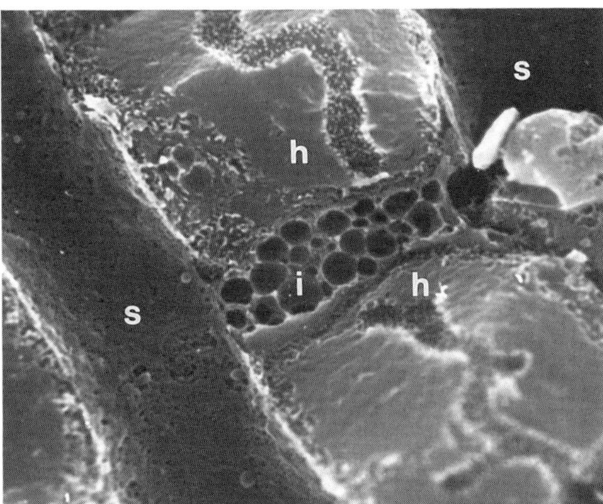

Fig. 15.3 Scanning electron micrograph of a fat-laden Ito cell bridging between two sinusoids (s) and flanked by hepatocytes (h). ×3400.

thus play a role in the paracrine stimulation of the Ito cells.

Endothelial porosity

Control of endothelial porosity

Although there has been much written on their structure and function, current interest encompasses the mechanism by which the endothelial cells alter fenestrae number and size. Recent studies of rat liver endothelial cells *in vitro* have shown that the contraction of fenestrae is enhanced by an increase in the intracellular calcium concentration, while dilatation is produced following depolarization of actin filaments, independent of intracellular calcium. Fenestrae of cultured endothelial cells contract either in the presence of a calcium ionophore inhibiting the binding of calcium to calmodulin, or following the addition of endothelin. From these studies, it is postulated that endothelin may be an endogenous modulator of fenestrael contractility via the calcium–calmodulin–actomyosin system (Arias *et al.* 1987; Oda *et al.* 1993). The microfilament-inhibiting drug, cytochalasin-B, increases the frequency of fenestrae in cultured mouse liver endothelial cells, via its effects on the cytoskeleton (Steffan *et al.* 1987).

Other recent studies have pointed to the importance of the extracellular matrix on the properties and function of the hepatic endothelium. The number and size of the fenestrae of endothelial cells cultured *in vitro* are regulated by the composition of the underlying matrix (McGuire *et al.* 1992). Cell surface receptors for extracellular matrix molecules, such as the "very late activation" (VLA) family of integrins, act as an interface between the intracellular cytoskeleton and the extracellular matrix, playing an important role in cell–cell and cell–matrix interactions (Hynes 1987; Volpes *et al.* 1991).

This evidence suggests that compounds affecting either the endothelial cell cytoskeleton or the extracellular matrix may promote defenestration or capillarization (Arthur 1990; Friedman 1992; Burt 1993).

Acute effects of ethanol on the "liver sieve"

The first drug shown to alter the diameter of fenestrae in the "liver sieve", and hence porosity, was alcohol. The dilatation of rat liver fenestrae from about 100 to 120 nm was shown to allow larger chylomicrons, and hence more dietary triacylglycerol, to be trapped in the liver (Fraser *et al.* 1980a). This might explain the finding that the fatty acid composition of triacylglycerols in the alcoholic fatty liver mirrors the dietary fatty acids (Lieber *et al.* 1966). Enlargement of the fenestrae following acute alcohol ingestion has been confirmed in the rat (Charels *et al.* 1986; Mori *et al.* 1991; Tanikawa *et al.* 1991) and baboon (Mak and Lieber 1984).

Chronic effects of ethanol on the "liver sieve"

Chronic ethanol ingestion in rats, however, causes large areas of the sinusoidal endothelium to lose fenestrae or defenestrate (Fraser *et al.* 1981; Charels *et al.* 1986; Tanikawa *et al.* 1991). This was suggested as an explanation of the patchy nature of steatosis sometimes seen in alcoholism (Fraser *et al.* 1981). A decrease in the frequency of fenestrae was also found in the ethanol-fed baboon (Mak and Lieber 1984), and the non-cirrhotic alcoholic human, concurrent with the deposition of a basement membrane underlying the endothelial cells (Horn *et al.* 1985). These latter workers more recently showed that defenestration occurred without the formation of a basement membrane in non-cirrhotic livers following alcohol abuse, implying that loss of endothelial fenestrae precedes the development of alcoholic cirrhosis (Horn *et al.* 1987). Capillarization of hepatic sinusoids and collagenization of the space of Disse had been seen previously in human alcoholic liver disease (Schaffner and Popper 1963; Orrego *et al.* 1979).

Defenestration and perisinusoidal fibrosis have been noted in an alcoholic human in conjunction with type V hyperlipoproteinaemia and elevated plasma triacylglycerols (Clark *et al.* 1988). It was proposed that defenestration (Fig. 15.4) prevented chylomicron remnants contacting the hepatocytes, so leading to an increase in their concentration in peripheral blood. Capillarization has been observed in a number of human liver biopsies concomitant with other causes of hepatic fibrosis (Bioulac-Sage *et al.* 1988).

Ethanol affects other sinusoidal cell functions as well as altering endothelial porosity. It influences Kupffer cells by modifying their phagocytotic activity (Sim and Earnest 1987) and also alters the endocytotic activity of endothelial cells (Baskin

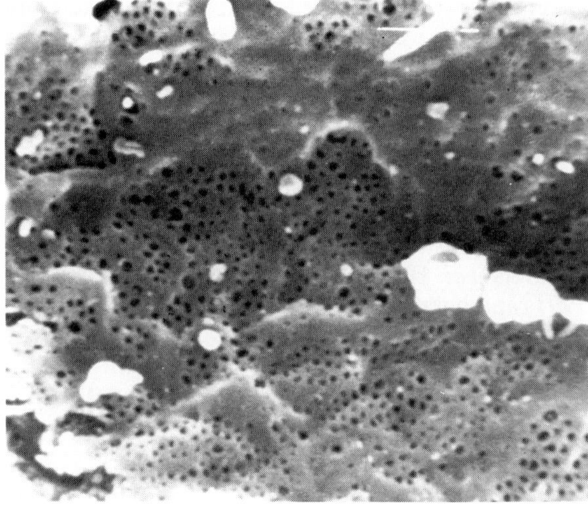

(a)

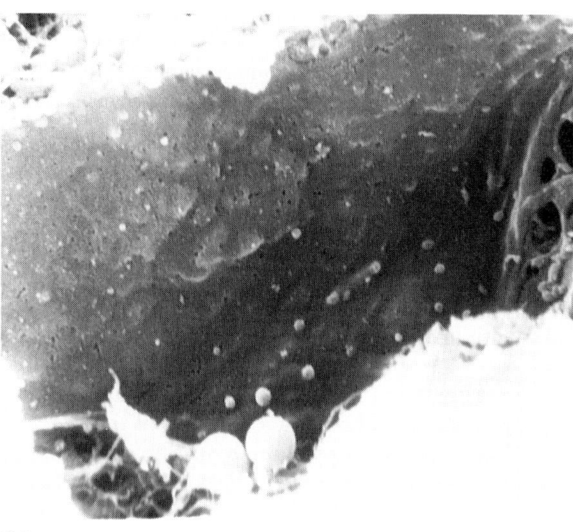

(b)

Fig. 15.4   (a) Scanning electron micrograph of a normally fenestrated human sinusoid. ×18,000. (b) Scanning electron micrograph of a defenestrated sinusoid from an alcoholic patient with type V hyperlipoproteinaemia. ×12,000.

1990). Ethanol may also stimulate Kupffer cells to release substances which might alter the endothelial cell cytoskeleton.

Other factors affecting endothelial porosity

Factors shown to alter the porosity of the hepatic endothelium within a species include: drugs and chemical hepatotoxins, portal venous pressure, hypoxia, viruses, hormones and endotoxins.

It is widely accepted that alcohol enhances the toxic effects of other *xenobiotics*, e.g. paracetamol (Edwards and Oliphant 1992), carbon tetrachloride (Hall *et al*. 1991), xylene (Elovaara *et al*. 1980), haloalkanes (including the anaesthetic agent, halothane), various drugs, the nitrosamines (including dimethylnitrosamine) and, curiously, vitamin A (Zimmerman 1986) and carotene (Leo *et al*. 1992) (see also Chapters 2 and 16). Many of these drugs and toxins injure endothelial cells as well as hepatocytes (see below).

Drugs such as nicotine reduce the diameter of fenestrae, consequently making rats susceptible to dietary cholesterol (Fraser *et al*. 1988). Pantethine, on the other hand, dilates rabbit fenestrae and makes these animals less susceptible to dietary cholesterol (Fraser *et al*. 1989). Paracetamol (acetaminophen) has been shown to induce ultrastructural changes to the sinusoidal endothelium in mice (Walker *et al*. 1983).

Exogenous chemical hepatotoxins produce even more drastic effects on the endothelium. Loss of endothelial fenestrae (defenestration) and capillarization occur after acute exposure of the liver to either dimethylnitrosamine or carbon tetrachloride, hepatotoxins used commonly in animal models of cirrhosis (Fraser *et al*. 1991; Martinez-Hernandez and Martinez 1991). Defenestration occurs well before the development of cirrhosis in the dimethylnitrosamine model (Fraser *et al*. 1991). When exposure to dimethylnitrosamine is ceased after acute dosing, fenestrae quickly reform (Tamba-Lebbie *et al*. 1993).

High portal pressure disrupts the normal endothelium, removing its ability to sieve or discriminate between large and small chylomicrons and their remnants (Fraser *et al*. 1980b). Hypoxia, due to hepatic venous outflow obstruction, has been shown to disrupt the endothelium resulting in an enlargement of fenestrae (Nopanitaya *et al*. 1976). Similar effects have been noted following ischaemia-reperfusion injury, which is important in organ transplantation (Caldwell-Kenkel *et al*. 1989).

Infection with some of the hepatitis viruses alters hepatic sinusoidal morphology. Mice, for example, infected with mouse hepatitis virus-3, develop hepatic steatosis with markedly reduced endothelial cell cholesterol content coinciding with the loss of fenestrae (Bingen *et al*. 1992). The possibility that defenestration, induced by a coexistent viral infection, contributes to the pathogenesis of alcohol-related liver injury merits consideration.

Hormones shown to alter the size of fenestrae include serotonin and adrenalin, both of which reduce fenestral diameter (Wisse *et al.* 1980; Arias *et al.* 1987). In similar studies performed in rats *in vivo*, the neurotransmitter acetylcholine and its analogue, bethanechol, caused an increase in fenestral diameter and dilatation of the sinusoidal lumen resulting in increased sinusoidal blood flow (Oda *et al.* 1984).

Endothelial and Kupffer cells are both involved in the uptake of bacterial endotoxin from portal blood and these interactions are considered to be of great importance in the pathogenesis of liver disease (Nolan and Cohen 1988). Exposure of rats to endotoxin induces a splenic release of TNFα, resulting in hepatic endothelial cell damage through an endocrine interaction (Tanaka *et al.* 1992). Recent studies in our laboratory have shown that in rats given endotoxin intravenously, the porosity of the "liver sieve" is reduced (Dobbs *et al.* 1994). During high ethanol intake, it is probable that portal venous endotoxin levels are elevated owing to increased intestinal permeability, that is an alcoholic "leaky gut" (Bjarnason *et al.* 1984). We suggest that defenestration due to endotoxinaemia may be a factor in alcoholic liver injury (see also Chapters 6 and 14).

Importance of the "liver sieve" in chylomicron metabolism

The frequency and diameter of endothelial fenestrae varies between species, altering sinusoidal porosity (Fraser *et al.* 1986a). For example, both rabbits and chickens have a porosity about half that of rats; in rabbits, this is due to small fenestrae of about 50 nm diameter compared with 100 nm in rats. Conversely, chickens have a much lower frequency of fenestrae (number of fenestrae per unit area of sinusoid) rather than a reduced diameter. This finding may explain the susceptibility of rabbits and chickens to dietary cholesterol resulting in hypercholesterolaemia and atherosclerosis, which does not occur in rats (Wright *et al.* 1983; Fraser *et al.* 1986b).

Chylomicron remnants, formed from parent dietary chylomicrons by the action of peripheral tissue lipoprotein lipase (Redgrave 1970), are rapidly removed from the circulation by the liver after recognition by specific receptors on the parenchymal cells (Beisiegel *et al.* 1991; Mahley and Hussain 1991). Floren (1984) showed that chylomicrons and their remnants derived from plasma bind equally well to adult human liver membranes *in vitro*, but

only remnants bind to hepatocytes *in vivo*. He proposed that other factors, such as "steric hindrance in the space of Disse", might be important in excluding chylomicrons from binding to liver membranes *in vivo*. We believe the "steric hindrance in the space of Disse" to be the "liver sieve" (Rogers *et al.* 1992).

The hypothesis that the fenestrated sinusoidal endothelium "sieved" chylomicrons of different sizes was tested by measuring the diameter of lipid particles both within the sinusoids and in the space of Disse (Fraser *et al.* 1978; Naito and Wisse 1978). Following a single-pass perfusion of rat liver with radiolabelled chylomicrons, a higher proportion of those less than 100 nm diameter was trapped than those of greater diameter (Fraser *et al.* 1978). The hypothesis was extended to explain the preferential uptake by the liver of chylomicron remnants, leading to the coining of the term "liver sieve" (Fraser *et al.* 1978). In addition, we have shown that the ability of the "liver sieve" to differentiate large from small chylomicrons is lost following disruption of the fenestrated endothelium by high-pressure portal perfusion (Fraser *et al.* 1980b).

Effects of ethanol on retinol metabolism

Retinol, absorbed from the diet by the small intestine, is transported in the core of chylomicrons and their remnants in the ester form. Retinyl esters within the remnants are taken up by the parenchymal cells of the liver and passed as free retinol to the Ito cells to be re-esterified for storage (Blomhoff *et al.* 1991; see also Chapter 4).

In rats the hepatic levels of retinol are known to decrease after chronic ethanol consumption (Norum *et al.* 1986). These workers previously demonstrated that the uptake of chylomicron retinyl esters was the same in ethanol-fed rats as in controls, but suggested that the metabolism of retinol was increased by ethanol (Rasmussen *et al.* 1985). In humans chronic ingestion of alcohol has been reported to decrease hepatic retinol content (Lieber 1988). Reduction of the retinol content of the Ito cells *in vitro* leads to their activation and multiplication (Davis and Vucic 1988).

Defenestration of the sinusoidal endothelium (loss of the "liver sieve") may trigger fibrogenesis by blocking the hepatic uptake of retinol. To test this hypothesis, we have used the dimethylnitrosamine-

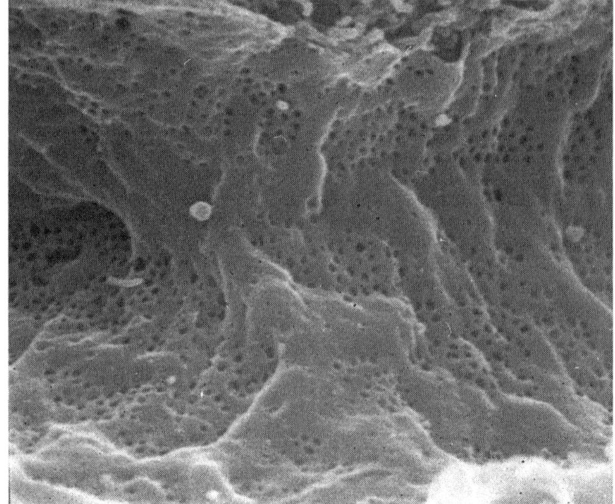

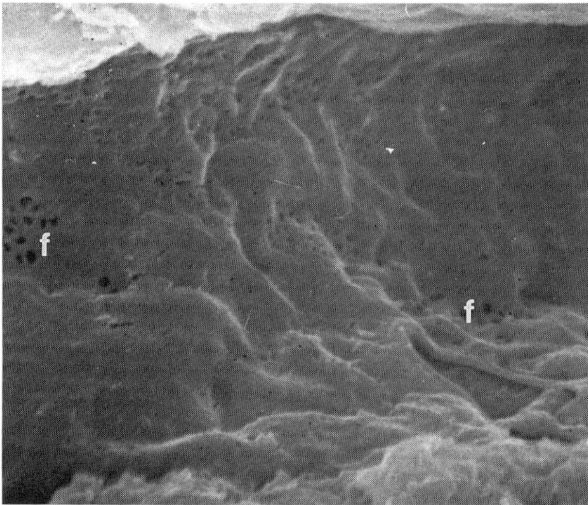

Fig. 15.5 (a) Scanning electron micrograph of a fenestrated sinusoid from a normal rat. ×11,000. (b) Scanning electron micrograph of sinusoid with few fenestrae (f) from a dimethylnitrosamine-treated rat. ×11,000.

fed rat, an animal model of micronodular cirrhosis closely resembling human alcoholic cirrhosis (Jenkins *et al.* 1985). In addition, the dimethylnitrosamine model has proven useful for studying the early changes occurring during the development of fibrosis in the rat (Jezequel *et al.* 1987). Marked defenestration occurs after acute dosing with dimethylnitrosamine, well before the onset of fibrosis (Fig. 15.5) (Fraser *et al.* 1991). This defenestration was shown to reduce severely the hepatic uptake of chylomicrons radiolabelled in either their cholesterol or retinol moieties (Rogers *et al.* 1992).

Recently, assessment of the plasma clearance rate of chylomicron retinyl esters has been suggested to be useful in the diagnosis of cirrhosis (Kasai *et al.* 1993).

On this evidence, one would predict that depleting Ito cells of dietary vitamin A should result in hepatic fibrogenesis. Recently, we have examined the hepatic sinusoidal ultrastructure of rats depleted of dietary retinol. In these rats we found periportal (zone 1) fibrosis, despite a normally fenestrated endothelium (Rogers *et al.* 1993).

Retinol is known to be important in the differentiation of cells, and low levels of retinol are correlated with the development of certain cancers (Lotan 1980; Peto *et al.* 1981). Although ethanol itself has not been shown to be carcinogenic, it has been suggested as being a "co-carcinogen" (Garro and Lieber 1990), and it may promote liver cancers in man via the depletion of retinol (Adachi *et al.* 1991; see also Chapters 2 and 16). Defenestration of the hepatic endothelium has been reported in both human and experimental primary hepatocellular carcinoma (Madarame *et al.* 1986). Defenestration, by interfering with retinol metabolism, could be a factor in the development of some carcinomas.

Summary

Ethanol acts on the "liver sieve" by inducing subtle changes in porosity. Acute and possibly chronic low-dose exposure to ethanol increases the porosity of the hepatic endothelium by dilatation of the fenestrae. We believe this enhances the hepatic clearance of dietary lipid, which is a factor in the pathogenesis of alcoholic steatosis, and may account in part for the protection from atherosclerosis ascribed to low-dose alcohol consumption.

Chronic alcohol abuse, on the other hand, results in a reduction in the porosity of the sinusoidal endothelium, and in the extreme leads to complete defenestration or capillarization. Rather than ethanol merely affecting the endothelium, defenestration and capillarization result from a complex sequence of events, which are as yet not clearly defined.

The Ito cell is the major cell involved in the production of extracellular matrix. Paracrine events between parenchymal and sinusoidal cells, and endocrine interactions between other organs and sinusoidal cells, are both important in the control of Ito cell function. During chronic alcohol abuse, defenestration may alter the balance of cytokines in the space of Disse, perturbing Ito cell function, and thus affecting the extracellular matrix and the "liver sieve".

Storage of retinol is a function of the normal Ito cell. Depletion of hepatic retinol, owing to decreased uptake following defenestration or loss of the "liver sieve", is correlated with transformation of Ito cells to myofibroblasts and changes in matrix composition.

In combination with ethanol, factors such as viruses, bacterial endotoxins and other hepatotoxins, may play a significant role in the pathogenesis of alcoholic cirrhosis by further affecting sinusoidal porosity.

To conclude, ethanol induces seemingly minor morphological changes to the hepatic sinusoidal endothelium or "liver sieve", culminating in profound effects on other sinusoidal and parenchymal cells. We believe defenestration occurs early in the development of cirrhosis and also plays a role in related pathological changes, such as hyperlipoproteinaemia and perhaps carcinogenesis. Much research in this field has concentrated on function and associated ultrastructure; future research will no doubt focus on the molecular mechanisms of these subtle events.

References

Adachi, S., Moriwaki, H., Muto, Y., Yamada, Y., Fukutomi, Y., Shimazaki, M., Okuno, M. and Ninomiya, M. (1991). Reduced retinoid content in hepatocellular carcinoma with special reference to alcohol consumption. *Hepatology* **14**, 776–780.

Arias, I.M., Peleg, Y., Gatmaitan, Z. and Adelstein, R.A. (1987). The mechanism whereby serotonin produces fenestrael contraction in rat hepatic endothelial cells. *Hepatology* **7**, 14A, 1026.

Arthur, M.J. (1990). Matrix degradation in the liver. *Seminars in Liver Disease* **10**, 47–55.

Aterman, K. (1979). "Kupffer" or "von Kupffer" cells? *Kupffer Cell Bulletin* **2**, 8–9.

Baskin, G. (1990). Ethanol and regulation of receptor-mediated endocytosis. *Hepatology* **12**, 1240–1245.

Beisiegel, U., Weber, W. and Bengtsson-Olivecrona, G. (1991). Lipoprotein lipase enhances the binding of chylomicrons to low density lipoprotein receptor-related protein. *Proceedings of the National Academy of Science, USA* **88**, 8342–8346.

Bingen, A., Martin, J.-P., Klein, F. and Pessah, M. (1992). Modification of the amount of cholesterol in hepatic steatosis induced in susceptible and resistant mice infected with MHV3: A biochemical and ultrastructural study. *Hepatology* **15**, 1137–1146.

Bioulac-Sage, P., Lafon, M.E., Le Bail, B., Boulard, A., Du Buisson, L., Quinton, A., Lamouliatte, H., Saric, J. and Balabaud, C. (1988). Ultrastructure of sinusoids in liver disease. In *Sinusoids in Human Liver: Health and Disease* (Edited by Bioulac-Sage, P. and Balabaud, C.), pp. 223–278. Kupffer Cell Foundation, Leiden.

Bjarnason, I., Ward, K. and Peters, T.J. (1984). The leaky gut of alcoholism: Possible route of entry for toxic compounds. *Lancet* **i**, 179–182.

Blomhoff, R., Green, M.H., Balmer Green, J., Berg, T. and Norum, K.R. (1991). Vitamin A metabolism: New perspectives on absorption, transport, and storage. *Physiological Reviews* **71**, 951–990.

Bouwens, L. and Wisse, E. (1988). Tissue localization and kinetics of pit cells or large granular lymphocytes in the liver of rats treated with biological response modifiers. *Hepatology* **8**, 46–52.

Bouwens, L., Baekeland, M. and Wisse, E. (1984). Importance of local proliferation in the expanding Kupffer cell population of rat liver after zymosan stimulation and partial hepatectomy. *Hepatology* **4**, 213–219.

Burt, A.D. (1993). C.L. Oakley Lecture: Cellular and molecular aspects of hepatic fibrosis. *Journal of Pathology* **170**, 105–114.

Caldwell-Kenkel, J.C., Currin, R.T., Tanaka, Y., Thurman, R.G. and Lemasters, J.J. (1989). Reperfusion injury to endothelial cells following cold ischemic storage of rat livers. *Hepatology* **10**, 292–299.

Charels, K., De Zanger, R.B., Van Bossuyt, H., Van Der Smissen, P. and Wisse, E. (1986). Influence of acute alcohol administration on endothelial fenestrae of rat livers: An *in vivo* and *in vitro* scanning electron microscopic study. In *Cells of the Hepatic Sinusoid* (Edited by Kirn, A., Knook, D.L. and Wisse, E.), Vol. 1, pp. 497–502. Kupffer Cell Foundation, Leiden.

Clark, S.A., Angus, H.B., Cook, H.B., George, P.M., Oxner, R.B.G. and Fraser, R. (1988). Defenestration of hepatic sinusoids as a cause of hyperlipoproteinaemia in alcoholics. *Lancet* **ii**, 1225–1227.

Davis, B.H. and Vucic, A. (1988). The effect of retinol on Ito cell proliferation *in vitro*. *Hepatology* **8**, 788–793.

Dobbs, B.R., Rogers, G.W.T., Xing, H.-Y. and Fraser, R. (1994). Endotoxin-induced defenestration of the hepatic sinusoidal endothelium: a factor in the pathogenesis of cirrhosis? *Liver* (in press).

Edwards, R. and Oliphant, J. (1992). Paracetamol toxicity in chronic alcohol abusers – a plea for greater consumer awareness. *New Zealand Medical Journal* **105**, 174–175.

Eguchi, H., McCuskey. P.A. and McCuskey, R.S. (1991). Kupffer cell activity and hepatic microvascular events after acute ethanol ingestion in mice. *Hepatology* **13**, 751–757.

Elovaara, E., Collan, Y., Pfaffli, P. and Vainio, H. (1980). The combined toxicity of technical grade xylene and ethanol in the rat. *Xenobiotica* **10**, 435–445.

Floren, C.H. (1984). Binding of apolipoprotein E-rich remnant lipoproteins to human liver membranes. *Scandinavian Journal of Gastroenterology* 19, 473–479.

Fraser, R., Cliff, W.J. and Courtice, F.C. (1968). The effect of dietary fat load on the size and composition of chylomicrons in thoracic duct lymph. *Quarterly Journal of Experimental Physiology* 53, 390–398.

Fraser, R., Bosanquet, A.G. and Day, W.A. (1978). Filtration of chylomicrons by the liver may influence cholesterol metabolism and atherosclerosis. *Atherosclerosis* 29, 113–123.

Fraser, R., Bowler, L.M. and Day, W.A. (1980a). Damage of rat liver sinusoidal endothelium by ethanol. *Pathology* 12, 371–376.

Fraser, R., Bowler, L.M., Day, W.A., Dobbs, B., Johnson, H.D. and Lee, D. (1980b). High perfusion pressure damages the sieving ability of sinusoidal endothelium in rat livers. *British Journal of Experimental Pathology* 61, 222–228.

Fraser, R., Day, W.A. and Wright, P.L. (1981). Fatty liver and the sinusoidal cells. In *Festschrift for F.C. Courtice* (Edited by Garlick, D.), pp. 139–144. University of New South Wales Press, Sydney.

Fraser, R., Day, W.A. and Fernando, N.S. (1986a). Review: The liver sinusoidal cells. Their role in disorders of the liver, lipoprotein metabolism and atherogenesis. *Pathology* 18, 5–11.

Fraser, R., Heslop, V.R., Murray, F.E.M. and Day, W.A. (1986b). Ultrastructural studies of the portal transport of fat in chickens. *British Journal of Experimental Pathology* 67, 783–791.

Fraser, R., Clark, S.A., Day, W.A. and Murray, F.E.M. (1988). Nicotine decreases the porosity of the rat liver sieve: A possible mechanism for hypercholesterolaemia. *British Journal of Experimental Pathology* 69, 345–350.

Fraser, R., Clark, S.A., Bowler, L.M., Murray, F.E.M., Wakasugi, J., Ishihara, M. and Tomikawa, M. (1989). The opposite effects of nicotine and pantethine on the porosity of the liver sieve and lipoprotein metabolism. In *Cells of the Hepatic Sinusoid* (Edited by Wisse, E., Knook, D.L. and Decker, K.), Vol. 2, pp. 335–338. Kupffer Cell Foundation, Leiden.

Fraser, R., Rogers, G.W.T., Bowler, L.M., Day, W.A., Dobbs, B.R. and Baxter, J.N. (1991). Defenestration and vitamin A status in a rat model of cirrhosis. In *Cells of the Hepatic Sinusoid* (Edited by Wisse, E., Knook, D.L. and McCuskey, R.S.), Vol. 3, pp. 195–198. Kupffer Cell Foundation, Leiden.

Friedman, S.L. (1992). "Cuts both ways": Collagenases, lipocyte activation and polyunsaturated lecithin. *Hepatology* 15, 549–551.

Fukui, H., Brauner, B., Bode, J.C. and Bode, C. (1991). Plasma endotoxin concentrations in patients with alcoholic and non-alcoholic liver disease: Reevaluation with an improved chromogenic assay. *Journal of Hepatology* 12, 162–169.

Garro, A.J. and Lieber, C.S. (1990). Alcohol and cancer. *Annual Reviews of Pharmacology and Toxicology* 30, 219–249.

Gressner, A.M. (1991). Major topics of fibrosis research: 1990 update. In *Cells of the Hepatic Sinusoid* (Edited by Wisse, E., Knook, D.L. and McCuskey, R.S.), Vol. 3, pp. 136–144. Kupffer Cell Foundation, Leiden.

Gressner, A.M., Lofti, S., Gressner, G. and Lahme, B. (1992). Identification and partial characterization of a hepatocyte-derived factor promoting proliferation of cultured fat-storing cells (parasinusoidal lipocytes). *Hepatology* 16, 1250–1266.

Hall, P. de la M., Plummer, J.L., Ilsley, A.H. and Cousins, M.J. (1991). Hepatic fibrosis and cirrhosis after chronic administration of alcohol and "low-dose" carbon tetrachloride vapor in the rat. *Hepatology* 13, 815–819.

Horn, T., Junge, J. and Christoffersen, P. (1985). Early alcoholic liver injury: Changes of the Disse space in acinar zone 3. *Liver* 5, 301–310.

Horn, T., Christoffersen, P. and Henriksen, J.H. (1987). Alcoholic liver injury: Defenestration in noncirrhotic livers – A scanning electron microscopic study. *Hepatology* 7, 77–82.

Hynes, R.O. (1987). Integrins: A family of cell surface receptors. *Cell* 48, 549–554.

Ito, T. (1973). Recent advances in the study on the fine structure of the hepatic sinusoidal wall: A review. *Gumna Reports of Medical Science* 6, 119–163.

Jenkins, S.A., Grandison, A., Baxter, J.N., Day, D.W., Taylor, I. and Shields, R. (1985). A dimethylnitrosamine-induced model of cirrhosis and portal hypertension in the rat. *Journal of Hepatology* 1, 489–499.

Jezequel, A.M., Mancini, R., Rinaldesi, M.L., Macarri, G., Venturini, C. and Orlandi, F. (1987). A morphological study of the early stages of hepatic fibrosis induced by low doses of dimethylnitrosamine in the rat. *Journal of Hepatology* 5, 174–181.

Kasai, T., Moriwaki, H., Okuno, M., Numaguchi, S., Murakami, N., Seishima, M., Ohnishi, H., Shidoji, Y. and Muto, Y. (1993). The clearance rate of chylomicron retinyl ester from plasma can be used to distinguish rats with cirrhosis from those with portacaval shunt. *Hepatology* 17, 125–130.

Kent, G., Inouye, T., Minick, O.T. and Bahu, R.M. (1977). Role of lipocytes (perisinusoidal cells) in fibrogenesis. In *Kupffer Cells and other Liver Sinusoidal Cells* (Edited by Wisse, E. and Knook, D.L.), pp. 73–82. Elsevier, Amsterdam.

Lafon, M.E., Bioulac-Sage, P., Le Bail, B., Saric, J., Quinton, A. and Balabaud, C. (1989). Nerves and perisinusoidal cells in human liver. In *Cells of the Hepatic Sinusoid* (Edited by Wisse, E., Knook, D.L. and Decker, K.), Vol. 2, pp. 230–234. Kupffer Cell Foundation, Leiden.

Laschi, R. and Casanova, S. (1969). Fenestrae closed by a diaphragm in the endothelium of liver sinusoids. *Journal of Microscopy* 8, 1037–1040.

Lautenschlager, I., Vaananen, H. and Kulonen, E. (1982). Qualitative study on the Kupffer cells in the liver of ethanol- and carbon tetrachloride-treated rats. *Acta Pathologica et Microbiologica Scandinavica* **90**, 347–351.

Lee, J.A., Ahmed, Q., Hines, J.E. and Burt, A.D. (1992). Disappearance of hepatic parenchymal nerves in human liver cirrhosis. *Gut* **33**, 87–91.

Leo, M.A., Kim, C., Lowe, N. and Lieber, C.S. (1992). Interaction of ethanol with β-carotene: Delayed blood clearance and enhanced hepatotoxicity. *Hepatology* **15**, 883–891.

Lieber, C.S. (1988). Biochemical and molecular basis of alcohol-induced injury to liver and other tissues. *New England Journal of Medicine* **319**, 1639–1650.

Lieber, C.S., Spritz, N. and De Carli, L.M. (1966). Role of dietary, adipose and endogenously synthesised fatty acids in the pathogenesis of the alcoholic fatty liver. *Journal of Clinical Investigation* **45**, 51–62.

Lotan, R. (1980). Effects of vitamin A and its analogs (retinoids) on normal and neoplastic cells. *Biochimica et Biophysica Acta* **605**, 33–91.

Madarame, T., Masuda, T., Suzuki, A., Satodate, R., Suzuki, K. and Sato, S. (1986). Ultrastructural features of the vascular channel of human and experimentally induced hepatocellular carcinoma. In *Cells of the Hepatic Sinusoid* (Edited by Kirn, A., Knook, D.L. and Wisse, E.), Vol. 1, pp. 399–402. Kupffer Cell Foundation, Rijswijk.

Mahley, R.W. and Hussain, M.M. (1991). Chylomicron and chylomicron remnant catabolism. *Current Opinion in Lipidology* **2**, 170–176.

Mak, K.M. and Lieber, C.S. (1984). Alterations in endothelial fenestrations in liver sinusoids of baboons fed alcohol: A scanning electron microscopic study. *Hepatology* **4**, 386–391.

Martinez-Hernandez, A. and Martinez, J. (1991). The role of capillarisation in hepatic failure: Studies in carbon tetrachloride-induced cirrhosis. *Hepatology* **14**, 864–874.

McCuskey, R.S. (1991). Responses of the hepatic sinusoid lining and microcirculation to combinations of endotoxin, cytokines and ethanol. In *Cells of the Hepatic Sinusoid* (Edited by Wisse, E., Knook, D.L. and McCuskey, R.S.), Vol. 3, pp. 1–5. Kupffer Cell Foundation, Leiden.

McCuskey, P.A., McCuskey, R.S. and Hinton, D.E. (1986). Electron microscopy of cells of the hepatic sinusoids in rainbow trout (*Salmo gairdneri*). In *Cells of the Hepatic Sinusoid* (Edited by Kirn, A., Knook, D.L. and Wisse, E.), Vol. 1, pp. 489–494. Kupffer Cell Foundation, Rijswijk.

McGee, J.O. and Patrick, R.S. (1972). The role of perisinusoidal cells in hepatic fibrogenesis: An electron microscopic study of acute carbon tetrachloride liver injury. *Laboratory Investigation* **26**, 429–440.

McGuire, R.F., Bissell, D.M., Boyles, J. and Roll, F.J. (1992). Role of extracellular matrix in regulating fenest-

rations of sinusoidal endothelial cells isolated from normal rat liver. *Hepatology* **15**, 989–997.

Mori, T., Okanoue, T., Sawa, Y., Itoh, Y., Kanaoka, H., Hori, N., Enjyo, F., Nakagawa, Y., Kagawa, K. and Kashima, K. (1991). Effect of ethanol on the sinusoidal endothelial fenestration of rat liver – *in vivo* and *in vitro* study. In *Cells of the Hepatic Sinusoid* (Edited by Wisse, E., Knook, D.L. and McCuskey, R.S.), Vol. 3, pp. 469–471. Kupffer Cell Foundation, Leiden.

Motta, P. and Porter, K.R. (1974). Structure of rat liver sinusoids and associated tissue spaces as revealed by scanning electron microscopy. *Cell and Tissue Research* **148**, 111–125.

Nagano, T., Kita, T. and Tanaka, N. (1992). The immunocytochemical localization of tumour necrosis factor and leukotriene in the rat liver after treatment with lipopolysaccharide. *International Journal of Experimental Pathology* **73**, 675–683.

Naito, M. and Wisse, E. (1978). Filtration effect of endothelial fenestrations on chylomicron transport in neonatal rat liver sinusoids. *Cell and Tissue Research* **190**, 371–382.

Nakano, M. and Lieber, C.S. (1982). Ultrastructure of initial stages of perivenular fibrosis in alcohol-fed baboons. *American Journal of Pathology* **106**, 145–155.

Nolan, J.P. and Cohen, S.A. (1988). Interaction of endotoxin with sinusoidal cells of the liver. In *Sinusoids in Human Liver: Health and Disease* (Edited by Bioulac-Sage, P. and Balabaud, C.), pp. 341–358. Kupffer Cell Foundation, Rijswijk.

Nopanitaya, W., Lamb, J.C., Grisham, J.W. and Carson, J.L. (1976). Effect of hepatic venous outflow obstruction on pores and fenestrations in sinusoidal endothelium. *British Journal of Experimental Pathology* **57**, 604–609.

Norum, K.R., Rasmussen, M., Blomhoff, R., Berg, T. and Nilsson, A. (1986). The influence of ethanol intake on the hepatic storage of retinol. In *Cells of the Hepatic Sinusoid* (Edited by Kirn, A., Knook, D.L. and Wisse, E.), Vol. 1, pp. 203–205. Kupffer Cell Foundation, Leiden.

Oda, M., Tsukada, N., Watanabe, N., Komatsu, H., Yonei, Y. and Tsuchiya, M. (1984). Functional implications of the sinusoidal endothelial fenestrae in the regulation of the hepatic microcirculation. *Hepatology* **4**, 17A, 754.

Oda, M., Kazemoto, S., Kaneko, H., Yokomori, H., Tsukada, N., Watanabe, N., Suematsu, M. and Tsuchiya, M. (1993). Involvement of Ca^{++}–calmodulin–actomyosin system in contractility of hepatic sinusoidal endothelial fenestrae. In *Cells of the Hepatic Sinusoid* (Edited by Wisse, E., Knook, D.L. and McCuskey, R.S.), Vol. 4, pp. 174–178. Kupffer Cell Foundation, Leiden.

Orci, L., Matter, A. and Rouiller, Ch. (1971). A comparative study of freeze-etch replicas and thin sections of rat liver. *Journal of Ultrastructural Research* **35**, 1–19.

Orrego, H., Medline, A., Blendis, L.M., Rankin, J.G.

and Kreaden, D.A. (1979). Collagenisation of the Disse space in alcoholic liver disease. *Gut* **20**, 673–679.

Peto, R., Doll, R., Buckley, J.D. and Sporn, M.B. (1981). Can dietary beta-carotene materially reduce human cancer rates? *Nature* **290**, 201–208.

Rasmussen, M., Blomhoff, R., Helgerud, P., Solberg, L.A., Berg, T. and Norum, K.R. (1985). Retinol and retinyl esters in parenchymal and nonparenchymal rat liver cell fractions after long-term administration of ethanol. *Journal of Lipid Research* **26**, 1112–1119.

Redgrave, T.G. (1970). Formation of cholesteryl ester-rich particulate lipid during metabolism of chylomicrons. *Journal of Clinical Investigation* **49**, 465–471.

Rogers, G.W.T., Dobbs, B.R. and Fraser, R. (1992). Decreased hepatic uptake of cholesterol and retinol in the dimethylnitrosamine rat model of cirrhosis. *Liver* **12**, 326–329.

Rogers, G.W.T., Dodeman, I., Azais-Braesco, V., Dobbs, B.R. and Fraser, R. (1993). Hepatic fibrosis in the vitamin A (retinol) deficient rat. *New Zealand Medical Journal* **106**, 291.

Rosenbaum, J., Mavier, P., Preaux, A.M., Lescs, M.C. and Dhumeaux, D. (1989). Mouse hepatic endothelial cells in culture secrete a growth inhibitor for hepatic lipocytes and Balb/c 3T3 fibroblasts. *Journal of Hepatology* **9**, 295–300.

Sano, A., Taylor, M.E., Leaning, M.S. and Summerfield, J.A. (1990). Uptake and processing of glycoproteins by isolated rat hepatic endothelial and Kupffer cells. *Journal of Hepatology* **10**, 211–216.

Schaffner, F. and Popper, H. (1963). Capillarization of hepatic sinusoids in man. *Gastroenterology* **44**, 239–242.

Shiratori, Y., Jin'nai, H., Teraoka, H., Matano, S., Matsumoto, K., Kamii, K., Tanaka, M. and Okano, K. (1989). Phagocytic properties of hepatic endothelial cells and splenic macrophages compensating for a decreased phagocytic function of Kupffer cells in the chronically ethanol-fed rat. *Experimental Cell Biology* **57**, 300–309.

Sim, W.W. and Earnest, D.L. (1987). Ethanol stimulates or inhibits Kupffer cell function dependent on its concentration in blood. *Hepatology* **7**, 77A, 1042.

Smedsrod, B., Pertoft, H., Gustafson, S. and Laurent, T.C. (1990). Scavenger functions of the liver endothelial cell. *Biochemical Journal* **266**, 313–327.

Steffan, A.-M., Gendrault, J.-L. and Kirn, A. (1987). Increase in the number of fenestrae in mouse endothelial liver cells by altering the cytoskeleton with cytochalasin B. *Hepatology* **7**, 1230–1238.

Tamba-Lebbie, B., Rogers, G.W.T., Dobbs, B.R. and Fraser, R. (1993). Defenestration of the hepatic sinusoidal endothelium in the dimethylnitrosamine fed rat: Is this process reversible? In *Cells of the Hepatic Sinusoids* (Edited by Knook, D.L. and Wisse, E.), Vol. 4, pp. 179–181. Kupffer Cell Foundation, Leiden.

Tanaka, S., Kumashiro, R. and Tanikawa, K. (1992). Role of the spleen in endotoxin-induced hepatic injury in chronic alcohol-fed rats. *Liver* **12**, 306–310.

Tanikawa, K., Noguchi, K. and Sata, M. (1991). Ultrastructural features of Kupffer cells and sinusoidal endothelial cells in chronic ethanol-fed rats. In *Cells of the Hepatic Sinusoid* (Edited by Wisse, E., Knook, D.L. and McCuskey, R.S.), Vol. 3, pp. 445–448. Kupffer Cell Foundation, Leiden.

Tsukamoto, H., Gaal, K. and French, S.W. (1990). Insights into the pathogenesis of alcoholic liver necrosis and fibrosis: Status report. *Hepatology* **12**, 599–608.

Volpes, R., Van den Oord, J.J. and Desmet, V.J. (1991). Distribution of the VLA family of integrins in normal and pathological human liver tissue. *Gastroenterology* **101**, 200–206.

Wake, K. (1971). "Sternzellen" in the liver: Perisinusoidal cells with special reference to the storage of vitamin A. *American Journal of Anatomy* **132**, 429–462.

Wake, K. (1982). The Sternzellen of von Kupffer – After 106 years. In *Sinusoidal Liver Cells* (Edited by Knook, D.L. and Wisse, E.), pp. 1–12. Elsevier, Amsterdam.

Wake, K. (1988). Liver perivascular cells revealed by gold and silver-impregnation methods and electron microscopy. In *Biopathology of the Liver: An Ultrastructural Approach* (Edited by Motta, P.M.), pp. 23–36. Kluwer Academic, Dordrecht.

Wake, K., Decker, K., Kirn, A., Knook, D.L., McCuskey, R.S., Bouwens, L. and Wisse, E. (1989). Cell biology and kinetics of Kupffer cells in the liver. *International Review of Cytology* **118**, 173–229.

Walker, R.M., Racz, W.J. and McElligott, T.F. (1983). Scanning electron microscopic examination of acetaminophen-induced hepatotoxicity and congestion in mice. *American Journal of Pathology* **113**, 321–330.

Wisse, E. (1970). An electron microscopic study of the fenestrated endothelial lining of rat liver sinusoids. *Journal of Ultrastructural Research* **31**, 125–150.

Wisse, E. (1972). An ultrastructural characterization of the endothelial cell in the rat liver sinusoid under normal and various experimental conditions, as a contribution to the distinction between endothelial and Kupffer cells. *Journal of Ultrastructural Research* **38**, 528–562.

Wisse, E., Van't Noordende, J.M., Van Der Meulen, J. and Daems, W.Th. (1976). The pit cell: Description of a new type of cell occurring in rat liver sinusoids and peripheral blood. *Cell and Tissue Research* **173**, 423–435.

Wisse, E., Van Dierendonck, J.H., De Zanger, R.B., Fraser, R. and McCuskey, R.S. (1980). On the role of the liver endothelial filter in the transport of particulate fat (chylomicrons and their remnants) to parenchymal cells and the influence of certain hormones on the endothelial fenestrae. In *Communications of Liver Cells* (Edited by Popper, H., Bianchi, L., Gudat, F. and Reutter, W.) MTP Press, Lancaster.

Wisse, E., De Zanger, R.B., Charels, K., Van Der Smissen, P. and McCuskey, R.S. (1985). The liver sieve: Considerations concerning the structure and function of endothelial fenestrae, the sinusoidal wall and the space of Disse. *Hepatology* **5**, 683–692.

Wright, P.L., Smith, K.F., Day W.A. and Fraser, R. (1983). Small liver fenestrae may explain the susceptibility of rabbits to atherosclerosis. *Atherosclerosis* **3**, 344–348.

Yamagishi, M. (1959). Electron microscope studies on the fine structure of the sinusoidal wall and fat-storing cells of rabbit livers. *Archives of Histology (Japan)* **18**, 223–261.

Zimmerman, H.J. (1986). Effects of alcohol on other hepatotoxins. *Alcoholism: Clinical and Experimental Research* **10**, 3–15.

16 Interactions between alcohol and other hepatotoxins

Michael K. Bay and Steven Schenker

Introduction

The purpose of this review is to discuss the interaction of ethanol (alcohol) and other hepatotoxins. As this is an extension of the interface of ethanol and other drugs generally in the liver, this area will also be considered. Moreover, the problem probably involves the unusual susceptibility of alcoholics to the adverse effects of some carcinogens. As some of the mechanisms of these effects of ethanol may be similar to the hepatotoxin issue, it too deserves mention (Lieber *et al.* 1986). Some elegant reviews of this general subject are available (Strubelt 1980; Zimmerman 1986; Lieber 1988, 1990).

There are two primary reasons for the importance of the liver in alcohol (drug)–drug interactions. First, the strategic location of the liver across the portal vein exposes this organ readily to absorbed xenobiotics. Second, the liver is the largest repository of enzymes which biotransform alcohol, drugs and other potentially hepatotoxic agents. This is important, because concomitant with metabolism which renders these substances more polar and thus more readily excretable in bile and urine, there is also sometimes formation of toxic metabolites. These biotransforming enzymes can be divided into various subtypes (isozymes), each of which is capable of metabolizing various xenobiotics at a rate dependent on the relative affinities of their binding to the various substrates. This provides opportunities for competition among the xenobiotics (i.e. inhibition of metabolism and elimination) or induction of the particular isozyme by one agent, thus promoting the metabolism of another. It is this interactive system, together with the passage of the xenobiotics through the liver, that defines the importance of drug–drug interactions in this organ.

Alcohol is, of course, ingested and rapidly absorbed in the upper gastrointestinal tract and is very largely metabolized by the liver (Lieber 1977; see also Chapter 2). While some alcohol degradation (at low concentrations) proceeds via the cytosolic alcohol dehydrogenase pathway, at higher concentrations (above 50 mg/dl) the metabolism is substantially via the microsomal ethanol oxidizing system (MEOS), wherein the cytochrome P4502E1 (CYP2E1) has a very major role (Lieber 1988; see also Chapter 2). This isozyme is also used by many other substrates (see below), hence the setting is ripe for drug–drug interaction with ethanol (Watkins 1990). As alcohol is not a regulated agent in individuals of legal age (i.e. is available over the counter), and in many instances is ingested on a chronic basis with acute exacerbations, there is a frequent and prolonged potential for it to affect the elimination and possible toxicity of other agents.

Alcohol could interact with other agents due to drug–drug (pharmacokinetic) effects or by summation at the target organ (pharmacodynamic) level. In terms of pharmacokinetics, alcohol–xenobiotic interactions which impact on the liver and the patient could occur sequentially at the level of drug absorption, drug binding in plasma, drug delivery to the liver via blood flow or metabolic interaction in the liver itself. As elegantly discussed by Lieber (1990), no important ethanol effects are exerted on the first three steps (above), hence our attention in this review will focus on metabolic interaction within the liver. An exception to this is the controversy which surrounds the effects of various H$_2$-receptor antagonists on gastric alcohol absorption (first pass), some reporting increased alcohol delivery into the circulation (Caballeria *et al.* 1989; see also Chapter 2) and others no significant clinical effects (Raufman *et al.* 1993). As regards the pharmacodynamics interaction, the most important examples relate to the use of sedatives and analgesics/narcotics in patients who also drink alcohol. In these individuals, there may be a sedative summation of these soporific agents on the brain with resultant greater risk of accidents and injury. The pharmacokinetic and pharmacodynamic contributions may coexist when alcohol inhibits the elimination of a given sedative and the resulting higher drug concentration summates with the cerebral or respiratory depressant effects of alcohol. Such combined effects have been documented for benzodiazepines, phenothiazines, tricyclic antidepressants, barbiturates and various narcotics (Lieber 1990).

General mechanisms of ethanol–xenobiotic oxidative microsomal interactions

Acute ethanol effects

As commented on briefly above, the primary intrahepatic interaction of ethanol with xenobiotics is at the level of microsomal ethanol oxidizing enzymes, especially CYP2E1 (Lieber 1990). With acute (brief) ethanol exposure, the major effect of ethanol is competitive (i.e. inhibitory) as regards other substrates of this isozyme (Rubin *et al.* 1970, 1971). This results in a slowing of the rate of metabolism and, thus, of elimination of a number of agents. Commonly used (or previously prescribed) drugs which are thus affected by acute alcohol administration include pentobarbital (Rubin *et al.* 1970), meprobamate (Rubin *et al.* 1971), various orally administered benzodiazepines (Hoyumpa *et al.*

1980), chlorpromazine (Forrest *et al.* 1971), amitriptyline (Dorian *et al.* 1983), chlormethiazole (Neuvonen *et al.* 1981), morphine (Bodd *et al.* 1985), methadone (Browsky and Lieber 1978), tolbutamide (Carulli *et al.* 1971) and warfarin (Coleman and Evans 1975). The bioavailability of propranolol, likewise, is enhanced by alcohol (Grabowski *et al.* 1980). This acute effect of ethanol may extend to various industrial solvents and has been well documented for xylene, which is used in the manufacture of glues, printing inks and pesticides (Riihimaki *et al.* 1982). The effects of such inhibition of drug elimination will have varying consequences, with potential toxicity dependent on the therapeutic index (margin between therapeutic and toxic level) of the drug and duration of its use. For instance, the risks of increased anticoagulation with higher warfarin concentration are more likely to be of clinical importance than a change in meprobamate level.

Much remains to be learned about the competitive effects of *acute* ethanol dosing and metabolism of other drugs, especially in man. Thus, the minimal inhibitory dose, a dose–response relationship between alcohol and other agents and the time needed for alcohol to compete with the other drugs remain to be defined for most agents. The inhibitory effects will also vary for various substrates, possibly related to different binding affinities of the competing substrates for various sites in CYP2E1 (Muhoberac *et al.* 1984). This inhibitory effect may also be enhanced by consumption of NADPH via microsomal ethanol degradation and may depend, in part, on the individual microsomal activity (phenotypism) of the patient.

Chronic ethanol effects

In contrast to the inhibitory (competitive) effects of acute ethanol exposure, chronic use of ethanol has a stimulatory (inducing) effect on the microsomal oxidizing system (Lieber 1990; see also Chapter 2). This is exerted primarily on the best studied cytochrome subtype, CYP2E1. This protein has been purified from rat and rabbit, as well as from human liver, has been reconstituted *in vitro* with NADPH-cytochrome P450 reductase, phospholipid and rat microsomal P450, and has been found to metabolize not only ethanol but also other alcohols and other substrates such as aniline, acetaminophen, possibly cocaine and isoniazid (Lieber 1988). It also catalyses the biotransformation of carbon tetrachloride, benzene and *N*-nitrosodimethylamine among various other hepatotoxins (Lieber 1988). The CYP2E1 gene (Nebert nomenclature: Nebert *et al.* 1987) has been localized to chromosome-7 in the rat and chromosome-10 in humans (Umeno *et al.* 1988a, b). There is discussion concerning the mechanism(s) of induction of hepatic CYP2E1 by ethanol. In one model system using the enteral nutrition system and wide alcohol level oscillations, chronic (subacute) administration of ethanol apparently induces the CYP2E1 protein by post-translational events at low ethanol concentrations and by stimulating transcription at high ethanol concentrations (Ronis *et al.* 1993). In the more common liquid diet studies, the main mechanism was increased enzyme synthesis (Tsutsumi *et al.* 1993) and the effect was seen within 3 days. It is uncertain whether there is polymorphism of the CYP2E1 as a possible explanation of varying hepatotoxicity related to its induction.

Another mechanism is induction by protein stabilization (Song *et al.* 1989). Recent work studying inhibition and induction of CYP2E1 by using isoniazid in a group of 10 slow acetylators showed that 2 days after stopping isoniazid, a 56 percent increase in chlorzoxazone clearance (a drug that is specifically metabolized by CYP2E1) over baseline occurs. In contrast, while taking isoniazid, chlorzoxazone clearance was decreased by 58 percent. The authors concluded that these data suggested a mechanism in which isoniazid has the dual effect of inducing and at the same time inhibiting CYP2E1. Isoniazid stabilizes CYP2E1, which also results in inhibition of catalytic activity while isoniazid is bound to the enzyme. Upon stopping isoniazid, increased enzymatic activity is seen as isoniazid is eliminated (Zand *et al.* 1993).

It is still not certain what constitutes the minimal period and quantity of ethanol exposure to induce CYP2E1, especially in humans, but carbon tetrachloride hepatotoxicity is not enhanced by 2 h exposure to ethanol, while by 8 h there is a five-fold increase in the toxicity of carbon tetrachloride (Zimmerman 1986). In another study, a week of ethanol administration to rats, equivalent to 40 g ethanol daily (about four highballs) in humans, enhanced carbon tetrachloride toxicity (Strubelt 1978). Anecdotal data imply that most reported cases involve at least 6–8 beers a day for a protracted time. The effect of ethanol is not related to its metabolism, can be reproduced with other alcohols and cannot be induced with acetaldehyde (Zimmerman 1986). In the presence of ethanol, the inducing effect is blunted, but still overrides the inhibitory effects of acute ethanol exposure (see above) (Altomare *et al.* 1984a). Experimentally, the largest inducing effect is seen after chronic (subacute) ethanol exposure, but when ethanol is not present in the circulation (Lieber 1988). This may correspond to the post-drinking (withdrawal) period in humans. The offset of the inducing effect is variable for different substrates, but probably is between several days and several (usually 2) weeks (Lieber 1990; Hetu and Joly 1985). The inducing effects of chronic ethanol affect not only CYP2E1, but also spill over to other components of the microsomal oxidizing system (other P450 isozymes and NADPH cytochrome P450–reductase activity). In fact, histologically, there is evidence of proliferation of the smooth endoplasmic reticulum (see Chapter 3). The recent availability of chlorzoxazone, a non-toxic substrate for CYP2E1 in humans, may provide a safe test agent for assessing the amount and duration of ethanol intake to induce this metabolic pathway and define the effect (Kharasch *et al.* 1993).

The importance of this enhanced microsomal activity by chronic (subacute) ethanol intake is that it also increases the conversion of various xenobiotics to potentially toxic metabolites. This has been demonstrated not only for the prototype toxin, carbon tetrachloride, but also for other substances such as bromobenzene, various anaesthetic agents, and commonly used therapeutic agents such as acetaminophen and isoniazid (Lieber 1988, 1990). These agents apparently are primarily metabolized to their toxic derivatives also by cytochrome CYP2E1. A list of main xenobiotics whose hepatotoxicity is increased by chronic (prolonged) alcohol use is given in Table 16.1.

The concern about greater hepatotoxicity of various xenobiotics with prolonged alcohol use extends to possible promotion of carcinogenesis (Lieber *et al.* 1986). There is a clear association between chronic alcohol consumption and higher incidence of cancer of the upper alimentary and respiratory tracts, of the liver and possibly other organs. While the mechanism(s) for this relationship are probably complex, some of the agents which function as hepatotoxins with long-term alcohol use are also carcinogenic in experimental animals. Some agents which may be rendered more carcinogenic by alcohol use are shown in Table 16.2. Perhaps the best studied examples are nitrosodimethylamine and vinyl chloride (Lieber *et al.* 1986; Lieber 1990; Anderson 1992a). The former has been reported to produce lung tumours in experimental animals (Hetu and Joly 1985) and the latter was associated

Table 16.1 Xenobiotics with ethanol-enhanced hepato-toxicity[a]

Definite

  Acetaminophen
  Aflatoxin B
  Carbon tetrachloride
  Chloroform
  Cocaine
  Dimethylnitrosamine
  1,1,2-Trichloromethane
  Trichloroethylene
  Trichlorobromoethane
  Vitamin A
  Vinyl chloride

Probable

  Allyl alcohol
  Bromobenzene
  Galactosamine
  Manganese
  Vinylidene chloride

---

[a]Modified with permission from Zimmerman (1986).

with the development of angiosarcoma and hepato-cellular carcinoma in rats, both apparently augmented by the administration of ethanol (Lieber *et al.* 1986). A major explanation of the potentiating effects of ethanol in general, with respect to hepatotoxicity, relate to increased microsomal formation of carcinogenic derivatives from the parent agents. In the case of nitrosodimethylamine, the effects of ethanol may not only be to enhance the formation of toxic/carcinogenic derivatives in the liver with long-term ethanol use, but also to inhibit first-pass metabolism of the parent drug in the liver (i.e. its clearance) with acute ethanol and to shunt the agent in higher concentrations to the organs (i.e. lung) where the toxic effect (i.e. methylation) may be exerted (Hetu and Joly 1985; Anderson *et al.* 1992b). Alcoholics are frequently heavy smokers and the two conditions may also interact in promoting cancer development, especially as the upper digestive and respiratory tracts are most vulnerable. Ethanol and tobacco products may use similar metabolic pathways in the liver as one explanation for this interaction (Lieber *et al.* 1986).

In addition to increased formation of carcinogenic metabolites by ethanol, other mechanisms may contribute to this interaction. As elegantly reviewed by Lieber *et al.* (1986), these may include effects of ethanol on DNA metabolism (especially impaired DNA repair), immunosuppression, local mucosal effects on the alimentary tract, deficiencies of key nutrients (i.e. iron, zinc, riboflavin and vitamin A) and possibly an effect of congeners. While the precise contributions of these factors are speculative and may vary among patients, the possible role of each has an experimental basis. Their effects may be exerted at the stage of initiation, promotion or progression of carcinogenesis as outlined recently (Garro *et al.* 1992).

Mechanisms of ethanol–xenobiotic cytosolic interactions

As indicated above, ethanol, especially at low concentrations, is metabolized to acetaldehyde by cytosolic alcohol dehydrogenase. This enzyme is not specific for ethanol and is used by a variety of substrates, including digitalis preparations, ethylene glycol and methanol (Lieber 1990). The toxic effects of the latter two agents depend on formation of active metabolites and inhibition of such conversion by ethanol has been used to advantage therapeutically (Lieber 1990; Wacker *et al.* 1965).

Other competitive enzymatic effects related to ethanol metabolism involve aldehyde dehydrogenase, wherein acetaldehyde is eliminated. A variety of therapeutic agents (sulphonylureas, metronidazole, quinacrine, furazolidone and some cephalosporins) serve as substrates for this enzyme and when used in conjunction with alcohol may result in the accumulation of acetaldehyde and a toxic (disulfiram-like) reaction (Lieber 1990). Hence, caution in the use of such agents in alcohol-consuming patients is warranted.

Generation of reduced nicotinamide adenine nucleotide (NADH) due to ethanol metabolism may secondarily inhibit the glucuronidation of some drugs and decrease their elimination. This is due not to an inhibition of glucuronyl transferases but to a decrease in the supply of uridine-5′-diphospho-glucuronic acid (Bodd *et al.* 1985; Moldeus *et al.* 1978). Accumulation of such agents (i.e. morphine) may result in toxic effects, depending on the therapeutic index of the drug. By contrast, there is evidence for enhanced acetylation of some drugs, presumably due to greater supply of acetyl CoA from ethanol metabolism (Olsen and Morland 1978).

Table 16.2   Association of alcohol abuse and cancer[a]

1. *Human data*

Mouth	World Health organization (1964), Wynder and Bross (1957), Wynder *et al.* (1957)
Pharynx	Wynder and Bross (1957), Flamant *et al.* (1964)
Larynx	Wynder *et al.* (1956)
Oesophagus/stomach	World Health Organization (1964), Tuyns (1983), MacDonald (1972) Keller (1978)
Liver	Lieber *et al.* (1979), Keller (1978)
Pancreas[b]	Burch and Ansari (1968), International Agency for Research on Cancer (1973)
Colon[b]	Williams and Horm (1977), Engstrom (1977), Kono and Ikeda (1979), Tuyns *et al.* (1982), Potter *et al.* (1982)

2. *Experimental data[c]*

Substance	*Cancer site*
7,12-Dimethylbenzanthracene	Cheek epithelium of hamsters (Elzay 1966, 1969)
	Skin of mice (Stenback 1969)
Diethylnitrosamine	Oesophagus in rats (Gibel 1967)
Vinyl chloride	Liver in rats (Radike *et al.* 1981)
Nitrosopyrolidine	Nasopharynx in hamsters (Gibel 1967)
Dimethylhydrazine	Rectum in rats (Seitz *et al.* 1984)

[a]Modified with permission from Lieber *et al.* (1986).
[b]Some data are conflicting or negative (Longnecker 1992).
[c]Negative data for alcohol and some carcinogens not cited.

General mechanisms of alcohol hepatotoxin-induced hepatic injury

The exact mechanism(s) of *ethanol*-induced liver injury is uncertain; however, it is likely that the mechanism is multifactorial. The subject has been well-reviewed (Lieber 1988; see also Chapters 2–6). Consideration of the interaction of alcohol with *other hepatotoxins* as to mechanism of liver damage adds another layer of complexity to the discussion. Each toxin may exert its pathogenetic effects via a number of mechanisms and the importance of these may vary (Lieber 1990). In many instances, the precise key mechanism is uncertain. While some important agents will be considered individually later, this section will address some general concepts.

Hepatotoxicity depends on a balance of toxifying and detoxifying factors (Kaplowitz *et al.* 1988; Schenker 1991). Increased production of toxic metabolites, as following induction with chronic ethanol, may cause hepatic injury by various reactive pathways. These are usually placed in three categories: electrophiles, free radicals and redox cyclic substances (Schenker 1991). As shown in Table 16.3, formation of these metabolites varies

with the drug. Hepatic parenchymal cell disruption may be via lipid peroxidation, thiol oxidation and/or covalent binding to various components of the liver. Other than induction, some individuals may show enhanced formation of toxic metabolites due to genetic alterations (polymorphism) of P450 enzymes, an example of metabolic idiosyncrasy (Watkins 1990; Larrey *et al.* 1989). The metabolites can be toxic *per se* or can combine with liver proteins, often at the metabolic site on the smooth endoplasmic reticulum, and function as an immunogenic haptene, most likely after migrating to the plasma membrane surface. The exact mechanisms by which the toxic metabolites (Table 16.3) disrupt cell integrity are uncertain. Some seem to affect primarily individual organelles (i.e. mitochondria in the acetaminophen–alcohol interaction), others affect membranes. The latter may be especially important with cholestatic injury in which transport of bile acids by canalicular (and/or basolateral) membranes is altered (King and Blitzer 1990). There may also be a secondary effect of cell injury on Kupffer and endothelial cells with release of cytokines and other inflammatory mediators. The final common denominator of hepatocellular injury may be disruption of cellular calcium regulation and

Table 16.3　Major pathways of action of hepatotoxins exerting their effect via metabolic activation

Toxic metabolic	Definition	Drug example	Metabolic activation	Consequences	Endogenous defence
Free radical	Substance with unpaired electron. Removes these from other substances changing these to free radicals and perpetuating reaction	CCL_4, halothane	Reductive-P450	Lipid peroxidation and covalent binding to membrane unsaturated fatty acids	Tocopherol? GSH
Electrophile	Compounds which take electrons from other substances. In this exchange the substances form a covalent bond. Bonding may be with thiols or amino acids	Acetaminophen, bromobenzene	Oxidative-P450	Covalent binding to protein-SH	GSH
Oxygen radicals	Transfer reactions with H_2O_2 formation. This forms hydroxyl radicals, which peroxidize (disrupt) lipids and other cell components	Adriamycin	Redox cycling	Lipid peroxidation, thiol oxidation	GSH Tocopherol?

Modified with permission from Kaplowitz *et al*. (1988).

subsequent disturbance of mitochondrial energy production. Much remains to be learned about these specific intracellular processes.

On the detoxifying side, the endogenous defence mechanisms include glutathione (critically important in the acetaminophen–alcohol interaction), various antioxidants (e.g. vitamin E) and likely membrane stabilizers (i.e. prostaglandins) (Kaplowitz *et al*. 1988; Schenker 1991). To the extent that ethanol (especially over a long period of time) inhibits hepatic glutathione stores, especially its transport into mitochondria, this detoxifying pathway has major relevance to hepatotoxicity of some drugs (e.g. acetaminophen). Other agents made more hepatotoxic by glutathione depletion are carbon tetrachloride, allyl alcohol and bromobenzene (Table 16.1). Moreover, nutrition may, importantly, affect glutathione and vitamin E concentrations in liver and may render it more susceptible to alcohol/hepatotoxin interaction (Young *et al*. 1993). It has been also suggested by some that ethanol increases hepatic oxygen consumption (see Chapter 19), and that this may promote greater centrilobular (zone 3) damage by many hepatotoxins (e.g. carbon tetrachloride). However, this localization of drug effect may simply reflect greater generation of toxic derivatives in zone 3, and indeed for

some agents (e.g. thioacetamide), hepatotoxicity is decreased with hypoxia (Strubelt 1980). Moreover, decreased centrilobular oxygenation with ethanol has not been uniformly accepted.

Interaction of ethanol and specific hepatotoxins

Carbon tetrachloride

This is probably the oldest known and best studied example of ethanol interaction with a specific hepatotoxin (Zimmerman 1986). The agent was initially used for treatment of hookworm infestation until its toxicity to patients became evident (Hall 1921). It has been well-studied in multiple animal species as well. Ethanol, both in humans and experimental animals, is well-documented to potentiate carbon tetrachloride toxicity. It is estimated that between 1939 and 1953, some 65 percent of reported cases of subacute carbon tetrachloride poisoning occurred in alcoholics (cited in Williams and Burk 1990).

It appears that as little as one ounce of carbon tetrachloride can be fatal to humans and the agent can be absorbed from the gastrointestinal tract, lungs and even the skin. In experimental animals ethanol can potentiate carbon tetrachloride-induced liver damage after only 3 h of *prior* ethanol exposure but this enhancement increases with the duration of ethanol use (Zimmerman 1986; Hall *et al.* 1991). Even small amounts of ethanol, equivalent to 40 g alcohol daily in humans, may augment the damage. *Concurrent* ethanol use may actually decrease carbon tetrachloride toxicity (Tesche *et al.* 1983). Other alcohols, as well as ethanol, share in this potentiating effect and it is not dependent on ethanol metabolism, i.e. the ethanol *per se* is responsible. In fact, other alcohols may enhance the carbon tetrachloride effect more than ethanol (Zimmerman 1986). The potentiating effect of ethanol is reflected in increased hepatocellular damage with greater release of liver enzymes, decrease in liver function as assessed by drug metabolism and evidence of histologic damage (Zimmerman 1986).

The mechanism(s) of carbon tetrachloride-induced liver injury is not fully worked out, but it is generally agreed that it is mediated by toxic metabolites (Williams and Burk 1990). It appears that ethanol use enhances this process by inducing cytochromes, especially the CYP2E1 isozyme. Increased formation of reactive metabolites will also be affected by the total pattern of other cytochrome P450 isozymes and the oxygen tension at the metabolic site. The free radicals generated by carbon tetrachloride metabolism are felt to react with and damage cell lipids and cell membranes. Protection is afforded by a high oxygen tension, glutathione and antioxidants such as vitamin E. A detailed discussion of the known mechanistic aspects of carbon tetrachloride toxicity to liver cells has recently been presented and served as a basis for some potential therapeutic manoeuvres such as the use of hyperbaric oxygen to decrease free radical formation (Williams and Burk 1990).

Vinyl chloride

Vinyl chloride has been included in this review as a prototype drug for several reasons. First, it is a halogenated aliphatic hydrocarbon, resembling various anaesthetics and trichloroethylene. Second, in humans it has been elegantly proven to cause both hepatic fibrosis (Marsteller *et al.* 1973) and angiosarcoma of the liver (Lee and Harry 1974) with chronic exposure. These carcinogenic effects have been reproduced in experimental animals (Radike *et al.* 1981). Third, the toxic effects of this agent are felt to

be due to its active metabolite(s), possibly an epoxide; moreover, the biotransformation of vinyl chloride is fairly well worked out (Berk *et al.* 1976; Tamburro 1984). At low levels of the drug (i.e. 50 ppm), it is metabolized by alcohol dehydrogenase and above this concentration by oxidation to chlorethylene oxide and then to chloracetaldehyde (Tamburro 1984; Hefner *et al.* 1975). The former may bind covalently to adenine and cytosine, and then to DNA with possible mutagenic effects (Basu *et al.* 1993). Chloracetaldehyde also binds to glutathione with subsequent elimination as cysteine derivatives in the urine (Tamburro 1984; Gitlin 1990). Finally, ethanol may compete for the metabolism of vinyl chloride via alcohol dehydrogenase and may theoretically drive more vinyl chloride into the oxidative (? toxic) pathway (Hultmark *et al.* 1979). Clearly, any ethanol (or other) induced decrease in hepatic glutathione concentration could also decrease the elimination of vinyl chloride. Thus, both in terms of an enhanced formation of toxic derivatives and a decrease in protective factors, ethanol theoretically could potentiate the toxicity of vinyl chloride.

In the clinical setting, it has been difficult to prove an association of alcohol exposure with vinyl chloride toxicity as the latter is rare and usually diagnosed retrospectively. In experimental animals, we are aware of one study wherein chronic pre-treatment of rats with alcohol potentiated the carcinogenic effects of vinyl chloride alone on the liver (Radike *et al.* 1981). Unfortunately, in this report there was a surprisingly high incidence of neoplastic lesions due to ethanol alone. In another report, pre-treatment for 7 days with 5 percent ethanol also enhanced the toxicity of vinylidene chloride, but concomitant administration of ethanol inhibited the toxic effect of vinylidene chloride (Siegers *et al.* 1983). Clearly, more research is necessary to determine if the above cited theoretical considerations of greater vinyl chloride hepatotoxicity with alcohol exposure are relevant to clinical medicine.

The recognition of vinyl chloride hepatotoxicity is a fine example of meticulous epidemiologic research which evolved into characterization of drug metabolism and improved patient care via preventive medicine. Stringent safeguards for industry have been established with mandatory reduction in vinyl chloride exposure to 1 ppm (Gitlin 1990; Griciute 1978). This is especially important as detection of early liver damage due to vinyl chloride may be difficult in the absence of liver biopsy (Berk *et al.* 1976). Indocyanine green clearance (Tamburro *et al.* 1978; Tamburro and Greenberg 1981) and fasting serum bile acid analysis (Liss *et al.* 1985) have been suggested as possible early non-invasive screening techniques.

Acetaminophen (paracetamol)

Acetaminophen (*N*-acetyl-*p*-aminophenol) is a common analgesic/antipyretic. A prescribed drug in the USA from 1955 to 1960, it received FDA approval for over-the-counter use in 1960 and since that time has achieved impressive widespread acceptance. In the 12 month period ending 1 September 1989, 249.8 million packages of acetaminophen-containing products were sold in the USA. Given the fact that alcohol is consumed by two-thirds of the American population with 12 percent considered to be heavy drinkers, significant potential exists for the concurrent consumption of these two substances.

The interactions between ethanol and acetaminophen can be divided into chronic and acute ethanol exposure. With chronic ethanol exposure there is excellent evidence from animal studies and some good data from human studies for the potentiation of hepatotoxicity. In contrast, acute ethanol exposure may actually serve to protect the liver from the toxicity of large doses of acetaminophen. Over the past two decades, animal and human studies have provided insight into the mechanism(s) that help explain this dual nature of ethanol.

Starting in the 1970s, several reports called attention to significant liver injury with unusually high transaminase levels in alcoholics who were taking moderate doses of acetaminophen (Emby and Frazer 1977; Barker *et al.* 1977; Goldfinger *et al.* 1978; Labrecque and Mitros 1980; McClain *et al.* 1980; Licht *et al.* 1980; Johnson *et al.* 1981; Levinson 1983). Strikingly high transaminase levels were a clue that hepatic injury other than that due to alcohol alone may be involved, since the aspartate aminotransferase (AST) levels greatly exceeded what would be expected (>1000 U/ml) in isolated alcoholic liver disease. In many patients, AST elevations even exceeded what would be considered consistent for viral hepatitis. Furthermore, many of these patients showed centrilobular (zone 3) necrosis on liver biopsy. The worrisome aspect of these reports was the significant liver injury after taking seemingly non-toxic amounts (<10 g/day) of acetaminophen.

In one series of 25 chronic alcoholics (16 males and nine females), all had evidence of severe hepatocellular necrosis and often strikingly high serum aminotransferase levels. The reported dosage of acetaminophen ranged from 2.6 to 16.5 g/24 h. In 11 patients, the reported dose was less than 6 g/24 h. In 22 patients, the serum AST was greater than 3000 IU/l and in six patients the value was greater than 10,000 IU/l. Five of the 25 patients died (20 percent mortality). One of these five reportedly took only 6 g/24 h of acetaminophen (Seeff *et al.* 1986).

Experimental studies confirmed increased acetaminophen toxicity in animals pretreated with ethanol. Chronic ethanol exposure in mice (Strubelt 1978, 1980; Strubelt *et al.* 1978; Walker *et al.* 1983), rats (Sato *et al.* 1981a) and hamsters (Rosen *et al.* 1983) was associated with increased acetaminophen hepatotoxicity. Studies using rat hepatocytes (Moldeus *et al.* 1980) and *in vivo* studies using mice (Peterson *et al.* 1980) and baboons (Altomare *et al.* 1984a) suggested that chronic ethanol exposure increased acetaminophen clearance to both reactive and glucuronidated metabolite. Subsequently, increased clearance of acetaminophen in alcoholic humans was reported supporting the previous observation (Girre *et al.* 1993; Dietz *et al.* 1984).

Acute ethanol exposure decreases the metabolism of acetaminophen to active metabolites and protects the liver from acetaminophen toxicity in mice (Wong *et al.* 1980; Altomare *et al.* 1984a; Tredger *et al.* 1986) and rats (Sato and Lieber 1981a; Sato *et al.* 1981b). Furthermore, acute ethanol exposure has been reported to result in decreased formation of oxidative metabolites in humans (Critchley *et al.* 1983; Hartnell *et al.* 1983). One mechanism that has been proposed suggests that the hepatoprotective effect of ethanol is due to direct inhibition of the cytochrome P450 that oxidizes acetaminophen to the toxic metabolite NAPQI (Wong *et al.* 1980; Sato and Lieber 1981a). An alternative or additional mechanism proposes indirect inhibition by depletion of free NADPH concentration in cytosol resulting in a decrease in the rate of mixed-function oxidation (Reinke *et al.* 1980; Thummel *et al.* 1988).

The major explanation proposed for the enhancement of acetaminophen hepatotoxicity with chronic ethanol exposure postulates induction of cytochrome P450 isozymes, primarily CYP2E1 by ethanol. This isozyme metabolizes acetaminophen to a toxic metabolite. Another mechanism postulates depletion of hepatic glutathione, especially mitochondrial glutathione stores (Fernandez-Checa *et al.* 1991), with chronic ethanol exposure resulting in increased acetaminophen toxicity. Glutathione

cocaine in mediating lethality. *Pharmacology, Biochemistry and Behavior* **31**, 531–533.

Hefner, R.E., Jr., Watanabe, P.G. and Gehring, P.G. (1975). Preliminary studies of the fate of inhaled vinyl chloride monomer in rats. *Annals of the New York Academy of Science* **246**, 135–148.

Hetu, C. and Joly, J.-G. (1985). Differences in the duration of the enhancement of liver mixed-function oxidase activities in ethanol-fed rats after withdrawal. *Biochemical Pharmacology* **34**, 1211–1216.

Hoyumpa, A.M., Desmond, P.V., Roberts, R.K., Nichols, S., Johnson, R.F. and Schenker, S. (1980). Effect of ethanol on benzodiazepine disposition in dogs. *Journal of Laboratory and Clinical Medicine* **95**, 310–322.

Hultmark, D., Sundh, K., Johannson, L. and Arhenius, F. (1979). Ethanol inhibition of vinyl chloride metabolism in isolated rat hepatocytes. *Chemico–Biological Interactions* **25**, 1–6.

Inaba, T., Stewart, D.J. and Kalow, W. (1978). Metabolism of cocaine in man. *Clinical Pharmacology and Therapeutics* **23**, 547–552.

International Agency for Research on Cancer (1973). *Alcohol and Cancer Report: Interim report*. IARC, Lyons, France.

Isner, J.M., Estes, N.A., III, Thompson, P.D., Castanzo-Nordin, M.R., Subramanian, R., Miller, G., Katsus, G., Sweeney, K. and Sturner, W.Q. (1986). Acute cardiac events temporally related to cocaine abuse. *New England Journal of Medicine* **315**, 1438–1443.

Israel, Y., Kalant, H., Orrego, H., Khanna, J.M., Videla, L. and Phillips, J.M. (1975). Experimental alcohol-induced hepatic necrosis: Suppression by propylthiouracil. *Proceedings of the National Academy of Sciences, USA* **72**, 1137–1141.

James, R.C., Schiefer, M.A., Roberts, S.M. and Harbison, R.D. (1987). Antagonism of cocaine-induced hepatotoxicity by the alpha-adrenergic antagonists phentolamine and yohimbine. *Journal of Pharmacology and Experimental Therapeutics* **242**, 726–732.

Jatlow, P., Elsworth, J.D., Bradberry, C.W., Winger, G., Taylor, J.R., Russel, R. and Roth, R.H. (1991). Cocaethylene: A neuropharmacologically active metabolite associated with concurrent cocaine–ethanol ingestion. *Life Sciences* **48**, 1787–1794.

Jindal, S.P. and Lutz, T. (1986). Ion cluster techniques in drug metabolism: Use of a mixture of labeled and unlabeled cocaine to facilitate metabolite identification. *Journal of Analytic Toxicology* **10**, 150–155.

Jindal, S.P., Lutz, T. and Vestergaard, P. (1978). Mass spectrometric determination of cocaine and its biologically active metabolite, norcocaine, in human urine. *Biomedical Mass Spectrometry* **5**, 658–663.

Johanson, C.E. and Fischman, M.W. (1989). The pharmacology of cocaine related to its abuse. *Pharmacology Review* **41**, 3–52.

Johnson, M.W., Friedman, P.A. and Mitch, W.E. (1981). Alcoholism, nonprescription drugs and hepatotoxicity: The risk from unknown acetaminophen ingestion. *American Journal of Gastroenterology* **76**, 530–533.

Jollow, D.J., Mitchell, J.R., Potter, W.Z., Davis, D.C., Gillette, J.R. and Brodie, B.B. (1973). Acetaminophen-induced hepatic necrosis: II. Role of covalent binding *in vivo*. *Journal of Pharmacology and Experimental Therapeutics* **187**, 195–202.

Jover, R., Ponsoda, X., Gomez-Lechon, M.J., Herrero, C., del Pino, J. and Castell, J.V. (1991). Potentiation of cocaine hepatotoxicity by ethanol in human hepatocytes. *Toxicology and Applied Pharmacology* **107**, 526–534.

Kanel, G.C., Cassidy, W., Shuster, L. and Reynolds, T.B. (1990). Cocaine-induced liver cell injury: Comparison of morphological features in man and experimental models. *Hepatology* **11**, 646–651.

Kaplowitz, N., Aw, T.-Y. and Stolz, A. (1988). Drug-induced hepatotoxicity. In *Gastrointestinal and Liver Diseases*. (Edited by Gitnick, G.), pp. 1089–1102. Elsevier, New York.

Keller, A.Z. (1978). Liver cirrhosis, tobacco, alcohol and cancer among blacks. *Journal of the National Medical Association* **70**, 575–580.

Kharasch, E.D., Thummel, K.E., Mhyre, J. and Lillibridge, J.H. (1993). Single-dose disulfiram inhibition of chlorzoxazone metabolism: A clinical probe for P4502E1. *Clinical Pharmacology and Therapeutics* **53**, 643–650.

King, P.D. and Blitzer, B.L. (1990). Drug-induced cholestasis: Pathogenesis and clinical features. *Seminars in Liver Disease* **10**, 316–321.

Kloss, M.W., Rosen, G.M. and Rauchman, E.J. (1982). Acute cocaine-induced hepatoxicity in DBA/2Ha male mice. *Toxicology and Applied Pharmacology* **65**, 75–83.

Kokko, J.P. (1990). Metabolic and social consequences of cocaine abuse. *American Journal of the Medical Sciences* **229**, 361–365.

Kono, S. and Ikeda, M. (1979). Correlation between cancer mortality and alcohol beverage in Japan. *British Journal of Cancer* **40**, 449–455.

Kopanoff, D.E., Snider, D.E. and Cavas, G.J. (1978). Isoniazid-related hepatitis. *American Review of Respiratory Disease* **117**, 991–1001.

Labrecque, D.R. and Mitros, F.A. (1980). Increased hepatotoxicity of acetaminophen in the alcoholic (abstract). *Gastroenterology* **78**, 1310.

Lambert, S.M. (1922). Carbon tetrachloride in the treatment of hookworm disease: Observations in twenty thousand cases. *Journal of the American Medical Association* **79**, 2055–2057.

Larrey, D., Berson, A., Habersetzer, F., Tinel, M., Castot, A., Babany, G., Letteron, P., Freneaux, E., Loeper, J., Dansette, P. and Pessayre, D. (1989). Genetic predisposition to drug hepatotoxicity: Role in hepatitis caused by amineptine, a tricyclic antidepressant. *Hepatology* **10**, 168–173.

Lautenburg, B.H., Davies, J. and Mitchell, J.R. (1984).

Ethanol suppresses hepatic glutathoine synthesis in rats *in vivo*. *Journal of Pharmacology and Experimental Therapeutics* **230**, 7–11.

Lee, F.I. and Harry, D.S. (1974). Angiosarcoma of the liver in a vinyl chloride worker. *Lancet* **1**, 1316–1318.

Leist, M.H., Gluskin, L.E. and Payne, J.A. (1985). Enhanced toxicity of acetaminophen in alcoholics: Report of 3 cases. *Journal of Clinical Gastroenterology* **7**, 55–59.

Leo, M.A. and Lieber, C.S. (1982). Hepatic vitamin A depletion in alcoholic liver injury in man. *New England Journal of Medicine* **37**, 597–601.

Leo, M.A. and Lieber, C.S. (1983). Interaction of ethanol with vitamin A. *Alcoholism: Clinical and Experimental Research* **7**, 15–21.

Leo, M.A. and Lieber, C.S. (1985). New pathway for retinol metabolism in liver microsomes. *Journal of Biological Chemistry* **260**, 5228–5231.

Leo, M.A., Sato, M. and Lieber, C.S. (1983). Effect of hepatic vitamin A depletion on the liver in men and rats. *Gastroenterology* **84**, 562–572.

Leo, M.A., Iida, S. and Lieber, C.S. (1984a). Retinol acid metabolism by a system reconstituted with cytochrome P450. *Archives of Biochemistry and Biophysics* **234**, 305–312.

Leo, M.A., Lowe, N. and Lieber, C.S. (1984b). Decreased hepatic vitamin A after drug administration in men and rats. *American Journal of Clinical Nutrition* **40**(6), 1131–1136.

Lesser, P.B., Vietti, M.D. and Clark, W.D. (1986). Lethal enhancement of therapeutic doses of acetaminophen by alcohol. *Digestive Diseases and Sciences* **31**, 103–105.

Lester, D. (1964). The acetylation of isoniazid in alcoholics. *Quarterly Journal on the Study of Alcohol* **25**, 541–543.

Levinson, M. (1983). Ulcer, back pain and jaundice in an alcoholic. *Hospital Practice* **18**, 481–485.

Licht, H., Seeff, L.B. and Zimmerman, H.J. (1980). Apparent potentiation of acetaminophen hepatotoxicity by alcohol. *Annals of Internal Medicine* **92**, 511.

Lieber, C.S. (1977). Metabolism of ethanol. In *Metabolic Aspects of Alcoholism* (Edited by Lieber, C.S.), pp. 1–29. University Park Press, Baltimore, MD.

Lieber, C.S. (1988). Biochemical and molecular basis of alcohol-induced injury to liver and other tissues. *New England Journal of Medicine* **319**, 1639–1650.

Lieber, C.S. (1990). Interactions of ethanol with drugs, hepatotoxic agents, carcinogens and vitamins. *Alcohol and Alcoholism* **25**, 157–176.

Lieber, C.S., Seitz, H.K., Garro, A.J. and Worner, T.M. (1979). Alcohol-related diseases and carcinogenesis. *Cancer Research* **39**, 2863–2886.

Lieber, C.S., Garro, A., Leo, M.A., Mak, K.M. and Worner, T. (1986). Alcohol and cancer. *Hepatology* **6**, 1005–1019.

Liss, G.M., Greenberg, R.A. and Tamburro, C.H. (1985). Use of serum bile acids in the identification of vinyl chloride hepatotoxicity. *American Journal of Medicine* **78**, 68–76.

Longnecker, M.P. (1992). Alcohol consumption in relation to risk of cancers of the breast and large bowel. *Alcohol Health and Research World* **16**, 223–229.

Lowry, W.T., Lomonte, J.N., Hatchett, D. and Garnott, J.C. (1979). Identification of two novel cocaine metabolites in bile by gas chromatography and gas chromatography/mass spectrometry in a case of acute intravenous cocaine overdose. *Journal of Analytic Toxicology* **3**, 91–95.

MacDonald, W.C. (1972). Clinical and pathological features of adenocarcinoma of the gastric cardia. *Cancer* **29**, 724–732.

Marsteller, H.J., Lelbach, W.K., Muller, R. *et al.* (1973). Chronischtoxische leberschaden bei arbeitern in der PVC-produktion. *Dtsch Med Wochenschr* **98**, 2311–2314.

McClain, C.J., Kromhout, J.P., Peterson, F.J. and Holtzman, J.L. (1980). Potentiation of acetaminophen hepatotoxicity by alcohol. *Journal of the American Medical Association* **244**, 251–253.

Mitchell, J.R., Long, M.W.W., Thorgeirsson, O.P. and Jollow, D.J. (1975a). Acetylation rates and monthly liver function tests during one year of isoniazid preventive therapy. *Chest* **68**, 181–190.

Mitchell, J.R., Thorgeirsson, U.P., Black, M., Timbrell, J.A., Snodgrass, W.R., Potter, W.Z., Jollow, H.R. and Keiser, H.R. (1975b). Increased incidence of isoniazid hepatitis in rapid acetylators: Possible relation to hydrazine metabolites. *Clinical Pharmacology and Therapeutics* **18**, 70–79.

Mitchell, J.R., Zimmerman, H.J., Ishak, K.G., Thorgeirsson, U.P., Timbrell, J.A., Snodgrass, W.R. and Nelson, S.D. (1976). Isoniazid liver injury: Clinical spectrum, pathology, and probable pathogenesis. *Annals of Internal Medicine* **84**, 181–192.

Moldeus, P., Andersson, B. and Norling, A. (1978). Interaction of ethanol oxidation with glucuronidation in isolated hepatocytes. *Biochemical Pharmacology* **27**, 2583–2588.

Moldeus, P., Andersson, B., Norling, A. and Ormstad, K. (1980). Effect of chronic ethanol administration on drug metabolism in isolated hepatocytes with emphasis on paracetamol activation. *Biochemical Pharmacology* **29**, 1741–1745.

Moulding, T.S., Redeker, A.G. and Kanel, G.C. (1989). Twenty isoniazid-associated deaths in one state. *American Review of Respiratory Diseases* **140**, 700–705.

Muhoberac, B., Roberts, R., Hoyumpa, A. and Schenker, S. (1984). State of the art: Mechanism(s) of ethanol–drug interaction. *Alcoholism: Clinical and Experimental Research* **8**, 583–593.

Murphy, R., Swartz, R. and Watkins, P.B. (1990). Severe acetaminophen toxicity in a patient receiving isoniazid. *Annals of Internal Medicine* **113**, 799–800.

Nebert, D.W., Adesnik, M., Coon, M.J., Estabrook, R.W., Gonzalez, F.J., Guengerich, F.P., Gunsalus,

I.C., Johnson, E.F., Kemper, B., Levin, W., Phillips, I.R., Sato, R. and Waterman, M.R. (1987). The P-450 gene superfamily: Recommended nomenclature. *DNA* **6**, 1–11.

Neuvonen, P.J., Pentikainen, P.J., Jostell, K.G. and Syvalahti, E. (1981). Effects of ethanol on the pharmacokinetics of chlormethiazole in humans. *International Journal of Clinical Pharmacology, Therapy and Toxicology* **19**, 552–560.

Odeleye, O.E., Watson, R.R., Cleamond, D.E. and Earnest, D. (1993). Enhancement of cocaine-induced hepatotoxicity by ethanol. *Drug and Alcohol Dependence* **31**, 253–263.

Olsen, H. and Morland, J. (1978). Ethanol-induced increase in drug acetylation in man. *British Medical Journal* **2**, 1260–1262.

Olsen, H. and Morland, J. (1982). Ethanol-induced increase in procainamide acetylation in man. *British Journal of Clinical Pharmacology* **13**, 203–208.

Perino, L.E., Warren, G.H. and Levine, J.S. (1987). Cocaine-induced hepatotoxicity in humans. *Gastroenterology* **93**, 176–180.

Peterson, F.J., Holloway, D.E., Erickson, R.R., Duquette, P.H., McClain, C.J. and Holtzman, J.L. (1980). Ethanol induction of acetaminophen toxicity and metabolism. *Life Sciences* **27**, 1705–1711.

Potter, J.D., McMichael, A.J. and Hartshorne, J.M. (1982). Alcohol and beer consumption in relation to cancers of bowel and lung: An extended correlation analysis. *Journal of Chronic Diseases* **35**, 833–842.

Potter, W.Z., Davis, D.C., Mitchell, J.R., Jollow, D.J., Gillette, J.R. and Brodie, B.B. (1973). Acetaminophen-induced heptic necrosis: II. Cytochrome P450-mediated covalent binding *in vitro*. *Journal of Pharmacology and Experimental Therapeutics* **187**, 203–210.

Radike, M.J., Stemmer, K.L. and Bingham, E. (1981). Effect of ethanol on vinylchloride carcinogenesis. *Environmental Health Perspective* **4**, 59–62.

Rauckman, E.J., Kloss, M.W. and Rosen, G.M. (1982). Involvement of nitroxide radicals in cocaine-induced hepatotoxicity. *Canadian Journal of Chemistry* **60**, 1614–1620.

Raufman, J.-P., Notar-Francesco, V., Raffaniello, R.D. and Straus, E.W. (1993). Histamine-2 receptor antagonists do not alter serum ethanol levels in fed, nonalcoholic men. *Annals of Internal Medicine* **118**, 488–494.

Reinke, L.A., Kaufmann, F.C., Belinsky, S.A. and Thurman, R.G. (1980). Interactions between ethanol metabolism and mixed-function oxidation in perfused rat liver: Inhibition of *p*-nitroanisole *o*-demethylation. *Journal of Pharmacology and Experimental Therapeutics* **213**, 70–78.

Riihimaki, V., Savolainen, K., Pfaffli, P., Pekari, K., Sippel, H.W. and Laine, A. (1982). Metabolic interaction between *n*-xylene and ethanol. *Archives of Toxicology* **49**, 253–263.

Ronis, M.J.J., Huang, J., Crouch, J., Mercado, C., Irby, D., Valentine, C.R., Lumpkin, C.K., Ingelman-Sundberg, M. and Badger, T.M. (1993). Cytochrome P450 CYP2E1 induction during chronic alcohol exposure occurs by a two-step mechanism associated with blood alcohol concentrations in rats. *Journal of Pharmacology and Experimental Therapeutics* **264**, 944–950.

Rosen, G.M., Singletary, W.V., Rauckman, E.J. and Killenberg, P.G. (1983). Acetaminophen hepatotoxicity: An alternative mechanism. *Biochemical Pharmacology* **32**, 2053–2059.

Rubin, E., Gang, H., Misra, P.S. and Lieber, C.S. (1970). Inhibition of drug metabolism by acute ethanol intoxication: An hepatic microsomal mechanism. *American Journal of Medicine* **49**, 801–806.

Rubin, E., Lieber, C.S., Alvares, A.P., Levin, W. and Kuntzman, R. (1971). Ethanol binding to hepatic microsomes: Its increase by ethanol consumption. *Biochemical Pharmacology* **20**, 229–231.

Sato, C. and Lieber, C.S. (1981a). Mechanism of the preventive effect of ethanol on acetaminophen-induced hepatotoxicity. *Journal of Pharmacology and Experimental Therapeutics* **218**, 811–815.

Sato, M. and Lieber, C.S. (1981b). Hepatic vitamin A depletion after chronic ethanol consumption in baboons and rats. *Journal of Nutrition* **111**, 2015–2023.

Sato, M. and Lieber, C.S. (1982). Changes in vitamin A status after actue ethanol administration in the rat. *Journal of Nutrition* **112**, 1188–1196.

Sato, C., Matsuda, Y. and Lieber, C.S. (1981a). Increased hepatotoxicity of acetaminophen after chronic ethanol consumption in the rat. *Gastroenterology* **80**, 140–148.

Sato, C., Nakano, M. and Lieber, C.S. (1981b). Prevention of acetaminophen-induced hepatotoxicity by acute ethanol administration in the rat: Comparison with carbon tetrachloride-induced hepatotoxicity. *Journal of Pharmacology and Experimental Therapeutics* **218**, 805–810.

Schenker, S. (1991). Toxic and drug-induced hepatitis. In *Hepatitis: Viral and Drug-Induced*, pp. 46–56. National Health Labs., Inc., La Jolla, CA.

Seeff, L.B., Cuccherihi, B.A., Zimmerman, H.J., Alder, E. and Benjamin S.B. (1986). Acetaminophen hepatotoxicity in alcoholics: A therapeutic misadventure. *Annals of Internal Medicine* **104**, 399–404.

Seitz, H.K., Czygan, P., Waldherr, R., Veith, S., Raedsch, R., Kassmodel, H. and Kommerell, B. (1984). Enhancement of 1,2-dimethylhydrazine-induced rectal carcinogenesis following ethanol consumption in the rat. *Gastroenterology* **86**, 886–891.

Sharkey, J., Ritz, M.C., Schenden, J.A., Hayson, R.C. and Kuhar, M.J. (1988). Cocaine inhibits muscarinic cholinergic receptors in heart and brain. *Journal of Pharmacology and Experimental Therapeutics* **246**, 1048–1055.

Shuster, L., Quimby, F., Bates, A. and Thompson, M.L. (1977). Liver damage from cocaine in mice. *Life Sciences* **20**, 1035–1042.

Shuster, L., Casey, E. and Welankiwar, S.S. (1983). Metabolism of cocaine and norcocaine to *N*-

hydroxynorcocaine. *Biochemical Pharmacology* **32**, 3045–3051.

Siegers, C.P., Heidbuchel, K. and Younes, M. (1983). Influence of alcohol, dithrocarb and (+)-catechin on the hepatotoxicity and metabolism of vinylidene chloride in rats. *Journal of Applied Toxicology* **3**, 90–95.

Smith, A.C., Freeman, R.W. and Harbison, R.D. (1981). Ethanol enhancement of cocaine-induced hepatotoxicity. *Biochemical Pharmacology* **30**, 453–458.

Song, B.J., Veech, R.L., Park, S.S., Gelboin, H.V. and Gonzalez, F.J. (1989). Induction of rat hepatic *N*-nitrosodimethylamine demethylase by acetone is due to protein stabilization. *Journal of Biological Chemistry* **264**, 3568–3572.

Stenback, F. (1969). The tumorigenic effect of ethanol. *Acta Pathologica et Microbiologica Scandinavica* **77**, 7325–7326.

Strubelt, O. (1978). Alcohol potentiation of liver injury. *Fundamental Applied Toxicology* **4**, 144–151.

Strubelt, O. (1980). Interactions between ethanol and other hepatotoxic agents. *Biochemical Pharmacology* **29**, 1445–1449.

Strubelt, O., Obermeier, R. and Siegers, C.P. (1978). The influence of ethanol pretreatment on the effects of nine hepatotoxic agents. *Acta Pharmacologica Toxicology* **43**, 211–218.

Suarez, K.A., Bhonsle, P. and Richardson, D.L. (1986). Protective effect of *N*-acetylcysteine pretreatment against cocaine induced hepatotoxicity and lipid peroxidation in the mouse. *Research Communications on Substance Abuse* **7**, 7–18.

Tabasco-Minguillan, J., Novick, D.M. and Kreek, M.J. (1990). Liver function tests in non-parenteral cocaine users. *Drug and Alcohol Dependence* **26**, 169–174.

Tamburro, C.H. (1984). Relationship of vinyl monomers and liver cancers: Angiosarcoma and hepatocellular carcinoma. *Seminars in Liver Disease* **4**, 158–169.

Tamburro, C.H. and Greenberg, R.A. (1981). Effectiveness of federally required laboratory screening in the detection of chemical liver injury. *Environmental Health Perspectives* **41**, 117–122.

Tamburro, C.H., Creech, J.J., Jr., Davis, A. and Greenberg, R.A. (1978). Indocyanine green clearance as the prospective indicator of hepatocellular chemical toxicity. *Gastroenterology* **75**, 989.

Tesche, R., Hauptmeier, K.H. and Frenzel, H. (1983). Effect of an acute dose of ethanol on the hepatotoxicity due to carbon tetrachloride. *Liver* **3**, 100–109.

Thompson, M.L., Shuster, L. and Shaw, K. (1979). Cocaine-induced hepatic necrosis in mice: The role of cocaine metabolism. *Biochemical Pharmacology* **30**, 453–458.

Thompson, M.L., Shuster, L., Casey, E. and Kanel G.C. (1984). Sex and strain differences in response to cocaine. *Biochemical Pharmacology* **33**, 1299–1307.

Thummel, K.E., Slattery, J.T. and Nelson, S.D. (1988). Mechanism by which ethanol diminishes the hepatotox-

icity of acetaminophen. *Journal of Pharmacology and Experimental Therapeutics* **245**, 129–136.

Tredger, J.M., Smith, H.M., Read, R.B. and Williams, R. (1986). Effects of ethanol ingestion on the metabolism of a hepatoxic dose of paracetamol in mice. *Xenobiotica* **16**, 661–670.

Tsutsumi, M., Lasker, J.M., Takahashi, T. and Lieber, C.S. (1993). *In vivo* induction of hepatic P4502E1 by ethanol: Role of increased enzyme synthesis. *Archives of Biochemistry and Biophysics* **304**, 209–218.

Tuyns, A.J. (1983). Oesophageal cancer in non-smoking drinkers and in non-drinking smokers. *International Journal of Cancer* **32**, 443–444.

Tuyns, A.J., Pequignot, G., Gignoux, M. and Valla, A. (1982). Cancers of the digestive tract, alcohol and tobacco. *International Journal of Cancer* **30**, 9–11.

Umeno, M., McBride, O.W., Yang, C.S., Gelboin, H.V. and Gonzalez, F.J. (1988a). Human ethanol-inducible P450IIEI: Complete gene sequence, promotes characterization, chromosome mapping and a DNA-directed expression. *Biochemistry* **27**, 9006–9013.

Umeno, M., Song, B.J., Kozak, C., Gelboin, H.V. and Gonzalez, F.J. (1988b). The rat P450IIEI gene: Complete nitron and exon sequence, chromosome mapping, and correlation of developmental expression with specific 5′cytosine demethylation. *Journal of Biological Chemistry* **263**, 4956–4962.

Wacker, W.E.C., Haynes, H., Druyan, R., Fisher, W. and Coleman, J.E. (1965). Treatment of ethylene glycol poisoning with ethyl alcohol. *Journal of the American Medical Association* **194**, 1231–1235.

Walker, R.M., McElligott, T.F., Power, E.M. and Racz, W.J. (1983). Increased acetaminophen induced hepatotoxicity after chronic ethanol consumption in mice. *Toxicology* **28**,193–206.

Wanless, I.R., Dore, S., Gopinath, N., Tan, J., Cameron, R., Heathcote, E.J., Blendis, L.M. and Levy, G. (1990). Histopathology of cocaine hepatotoxicity: Report of four patients. *Gastroenterology* **98**, 497–501.

Watkins, P.B. (1990). Role of cytochrome P-450 in drug metabolism and hepatotoxicity. *Seminars in Liver Disease* **10**, 2335–2350.

Wiener, H.L. and Reith, M.E.A. (1990). Differential effects of daily administration of cocaine on hepatic and cerebral glutathione in mice. *Biochemical Pharmacology* **40**, 1763–1768.

Williams, A.T. and Burk, R.F. (1990). Carbon tetrachloride hepatotoxicity: An example of free radical-mediated injury. *Seminars in Liver Disease* **10**, 279–284.

Williams, R.R. and Horm, W.J. (1977). Association of cancer sites with tobacco and alcohol consumption and socioeconomic status of patients: Interview study from the Third National Cancer Survey. *Journal of the National Cancer Institute* **58**, 525–547.

Wong, L.T., Whitehouse, L., Solomonraj, G. and Paul, C.J. (1980). Effect of a concomitant single dose of ethanol on the hepatotoxicity and metabolism of acetaminophen in mice. *Toxicology* **17**, 297–309.

World Health Organization (1964). Cancer agents that surround us. *World Health* **9**, 16–17.

Wrighton, S.A., Thomas, P.E., Molowa, D.T., Haniu, M., Shively, J.E., Maines, S.L., Watkins, P.B., Parker, G., Mendez-Picon, G., Levin, W. and Guzelian, P.S. (1986). Characterization of ethanol-inducible human liver *N*-nitrodimethylamine demethylase. *Biochemistry* **25**, 6731–6735.

Wynder, E.L. and Bross, I.J. (1957). Aetiological factors in mouth cancer: An approach to its prevention. *British Medical Journal* **1**, 1137–1143.

Wynder, E.L., Bross, I.J. and Day, E.A. (1956). Epidemiological approach to the etiology of cancer in the larynx. *Journal of the American Medical Association* **160**, 1384–1391.

Wynder, E.L., Bross, I.J. and Feldmann, R.M. (1957). A study of etiological factors in cancer of the mouth. *Cancer* **10**, 1300–1323.

Young, E.A., Harris, M.M., Cantu, T.L. and Schenker, S. (1993). Hepatic response to very low calorie diets (VLCD) as assessed by the aminopyrine breath test (ABT). *American Journal of Clinical Nutrition* **57**, 863–867.

Zand, R., Nelson, S.D., Slattery, J.T., Thummel, K.E., Kalhorn, T.F., Adams, S.P. and Wright, J.M. (1993). Inhibition and induction of cytochrome P4502E1-catalyzed oxidation by isoniazid in humans. *Clinical Pharmacology and Therapeutics* **54**, 142–149.

Zimmerman, H.J. (1986). Effects of alcohol on other hepatotoxins. *Alcoholism: Clinical and Experimental Research* **10**, 3–15.

17 Animal models of alcohol-associated liver injury

Samuel W. French, Michio Morimoto and Hidekazu Tsukamoto

Introduction

The variation in the animal models used in the study of alcoholic liver disease is testimony to the fact that no one model exactly replicates the human prototype. Rather, each model emphasizes one or more of the features seen in humans. In this way, each model makes a contribution to some aspect of our understanding of the pathogenesis of alcoholic liver disease.

In a review of the animal models of alcoholic liver disease it is important to have a clear view of the pathology of the three main stages of this disease, namely fatty liver, alcoholic hepatitis and cirrhosis. This is important because each stage probably involves different pathologic processes and may have different consequences. Thus, different animal models are used to produce either fatty liver or cirrhosis. Consequently, in this review, the animal models will be evaluated according to the stage of alcoholic liver disease that is to be replicated.

Many reports of the pathogenesis of alcohol-associated liver disease in animal models do not include an assessment of the liver pathology, but rather involve short-term studies of a single parameter which has not correlated with any morphologic feature. For this reason, it is well to review the salient features of the pathology of alcoholic liver disease in the hope that future investigations will employ an experimental design which includes an

assessment of the liver pathology, and correlation of factors contributing to liver injury with the particular types of liver injury.

A recent review of the pathology of alcoholic liver disease in humans (French *et al.* 1993a) highlighted the following features: (1) moderate elevation of serum aspartate aminotransferase (AST) and alanine aminotransferase (ALT) with AST greater than ALT; (2) cholestasis; (3) fatty liver; (4) hepatocellular ballooning degeneration with loss of normal cytokeratin immunostaining; (5) Mallory body formation; (6) bile ductular metaplasia of hepatocytes at the limiting plate; (7) periportal Ito cell proliferation, transformation and fibrosis; (8) perivenular Ito cell proliferation, transformation and fibrosis; (9) megamitochondria; (10) acinar inflammation; (11) apoptosis; (12) spotty necrosis; (13) zonal necrosis; and (14) cirrhosis. These features should be evaluated as markers of alcohol-associated liver injury in experimental models. The features of alcoholic liver disease that have been reported in the various animal models are summarized in Table 17.1.

Historical review: Rabbits, dogs

The first comprehensive description of an animal model of alcoholic liver disease was published by Friedenwald (1905). In these studies, the rabbits were fed ethanol for prolonged periods with a poorly characterized diet. Fatty liver and cirrhosis developed. Unfortunately, no controls were studied. Connor (1940) improved the rabbit model using a high protein (40 percent), high fat (48 percent) and lecithin (3.8 percent) diet with vitamin supplements; controls were included. Alcohol was fed by

Table 17.1 Experimental animal models of alcoholic liver disease

Authors	Animal	Fatty liver	Alcoholic hepatitis	Cirrohsis	Metaplasia ductular	MB	Centrilobular fibrosis	Balloon cells	Apoptosis	Elevated serum enzyme	Cholestasis	Megamito-chondria	Inflammation	Necrosis spotty	Necrosis zonal	Duration
Friedenwald (1905)	Rabbit	X		X										X		10 mo–5 yrs
Connor (1940)	Rabbit	X		X	X										X	93–224 days
Connor and Chaikoff (1939)	Dog	X		X	X		X				X		X			106 days
Chey et al. (1971)	Dog	X	X				X	X		X	X	X	X	X	X	10–18 months
Lieber et al. (1963)	Rat	X														1 month
Lindros et al. (1983)	Rat	X											X	X		12 weeks
Takada et al. (1986)	Rat	X						X						X		12 weeks
Tsukamoto et al. (1986)	Rat	X					X		X	X			X	X	X	4 months
French et al. (1986)	Rat	X					X	X		X			X	X		6 months
Rubin and Lieber (1973)	Baboon	X	X	X		X	X			X	X	X	X		X	8–22 months
Ainley et al. (1988)	Baboon	X					X			X	X	X	X			18 mo–5 yrs
McGee et al. (1992)	Micropig	X					X									12 months
Smith and Hoy (1990)	Mice	X														4–10 weeks
Yunice et al. (1984)	Guinea-pig	X														8 weeks

stomach tube at a maximum dose which supported weight gain. Fifty-one rabbits survived. Thirty-eight rabbits fed the soybean diet survived 19–304 days and the average weight loss was 16 percent. Fatty liver (20/38), atrophy (16/38), necrosis (4/38) and periportal fibrosis (7/38) developed. Fibrosis was periportal and necrosis was zonal judging from the photomicrographs. Cirrhosis was formed by portal–portal bridging fibrosis. The problem with the experimental design in this study was that alcohol intoxication prevented adequate intake of the diet which was fed *ad lib*.

In the same laboratory, cirrhosis was also produced in a dog model of alcoholic liver disease (Connor and Chaikoff 1939; Chaikoff *et al.* 1948). Alcohol was fed with a diet high in lean meat alternating with a high fat (lard) diet given by stomach tube; vitamins and minerals were supplemented. All alcohol-fed animals developed fatty liver. Some livers were green, indicating cholestasis. Atrophy and "hyaline" degeneration were observed. Some dogs (4/16) developed cirrhosis similar to that seen in alcoholic patients. In a second study in which dogs were fed a high protein diet with alcohol by forced feeding, 2/12 developed cirrhosis, one after 72 and the other after 130 weeks of treatment. In another study dogs, fed the high fat diet continuously without alcohol also went on to develop cirrhosis (Chaikoff *et al.* 1943); depancreatized dogs also developed cirrhosis (Chaikoff *et al.* 1938), perhaps in the same way as non-alcoholic steatohepatitis and cirrhosis develop in obese and diabetic patients (French *et al.* 1989).

Chey *et al.* (1971) performed studies on dogs fed alcohol and a beef diet through a gastric fistula 5 days a week, for 10–18 months, achieving blood alcohol levels of 315–477 mg percent. The dogs received an enriched diet, including choline supplement, *ad lib*. Serial biopsies of the liver showed fatty liver, megamitochondria (our interpretation), ballooning degeneration, zonal necrosis, cholestasis, spotty necrosis, inflammation and centrilobular fibrosis accompanied by elevated serum enzymes. The findings are quite comparable to those seen in pre-cirrhotic alcoholic liver disease in humans. Controls were normal. The defects in the experimental design were that the treatment was not given at the weekends and the dogs lost weight. These studies set the stage for future tube-feeding models where the intake of alcohol and a nutritious diet are assured, and blood alcohol levels are maintained at a high level. This kind of dietary control has proved to be necessary in order to achieve liver pathology which resembles that seen in alcoholic liver disease in humans.

Current animal models for alcohol-associated liver disease

Mammalian models of alcoholic liver disease are numerous and include the rat, the mouse, the mini pig, the guinea-pig, the hamster, the ferret and various primates. None of these models fulfils all the criteria of alcoholic liver disease as seen in the human liver and many only develop fatty liver or minimal abnormalities.

Rat models

The rat model of alcoholic liver disease began with the studies of Ashworth (1947), who fed alcohol by stomach tube and the diet was fed orally *ad lib*. This model produced a fatty liver. However, this model was not controlled for nutrient replacement by calories derived from alcohol and the rats lost weight. Best *et al.* (1949) then introduced isocaloric pair-feeding to control for calorie replacement by ethanol, adding sucrose to the control diet in amounts equal calorically to the alcohol consumed by the experimental rats. The ethanol-fed rats developed a fatty liver as did the sucrose pair-fed controls, except that if the basal diet was supplemented with either methionine, choline or casein (all methyl donors) fatty liver was prevented. The concept that alcohol was not a direct liver toxin developed as a result of these findings. Rather, alcohol was thought to damage the liver by increasing the requirement for choline and other nutrients. Cirrhosis can be easily produced in the rat fed ethanol and a choline-deficient diet (Fig. 17.1). Subsequently, numerous studies using a solid diet fed *ad lib* and separately from the alcohol, which was also fed *ad lib*, substantiated this concept (Klatskin *et al.* 1954; Porta *et al.* 1965, 1967, 1968, 1969, 1972; French 1966; Takada *et al.* 1967; Hartroft and Porta 1968; Takeuchi *et al.* 1968; Porta and Gomez-Dumm 1968; Gomez-Dumm *et al.* 1968; Koch *et al.* 1969; Barak *et al.* 1971; Thompson and Reitz 1976, 1979). Prophetically, choline deficiency has recently been documented in humans (Zeisel *et al.* 1991), suggesting that choline deficiency may be important in the pathogenesis of alcoholic liver disease in humans. However, there are dietary studies where ethanol

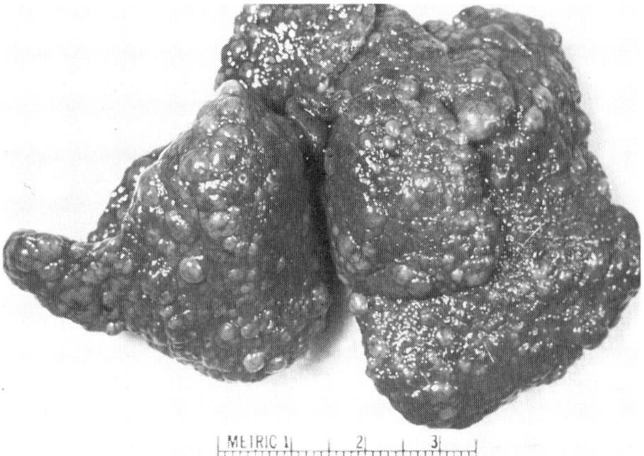

Fig. 17.1   Cirrhotic liver from a rat fed ethanol and a choline and methyl donor deficient diet *ad lib*.

was found to ameliorate the effects of choline deficiency on the liver (Takada *et al.* 1972; Patek *et al.* 1973).

In order to overcome the confounding nutritional problems inherent in separately feeding rats a solid diet and alcohol *ad lib*, Lieber *et al.* (1963) designed a liquid diet in which the ethanol and the diet were mixed together. This regimen ensured that the rats received adequte amounts of a balanced diet as well as ethanol in amounts which would induce a fatty liver after 1 month of feeding. The severity of the fatty change was dependent on the percent of calories derived from fat (Lieber and DeCarli 1970). Ten percent of calories derived from fat achieved a doubling of the liver fat stores, whereas 45 percent of calories as fat achieved a seven-fold increase in fat stores. Using this technique, a daily alcohol ingestion of 12–18 g/kg and blood alcohol levels ranging from 100 to 150 mg/dl can be achieved. The possibility of loss of alcohol by spillage and evaporation must be considered in these experiments.

The liquid diet used by Lieber and DeCarli has been criticized for not being nutritionally adequate and not supporting optimum growth rates in young growing rats (Rao and Larkin 1985). The addition of ethanol to the diet causes the rats to reduce their total calorie intake (Lieber and DeCarli, 1989a). This is controlled for by pair-feeding the controls an isocaloric diet substituting carbohydrate for ethanol calories. Numerous dietary ingredients become suboptimal in concentration when the amount of diet consumed is reduced by adding ethanol. These include calcium, copper, iron, manganese, phosphorous, vitamin B6 and choline (Rao and Larkin 1975; Derr 1989). However, Lieber and DeCarli

(1989b) showed that supplementing their diet with minerals and vitamins (increased × 2.5) failed to prevent the alcohol-induced fatty liver. Furthermore, Lieber and DeCarli (1989c) point out that the studies by Derr (1989), in which rats were fed ethanol and diet *ad lib*, did not induce fatty liver. In these studies, the rats ingested about 25 percent less alcohol/kg body weight, and significant blood alcohol levels were not achieved, so that the toxic effects of ethanol on the liver which result in fatty change were not manifested. Failure to produce alcoholic liver disease with the Porta *et al.* model (Azzalis *et al.* 1992), where the alcohol was fed with sugar *ad lib*, might have been due in part to the fact that a high carbohydrate diet prevents the induction of cytochrome P450 as discussed below. It can be concluded that the Lieber–DeCarli alcohol liquid diet in the rat model provides a useful model for the study of the pathogenesis of alcohol-induced fatty liver but does not maintain a sustained high blood alcohol level, nor are the more severe and advanced stages of alcoholic liver disease achieved.

Pyrazole model

Sustained higher blood alcohol levels seemed necessary to induce significant liver pathology, and therefore Lindros *et al.* (1983) devised a method for maintaining high blood alcohol levels using 4-methylpyrazole (4-MP), which inhibits alcohol dehydrogenase. Blood alcohol levels were 60–80 mM (260–350 mg percent) but fell to zero just before feeding. After 12 weeks of this dietary regimen, fatty liver and degenerative changes developed, including spotty necrosis, and a granulocytic and lymphocytic infiltration. The administration of pyrazole with alcohol also resulted in ballooning degeneration of hepatocytes (Matsuda *et al.* 1985). A high fat diet increased the severity of the ethanol/pyrazol-induced liver injury; the features included ballooning degeneration and necrosis of hepatocytes in the centrilobular areas, and elevated serum AST levels (Takada *et al.* 1986). This accentuation of the severity of centrilobular injury is probably due to an increase in the cytochrome P4502E1 (CYP2E1) oxidation of ethanol, since CYP2E1 is induced by both ethanol and pyrazole (Dicker and Cederbaum 1991). Thus, this model is complicated by the effect of pyrazole on the alternate routes of metabolism of ethanol. Alternatively, alcohol may enhance the cytotoxicity of pyrazole in a way analogous to the enhancement of metabolism of other drugs and toxins induced by ethanol (Hasumura *et al.* 1974; Sato *et al.* 1981; Bosma *et al.* 1988; Tsutsumi *et al.*

1990; Hall *et al.* 1991) because of the marked induction of CYP2E1 (see also Chapter 16).

Intragastric tube feeding model

The development of the intragastric tube feeding of ethanol and liquid diet by the continuous infusion method for the induction of alcoholic liver disease (Tsukamoto *et al.* 1986, 1990; French *et al.* 1986) was based on the early methods of drug administration via this route (Lukas and Moreton 1979). This method of alcohol feeding was initially developed in order to study alcohol withdrawal in the rat following a short-term alcohol intoxication (Pettit *et al.* 1980). With this model, the rat rapidly develops a high degree of central nervous system tolerance and physical dependence, tolerating a blood alcohol level up to 700 mg percent before dying. Forssell (1981) subsequently developed a similar method of continuous intragastric tube feeding of alcohol, but fed the solid diet *ad lib*. Both methods allow control of the blood alcohol level, but the latter does not control for adequate nutrition and the liver pathology has not been reported.

Initially, we fed ethanol and liquid diet through a single cannula but alternated the diet and ethanol over a 24 hour period so that the diet was infused 08:00 to 16:00 and ethanol was infused 16:00 to 08:00. This allowed adequate nutrition, high blood alcohol levels (400–500 mg percent) and adequate growth, and the development of severe fatty liver – with apoptosis and inflammation – developing over 4 months of feeding (French *et al.* 1984). When exposed to hypoxia, these animals developed central necrosis and high serum enzyme levels, which suggested that hypoxia may play a role in the pathogenesis of alcoholic liver disease.

We then further perfected the intragastric cannula model to deliver ethanol and liquid diet simultaneously so that both the amount of alcohol and the diet could be varied independently (Tsukamoto *et al.* 1984, 1985a). Thus, an adequate intake of calories could be maintained while at the same time the dose of alcohol could be titrated to achieve continuously high blood alcohol levels. The blood alcohol was measured daily through a jugular sampling method; the blood that was removed was retransfused, as packed red blood cells, into the jugular cannula so as not to induce anaemia. The blood alcohol cycled high and low over a 5–6 day period, as long as animals were challenged with doses of ethanol to raise the blood alcohol level above 210 mg/dl (Tsukamoto *et al.* 1985c). The cyclic phenomenon has recently been shown to correlate with CYP2E1

induction and mRNA fluctuation in response to the level of the blood alcohol (Ronis *et al.* 1993). The degree of fluctuation of the blood alcohol level (SD) correlated with the liver pathology score, suggesting that a high degree of fluctuation worsened the liver damage caused by alcohol (Tsukamoto *et al.* 1985b).

The pathology of alcoholic liver disease induced by the intragastric tube feeding of ethanol and a low fat diet (5 percent of calories) was impressive and included fatty liver, focal necrosis and inflammation, and elevated serum enzymes (Tsukamoto *et al.* 1985a). The blood alcohol levels were maintained on average above 200 mg percent. The blood alcohol levels achieved correlated with the degree of fatty liver, and the serum enzyme levels correlated with the duration of alcohol feeding.

When the dietary fat was increased to 25 percent of calories, using the same basic intragastric tube feeding model, alcohol induced a more severe form of liver injury, which more closely resembled that seen in humans in that focal central fibrosis, necrosis and inflammation were seen with elevated serum enzymes (Tsukamoto *et al.* 1986; French *et al.* 1986). The amount of ethanol needed to maintain high blood alcohol levels was 47 percent of calories after 4 months of feeding. Weight gain was 20 g/ week, and was the same as the rats fed chow *ad lib*.

When a diet marginal in nutrients such as protein, vitamins and choline was fed with ethanol and a high fat diet, the liver damage was more severe and the pathology score higher (French *et al.* 1986, 1988a), especially the centrilobular fibrosis, although morphometric studies indicated an increase in collagen in both the centrilobular areas and the portal areas. Pericellular fibrosis was also seen and bridging fibrosis was prominent. Focal scarring appeared after 2–3 months feeding and continued up to 5 months as indicated in monthly liver biopsies. Ito cell activation, as indicated by an increase in rough endoplasmic reticulum, was noted in the perisinusoidal location as well as in the scars. In these rats, 12.5 g/kg body weight/day of alcohol was needed to maintain high blood alcohol levels (329 $\pm$ 109 mg/ dl). Weight gain over 6 months was 105 percent for the ethanol-fed and 150 percent in the control rats. Eight pairs of animals lived 8 weeks, six pairs lived 12 weeks, five pairs lived 16 weeks, three pairs lived 20 weeks and two pairs lived 24 weeks. Death occurred for a variety of reasons, including plugged cannulas, convulsions, postoperative state and ethanol overdose. Infection of the wound where the tube entered the skin in the rat's back was occasionally encountered. We currently prevent this by using a

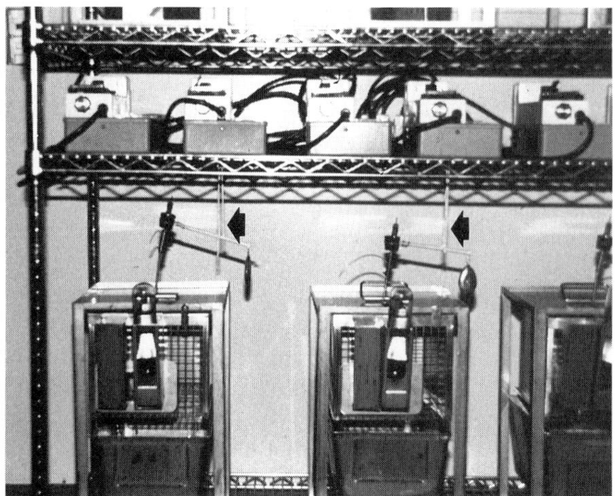

Fig. 17.2 Photograph of cages and pumps used to pair-feed rats ethanol and diet by intragastric tube. Note the fulcrum suspended by a string (arrows) which acts as a gentle spring to prevent tugging by the tube where it is attached to the back of the rat. The tube is balanced by a weight attached at the opposite end of the stick.

lever spring which minimizes the tension on the tube when the rat moves in its cage (Fig. 17.2). Alternatively, the small amount of ampicillin powder or betadine can be sprinkled around the anchoring button which is covered with Dacron felt to prevent ascending infection. When one of the pair-fed rats died, its partner was killed. The rats developed depressed levels of liver ATP and increased adenosine as further evidence of the role of hypoxia in the pathogenesis of the liver injury (Miyamoto and French 1988a, b).

When using the intragastric tube feeding model in younger rats, where the starting weight was around 200 g, the calorie content of the diet and ethanol had to be increased 1.5 times to sustain normal growth and high blood alcohol levels. The liver injury in these rapidly growing rats was more severe, with focal centrilobular fibrosis and bridging fibrosis sometimes observed as early as 1 month but commonly after 12 weeks of feeding (Takahashi *et al.* 1990). The pathology score correlated with the duration of ethanol feeding up to 24 weeks. The energy stores in the liver were decreased as indicated by a ^{31}P nuclear magnetic resonance spectroscopy detected increase in the Pi/β-ATP ratio, again supporting the role of hypoxia in the pathogenesis of alcoholic liver disease. Further evidence for this hypothesis was found in the intragastric tube feeding model in older rats, which had decreased O_2

tension in the hepatic venous blood at the time when centrilobular liver necrosis was induced (Tsukamoto and Xi 1989). This central venous hypoxaemia was attributable to incomplete compensation of markedly enhanced hepatic oxygen consumption due to a limited increase in hepatic oxygen delivery (Tsukamoto and Xi 1989). Rats fed by intragastric tube feeding were more vulnerable to the decreased O_2 transport due to carboxy haemoglobin induced by carbon monoxide inhalation over a 4 month period, as indicated by the marked elevation of serum enzymes (Nanji *et al.* 1989a). The focal hepatocyte necrosis caused by hypoxia observed with this model can be explained by the observation that high blood alcohol levels induce vasoconstriction in the liver microcirculation *in vitro* (Oshita *et al.* 1992a). The vasoconstriction was inhibited by sodium nitroprusside, a vasodilator. This implies that ethanol alters the endothelin–nitric oxide controlled microcirculation by causing an increased tone of the Ito cells, which may cause local ischaemia and necrosis during reflow (Oshita *et al.* 1992a, b; Sakamoto 1991; see also Chapter 14).

The intragastric tube feeding model lends itself well to studies of the sequential relationship of Ito cell activation to focal fibrosis, and variations in dietary fatty acid composition. For instance, using the intragastric tube feeding model where blood alcohol levels were kept at comparable levels, two diets were compared, in which the fatty acid composition was either rich or relatively devoid of linoleic acid (Nanji *et al.* 1989b; Nanji and French 1989). Using this experimental design, in which high blood alcohol levels were maintained for 6 months, we showed that no liver injury or Ito cell activation was induced by intragastric feeding of ethanol and a diet low in linoleate (tallow), whereas a diet rich in linoleic acid (corn oil) led to the development of alcoholic liver disease with features including activation of Ito cells and focal fibrosis (Takahashi *et al.* 1991). This result implies that Ito cell activation is not a direct effect of ethanol or acetaldehyde; rather, it appears to be mediated by an intermediate dependent on linoleate metabolism. Studies by Matsuoka *et al.* (1990) and Matsuoka and Tsukamoto (1990) using Ito cells and Kupffer cells isolated from the intragastric infusion model revealed the following:

1. Ito cells isolated from ethanol-fed rats have higher DNA and collagen synthesis rates compared with those from pair-fed controls.
2. Autologous Kupffer cells release *in vitro* factors

which further increase Ito cell DNA and collagen synthesis.
3. TGFβ-1 is a major Kupffer cell-derived fibrogenic cytokine.
4. The diet high in polyunsaturated fat sensitizes Ito cells to Kupffer cell stimulation.

Vitamin A supplements appear to inhibit Ito cell activation and scar formation (Senoo and Wake 1985; Davis and Madri 1987); thus, in this model a decrease in hepatic vitamin A, induced by ethanol, may be involved in Ito cell activation (French *et al.* 1989). In fact, Ito cells appear to undergo two stages of activation in our model, the early mitogenic response and the late fibrogenic response – vitamin A depletion accompanies or precedes the early activation (Tsukamoto *et al.* 1991). The effects of ethanol on Ito cell activation in scars is similar in both rats fed ethanol in the intragastric tube feeding model, and in human alcoholic liver disease (Okanoue *et al.* 1983; French *et al.* 1988a, b, c, 1991; Minato *et al.* 1983; Horn *et al.* 1986).

The ability to alter the composition of the diet but maintain caloric and ethanol levels that support both good growth and the induction of alcoholic liver disease pathology is a major advantage of the intragastric tube feeding model. With this approach, it is possible to vary both the amount and type of the fatty acid content of the diet and induce either severe alcoholic liver disease, mild injury or no liver injury (Nanji *et al.* 1989b; Nanji and French 1989; French 1993). Thus beef fat and alcohol fed by intragastric tube does not induce alcoholic liver disease, whereas pork fat, olive oil, corn oil, safflower oil and sunflower oil all support ethanol-induced liver injury (Figs 17.3, 17.4). Saturated fatty acids do not support the induction of alcoholic liver disease (Mak and Lieber 1988) because it is necessary to have linoleic acid above 0.7 percent of fat in the diet to induce alcoholic liver disease in the intragastric tube feeding model (Nanji and French 1989). An exception to this is fish oil, which is very low in linoleic (1.8 percent) but high in eicosapentaenoic and docasahexaeonic acids, which are polyunsaturated fatty acids (French 1993; Nanji *et al.* 1992c). Therefore, fish oil, like corn oil, supports ethanol-induced liver disease when administered by the intragastric tube-feeding model (Degli Esposti *et al.* 1991; French 1993).

In addition to studies of dietary factors contributing to alcoholic liver disease, the intragastric feeding model is ideal for studies of pathogenic mechanisms associated with alcohol-induced liver

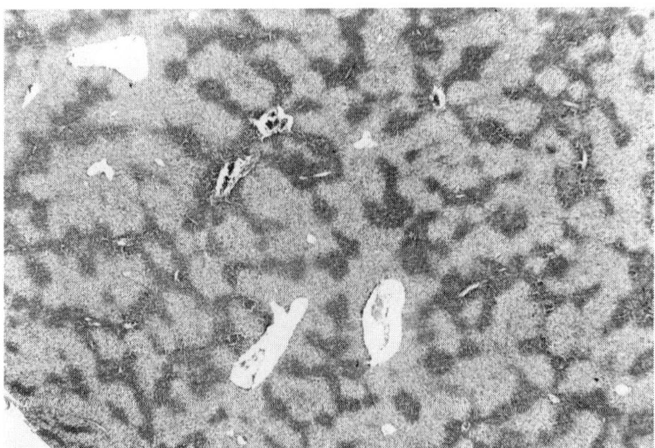

Fig. 17.3 Liver biopsy from a rat fed alcohol and 35 percent of calories as corn oil using the intragastric tube feeding model of alcoholic liver disease. The diet was fed for 30 days. The liver shows severe centrilobular fatty change (the pale areas). H&E, $\times$ 20.

pathology. In addition, the model can be used to discriminate between significant mechanisms and epiphenomena.

By using the two diets, one which enhances the development of ethanol-induced liver disease and the other which does not, we have shown that CYP2E1 levels were twice as high when corn oil was fed with ethanol compared with beef fat, indicating that CYP2E1 induction may be important in the pathogenesis of alcoholic liver disease (Takahashi *et al.* 1992). Nanji *et al.* (1992b), using the same approach, reported that CYP2E1 induction correlated with the production of alcoholic liver disease. In the intragastric feeding model, alcohol feeding also decreased arachidonic acid measured in liver microsomes, whereas diene conjugates increased (Nanji *et al.* 1992c). The three changes are significantly correlated with each other, suggesting that free radicals generated by the CYP2E1 system during ethanol oxidation caused the reduction of arachidonic acid, and lipid peroxidation-mediated damage to the hepatocytes. Others have confirmed this phenomenon using variations on the intragastric tube feeding model (Kamimura *et al.* 1992; French *et al.* 1993b; Badger *et al.* 1993; Castillo *et al.* 1992).

It is important to emphasize that the diet must be low in carbohydrate if ethanol is to induce cytochrome P450 and lipid peroxidation. The use of a high carbohydrate diet with ethanol may explain why alcohol-feeding studies by some investigators failed to cause any liver injury, cytochrome P450 induction or lipid peroxidation (Azzalis *et al.* 1992). CYP2E1 induction, in addition to increasing lipid

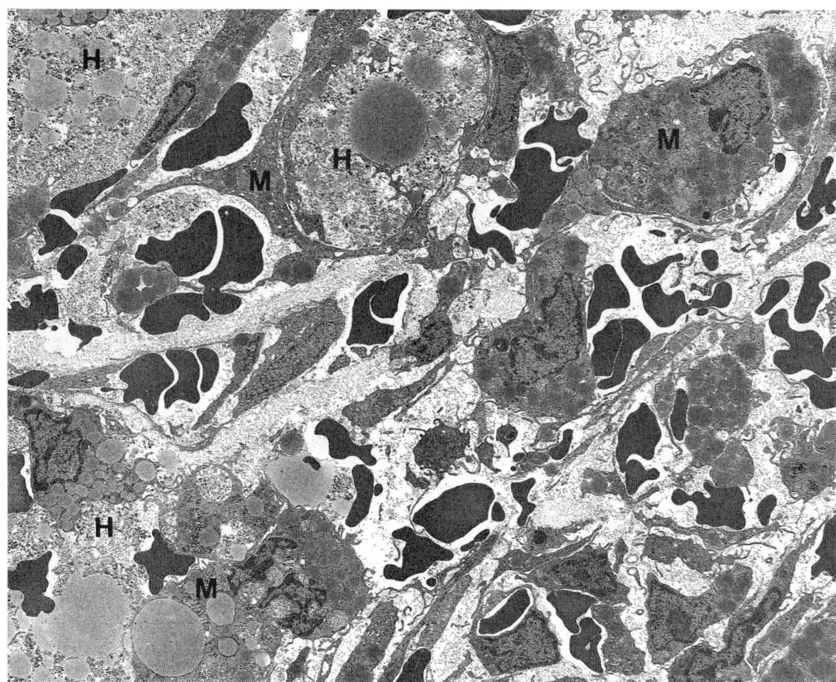

Fig. 17.4   Electron micrograph of a liver from a rat fed alcohol and 35 percent of calories as sunflower oil for 6 months using the intragastric tube feeding model. The serum ALT was 124 U/l and the blood alcohol level was 234 mg percent. Note the necrotic hepatocytes (H), collapsed sinusoids and macrophages (M). × 1860.

peroxidation, could damage the liver by altering eicosanoid metabolism to increase the synthesis of thromboxane (Nanji *et al.* 1993a). Studies in which inhibitors of the two pathways (i.e. cimetidine and quinone) were fed intragastrically along with the diet and ethanol showed that both drugs inhibited the development of alcoholic liver disease (Nanji *et al.* 1993b, c). Similarly, when an oral iron chelator was fed, hepatic non-haem iron was reduced and this correlated with a reduction of the levels of lipid peroxidation (Sadrzadeh *et al.* 1993a). By reducing the level of CYP2E1 induction by ethanol by feeding diallyl sulphide intragastrically, we showed that both lipid peroxidation and serum ALT elevation were ameliorated (Morimoto *et al.* 1993). Thus, using the intragastric tube feeding model, it was possible to demonstrate that lipid peroxidation may be an important mechanism of ethanol-induced liver damage.

Finally, the intragastric tube feeding model is ideal for studying the effect of dietary enhancement on the alcohol-associated liver pathology. This approach has also provided some insight into the pathogenesis of alcoholic liver disease. For instance,

if free radical production and lipid peroxidation play a role in the development of alcoholic liver disease, then depletion of dietary antioxidants such as vitamin E, or an increase in oxidants such as non-haem iron in the liver, should enhance the ethanol-induced liver damage. Such has been shown to be the case; for example, a diet deficient in vitamin E has been shown to reduce hepatic vitamin E stores, increase lipid peroxidation and increase serum ALT in ethanol-fed rats (Sadrzadeh *et al.* 1993b). Vitamin E stores were also reduced by ethanol feeding even when the diet contained vitamin E. Likewise, rats fed ethanol and a diet supplemented with iron markedly increased ethanol-induced serum ALT levels, lipid peroxidation and fibrosis to the point that micronodular cirrhosis was observed after 4 months of feeding (Tsukamoto *et al.* 1992; see Fig. 17.5). The specific and direct role of enhanced oxidative stress in the pathogenesis of fibrosis in alcoholic liver disease was supported by significant correlations between the parameters of hepatic lipid peroxidation in our intragastric infusion model both with (Tsukamoto *et al.* 1993) and without (Kamimura *et al.* 1992) iron supplementation. Further-

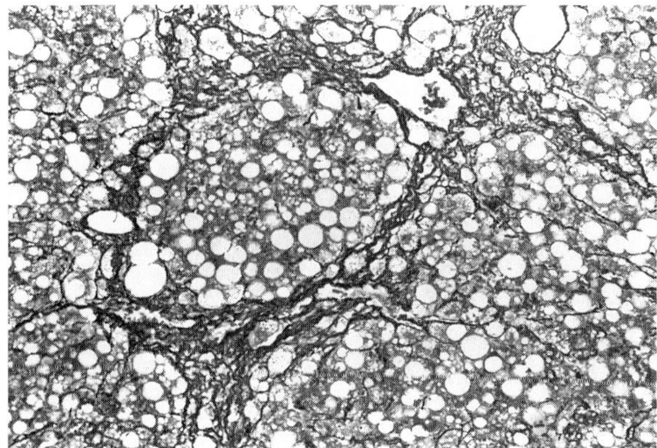

Fig. 17.5 Liver from a rat fed ethanol and a high fat (25 percent) diet supplemented with carbonyl iron for 16 weeks. Note the development of micronodular cirrhosis and steatosis. Reticulin stain, × 70.

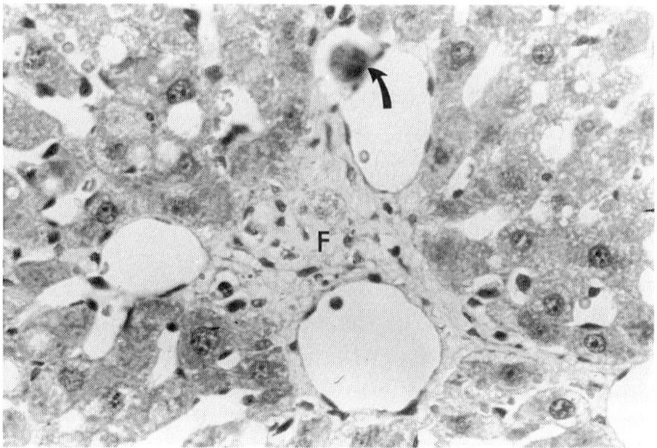

Fig. 17.6 Liver from a rat fed ethanol, 35 percent of calories as corn oil and isoniazid 3.5 mg/kg/day for 72 days, using the intragastric tube feeding model. Note the fibrosis (F) around the central vein and the apoptotic hepatocyte (arrow). H&E, × 290.

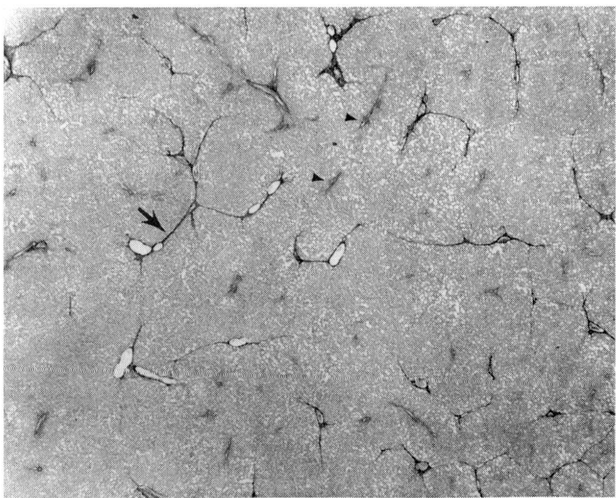

Fig. 17.7 Liver from a rat treated similarly to the rat shown in Fig. 17.6 showing the focal nature of the central–central bridging fibrosis (arrows). There is moderate fatty change. The portal tracts are normal (arrow heads). Sirius red, × 20.

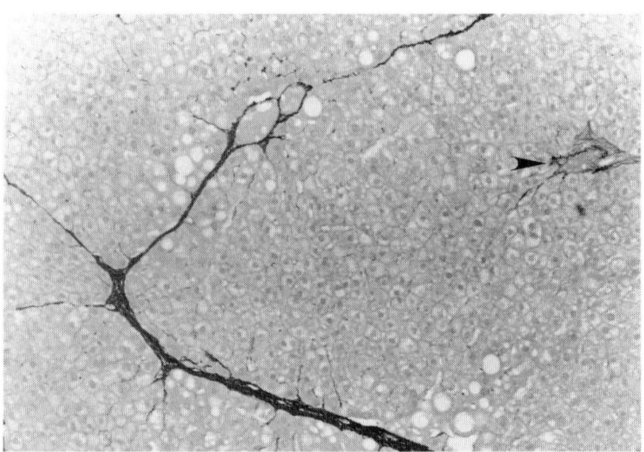

Fig. 17.8 Liver from a rat treated similarly to the rat shown in Fig. 17.6. Note the central–central bridging fibrosis, mild fatty change and normal portal tract (arrow head). Sirius red, × 80.

more, the demonstration of direct stimulation of Ito cells, resulting in collagen synthesis, by malondialdehyde and 4-hydroxynonenal (major aldehydric products of lipid peroxidation) provides additional support for this hypothesis (Tsukamoto *et al.* 1993).

Drugs which are metabolized by CYP2E1, with the production of free radicals, would be expected to enhance ethanol-induced liver damage (see Chapter 16). For instance, when ethanol and diet were fed with a therapeutic dose of isoniazid, fibrosis was found to be enhanced (French *et al.* 1993b; see Figs 17.6–17.10). Thus, ethanol fed with the diet supplemented with a drug can be precisely administered in a controlled and reproducible way using the intragastric feeding model.

Primate models

The problem with primate models of alcoholic liver disease is that they all involve voluntary ingestion of the diet and ethanol, which reduces the control over

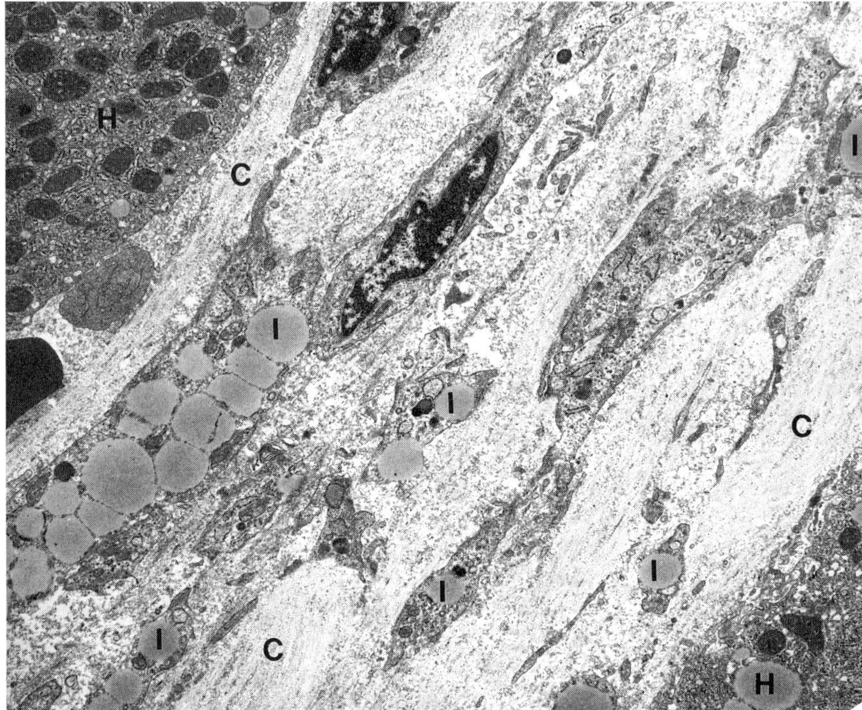

Fig. 17.9   Electron micrograph of a centrilobular scar from the same rat as in Fig. 17.7. Note the hepatocytes (H), the Ito cells (I) and the large amounts of collagen (C). × 5600.

the intake of the nutritients and the maintenance of high blood ethanol levels. Some animals stop ingesting the diet and will not resume eating until ethanol is removed. Thus the dietary control can be temporarily lost for individual animals. Less serious, but nevertheless significant, is the voluntary reduction in caloric intake with reduction in weight gain or even weight loss resulting. This may explain why, as reviewed below, the results vary between laboratories.

Monkey models

The *Macaca mulatta* monkey (Rhesus) developed fatty liver, fibrosis, cirrhosis and oesophageal varices when fed a high fat, low choline, low protein diet in biscuit form with ethanol given by lavage three times a week for 8 months (Cueto *et al.* 1967). However, weight loss occurred and cirrhosis was also seen in the animals fed the same diet without ethanol. No pathology was observed in control monkeys fed the diet supplemented with choline. Since choline deficiency induces cirrhosis in the Rhesus monkey with or without ethanol in the diet (Ruebner *et al.* 1969), and ethanol fed with a nutriti-

ous diet caused no abnormalities, this model was not useful in the study of the pathogenesis of alcoholic liver disease. These results and others (Rogers *et al.* 1981) confirm that alcohol and a nutritious diet do not cause significant liver pathology in the Rhesus monkey. However, in another study, monkeys fed by nasogastric tube to provide 41 percent of calories as ethanol, fatty liver developed in 10 days, and serum enzymes doubled (Ruebner *et al.* 1972). Choline supplement did not prevent these changes. Finally, *Macaca radiata* monkeys fed ethanol in the Lieber–DeCarli liquid diet for 4 years developed fatty liver and megamitochondria (French *et al.* 1983) but no fibrosis (Mezey *et al.* 1983), and blood alcohol levels averaged 82 ± 27 mg/dl 3 h after initiating the morning feeding. Similar findings have been reported for *Macaca nemestrina* fed ethanol and a high cholesterol diet for 18 months (Leathers *et al.* 1981).

Baboon model

In a series of reports, Lieber and his associates (Rubin and Lieber 1973, 1974; Lieber *et al.* 1975; Lieber and DeCarli 1974; Popper and Lieber 1980)

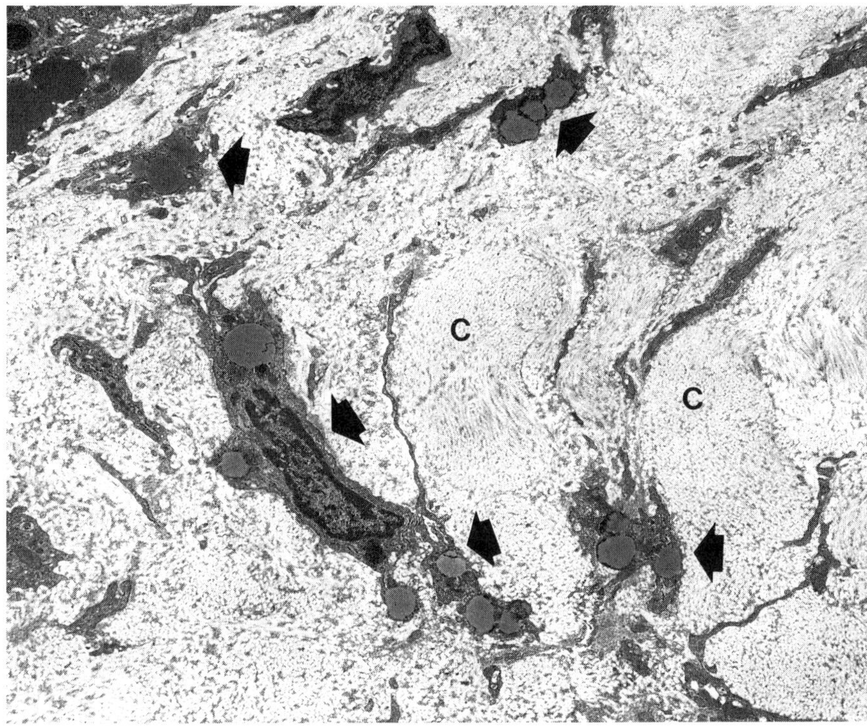

Fig. 17.10   Electron micrograph of a centrilobular scar from the rat liver shown in Fig. 17.7. Note the extensive collagen (C) deposition in which numerous Ito cells (arrows), containing lipid droplets, are embedded. × 5600.

described an alcoholic hepatitis-like liver lesion and cirrhosis in baboons fed ethanol and a liquid diet rich in nutrients where body weight was maintained. The features included fatty change, necrosis, inflammation, fibrosis and central hyaline sclerosis (Lieber *et al.* 1975); although the original reports documented the presence of alcoholic hyaline, this has never been validated by immunohistochemistry or electron microscopy and on review the eosinophic masses were probably giant mitochondria. Blood alcohol levels reached as high as 376 mg percent in some animals. In a later report, cirrhosis was observed in these animals (Lieber and DeCarli 1974; Rubin and Lieber 1974). Review of serial liver biopsies from the alcohol-fed baboons which developed cirrhosis led to the observation that perivenular fibrosis at the fatty liver stage, and not alcoholic hepatitis, preceded the development of cirrhosis (Van Waes and Lieber 1977; Popper and Lieber 1980).

Two problems have developed with the baboon model. The first is that studies in other laboratories of baboons fed ethanol in the Lieber–DeCarli liquid diet did not result in cirrhosis (Ainley *et al.* 1988;

Porto *et al.* 1988). In the Porto *et al.* (1988) study, in which baboons were fed ethanol and diet for 3 years (ethanol constituted 45 percent, protein 27 percent, fat 14 percent and carbohydrate 14 percent of calories), fatty change and megamitochondria were the predominant changes observed in the liver in all biopsies. Inflammation and necrosis were also seen. No classic features of alcoholic hepatitis or cirrhosis or extensive fibrosis were seen. Fibrosis was found in the perivenular zone, predominantly affecting the terminal hepatic venule and causing thickening of the perisinusoidal space of zone 3. Pericellular or perisinusoidal fibrosis was associated with inflammation or fibrosis of the central vein. This central fibrotic process was not progressive over time and in one case it was reversible. In another report, in which eight baboons were fed ethanol and a semiliquid diet (Mazuri diet) with or without zinc supplement for up to 5 years, eight animals were fed ethanol at a dose of 70 percent of calories which left no room for adequate nutrition from dietary calories (i.e. 5.5 percent fat, 17.4 percent carbohydrate and 7.1 percent protein calories) (Ainley *et al.* 1988). This could explain why liver biopsies done up to 30 months of feeding showed only mild fatty change. In the Lieber–DeCarli liquid diet, 21 percent of calories derive from fat. This is needed for ethanol to induce fatty liver (Lieber and DeCarli 1970). However, these authors fed the diet to provide 25 g ethanol/kg/day, which is far higher than baboons can metabolize (French 1989). For instance, the Lieber–DeCarli diet provides 4.5–8.3 g/kg/day of ethanol in the baboon model and this achieved a blood alcohol of 92–184 mg percent (Lieber *et al.* 1985). Despite these dietary discrepancies, the ethanol-fed baboons gained weight (Ainley *et al.* 1988). The mean blood alcohol levels ranged from 155 to 311 mg percent 1 h after feeding. Only one liver showed any suggestion of pericellular fibrosis and none of the animals developed cirrhosis.

Second, the caloric adequacy of the Lieber–DeCarli baboon model has been questioned on the grounds that the ethanol-fed baboons failed to ingest adequate calories and failed to gain weight (Rao *et al.* 1992). The Lieber–DeCarli liquid diet adjusted to meet the nutritional requirements of baboons contained 18 percent of total calories as protein, 60 percent as carbohydrate and 21 percent as fat (Portman 1970; Lieber *et al.* 1989). The alcohol-containing diet replaces carbohydrate to provide up to 50 percent of total calories. To rule out choline deficiency as a cause of ethanol-induced cirrhosis, baboons were fed a diet supplemented with choline (Lieber *et al.* 1985). This failed to prevent cirrhosis and instead was found to be toxic. Paradoxically, when the diet was supplemented with lecithin with polyunsaturated fatty acids, cirrhosis was prevented (Lieber *et al.* 1990), suggesting that choline supplemented in this way may have prevented fibrosis in the baboon model as it did in the rat model. However, it is possible that dilinoleate phosphatidyl choline provided in the diet prevented the ethanol-induced liver injury by restoring membrane phospholipids towards normal (Lieber *et al.* 1993).

Other animal models

Pig models

The Hanford miniature pig was studied for alcoholic liver disease by feeding lab chow in which 10 percent of calories were provided as protein, 25 percent as carbohydrate and 5 percent as fat, 4 g ethanol/kg or 60 percent of total calories, for 11 months. The pigs did not gain weight. The average peak blood ethanol was 130 mg/dl and serum transaminase levels were elevated but liver histology was not different from

controls (Zidenberg-Cherr *et al.* 1990). Using the same regimen but increasing the fat as corn oil to 12 percent of total calories fed for 20 months, Zidenberg-Cherr *et al.* (1991) also found no weight gain. Peak blood alcohol levels were 229 ± 14 mg/dl at 7 months and 195 ± 19 mg/dl at 20 months. The liver histopathology did not differ between the ethanol-fed pigs and the controls. There was no increase in the products of lipid peroxidation in either experiment. However, when the dietary fat was increased to 33 percent of dietary fat, with an increase in polyunsaturated fats in the diet, fatty liver and fibrosis were observed (McGee *et al.* 1992). The peak blood alcohol levels with this model (Yucatan micropigs) averaged 184 mg percent. Thus the micropig, like the rat and baboon, must have a high polyunsaturated fat diet before ethanol induces significant liver pathology.

Mouse models

Although mice have often been used for biomedical, immunological and pharmacological dependency studies on alcohol, there are only a small number of studies on alcohol-associated liver injury. In one study, in which mice were fed a liquid diet mixed with ethanol (30 percent of calories were derived from ethanol), weight loss on alcohol varied with the sex and strain of mice studied, and the livers showed mild to moderate fatty change (Smith and Hoy 1990). Mice have not proved useful in the study of alcoholic liver disease, probably because they have a very high metabolic rate which requires a high dose of alcohol (i.e. 25 g/kg/day) to be administered in order to maintain a high blood alcohol level. Such a dose of alcohol displaces the calories derived from nutrients and thus induces a malnourished state.

Ferret model

There is one report where ferrets were used to study alcohol-associated liver disease (Roselle *et al.* 1986). In this study, where ethanol was fed in the Lieber–DeCarli liquid diet, 21 percent of calories were derived from ethanol. Liver degeneration, fatty liver and "Mallory body-like" material was observed after 11 weeks. Bone marrow toxic changes and anaemia complicated the interpretation of the results and limited the duration of feeding.

Guinea-pig models

Guinea-pigs have been studied by feeding ethanol (40 percent of total calories) and diet (17.5 percent protein and 9.2 percent fat calories) in a solid form *ad lib* for 8 months (Wallerstedt *et al.* 1975). Although the controls gained weight, the alcohol-fed pigs did not. The liver pathology consisted of fatty change exclusively. Similar results were reported where guinea-pigs were given ethanol intravenously at 30 percent of total calories for 8 weeks (Yunice *et al.* 1984). Unless the diet was supplemented with ascorbate, the ethanol-infused pigs lost weight compared with the controls. Blood alcohol levels averaged 270 mg percent 3 h post-infusion. Centrilobular fatty liver was observed in the ethanol-infused pigs. The fatty change was essentially prevented by ascorbate but a product of lipid peroxidation was increased in both ethanol-infused groups.

Hamster models

Golden Syrian hamster have a strong preference to drink ethanol solutions compared with water. Hamsters fed ethanol and pelleted Purina rodent chow *ad lib* developed fatty livers (Cunnane *et al.* 1985). Rats fed 15 percent ethanol for 8 weeks ingested 19 percent of their total calories as ethanol. Weight gain was not significant in either the ethanol-fed or control hamsters. Extending these studies to 54 weeks apparently did not lead to progression of the liver disease (Cunnane *et al.* 1987). Interpretation of these results is difficult because ethanol and a solid diet were fed separately and the percent of calories derived from fat in the diet is not known.

Conclusion

Experimental models in which ethanol is administered in accordance with the following guidelines can be expected to induce significant liver pathology resembling the alcoholic liver disease seen in humans:

1. High blood ethanol levels are maintained.
2. The diet is rich in polyunsaturated fatty acids or linoleic acid.
3. The diet is high in fat and low in carbohydrate.
4. The diet can include other nutritional or pharmacological factors which produce synergistic effects with ethanol on oxidative stress.
5. The controls should be pair-fed a dietary regimen which varies in only one constituent (i.e. calories derived from glucose are substituted for calories derived from ethanol).

References

Ainley, C.C., Senapti, A., Brown, I.M.H., Iles, C.A., Slavin, B.M., Mitchell, W.P., Davies, D.R., Keeling, P.W.N. and Thompson, R.P.H. (1988). Is alcohol hepatoxic in the baboon? *Journal of Hepatology* **7**, 85–92.

Ashworth, C.T. (1947). Production of fatty infiltration of liver in rats by alcohol in spite of adequate diet. *Proceedings of the Society for Experimental Biology and Medicine* **66**, 382–385.

Azzalis, L.A., Pimentel, R., Simizu, K., Barros, S.B.M., Junqueria, V.B.C. and Porta, E.A. (1992). Hepatic effects of acute lindane treatment in rats chronically fed a high ethanol regimen. *Biochemical Archives* **8**, 45–67.

Badger, T.M., Ronis, M.J.J., Lumpkin, C.K., Valentine, C.R., Shahare, M., Irby, D., Huang, J., Mercado, C., Thomas, P. and Ingelman-Sundberg, M. (1993). Effects of chronic ethanol on growth hormone secretion and hepatic cytochrome P450 isozymes of the rat. *Journal of Pharmacology and Experimental Therapeutics* **264**, 438–447.

Barak, A.J., Tuma, D.J. and Beckenhauer, H.C. (1971). Ethanol feeding and choline deficiency as influences on hepatic choline uptake. *Journal of Nutrition* **101**, 533–538.

Best, C.H., Hartroft, W.S., Lucas, C.C. and Ridout, J.H. (1949). Liver damage produced by feeding alcohol or sugar and its prevention by choline. *British Medical Journal* **2**, 1001–1006.

Bosma, A., Brouwer, A., Seifert, W.F. and Knook, D.L. (1988). Synergism between ethanol and carbon tetrachloride in the generation of liver fibrosis. *Journal of Pathology* **156**, 15–21.

Castillo, T., Koop, D.R., Kamimura S., Triadafilopoulus, G. and Tsukamoto, H. (1992). Role of cytochrome P450 2E1 in ethanol–carbon tetrochloride and iron dependent microsomal lipid peroxidation. *Hepatology* **16**, 992–996.

Chaikoff, I.L., Connor, C.L. and Biskind, G.R. (1938). Fatty infiltration and cirrhosis of the liver in depancreatized dogs maintained with insulin. *American Journal of Pathology* **14**, 101–110.

Chaikoff, I.L., Eichorn, K.B., Connor, C.L. and Entenman, C. (1943). The production of cirrhosis in the liver of the normal dog by prolonged feeding of a high-fat diet. *American Journal of Pathology* **19**, 9–19.

Chaikoff, I.L., Entenman, C., Gillman, T. and Connor, C.L. (1948). Pathologic reactions in the livers and kidneys of dogs fed alcohol while maintained on a high protein diet. *Archives of Pathology* **45**, 435–446.

Chey, W.Y., Kosay, S. and Siplet, H. (1971). Observations on hepatic histology and function in alcoholic dogs. *American Journal of Digestive Diseases* **16**, 825–838.

Connor, C.L. (1940). Some effects of chronic alcohol poisoning in rabbits. *Archives of Pathology* **30**, 165–179.

Connor, C.L. and Chaikoff, I.L. (1939). Production of cirrhosis in fatty liver with alcohol. *Proceedings of the Society of Experimental Medicine and Biology* **39**, 356–359.

Cueto, J., Tajen, N., Gilbert, E. and Currie, R.A. (1967). Experimental liver injury in the Rhesus monkey: I. Effects of cirrhogenic diet and ethanol. *Annals of Surgery* **166**, 19–28.

Cunnane, S.C., Manku, M.S. and Horrobin, D.F. (1985). Effect of ethanol on liver triglycerides and fatty acid composition in the golden Syrian hamster. *Annals of Nutrition and Metabolism* **29**, 246–252.

Cunnane, S.C., McAdoo, K.R. and Horrobin, D.F. (1987). Long-term ethanol consumption in the hamster: Effects on tissue lipids, fatty acids and erythrocyte hemolysis. *Annals of Nutrition and Metabolism* **31**, 265–271.

Davis, B.H. and Madri, J.A. (1987). Vitamin A administration diminishes type I and II collagen production during carbon tetrachloride-induced hepatic fibrosis. *Hepatology* **7**, 1091A.

Degli Esposti, S., Frizell, E., He, A., Abraham, A., French, S.W. and Zern, M.A. (1991). Improved rat model of alcoholic liver disease: Omega-3 fatty acids (W3FAs) plus ethanol administration. *Hepatology* **14**, 132A.

Derr, R.F. (1989). The quantities of nutrients recommended by the NRC abate the effects of toxic alcohol dose administered to rats. *Journal of Nutrition* **119**, 1228–1230.

Dicker, E. and Cederbaum, A.I. (1991). Increased oxidation of dimethyl nitrosamine in pericentral microsomes after pyrozole induction of cytochrome P450–2E1. *Alcoholism: Clinical and Experimental Research* **15**, 1072–1076.

Forssell, L. (1981). Metabolic effects of ethanol in rats as studied with an intragastric infusion technique. I. Animal model. *Substance and Alcohol Actions/Misuse* **2**, 25–30.

French, S.W. (1966). Effect of chronic ethanol ingestion on liver enzyme changes induced by thiamine, riboflavin, pyridoxine or choline deficiency. *Journal of Nutrition* **88**, 291–302.

French, S.W. (1989). Alcoholic hepatotoxicity. *Journal of Hepatology* **9**, 134–135.

French, S.W. (1993). Nutrition in the pathogenesis of alcoholic liver disease. *Alcohol and Alcoholism* **28**, 97–100.

French, S.W., Ruebner, B.H., Mezey, E., Tamura, T. and Halsted, C.H. (1983). Effect of chronic ethanol feeding on hepatic mitochondria in the monkey. *Hepatology* **3**, 34–40.

French, S.W., Benson, N.C. and Sun, P.S. (1984). Centrilobular liver necrosis induced by hypoxia in chronic ethanol-fed rats. *Hepatology* **4**, 912–917.

French, S.W., Miyamoto, K. and Tsukamoto, H. (1986). Ethanol-induced hepatic fibrosis in the rat: Role of the amount of dietary fat. *Alcoholism: Clinical and Experimental Research* **10**, 13S–19S.

French, S.W., Miyamoto, K., Ohta, Y. and Geoffrion, Y. (1988a). Pathogenesis of experimental alcoholic liver disease in the rat. *Methods and Achievement in Experimental Pathology* **13**, 181–207.

French, S.W., Miyamoto, K., Wong, K., Jui, L. and Briere, L. (1988b). Role of the Ito cell in liver parenchymal fibrosis in rats fed alcohol and a high fat–low protein diet. *American Journal of Pathology* **132**, 73–85.

French, S.W., Wong, K., Nanji, A., Arseneault, R. and Mendenhall, C. (1988c). The role of the Ito cell in fibrogenesis in alcoholic liver disease. In *Biomedical and Social Aspects of Alcohol and Alcoholism* (Edited by Kuriyama, K., Takada, A. and Ishii, H.), pp. 767–773. Elsevier, Amsterdam.

French, S.W., Nanji, A.A. and Mobarham, S. (1989). Dietary fats modulate the effect of ethanol on hepatic vitamin A. *Hepatology* **10**, 702A.

French, S.W., Takahashi, H., Wong, K. and Mendenhall, C. (1991). Ito cell activation induced by chronic ethanol feeding in the presence of different dietary fats. *Alcohol and Alcoholism* **1**, 357–361 (suppl.).

French, S.W., Nash, J., Shitabata, P., Kachi, K., Hara, C., Chedid, A. and Mendenhall, C.L. (1993a). Pathology of alcoholic liver disease. *Seminars in Liver Disease* **13**, 154–169.

French, S.W., Wong, K., Jui, L., Albano, E., Hagbjork, A.-L. and Ingelman-Sundberg, M. (1993b). Effect of ethanol on cytochrome P450 2E1 (CYP 2E1), lipid peroxidation and serum protein adduct formation in relation to liver pathology pathogenesis. *Experimental and Molecular Pathology* **58**, 61–75.

Friedenwald, J. (1905). The pathologic effects of alcohol on rabbits: An experimental study. *Journal of the American Medical Association* **45**, 780–784.

Gomez-Dumm, C.L.A., Porta, E.A., Hartroff, W.S. and Koch, O.R. (1968). A new experimental approach in the study of chronic alcoholism. II. Effects of high alcohol intake in rats fed diets of various adequacies. *Laboratory Investigation* **18**, 365–378.

Hall, P. de la M., Plummer, J.L., Ilsley, A.H. and Cousins, M.J. (1991). Hepatic fibrosis and cirrhosis after carbon tetrachloride vapor in the rat. *Hepatology* **13**, 815–819.

Hartroft, W.S. and Porta, E.A. (1968). Alcohol, diet, and experimental hepatic injury. *Canadian Journal of Physiology and Pharmacology* **46**, 463–473.

Hasumura, Y., Teschke, R. and Lieber, C.S. (1974). Increased carbon tetrachloride hepatotoxicity, and its mechanism, after chronic ethanol consumption. *Gastroenterology* **66**, 415–422.

Horn, R., Junge, J. and Christoffersen, P. (1986). Early alcoholic liver injury: Activation of lipocytes in acinar zone 3 and correlation to degree of collagen formation in the Disse space. *Journal of Hepatology* **3**, 333–340.

Kamimura, S., Gaal, K., Britton, R.S., Bacon, B.R., Triadafilopoulos, G. and Tsukamoto, H. (1992).

Increased 4-hydroxynonenal levels in experimental alcoholic liver disease: Association of lipid peroxidation with liver fibrogenesis. *Hepatology* **16**, 448–453.

Klatskin, G., Krehl, W.A. and Corn, H. (1954). Effect of alcohol on choline requirement. I. Changes in rat liver following prolonged ingestion of alcohol. *Journal of Experimental Medicine* **100**, 605–614.

Koch, O.R., Porta, E.A. and Hartroft, W.S. (1969). A new experimental approach in the study of chronic alcoholism. V. Super diet. *Laboratory Investigation* **21**, 298–303.

Leathers, C.W., Bond, M.G., Bullock, B.C. and Rudel, L.L. (1981). Dietary ethanol and cholesterol in *Macaca nemestrina* scrum lipid and hepatic changes. *Experimental and Molecular Pathology* **35**, 285–299.

Lieber, C.S. and DeCarli, L.M. (1970). Quantitative relationship between the amount of dietary fat and the severity of the alcoholic fatty liver. *American Journal of Clinical Nutrition* **23**, 474–478.

Lieber, C.S. and DeCarli, L.M. (1974). An experimental model of alcohol feeding and liver injury in the baboon. *Journal of Medical Primatology* **3**, 153–163.

Lieber, C.S. and DeCarli, L.M. (1989a). Liquid diet technique of ethanol administration: 1989 update. *Alcohol and Alcoholism* **24**, 197–211.

Lieber, C.S. and DeCarli, L.M. (1989b). Effects of mineral and vitamin supplementation on alcohol-induced fatty liver and microsomal induction. *Alcoholism: Clinical and Experimental Research* **13**, 142–143.

Lieber, C.S. and DeCarli, L.M. (1989c). Recommended amounts of nutrients do not abate the toxic effects of an alcohol dose that sustains significant blood levels of ethanol. *Journal of Nutrition* **119**, 2038–2040.

Lieber, C.S., Jones, D.P., Mendelson, J. and DeCarli, L.M. (1963). Fatty liver, hyperlipemia and hyperuricemia produced by prolonged alcohol consumption, despite adequate dietary intake. *Transactions of the Association of American Physicians* **76**, 289–300.

Lieber, C.S., DeCarli, L.M. and Rubin, E. (1975). Sequential production of fatty liver, hepatitis, and cirrhosis in sub-human primates fed ethanol with adequate diets. *Proceedings of the National Academy Sciences, USA* **72**, 437–441.

Lieber, C.S., Leo, M.A., Mak, K.M., DeCarli, L.M. and Sato, S. (1985). Choline fails to prevent liver fibrosis in ethanol-fed baboons but causes toxicity. *Hepatology* **5**, 561–572.

Lieber, C.S., DeCarli, L.M. and Sorrell, M.F. (1989). Experimental methods of ethanol administration. *Hepatology* **10**, 501–510.

Lieber, C.S., DeCarli, L.M., Mak, K.M., Kim, C.I. and Leo, M.A. (1990). Attenuation of alcohol-induced hepatic fibrosis by polyunsaturated lecithin. *Hepatology* **12**, 1390–1398.

Lieber, C.S., Leo, M.A., Robins, S. and DeCarli, L.M. (1993). Ethanol decreases hepatic phosphatidyl methyl transferase activity whereas phosphatidyl choline in-

creases it with protection against cirrhosis. *FASEB Journal* **7**, 842A.

Lindros, K.O., Stowell, L., Vaananen, H., Sipponen, P., Lamminsivu, U., Pikkarainen, P. and Salaspuro, M. (1983). Uninterrupted prolonged ethanol oxidation as a main pathogenetic factor of alcoholic liver damage: Evidence from a new liquid diet animal model. *Liver* **3**, 79–91.

Lukas, S.E. and Moreton, J.E. (1979). A technique for chronic intragastric drug administration in the rat. *Life Sciences* **25**, 593–600.

McGee, C.D., Wong, T., Halsted, C.H., Villanueva, J., Peterson, C.M. and Rucker, R.B. (1992). Association between collagen expression, hydroxyproline and acetaldehyde levels in micropigs. *FASEB Journal* **6**, 1857A.

Mak, K.M. and Lieber, C.S. (1988). Lipocytes and transitional cells in alcoholic liver disease: A morphometric study. *Hepatology* **8**, 1027–1033.

Matsuda, Y., Takase, S., Takada, A., Sato, H. and Yashuhara, M. (1985). Comparison of ballooned hepatocytes in alcoholic and non-alcoholic liver injury in rats. *Alcohol* **2**, 303–308.

Matsuoka, M. and Tsukamoto, H. (1990). Stimulation of hepatic lipocyte collagen production by Kupffer cell-derived transforming growth factor β: Implication for a pathogenetic role in alcoholic liver fibrogenesis. *Hepatology* **11**, 599–605.

Matsuoka, M., Zhang, M. and Tsukamoto, H. (1990). Sensitization of hepatic lipocytes by high-fat diet to stimulatory effects of Kuppfer cell-derived factors: Implication in alcoholic liver fibrogenesis. *Hepatology* **11**, 173–182.

Mezey, E., Potter, J.J., French, S.W., Tamura, T. and Halsted, C.H. (1983). Effect of chronic ethanol feeding on hepatic collagen in the monkey. *Hepatology* **3**, 41–44.

Minato, Y., Hasumura, Y. and Takeuchi, J. (1983). The role of fat-storing cells in Disse space fibrogenesis in alcoholic liver disease. *Hepatology* **3**, 359–566.

Miyamoto, K. and French, S.W. (1988a). Hepatic adenine nucleotide metabolism measured *in vivo* in rats fed ethanol and a high fat–low protein diet. *Hepatology* **8**, 53–60.

Miyamoto, K. and French, S.W. (1988b). Hepatic adenosine in rats fed ethanol: Effect of acute hyeroxia or hypoxia. *Alcoholism: Clinical and Experimental Research* **12**, 512–515.

Morimoto, M., Hagbjork, A.-L., Nanji, A.A., Ingelman-Sundberg, M., Lindros, K.O., Fu, P.C., Albano, E. and French, S.W. (1993). Role of cytochrome P4502E1 in alcohol liver disease pathogenesis. *Alcohol* **10**, 459–464.

Nanji, A.A. and French, S.W. (1989). Dietary linoleic acid is required for development of experimentally induced alcoholic liver injury. *Life Sciences* **44**, 223–227.

Nanji, A.A., Jui, L.T. and French, S.W. (1989a). Effect

of chronic carbon monoxide exposure on experimental alcoholic liver injury in rats. *Life Sciences* **45**, 885–890.

Nanji, A.A., Mendenhall, C.L and French, S.W. (1989b). Beef fat prevents alcoholic liver disease in the rat. *Alcoholism: Clinical and Experimental Research* **13**, 15–19.

Nanji, A.A., Miller-Cassman, R., Kettry, U., Sadrzadeh, S.M.H., Thomas, P. and Yamanaka, T. (1992a). Relationship between development of experimental alcoholic liver injury and plasma levels of endotoxin and eicosanoids and Kuppfer cell supernatant levels of interleukin 1, tumor necrosis factor and eicosanoids. *Gastroenterology* **102**, 859A.

Nanji, A.A., Zhao, S., Sadrzadeh, S.M.H. and Waxman, D.J. (1992b). Serial changes in cytochromes P450 2E1 4A and -2B1 in experimental alcoholic liver injury. *Hepatology* **16**, 112A.

Nanji, A.A., Zhao, S., Sadrzadeh, S.M.H., Dannenberg, A. and Wayman, D.J. (1992c). Microsomal fatty acid changes in experimental alcoholic liver injury: Relationships to levels of cytochrome P450 2E1 (CYP 2E1) and in microsomal conjugated dienes. *Gastroenterology* **102**, 859A.

Nanji, A.A., Khettry, U., Sadrzadeh, S.M.H. and Yamanaka, T. (1993a). Severity of liver injury in alcoholic liver disease: Correlation with plasma endotoxin, prostaglandin E2, leukotriene B$_4$ and thromboxane B$_2$. *American Journal of Pathology* **142**, 367–373.

Nanji, A.A., Zhao, S., Sadrzadeh, S.M.H., Khettry, U. and Waxman, D.J. (1993b). Cimetidine prevents experimental alcoholic liver injury in the intragastric feeding rat model. *Gastroenterology* **104**, 962A.

Nanji, A.A., Sadrzadeh, S.M.H., Khettry, U., Thomas, P. and Yamanaka, T. (1993c). A novel hepatoprotective quinone derivative ameliorates experimental alcoholic liver injury. *Gastroenterology* **104**, 962A.

Okanoue, T., Burbige, E.J. and French, S.W. (1983). The role of the Ito cell in perivenular and intralobular fibrosis in alcoholic hepatitis. *Archives of Pathology and Laboratory Medicine* **107**, 459–463.

Oshita, M., Sato, N., Yoshihara, H., Takei, Y., Hijioka, T., Fukui, H., Goto, M., Matsunaga, T., Kashiwaga, T., Kawano, S., Fusamoto, H. and Kamada, T. (1992a). Ethanol-induced vasoconstriction causes focal hepatocellular injury in the isolated perfused rat liver. *Hepatology* **16**, 1007–1013.

Oshita, M., Takei, Y., Kawano, S., Hijioka, T., Fukui, H., Nishimura, Y., Fusamoto, H. and Kamada, T. (1992b). Nitric oxide attenuates ethanol-induced hepatic injury. *Hepatology* **16**, 109A.

Patek, A.J., Bowry, S.C. and Anuras, S. (1973). Alcohol and sucrose in choline deficiency cirrhosis in the rat. *Archives of Pathology* **96**, 377–382.

Pettit, N.B., Ihrig, T.J. and French, S.W. (1980). An intragastric pair-feeding model for ethanol administration. *Federation Proceedings* **39**, 1299A.

Popper, H. and Lieber, C.S. (1980). Histogenesis of alcoholic fibrosis and cirrhosis in the baboon. *American Journal of Pathology* **98**, 695–716.

Porta, E.A. and Gomez-Dumm, C.L.A. (1968). A new experimental approach in the study of chronic alcoholism. I. Effect of high alcohol intake in rats fed a commerical laboratory diet. *Laboratory Investigation* **18**, 352–364.

Porta, E.A., Hartroft, W.S. and De La Iglesia, F.A. (1965). Hepatic changes associated with chronic alcoholism in rats. *Laboratory Investigation* **14**, 1437–1455.

Porta, E.A., Hartroft, W.S., Gomez-Dumm, C.L.A. and Koch, O.R. (1967). Dietary factors in the progression and regression of hepatic alterations associated with experimental chronic alcoholism. *Federation Proceedings* **62**, 1449–1457.

Porta, E.A., Koch, O.R., Gomez-Dumm, C.L.A. and Hartroff, W.S. (1968). Effects of dietary protein on the liver of rats in experimental chronic alcoholism. *Journal of Nutrition* **94**, 437–446.

Porta, E.A., Koch, O.R. and Hartroft, W.S. (1969). A new experiment of alcoholic cirrhosis in rats and the role of lipotropes versus vitamins. *Laboratory Investigation* **20**, 562–572.

Porta, E.A., Koch, O.R. and Hartroft, W.S. (1972). Recovery from chronic hepatic lesions in rats fed alcohol and a solid super diet. *American Journal of Clinical Nutrition* **25**, 881–896.

Portman, O.W. (1970). Nutritional requirments of nonhuman primates. In *Feeding and Nutrition of Nonhuman Primates* (Edited by Harris R.S.), pp. 87–115. Academic Press, New York.

Porto, L.C., Chevallier, M. and Grimaud, J.-A. (1988). Morphometry of terminal hepatic veins. 2. Follow up in chronically alcohol-fed baboons. *Virchows Archives A* **414**, 299–307.

Rao, G.A. and Larkin, E.C. (1985). Inadequate intake by growing rats of essential nutrients from liquid diets used for chronic alcohol consumption. *Nutrition Research* **5**, 789–796.

Rao, G.A., Larkin, E.C., Derr, R.F. and Sankaran, H. (1992). Animal models show nutritional modulation of alcoholic liver disease. In *Nutrition and Alcohol* (Edited by Watson, R.R. and Watzl, B.), pp. 309–335. CRC Press, Boca Raton, FL.

Rogers, A.E., Fox, J.G. and Murphy, J.C. (1981). Ethanol and diet interactions in male Rhesus monkeys. *Drug–Nutrient Interactions* **1**, 3–14.

Ronis, M.J.J., Huang, J., Crouch, J., Mercado, C., Irby, D., Valentine, C.R., Lumpkin, C.K., Ingelman-Sundberg, M. and Badger, T.M. (1993). Cytochrome P450 CYP 2E1 induction during chronic alcohol exposure occurs by a two-step mechanism associated with blood alcohol concentrations in rats. *Journal of Pharmacology and Experimental Therapeutics* **264**, 944–950.

Roselle, G.A., Mendenhall, C.L., Muhleman, A.F. and Chedid, A. (1986). The ferret: A new model of oral ethanol injury involving the liver, bone marrow, and peripheral blood lymphocytes. *Alcoholism: Clinical and Experimental Research* **10**, 279–284.

Rubin, E. and Lieber, C.S. (1973). Experimental alcoholic hepatitis: A new primate model. *Science* **182**, 712–713.

Rubin, E. and Lieber, C.S. (1974). Fatty liver, alcoholic hepatitis and cirrhosis produced by alcohol in primates. *New England Journal of Medicine* **290**, 128–135.

Ruebner, B.H., Moore, J., Rutherford, R.B., Seligman, A.M. and Zuidema, G.D. (1969). Nutritional cirrhosis in Rhesus monkeys: Electron microscopy and histochemistry. *Experimental and Molecular Pathology* **11**, 53–70.

Ruebner, B.H., Brayton, M.A., Freeland, R.A., Kanayama, R. and Tsao, M. (1972). Production of a fatty liver by ethanol in Rhesus monkeys. *Laboratory Investigation* **27**, 71–75.

Sadrzadeh, S.M.H., Nanji, A.A., Price, P.L. and Meydani, M. (1993a). Oral iron chelators, L_1, lowers hepatic non-heme iron in ethanol-fed rats. *Gastroenterology* **104**, 982A.

Sadrzadeh, S.M.H., Nanji, A.A., Price, P.L. and Meydani, M. (1993b). The effect of chronic ethanol feeding on serum and liver alpha and gamma tocopherol levels in normal and vitamin E deficient rats. *Gastroenterology* **104**, 982A.

Sakamoto, M. (1991). Effect of endothelin on the contraction of Ito cells (fat-storing cells). *Acta Hepatologica Japonica* **32**, 1027–1033.

Sato, C., Matsuda, Y. and Lieber, C.S. (1981). Increased hepatoxicity of acetaminophen after chronic ethanol consumption in the rat. *Gastroenterology* **80**, 140–148.

Senoo, H. and Wake, K. (1985). Suppression of experimental hepatic fibrosis by administration of vitamin A. *Laboratory Investigation* **52**, 182–194.

Smith, S.M. and Hoy, H.E. (1990). *Ad libitum* alcohol ingestion does not induce renal IgA deposition in mice. *Alcoholism: Clinical and Experimental Research* **14**, 184–186.

Takada, A., Porta, E.A. and Hartroft, W.S. (1967). Regress of dietary cirrhosis in rats fed alcohol and a "sugar diet". *American Journal of Clinical Nutrition* **20**, 213–225.

Takada, A., Ohara, N., Matsuda, Y., Sawae, G. and Takeuchi, J. (1972). Effects of long-term alcohol administration on the development of fatty cirrhosis in choline-deficient rats. *Digestion* **6**, 83–93.

Takada, A., Matsuda, Y. and Takase, S. (1986). Effects of dietary fat on alcohol-pyrazole hepatitis in rats: The pathogenetic role of the alcohol dehydrogenase pathway in alcohol-induced hepatic cell injury. *Alcoholism: Clinical and Experimental Research* **10**, 403–411.

Takahashi, H., Geoffrion, Y., Butler, K.W. and French, S.W. (1990). *In vivo* hepatic energy metabolism during the progression of alcoholic liver disease: A non-invasive ^{31}P nuclear magnetic resonance study in rats. *Hepatology* **11**, 65–73.

Takahashi, H., Wong, K., Jui, L. and French, S.W. (1991). Effect of dietary fat on Ito cell activation by chronic ethanol intake: A long term serial morphometric study on alcohol-fed and control rats. *Alcoholism: Clinical and Experimental Research* **15**, 1060–1066.

Takahashi, H., Johansson, I., French, S.W. and Ingelman-Sundberg, M. (1992). Effects of dietary fat composition on activities of the microsomal ethanol oxidizing system and ethanol-inducible cytochrome P450 (CYP 2E1) in the liver of rats chronically fed ethanol. *Pharmacology and Toxicology* **70**, 347–351.

Takeuchi, J., Takada, A., Ebata, K., Sawae, G. and Okumura, Y. (1968). Effect of alcohol on the livers of rats. I. Effect of a single intoxicating dose of alcohol on the livers of rats fed a choline-deficient diet or a commercial ration. *Laboratory Investigation* **19**, 211–217.

Thompson, J.A. and Reitz, R.C. (1976). Studies on the acute and chronic effects of ethanol ingestion on choline oxidation. *Annals of the New York Academy of Science* **273**, 194–204.

Thompson, J.A. and Reitz, R.C. (1979). A possible mechanism for the increased oxidation of choline after chronic ethanol ingestion. *Biochimica et Biophysica Acta* **545**, 381–397.

Tsuji, S., Kawano, S., Michida, E., Masuda, E., Nagano, K., Takei, Y., Fusamoto, H. and Kamada, T. (1992). Ethanol stimulates immunoreactive endothelin-1 and -2 released from cultured human umbilical vein endothelial cells. *Alcoholism: Clinical and Experimental Research* **16**, 347–349.

Tsukamoto, H. and Xi, X.P. (1989). Incomplete compensation of enhanced hepatic oxygen consumption in rats with alcoholic centrilobular liver necrosis. *Hepatology* **9**, 302–306.

Tsukamoto, H., Reidelberger, R.D., French, S.W. and Largman, C. (1984). Long-term cannulation model for blood sampling and intragastric infusion in the rat. *American Journal of Physiology* **247**, R595–599.

Tsukamoto, H., French, S.W., Benson, N., Delgado, G., Rao, G.A., Larkin, E.C. and Largman, C. (1985a). Severe and progressive steatosis and focal necrosis in rat liver induced by continuous intragastric infusion of ethanol and low fat diet. *Hepatology* **5**, 224–232.

Tsukamoto, H., French, S.W. and Largman, C. (1985b). Correlation of cyclical blood alcohol levels with progression of alcoholic liver injury. *Biochemical Archives* **1**, 215–220.

Tsukamoto, H., French, S.W., Reidelberg, R.D. and Largman, C. (1985c). Cyclic pattern of blood alcohol levels during continuous intragastric ethanol infusion in rats. *Alcoholism: Clinical and Experimental Research* **9**, 31–37.

Tsukamoto, H., Towner, S.J., Ciofalo, L.M. and French, S.W. (1986). Ethanol-induced liver fibrosis in rats fed high-fat diet. *Hepatology* **6**, 814–822.

Tsukamoto, H., Gaal, K. and French, S.W. (1990). Insights into the pathogenesis of alcoholic liver necrosis and fibrosis: Status report. *Hepatology* **12**, 599–608.

Tsukamoto, H., Matsuoka, M., Blauer, W. and Chang,

S. (1991). Ito cell activation during progression of alcoholic liver fibrosis. In *Cells of the Hepatic Sinusoid* (Edited by Wisse E., Knook D.L. and McCluskey R.S.), Vol. 3, pp. 453–456. Kupffer Cell Foundation, Leiden.

Tsukamoto, H., Kamimura, S., Yeager, S., Chen, H.Y., Highman, T.J., Luo, Z.Z., Kim, C.M. and Brittenham, G.M. (1992). Hepatic cirrhosis in rats fed a diet with added alcohol and iron. *Hepatology* **16**, 113A.

Tsukamoto, H., Kim, C.W., Luo, Z.Z., Horn, W., Su, L.-C. and Brittenham, G.M. (1993). Role of lipid peroxidation in *in vivo* and *in vitro* models of liver fibrogenesis. *Gastroenterology* **104**, 1012A.

Tsutsumi, R., Leo, M.A., Cho-il, K., Tsutsumi, M., Lasker, J., Lowe, N. and Lieber, C.S. (1990). Interaction of ethanol with enflurane. *Alcoholism: Clinical and Experimental Research* **14**, 174–179.

Van Waes, L. and Lieber, C.S. (1977). Early perivenular sclerosis in alcoholic fatty liver: An index of progressive liver injury. *Gastroenterology* **73**, 646–650.

Wallerstedt, S., Olsson, R. and Korsan-Bengtsen, K.

(1975). Effects on lipids, coagulation factors and liver histology of long-term ethanol administration to guinea-pigs. *Acta Hepato-Gastroenterology* **22**, 236–241.

Yunice, A.A., Hsu, J.M., Fahmy, A. and Henry, S. (1984). Ethanol–ascorbate interrelationship in acute and chronic alcoholism in the guinea pig. *Proceedings of the Society for Experimental Biology and Medicine* **177**, 262–271.

Zeisel, S.H., DaCosta, K.-A., Franklin, P.D., Alexander, E.A., Lamont, J.T., Sheard, N.F. and Beiser, A. (1991). Choline, an essential nutrient for humans. *FASEB Journal* **5**, 2093–2098.

Zidenberg-Cherr, S., Halsted, C.H., Olin, K.L., Reisenauer, A.M. and Kleen, C.L. (1990). The effect of chronic alcohol ingestion on free radical defense in the minature pig. *Journal of Nutrition* **120**, 213–217.

Zidenberg-Cherr, S., Olin, K.L., Villanueva, J., Tang, A., Phinney, S.D., Halsted, C.H. and Keen, C.L. (1991). Ethanol-induced changes in hepatic free radical defense mechanisms and fatty-acid composition in the miniature pig. *Hepatology* **13**, 1185–1192.

Part VII
Clinical Implications

18 Factors influencing individual susceptibility to alcoholic liver disease

Pauline de la M. Hall

Introduction

The direct hepatotoxic effects of alcohol were demonstrated by Lieber and colleagues in the 1960s and 1970s in both animal studies (Lane and Lieber 1966; Rubin and Lieber 1974; Lieber *et al.* 1975) and in human volunteers (Rubin and Lieber 1967, 1968), and more recently in rats using the intragastric tube method for feeding alcohol (French *et al.* 1986, 1988; Tsukamoto *et al.* 1990). The acute changes – including structural and functional mitochondrial alterations, proliferation of smooth endoplasmic reticulum and the accumulation of fat droplets – are associated with the various metabolic disturbances that occur as a consequence of the metabolism of alcohol (see Chapter 2); these changes are rapidly reversible upon alcohol withdrawal. The response to acute alcohol feeding is fairly uniform, although there may be some individual variation in the severity of hepatocellular injury. This is in marked contrast to the effects of chronic alcohol consumption, as outlined below.

A prospective study by Sorensen *et al.* (1984) of the amount of alcohol consumed, and the rate of development of cirrhosis per unit time, suggested that "above a low but precisely determined level of alcohol consumption the risk of development of cirrhosis is not further influenced by the amount of alcohol consumed". Sorensen (1989) suggested that "alcohol abuse has a *permissive* rather than *dose-*

dependent role in the development of alcoholic liver injury". In addition, he suggested that the risk of development of cirrhosis, at a given level of alcohol consumption, may depend on the action of other factors which could change the hepatotoxic threshold for alcohol-associated injury. The observation by Sorensen that cirrhosis develops at a constant rate of 2 percent per year implies that such a factor(s) affects approximately one in every 50 drinkers each year (Sorensen 1989).

This chapter will collate the data relating to the various genetic and acquired factors that may influence the susceptibility of the individual to alcohol-associated liver injury (many of these factors have been discussed in detail elsewhere in this book); some of the interactions between alcohol and other agents will be illustrated.

Direct hepatotoxic effects of alcohol

In Western countries, alcohol is the most common cause of cirrhosis. Dufour *et al.* (1993) recently reviewed trends in cirrhosis morbidity and mortality in the USA; in 1988 cirrhosis was the ninth leading cause of death and 40 percent of cirrhosis deaths were alcohol-related (Grant *et al.* 1991). There is no doubt that chronic alcohol ingestion is aetiologically associated with cirrhosis. However, numerous epidemiological studies, such as those reviewed in Hall (1985), have shown that many of the heaviest drinkers do not develop liver injury despite a lifetime of heavy drinking. When considering the direct hepatotoxic effects of chronic alcohol ingestion, the following variables need to be evaluated – the daily alcohol intake, the duration of alcohol intake, the pattern of drinking (e.g. daily *vs* binge drinking with periods of abstinence) and the age at which drinking commenced.

Dose and duration of alcohol consumption

One of the main difficulties in determining the toxic threshold for alcohol (i.e. the lowest daily dose of alcohol that can cause chronic liver injury) is the acknowledged unreliability of the history of the amount of alcohol consumed. As discussed by Gavaler and Arria in Chapter 7, the alcohol history is just as likely to be unreliable in men as in women.

However, numerous epidemiological studies have shown that there is a relationship between the volume of alcohol consumed and the risk of developing cirrhosis (Lelbach 1975, 1985; Pequinot *et al.* 1978; Morgan 1985; Rankin *et al.* 1985). In most of the published series, the overall incidence of cirrhosis in chronic drinkers is only 10–15 percent (Lelbach 1975; Anthony *et al.* 1978). A lifetime of heavy drinking does not necessarily result in cirrhosis; for example, a mean daily alcohol intake of 227 g for a mean of 21.6 years resulted in cirrhosis in only 50 percent of drinkers (Lelbach 1975). In contrast, Pequignot *et al.* (1978) and Tuyns and Pequignot (1984) reported cirrhosis occurring in association with an alcohol intake as low as 20 g/day (e.g. two glasses of wine) in women and 40 g/day in men. This observation was confirmed by Batey *et al.* (1990), who studied the risk levels of alcohol consumption in men and found that the risk of developing cirrhosis increased significantly above the baseline when the alcohol intake exceeded 40 g/day.

The duration of alcohol consumption is also a factor that influences the risk of hepatic injury (Pares *et al.* 1986). In general, the longer the duration of chronic alcohol consumption, the greater the risk of liver injury (Pares *et al.* 1986); however, severe liver injury has been reported with alcohol abuse of only 3 months duration (Lischner *et al.* 1971).

A long duration and a high dose of alcohol are acknowledged as factors that increase the risk of liver injury (see Chapter 7). However, recent studies by Sorensen *et al.* (1984) suggest that cirrhosis can develop independently of the dose and duration of alcohol consumption. Sorensen used serial liver biopsies to monitor liver injury in 258 men, with an average daily alcohol consumption greater than 50 g over a period of 10–13 years. The initial liver biopsies, taken at the beginning of the study, did not show cirrhosis in any of the subjects but 38 (about 15 percent) developed cirrhosis during the period of the study. The risk of cirrhosis was nine times greater in those who developed alcoholic hepatitis than in those who did not show even steatosis.

A carefully conducted case-control study by Corrao *et al.* (1993), involving 320 patients with symptomatic liver disease and 320 pair-matched control individuals, utilized a standardized and reproducible questionnaire to determine the lifetime daily alcohol consumption and the duration of alcohol consumption. The odds ratio for cirrhosis, estimated by the conditional logistic regression, increased from 1.0 for lifetime abstainers to 4.2 for a lifetime daily alcohol intake of 225 g or more. Interestingly, there was a negative correlation between the duration of alcohol consumption and the development of cirrhosis. The authors suggest that factors influencing the degree of individual susceptibility to liver injury by alcohol may account for this unexpected finding. Thus individuals who are more susceptible, due to the presence of one or more risk factors, may develop liver injury that progresses to cirrhosis after a shorter period of alcohol consumption than those who are less susceptible. Perhaps factors in addition to alcohol are obligatory for the development of cirrhosis – the absence of such factors may account for the puzzling observation that only a minority of heavy drinkers develop cirrhosis despite a lifetime of drinking.

Pattern of drinking

Sorensen *et al.* (1984) reported a lower rate of development of cirrhosis in intermittent drinkers compared with daily drinkers even though they failed to demonstrate a correlation between the average daily alcohol consumption and the rate of development of cirrhosis.

Wodak *et al.* (1983) reported the development of alcoholic liver disease in only 18 percent of patients with severe alcohol dependence, compared with 56 percent of those who escaped the florid symptoms of alcohol addiction. Drinkers who seek treatment for alcohol addiction frequently have prolonged periods of abstinence. In contrast, drinkers who are not alcohol-dependent are able to maintain a more moderate but continuous consumption of alcohol over many years; this pattern of drinking may be associated with liver injury which is frequently asymptomatic. Thus, the lower prevalence of liver injury in people with alcohol dependence, compared with people who drink more moderately but continuously, may be associated with the beneficial effects of the periods of alcohol withdrawal e.g. improved hepatocyte regeneration (see Chapter 3).

A similar suggestion was made by Yates *et al.* (1987), who studied 100 men admitted to an alcohol treatment unit. Fifty men with elevated liver enzymes were matched by age and time of last drink with 50 men with normal enzymes. Those with elevated liver enzymes showed a trend towards a less severe pattern of alcohol dependence, and were less likely to be binge drinkers or to have blackouts, but were more likely to be daily drinkers. However, the conclusions of this study are weakened by the lack of biopsy confirmation of the presence or absence of liver injury; the authors acknowledged the possibility that some of the patients with normal liver enzymes may also have had liver injury.

Age of onset of drinking

Corrao *et al.* (1993) found a positive correlation between the age that drinking started and the risk of liver injury. Similarly, animal studies have demonstrated more severe and more rapidly progressive liver damage in young, rapidly growing rats compared with adult rats fed alcohol (Jahn *et al.* 1993 and personal observation).

The finding of established cirrhosis in both men and women, but particularly in women, in their 20s and early 30s is becoming increasingly common (personal observation) (Fig. 18.1). In most of the cases, heavy alcohol consumption began in early adolescence. Other risk factors, such as illicit drug use, hepatitis B and/or C are frequently present (Novick *et al.* 1985; to be discussed below). Novick *et al.* (1985) studied patients aged under 35 years admitted for treatment of alcohol and drug abuse. Forty-five percent of those with cirrhosis had been drinking for less than 7 years.

An intriguing observation by Friedman and colleagues (1988) was the presence of an elevated serum iron concentration and transferrin saturation in male adolescent drinkers, and also in female adolescent drinkers if they were oral contraceptive users. These abnormalities may be precursors of the siderosis seen in alcoholic liver disease. The possibility that iron overload potentiates alcohol-related liver injury is mentioned below and discussed in detail in Chapter 12.

Alcoholic beverages are relatively inexpensive

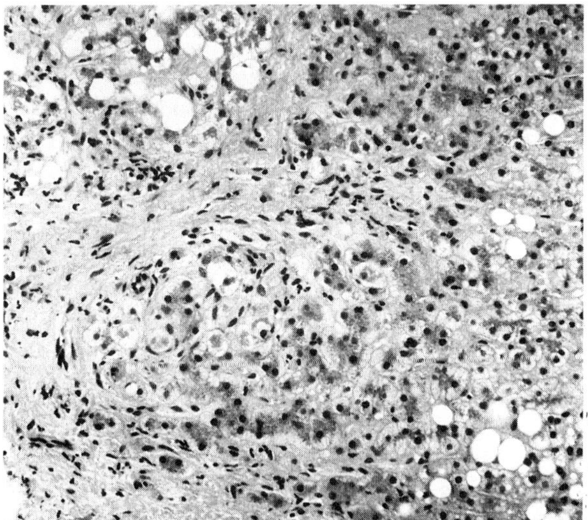

Fig. 18.1 Micronodular cirrhosis. Liver biopsy from a woman aged 28 years who had been drinking heavily since her early teens. Heavy drinking continued and she died several years later of bleeding oesophageal varices. The liver shows an established micronodular cirrhosis and mild alcoholic hepatitis. H&E, × 140.

and are now readily available. Consequently, many young people throughout the world are drinking on a regular basis. In addition, the current obssession of many young people, particularly young women in western countries, about being overweight frequently results in diets deficient in essential nutrients, which could further add to the risk of alcoholic liver disease (see below and Chapter 8). The suggestion that heavy and/or continuous alcohol consumption commencing during adolescence is itself a risk factor for liver injury merits careful investigation.

Genetic factors

The increased susceptibility of women to alcoholic liver disease (discussed in detail in Chapter 7), the growing knowledge of the genetic polymorphisms of alcohol-metabolizing enzymes and racial differences in alcohol metabolism (Chapter 2), the role of immune mechanisms, some aspects of which are genetically determined (Chapter 6), and the recognition of a genetic predisposition to alcohol addiction (Blum *et al.* 1990) have helped focus attention on a possible role of genetic factors in individual susceptibility to alcoholic liver disease.

Genetic polymorphism of alcohol-metabolizing enzymes

The enzymes involved in the metabolism of alcohol are discussed in detail in Chapter 2. Molecular studies have focused on the genes that code for the oxidative pathway in ethanol metabolism, that is alcohol dehydrogenase, acetaldehyde dehydrogenase and formaldehyde dehydrogenase (Li and Bosron 1987; Bosron *et al.* 1988). Alcohol dehydrogenase (ADH) catalyses the major rate-limiting step in the oxidation of alcohol to acetaldehyde. Polymorphism has been observed in ADH_2 (producing three β subunits) and ADH_3 (producing two τ subunits) on chromosome 4, the isoenzymes showing considerable variation in their kinetic properties. Day *et al.* (1991) studied 59 biopsy-proven alcoholic cirrhotics and 80 healthy controls, but unfortunately did not include a group of drinkers who did not have liver disease. The polymerase chain reaction was used to amplify extracts of leucocyte DNA, and the different allelic forms of the ADH_2 and ADH_3 genes were detected with allele-specific oligonucleotide probes. The ADH_3 allele frequencies were different in the patients and the controls; ADH_3^1 in controls (55.1 percent) differed significantly from that in alcoholic cirrhotics (62.7 percent). The authors suggested that the genetically determined differences in alcohol metabolism might help explain individual susceptibility to alcohol-associated diseases. In contrast, studies by Couzigou *et al.* (1990) and Poupon *et al.* (1992) concluded that polymorphism at the ADH_3 locus is not a genetic factor for alcoholic cirrhosis in France. Clearly, further studies in other countries are required in order to determine whether polymorphism of ADH is one of the factors that influences individual susceptibility.

Genetic polymorphisms of cytochrome P4502E1 (CYP2E1) – to date three types (A, B, C) have been identified by the restriction fragment length polymorphisms technique – may also be related to the development of alcoholic liver disease; the prevalence of the type A (homozygous for the c2 gene) has been shown to be significantly higher in patients with alcoholic liver disease (Tsutsumi *et al.*1993).

Racial differences in alcohol metabolism

Genetic polymorphisms of two alcohol-metabolizing enzymes – the cytosolic ADH_2 and the mitochondrial aldehyde dehydrogenase ($ALDH_2$) –

exist in Japanese and other Orientals. Ricciardi *et al.* (1983) developed a method for detecting ADH_{1-4} and the five ALDH isoenzymes, in liver biopsy cores, using starch gel electrophoresis. Only 4 percent of English controls had the atypical ADH_2 variant, which was in marked contrast to its occurrence in 84 percent of Chinese subjects. The rapidly migrating mitochondrial isoenzyme of ALDH was present in all the English subjects but was absent in 54 percent of the Chinese in the study. The "sensitivity" of many Orientals to alcohol is attributed to the rapid and sustained elevation of acetaldehyde by the more active, atypical ADH_2 isoenzymes. The high levels of acetaldehyde in the blood result in facial flushing, sweating, headache, elevation of skin temperature and increased pulse rate.

Shibuya and Yoshida (1988) used hybridization of genomic DNA samples with allele-specific synthetic oligonucleotide probes to determine the genotypes of ADH_2 and $ALDH_2$ loci of 23 Japanese with alcoholic liver disease and 49 healthy, unrelated Japanese. There was no significant difference in the ADH_2 genotypes in those with alcoholic liver disease and the control group; however, there was a marked difference between the two groups at the $ALDH_2$ locus. In the controls the frequency of the typical "Caucasian-type" $ALDH_2^1$ gene was found to be 0.65, compared with a frequency of 0.35 for the atypical "Oriental-type" $ALDH_3^2$ gene; whereas in the alcoholic liver disease group the frequencies were 0.93 and 0.07, respectively. Twenty of the 23 Japanese with alcoholic liver disease were homozygous Caucasian type $ALDH_2^1/ALDH_2^1$, and none of the patients was of the homozygous Oriental type $ALDH_2^2/ALDH_2^2$. This study suggests that Japanese who are "sensitive" to alcohol due to the presence of the atypical $ALDH_2^2$ allele are at less risk of developing alcoholic liver disease than those with the Caucasian type $ALDH_2^1/ALDH_2^1$ allele. In other words, this "sensitivity" to alcohol may be a deterrent to drinking, thus reducing the risk of alcohol-related disease, including liver disease.

Female gender

Review of the published data supports the widely held belief that women are more prone to alcoholic liver disease than men (see Chapter 7). This increased susceptibility manifests in a number of ways:

1. Women tend to present with more severe liver

disease after a shorter duration of consumption and a lower daily intake (Pequignot *et al.* 1978; Rankin *et al.* 1985; Loft *et al.* 1987; Norton *et al.* 1987) (Fig. 18.1).
2. Women (particularly < 45 years) have a higher incidence of alcoholic hepatitis and a worse long-term prognosis even if they abstain (Pares *et al.* 1986; Krasner *et al.* 1977).
3. Black women in the USA appear even more susceptible to alcoholic hepatitis than Caucasian women and have a poor prognosis (Galambos 1972).
4. Women with alcoholic cirrhosis have a higher mortality than men (Berglund 1984).

The current Australian National Health and Medical Research Council (1987) recommendation is that men should not drink more than 40 g alcohol per day (four glasses of wine, beer, etc.) and advises women to drink no more than half the daily amount recommended for men, for example no more than two glasses of wine per day. It is important to point out that Pequignot *et al.* (1978) consider that daily consumption of 20 g alcohol constitutes a significant cirrhotogenic risk for some women. It is also necessary to stress that the recommendation is not advising men and women to drink this amount of alcohol on a daily basis, but rather it advises that those who do drink should not exceed these amounts.

Frezza *et al.* (1990) have shown that women, both non-alcoholic and alcoholic, after consuming equal amounts of alcohol, have higher blood alcohol concentrations than men, even allowing for differences in body size. In non-alcoholic women, "first-pass" metabolism of alcohol (due to its oxidation in the stomach) and gastric ADH activity were 23 and 59 percent respectively of those in men. These differences were even more pronounced in alcoholic women when compared with alcoholic men, the first-pass metabolism being virtually absent in women. The authors concluded "that the increased bioavailability of ethanol resulting from decreased gastric oxidation of ethanol may contribute to the enhanced vulnerability of women to acute and chronic complications of alcohol". This study also confirmed the observation of Marshall *et al.* (1983) that the male–female differences in alcohol pharmacokinetics were closely associated with sex differences in body water content; oral alcohol results in a lower mean volume distribution of alcohol and a higher mean area under the curve of blood ethanol concentration in women.

Studies in rats (Caballeria *et al.* 1989a) and hu-mans (Caballeria *et al.* 1989b) have shown that first-pass metabolism of alcohol occurs in the stomach but not the duodenum, and does not occur after subtotal gastrectomy. The magnitude of first-pass metabolism can be reduced by fasting (Di Padova *et al.* 1987) and is significantly decreased by cimetidene in both humans and rats (Caballeria *et al.* 1989a).

A study by Thuluvath *et al.* (1993) showed no sex differences in gastric ADH activity but found a lower ADH activity in the gastric antrum of patients, in particular older males, with chronic active gastritis and *Helicobacter pylori* infection, thus identifying yet another factor that may contribute to sex- and age-related differences in susceptibility to alcoholic liver disease.

Thus, after a given oral dose of alcohol, women have a higher blood alcohol level than men, which persists for a longer period of time; this difference is even more pronounced in regular drinkers. Fasting and drugs such as cimetidene further impair first-pass metabolism of alcohol and may contribute to the susceptibility of women to liver injury.

Histocompatibility antigens

Numerous studies of the prevalence of particular histocompatibility (HLA) antigens in patients with alcoholic liver disease and in control populations have yielded various and sometimes conflicting results. The lack of standardized methods of analysis of the results obtained in the various studies makes it difficult to compare the results. The following are examples of some of the confusing results:

1. *HLA antigens and susceptibility to alcohol-associated liver injury.* Monteiro and colleagues (1988) concluded that the presence of HLA-Bw35 and A28 appear to mark susceptibility to all the histopathological manifestations of alcohol-induced liver injury, as well as being a marker, along with A1 and A9, for an increased risk of cirrhosis in particular.
2. *HLA antigens and risk of alcoholic cirrhosis.* Studies in the UK by Bailey *et al.* (1976) found an increased frequency of HLA-B8 in alcoholic cirrhotics with and without alcoholic hepatitis, while Morgan *et al.* (1980) found an increased frequency of HLA-B8 in men with alcoholic hepatitis, with and without cirrhosis. A study in France by Doffoel *et al.* (1986) found a significantly higher frequency of HLA-B15 and HLA-

DR4 in subjects with alcoholic cirrhosis compared with controls. Monteiro *et al.* (1988) studied 88 Portuguese alcohol abusers and showed that the presence of HLA-A1, A9, A28 and Bw35 marked a significant 2.5- to 3-fold increased estimated risk for the development of alcoholic cirrhosis, while the presence of HLA-B5 was associated with a significantly decreased risk of cirrhosis.

3. *HLA antigens and rate of development of cirrhosis.* Saunders *et al.* (1982) suggested that the presence of HLA-B8 is associated with an enhanced rate of development of alcoholic cirrhosis. Marbet *et al.* (1988) also showed that the presence of HLA-Bw35 appeared to be a marker for a more rapid progression to cirrhosis as well being associated with an increased incidence of alcoholic cirrhosis.

In contrast to the studies mentioned above a study of HLA Gm systems (HLA-A, -B, -C and DR antigens) in 51 mixed-race (Negroid–Caucasian) individuals of the French West Indies did not identify an association between HLA antigens and alcoholic cirrhosis (Poupon *et al.* 1991).

Further, carefully designed studies of various races, with the inclusion of appropriate controls, and standardized methods of analysis of results are required in order to overcome the current confusion about the possible value of HLA antigens as markers of susceptibility to alcoholic liver disease.

Immunological factors

The role of immunological factors in the pathogenesis of alcoholic liver disease has been discussed in detail in Chapter 6. Cellular and humoral abnormalities certainly occur in patients with alcoholic hepatitis and alcoholic cirrhosis. While some of these disturbances in immune function may be secondary to the liver disease, the possibility that some genetically determined aspects of immune function may contribute to individual susceptibility to alcoholic liver disease merits consideration. MacSween and Anthony (1985) suggested that increased susceptibility to alcoholic liver disease could, in some instances, be mediated by an enhanced immune response associated with the presence of HLA-B8; while Doffoel *et al.* (1986) observed a higher incidence of hepatitis B antibodies in B15-positive and DR4-positive alcoholic patients and suggested that this could be the result of differ-ences in their immune responsiveness when compared to B15-negative and DR4-negative patients.

Genetic predisposition to alcohol addiction

Both familial and non-familial (environmental) forms of alcoholism are thought to exist. Epidemiological studies of adoptees, siblings and twins have provided support for a genetic component to alcohol addiction (Jellinek and Joliffe 1940; Bohman 1978; Hrubec and Omenn 1981; Schuckit 1985). A four-fold higher risk of alcoholism was demonstrated in children of alcoholics, even when adopted out at birth. Also, a significantly higher concordance rate was found in identical (monozygotic) than fraternal (dizygotic) twins.

Recent reviews of the genetic transmission of alcoholism include those by Devor *et al.* (1988), Noble (1993), Saunders and Phillips (1993) and Bosron *et al.* (1993). It seems likely that a number of genetic factors are involved in alcoholism, as well as in alcohol metabolism and alcohol-related organ damage. Blum *et al.* (1990) reported a strong association between an allele of the dopamine D_2 receptor and alcoholism. They carried out a sex- and race-matched study of autopsy samples of the cerebral cortex from 35 alcoholics and 35 non-alcoholics using restriction fragment length polymorphism analysis and showed that the presence of the A_1 allele of the dopamine D_2 receptor gene correctly classified 77 percent of alcoholics, while the absence of the allele classified 72 percent of non-alcoholics. The authors suggested that the presence of the dopamine D_2 receptor gene (located on the q22–q23 region of chromosome 11) may confer susceptibility to at least one form of alcoholism. This study revealed a surprisingly strong association (77 percent) between the A_1 allele and alcoholism. The results suggest that several genes confer vulnerability to alcoholism and/or that the gene(s) for alcoholism may display incomplete penetrance, since 31 percent of the alcoholics studied did not associate with dopamine D_2 receptor gene polymorphism; alternatively, the alcoholism in these subjects may be environmental rather than genetic.

Since the initial observation by Blum *et al.* (1990) that the dopamine D_2 receptor gene was associated with alcoholism, a number of studies from a number of different countries have attempted to reproduce this finding (for details see the review by Noble 1993). The overall result of eight independent studies, which included a total of 176 severe alcoholics and 176 controls free of alcoholism, was that the prevalence of the A_1 allele was 45.5 percent in the alcoholics and 17.0 percent in the controls.

Current evidence suggests that the DRD_2 A_1 allele may be the most important single gene determinant of severe alcoholism. However, since calculations by Pickens *et al.* (1991) based on the prevalence of DRD_2 gene variants in various studies suggest that only 27 percent of the associated risk for severe alcoholism can be attributed to the A_1 allele, it is likely that environmental factors and/or other genes determine the majority of variance in vulnerability to alcoholism.

In summary, genetic factors that merit further investigation include: polymorphisms of alcohol-metabolizing enzymes that influence the rate of alcohol metabolism; gender-related differences in alcohol metabolism that appear to be associated with a greater risk of liver disease in women; HLA antigens – possibly HLA-B8 and HLA-Bw35 – that may be markers for both the risk and the rate of progression to cirrhosis; and the genes involved in alcohol addiction, although the risk of liver injury appears greater in non-alcohol-dependent drinkers.

Acquired factors

Several recent review articles (Johnson and Williams 1985; Hall 1992) have discussed the contribution of acquired or "environmental" factors to individual susceptibility to alcoholic liver disease. Important factors such as nutritional deficiencies (Chapter 8), chronic viral infections (Chapter 9), drugs and toxins (Chapter 16) are discussed in detail elsewhere in this book; consequently, only a brief discussion of these factors will be included in this chapter.

Nutritional factors

Nutritional deficiencies and excesses

Historically, liver injury associated with excess alcohol consumption was termed "nutritional cirrhosis". However, the studies in both animals (Rubin and Lieber 1974; Lieber *et al.* 1975) and humans (Lane and Lieber 1966; Rubin and Lieber 1967, 1968) clearly demonstrated that alcohol is a direct hepatotoxin. Nevertheless, it now appears that various nutritional deficiencies may contribute to the alcohol-associated liver injury (see Chapter 8 and the

following reviews: Mezey 1980; Morgan 1982; Sherlock 1984; French 1993; Schenker and Halff 1993). Causes for the various deficiencies include poor diet leading to an inadequate intake of essential nutrients such as vitamins and minerals (Mendenhall *et al.* 1984), impaired absorption due to the toxic effect of alcohol on enterocytes (Krasner *et al.* 1976), impaired hepatic metabolism of carbohydrates, proteins and vitamins, and increased catabolic loss of zinc, magnesium and calcium (Patek 1979). The role of dietary deficiencies and excesses in individual susceptibility to alcoholic liver disease is complex and multifactorial (see Chapter 8); for example, deficiencies of vitamin E have been described in drinkers (Kalvaria *et al.* 1986; Tanner *et al.* 1986). Vitamin E is an antioxidant which provides protection against ethanol-induced oxidative stress in the liver. Animal studies have shown increased lipid peroxidation in the livers of rats fed alcohol in a vitamin E-deficient diet. Enhanced lipid peroxidation could be the explanation for the potentiation of liver injury in vitamin E-deficient humans and animals consuming alcohol (Kawase *et al.* 1989). Our own studies using the alcohol/"low-dose" carbon tetrachloride model of cirrhosis vitamin E supplementation appear to suggest a lessening of the severity of liver injury and a slowing down of the rate of progression to cirrhosis.

Similarly, as discussed in Chapters 2, 4, 8 and 17, vitamin A depletion, which is not uncommon in drinkers, may contribute to alcohol-related liver injury. Vitamin A is important in the maintenance of the structure and function of Ito cells; depleted levels of hepatic vitamin A may contribute to Ito cell activation with transformation into a collagen-producing cell (Chapter 4). On the other hand, several studies have reported that the administration of excess vitamin A is associated with the development of hepatic fibrosis in alcohol-fed rats (Leo *et al.* 1982; Leo and Lieber 1983). Excess vitamin A has been observed to accelerate the rate of development of fibrosis and cirrhosis in the alcohol/ "low-dose" carbon tetrachloride model of cirrhosis (Hall *et al.* 1994).

Composition of diet

Both human and animal studies suggest that the type of diet consumed in association with excess alcohol may have a bearing on the pattern and severity of the liver injury. For example, in both humans and animals, fructose given simultaneously with ethanol accelerates the rate of ethanol metabolism (Crownover *et al.* 1986). Keegan and Batey

(1993), in a study using female rats, showed that dietary carbohydrate, given either as glucose or fructose, accelerates ethanol elimination. The authors suggest that the pathological consequences of alcohol consumption may be modified by dietary carbohydrate as a consequence of this alteration in ethanol metabolism.

Other studies have examined the effect of different dietary fats on alcohol metabolism and liver injury and found that pork fat, olive oil, corn oil, safflower oil and sunflower oil, but not beef fat, support the development of ethanol-induced liver injury (Nanji and French 1989; Nanji *et al.* 1989). Possible mechanisms for the effects of different fats are discussed in Chapter 17. One mechanism is the enhanced induction of CYP2E1 when alcohol is administered with corn oil rather than beef fat (Takahashi *et al.* 1992); while another mechanism relates differences in Ito cell activation associated with the types of dietary lipid (Mak and Lieber 1988; Takahashi *et al.* 1991).

Chronic viral infections

Hepatitis B virus
Numerous studies from different geographic regions have reported an increased prevalence of serological markers for the hepatitis B virus (HBV) in people with alcoholic liver disease (Mills *et al.* 1979; Hislop *et al.* 1981; Brechot *et al.* 1982; Saunders *et al.* 1983; Ohnishi *et al.* 1982; Nalpas *et al.* 1985; Ohnishi and Okuda 1985; Fong *et al.* 1988). There is, however, some uncertainty about the role of HBV in the progression of alcohol-related liver injury, not withstanding that some studies suggest that the presence of the virus accelerates the rate of progression of the liver injury (Villa *et al.* 1982; Ohnishi *et al.* 1982; and see Chapter 9).

Novick *et al.* (1985) found serological markers for HBV in almost 94 percent of a group of young (<35 years) people with alcoholic cirrhosis, 98 percent of whom had a history of heroin abuse. Forty-five percent of those with cirrhosis had been drinking alcohol for less than 7 years. The authors suggest that multiple factors contributed to the development of cirrhosis at a relatively young age. Such factors might include the adolescent onset of alcohol and parenteral heroin abuse as well as HBV infection occurring as a complication of intravenous drug use.

Chronic alcohol ingestion has been shown to increase the risk of hepatocellular carcinoma in people who are hepatitis B surface antigen positive (Ohnishi *et al.* 1982; Nonomura *et al.* 1986; see also Chapter 9).

Although the role of HBV in alcoholic liver disease is unclear, studies of the efficacy of hepatitis B vaccination in alcoholics are in progress (Degos *et al.* 1986).

Hepatitis C virus
Both morphological and serological studies have suggested that hepatitis C virus (HCV) infection has a role in liver injury in drinkers.

Morphological studies
Numerous studies have described the features of chronic persistent or chronic active hepatitis in liver biopsies from HBsAg-negative alcoholics (Ohnishi and Okuda 1985; Goldberg *et al.* 1977; Crapper *et al.* 1983; Nei *et al.* 1983; Sugimoto *et al.* 1985). For example, Sugimoto *et al.* (1985) studied 94 liver biopsies from patients drinking over 80 g alcohol daily for at least 5 years; 14 percent of the liver biopsies showed chronic hepatitis and in 77 percent of these the features were those of chronic active hepatitis. In some of these studies, the chronic active hepatitis was attributed to alcohol (Goldberg *et al.* 1977; Nei *et al.* 1983); however, more recent studies – since the advent of serological tests for HCV – have frequently incriminated HCV as the aetiological agent responsible for this pattern of injury in drinkers (Bruix *et al.* 1989; Pares *et al.* 1990). The notion that alcohol alone can cause chronic hepatitis is now being questioned (Takase *et al.* 1991). The identification of further non-A, non-B viruses should help clarify this problem.

In many instances, the histological features in liver biopsies from drinkers are highly suggestive of HCV infection. These features include the presence of lymphoid aggregates, often with well-formed lymphoid follicles and germinal centres, in the portal tracts and damage to small and medium-sized bile ducts; "activated" sinusoidal lymphocytes, and features of chronic persistent, chronic active and chronic acinar (lobular) hepatitis (Gerber *et al.* 1992; Scheuer *et al.* 1992; Lefkowitch *et al.* 1993; see Fig. 18.2). Since features of alcoholic liver disease are also present in these biopsies, it is difficult to determine whether the fatty change seen in many cases of HCV hepatitis is a viral effect or a manifestation of concomitant alcoholic injury (Fig. 18.3).

Serological studies
Pares *et al.* (1990) found HCV antibodies in 24.3 percent of chronic alcoholic patients and the preva-

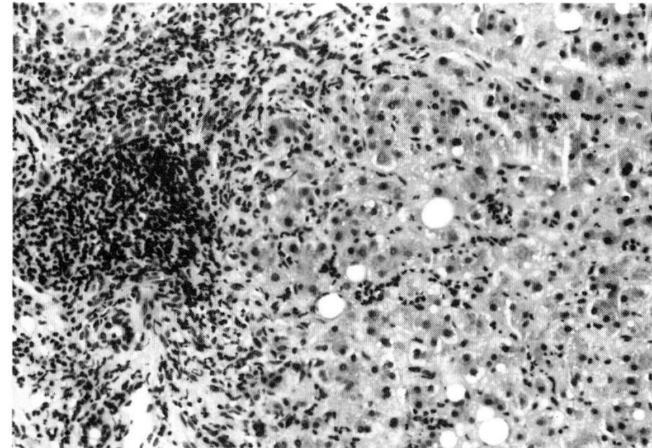

Fig. 18.2 Chronic hepatitis C virus infection in a heavy drinker. The liver shows chronic active hepatitis with a large lymphoid aggregate in a portal tract, also minor fatty change. H&E, × 100.

lence of those antibodies correlated with the severity of disease: 2.2 percent in patients without liver disease, 20 percent in those with steatofibrosis, 21.4 percent in those with alcoholic hepatitis and 42.6 percent in those with cirrhosis. A large multicentre study of the prevalence and clinical relevance of HCV in drinkers, with and without liver disease, provided similar results (Mendenhall *et al.* 1991), and also showed that survival at 24 months was significantly less in those who were antibody-positive. This prognostic disadvantage may be

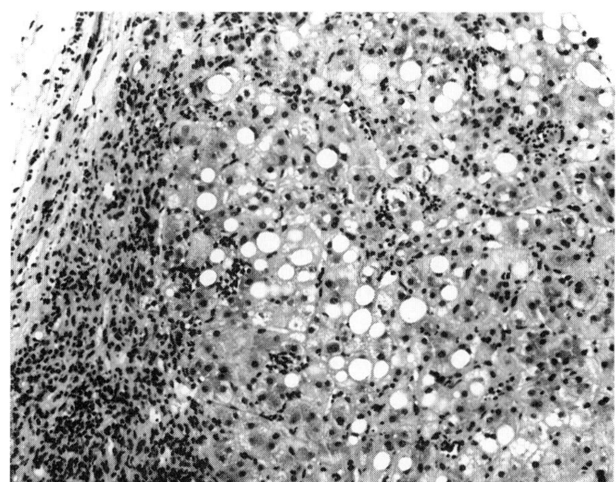

Fig. 18.3 Chronic hepatitis C and alcoholic hepatitis. The liver shows both chronic active hepatitis, and alcoholic hepatitis with focal hepatocyte necrosis, a neutrophil polymorph infiltrate and fatty change. H&E, × 100.

caused in part by a greater risk of malignancy. A retrospective serological study by Bruix *et al.* (1989) revealed a significantly higher prevalence (76 percent) of anti-HCV in patients with alcoholic cirrhosis and hepatocellular carcinoma than in patients with alcoholic cirrhosis alone (38.7 percent).

The increased prevalence of HCV infection in studies of drinkers hospitalized because of liver disease does not necessarily reflect the association between HCV and chronic alcohol consumption in the general community. Nevertheless, unlike the uncertainty relating to the prevalence and significance of HBV in alcoholic liver disease, HCV appears to influence the severity and rate of progression of alcohol-related injury, and to increase the risk of hepatocellular carcinoma. For a more detailed discussion of the role of viruses in alcoholic liver disease, see Chapter 9.

Drugs and toxins

Acute alcohol–drug or alcohol–toxin interactions

As discussed in Chapters 2 and 16, chronic alcohol consumption can potentiate the acute toxicity of a wide variety of drugs and toxins. The most commonly studied agents include carbon tetrachloride, paracetamol (acetaminophen) and vitamin A (see reviews by Strubelt 1980; Zimmerman 1986; Lieber 1988). Other agents reported to interact with alcohol include opioids (heroin, morphine and methadone) (Kreek 1984), cocaine (Conners *et al.* 1989), halothane (Takagi *et al.* 1983) and aflatoxin B_1 (Glinsukon *et al.* 1978). The basis for alcohol–drug/alcohol–toxin interactions is complex and is discussed in detail by Bay and Schenker in Chapter 16. In many instances, alcohol induction of the isoenzyme CYP2E1 (Koop *et al.* 1982; Umeno *et al.* 1988) enhances the metabolism of other agents that are also metabolized by this enzyme (Lieber 1988; Watkins 1990).

I am unaware of any published studies that have specifically addressed the rate of progression to cirrhosis in drinkers who have had one or more episodes of acute drug-related hepatitis. However, it is conceivable that acute alcohol–drug interactions could have long-term sequelae.

Chronic interactions

The enhanced metabolism of a variety of drugs and toxins that occurs as a result of alcohol induction of CYP2E1 can lower the toxic threshold of that drug

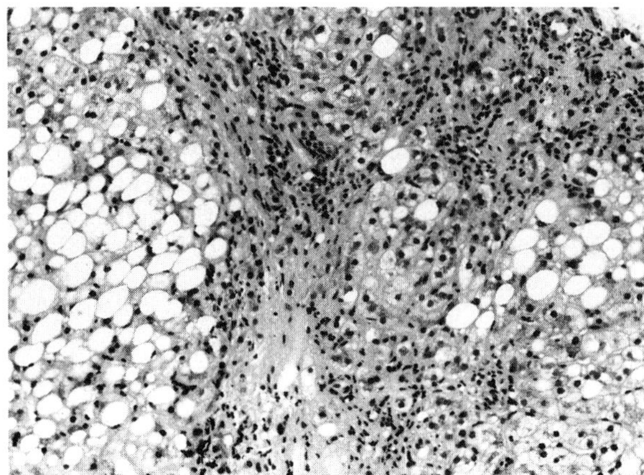

Fig. 18.4 Non-alcoholic steatohepatitis. Liver biopsy from a 50-year-old obese, diabetic woman who did not drink. The liver shows an alcoholic-type hepatitis, moderate fatty change and cirrhosis. H&E, × 100.

or toxin. Consequently, chronic alcohol consumption together with low doses of such a drug or toxin could potentiate alcohol-related injury by causing mild, and frequently subclinical, hepatitis accompanied by slowly progressive hepatic fibrosis. Chronic liver injury may occur even when the dose of each agent is selected so that, when given alone, it results in little or no hepatocyte necrosis and no fibrosis; for example, the rat model for cirrhosis in which alcohol is administered in the Lieber–De Carli liquid diet together with "low-dose" CCL_4 vapour (Hall *et al.* 1991).

The term non-alcoholic steatohepatitis (NASH) or "pseudoalcoholic liver disease" is used to describe liver injury which morphologically resembles alcoholic hepatitis but occurs in non-drinkers (Fig. 18.4). See Chapter 11 for a detailed review of NASH. Many reports of NASH included patients, usually women, who had been drinking small amounts of alcohol; the liver injury in these patients could be the result of interactive hepatotoxicity even though the dose of alcohol was insufficient to be incriminated as the sole cause of the liver injury. All patients with NASH, irrespective of the nature of the factors contributing to the liver injury (drugs, obesity, diabetes mellitis, etc.), should be advised to become totally abstinent.

Methotrexate, a drug that is currently being used widely in the treatment of chronic joint disease, is thought to interact with alcohol (Kevat *et al.* 1988; O'Keefe *et al.* 1991). Methotrexate given in a low weekly dose for rheumatoid arthritis appears to be

less toxic than the rather higher doses given 2–3 times weekly for psoriasis. Nevertheless, progressive hepatic fibrosis, and occasionally cirrhosis, has been observed in rheumatoid arthritis patients, particularly when advice to abstain from alcohol has not been heeded (O'Keefe *et al.* 1991; Chandran *et al.* 1994) (see Figs. 18.5a, b). Thus, alcohol is probably

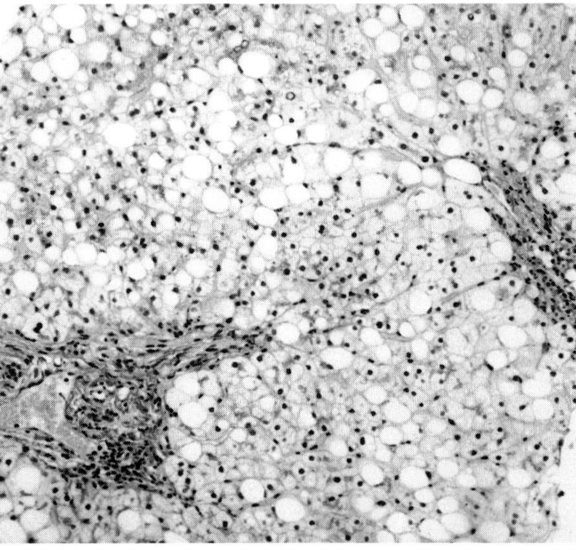

(a)

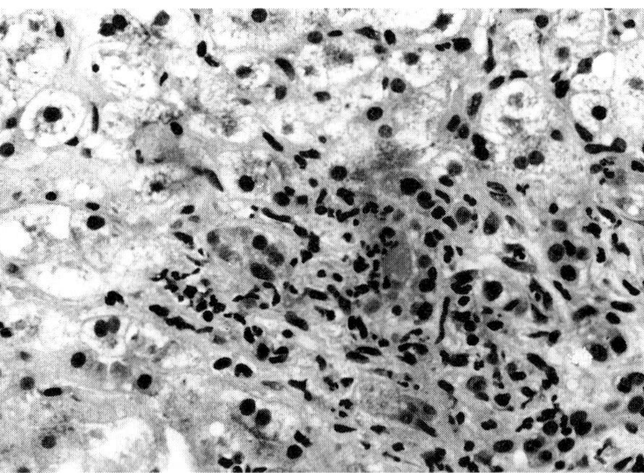

(b)

Fig. 18.5 Alcohol/methotrexate (MTX) hepatotoxicity. (a) Liver biopsy from an elderly man taken after several years of low-dose MTX for rheumatoid arthritis. The liver shows mild portal fibrosis and moderate fatty change. H&E, × 100.
(b) Liver biopsy from the same patient who continued to drink despite advice to abstain while on MTX. The liver shows alcoholic hepatitis with focal hepatocyte necrosis, a neutrophil polymorph infiltrate and Mallory bodies. H&E, × 200.

a risk factor for methotrexate hepatotoxicity and the reverse may also be true: i.e. methotrexate may potentiate alcohol-related liver injury. The presence of alcoholic hepatitis in a liver biopsy, taken from a patient receiving or about to receive methotrexate, should be regarded as an absolute contraindication to methotrexate usage (Fig. 18.5b). Rapid progression to cirrhosis has been observed when this recommendation is not heeded (Chandran *et al.* 1994). Ideally, methotrexate should not be prescribed for patients who are not prepared to abstain from alcohol.

Thus, a variety of agents may interact with alcohol, including therapeutic doses of prescription drugs, non-prescription agents, some illicit drugs and environmental toxins. Interaction on a long-term basis can result in chronic liver disease. The possibility that such chronic alcohol/drug or toxin interactions might occur even when the daily alcohol intake is within the Australian National Health and Medical Research Council's (1987) guidelines of 20 g for women (e.g. two glasses of wine) and 40 g for men per day, merits investigation. These low doses of alcohol, if consumed on a daily basis, may be sufficient to cause CYP2E1 induction, thus setting the scene for interactive hepatotoxicity.

The prevalence of chronic alcohol-associated liver disease due to alcohol–drug/alcohol–toxin interactions remains to be determined; this type of interactive hepatotoxicity may explain some cases of cryptogenic cirrhosis where there is a history of only mild or moderate alcohol consumption at an earlier age.

Hepatic iron overload

Mild siderosis (grade I to II) is not uncommon in alcoholic liver disease (see Chapters 3 and 12). For example, one study found mild siderosis in 57 percent of cases (Jakabovitis *et al.* 1979). Both clinical studies of genetic haemochromatosis and some studies in animal models of iron overload suggest that alcohol potentiates iron-related hepatotoxicity (Irving *et al.* 1988). Bassett *et al.* (1986) raised the possibility that chronic alcohol consumption might lower the threshold for iron-related hepatic fibrosis in patients with homozygous haemochromatosis (Fig. 18.6). However, the possibility that low-grade siderosis could potentiate alcoholic liver disease has been considered unlikely; consequently, venesection has not been recommended for low-grade iron

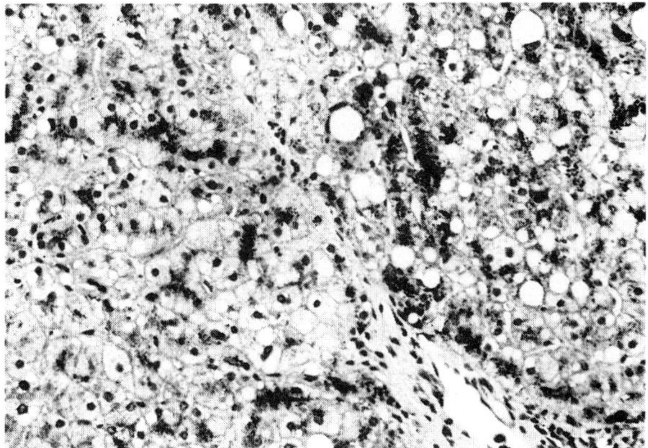

Fig. 18.6 Genetic haemochromatosis in a 40-year-old man who drank moderate amounts of alcohol. The liver shows grade 3 siderosis, also fatty change, heavy iron deposition in Kupffer cells and portal tract macrophages, and portal fibrosis. Perls' method for iron, × 190.

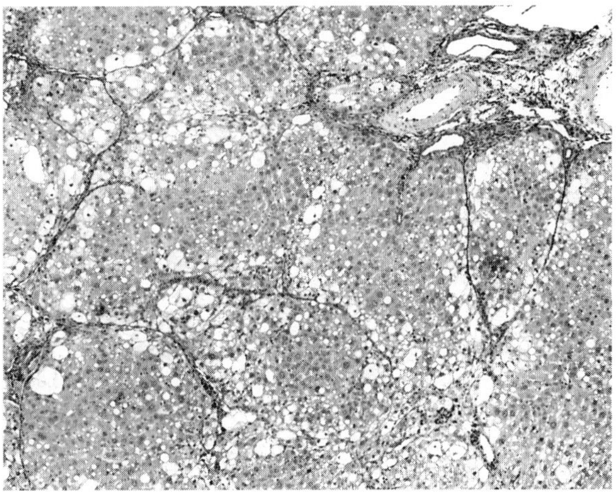

Fig. 18.7 Micronodular cirrhosis, in an iron-loaded rat. The cirrhosis was induced by 10 weeks of exposure to alcohol and CCl_4 vapour (the dose of alcohol plus CCl_4 caused only minimal fibrosis in the absence of iron overload). Sirius red, × 70.

overload in drinkers (Grace 1978). Mackinnon *et al.* (1993) found that iron-loading potentiates hepatic fibrosis and the rate of development of cirrhosis in the alcohol/"low-dose" model of cirrhosis, thus establishing a model in which the pathogenesis of iron–alcohol interaction can be pursued (Fig. 18.7).

Conclusion

The development of cirrhosis after a lifetime of heavy drinking is largely due to a dose-related direct hepatotoxic effect of alcohol, but it is interesting to speculate that such individuals are relatively less susceptible than those who develop cirrhosis in association with lower doses of alcohol for a shorter duration; for example, women as discussed by Gavaler and Arria in Chapter 7, and possibly people who begin drinking heavily in adolescence.

The realization that alcohol consumption may also have an indirect or "permissive" role in the development of cirrhosis has focused attention on the identification of the factors that contribute to individual susceptibility to alcohol-related liver disease. Once these factors have been identified, the next challenge will be the elucidation of the mechanisms of interaction between the various genetic and environmental factors. Ultimately, it may be possible to moderate some of the contributing factors, such as by vaccination against a range of viruses, avoidance of drugs that interact with alcohol and elimination of environmental toxins. By so doing, the risk of liver injury could be reduced while still allowing the enjoyment of modest amounts of alcohol. However, as more is learned about genetic susceptibility to alcoholic liver disease, some people will need to be advised to abstain from alcohol.

Acknowledgement

Several of my studies referred to in this chapter were supported by the National Health and Medical Research Council of Australia and the University Research Budget, Flinders University of South Australia.

References

Ashely, M.J., Olin, J.S., Le Riche, W.H., Kornaczewski, A., Schmidt, W. and Rankin, J.G. (1977). Morbidity in alcoholics: Evidence for accelerated development of physical disease in women. *Archives of Internal Medicine* **137**, 883–887.

Anthony, P.P., Ishak, K.G., Nayak, N.C., Poulsen, H.E., Scheuer, P.J. and Sobin, L.H. (1978). The morphology of cirrhosis: Recommendations on definition, nomenclature, and classification by a working group sponsored by the World Health Organization. *Journal of Clinical Pathology* **31**, 395–414.

Bach, N., Swan, N.T. and Schaffner, F. (1991). The histological features of chronic hepatitis C and auto-immune chronic hepatitis: A comparative analysis. *Hepatology* **4**, 572–577.

Bailey, R.J., Krasner, N., Eddleston, A.L.W.F., Williams, R., Tee, D.E.H., Doniach, D., Kennedy, L.A. and Batchelor, J.R. (1976). Histocompatibility antigens, autoantibodies and immunoglobulins in alcoholic liver disease. *British Medical Journal* **2**, 727–729.

Baptista, A., Bianchi, L., De Groote, J., Desmet, V.J., Gedigk, P., Korb, G., MacSween, R.N.M., Popper, H., Poulsen, H., Scheuer, P.J., Schmidt, M., Thaler, H. and Welper, W. (1981). Alcoholic liver disease: Morphological manifestations. Review by an International Group. *Lancet* **i**, 707–711.

Baraona, E., Jauhonen, P., Miyakawa, H. and Lieber, C.S. (1983). Zonal redox changes as a cause of selective perivenular hepatotoxicity of alcohol. *Pharmacology, Biochemistry and Behaviour* **18**, 449–454.

Bassett, M.L., Halliday, J.W. and Powell, L.W. (1986). Value of hepatic iron measurements in early haemochromatosis and determination of the critical iron level associated with fibrosis. *Hepatology* **6**, 24–29.

Batey, R.G., Burns, T., Benson, R.J. and Blyth, K. (1990). Alcohol consumption and the risk of cirrhosis. *Medical Journal of Australia* **156**, 413–416.

Bell, H. and Nordhagen, R. (1980). HLA antigens in alcoholics, with special reference to alcoholic cirrhosis. *Scandinavian Journal of Gastroenterology* **15**, 453–456.

Berglund, M. (1984). Mortality in alcoholics related to clinical state at first admission: A study of 537 deaths. *Acta Psychiatrica Scandinavica* **70**, 407–416.

Blum, K., Noble, E.P., Sheridan, P.J., Montgomery, A., Ritchie, T., Jagadeeswaren, P., Nogami, H., Briggs, A.H. and Cohn, J.B. (1990). Allelic association of human dopamine D_2 receptor gene in alcoholism. *Journal of the American Medical Association* **263**, 2055–2060.

Bohman, M. (1978). Some genetic aspects of alcoholism and criminality: A population of adoptees. *Archives of General Psychiatry* **35**, 269–276.

Bosron, W.F., Lumeng, L. and Li, T.-K. (1988). Genetic polymorphism of enzymes of alcohol metabolism and susceptibility to alcoholic liver disease. *Molecular Aspects of Medicine* **10**, 147–158.

Bosron, W.F., Ehrig, T. and Li, T.-K. (1993). Genetic factors in alcohol metabolism and alcoholism. *Seminars in Liver Disease* **13**, 126–135.

Brechot, C., Nalpas, B., Courouce, A.-M., Duhamel, G., Callard, P., Carnot, F., Tiollais, P. and Berthelot, P. (1982). Evidence that hepatitis B virus has a role in liver-cell carcinoma in alcoholic liver disease. *New England Journal of Medicine* **306**, 1384–1387.

Bruix, J., Barrera, J.M., Calvet, X., Ercilla, G., Costa, J., Sanchez-Topias, J.M., Verlura, M., Vall, M., Bruguera, M., Bra, C., Castillo, R. and Rodes, J. (1989). Prevalence of antibodies of hepatitis C virus in Spanish patients with hepatocellular carcinoma and hepatic cirrhosis. *Lancet* **ii**, 1004–1006.

Caballeria, J., Baraona, E., Rodamilans, M. and Lieber, C.S. (1989a). Effects of cimetidine on gastric alcohol dehydrogenase activity and blood ethanol levels. *Gastroenterology* **96**, 388–392.

Cabelleria, J., Frezza, M., Hernandez-Munoz, R., Di Padova, C., Korsten, M.A., Baraona, E. and Lieber, C.S. (1989b). Gastric origin of the first-pass metabolism of ethanol in humans: Effect of gastrectomy. *Gastroenterology* **97**, 1205–1209.

Chandran, G., Ahern, M.J., Hall, P. de la M., Hill, W., Geddes, R. and Harley, H. (1994). Cirrhosis in patients with rheumatoid arthritis receiving methotrexate. *British Journal of Rheumatology*, in press.

Coates, R.A., Halliday, M.L., Rankin, J.G., Feinman, S. and Fisher, M.M. (1986). Risk of fatty infiltration or cirrhosis of the liver in relation to ethanol consumption: A case-control study. *Clinical and Investigative Medicine* **9**, 26–32.

Conners, S., Rankin, D.R., Krumdieck, C.L. and Brendel, K. (1989). Interactive toxicity of cocaine with phenobarbital, morphine and ethanol in organ cultured human and rat liver slices. *Proceedings of the Western Pharmacology Society* **32**, 205–208.

Corrao, G., Arico, S., Lepore, R., Valenti, M., Torchio, P., Galatola, G., Tabone, M. and Di Orio, F. (1993). Amount and duration of alcohol as risk factors of symptomatic liver cirrhosis. A case-control study. *Journal of Clinical Epidemiology* **46**, 601–617.

Couzigou, P., Fleury, B., Groppi, A., Cassaigne, A., Begueret, J., Iron, A. and the French Group for Research on Alcohol and the Liver (1990). Genotyping study of alcohol dehydrogenase class I polymorphism in French patients with alcoholic liver cirrhosis. *Alcohol and Alcoholism* **25**, 623–626.

Crapper, R.M., Bhathal, P.S. and Mackay, I.R. (1983). Chronic active hepatitis in alcoholic patients. *Liver* **3**, 327–337.

Crownover, B.P., LaDine, J., Bradford, B., Glassman, E., Forman, D., Schnieder, H. and Thurman, R.G. (1986). Activation of ethanol metabolism in humans by fructose: Importance of experimental design. *Journal of Pharmacology and Experimental Therapeutics* **236**, 574–579.

Dalke, D.D., Sorrell, M.F., Casey, C.A. and Tuma, D.J. (1990). Chronic ethanol administration impairs receptor-mediated growth factor by rat hepatocytes. *Hepatology* **12**, 1085–1091.

Day, C.P., Bashir, R., James, O.F.W., Bassendine, M.F., Li, T.K. and Edenberg, H.J. (1991). Investigation of the role of polymorphisms at the alcohol and aldehyde dehydrogenase loci in genetic predisposition to alcohol-related end-organ damage. *Hepatology* **14**, 798–801.

Degos, F., Duhamel, G., Brechot, C., Nalpas, B., Courouce, A.M., Tron, F. and Berthelot, P. (1986). Hepatitis B vaccination in chronic alcoholics. *Journal of Hepatology* **2**, 402–409.

Devor, E.J., Reich, T. and Cloninger, C.R. (1988). Genetics of alcoholism and related end-organ damage. *Seminars in Liver Disease* **8**, 1–11.

Di Padova, C., Worner, T.M., Julkunen, R.J. and Lieber, C.S. (1987). Effects of fasting and chronic alcohol consumption on the first-pass metabolism of ethanol. *Gastroenterology* **92**, 1169–1173.

Doffoel, M., Tongio, M.M., Gut, J.-P., Ventre, G., Charrault, A., Vetter, D., Ledig, M., North, M.L., Mayer, S. and Bockel, R. (1986). Relationships between 34 HLA-A and HLA-DR antigens and the serological markers of viral infections in alcoholic cirrhosis. *Hepatology* **6**, 457–463.

Dufour, M.C., Stinson, F.S. and Caces, M.F. (1993). Trends in cirrhosis morbidity and mortality: United States, 1979–1988. *Seminars in Liver Disease* **13**, 109–125.

Duguay, L., Coutu, D., Hetu, C. and Joly, J.-G. (1982). Inhibition of liver regeneration by chronic alcohol administration. *Gut* **23**, 8–13.

Fong, T.-L., Govindarijan, S., Valinluck, B. and Redeker, A.G. (1988). Status of hepatitis B virus DNA in alcoholic liver disease: A study of a large urban population in the United States. *Hepatology* **8**, 1602–1604.

French, S.W. (1993). Nutrition in the pathogens of alcoholic liver disease. *Alcohol and Alcoholism* **28**, 97–109.

French, S.W., Miyamoto, K. and Tsukamoto, H. (1986). Ethanol-induced hepatic fibrosis in the rat: Role of the amount of dietary fat. *Alcoholism: Clinical and Experimental Research* **10**, 13S–19S.

French, S.W., Miyamoto, K., Ohta, Y. and Geoffrion, Y. (1988). Pathogenesis of experimental alcoholic liver disease in the rat. *Methods and Achievement in Experimental Pathology* **13**, 181–207.

French, S.W., Wong, K., Jui, L., Albano, E., Hagbjork, A.-L. and Ingelman-Sundberg, M. (1993). Effect of ethanol on cytochrome P450 2E1 (CYP 2E1), lipid peroxidation and serum protein adduct formation in relation to liver pathology pathogenesis. *Experimental and Molecular Pathology* **58**, 61–75.

Frezza, M., Di Padova, C., Pozzato, G., Terpin, M., Baraona, E. and Lieber, C.S. (1990). High blood alcohol levels in women: The role of decreased gastric alcohol dehydrogenase activity and first-pass metabolism. *New England Journal of Medicine* **322**, 95–99.

Friedman, I.M., Kraemer, H.C., Mendoza, F.S. and Hammer, L.D. (1988). Elevated serum iron concentration in adolescent alcohol users. *American Journal of Diseases in Children* **142**, 156–158.

Friedman, S.L. and Arthur, M.J.P. (1989). Activation of lipocytes by Kupffer cell-conditioned medium: Direct enhancement of matrix production and stimulation of proliferation via expression of PDGF receptors. *Journal of Clinical Investigation* **84**, 1780–1785.

Friedman, S.L., Roll, F.J., Boyles, J. and Bissell, D.M. (1985). Hepatic lipocytes: The principal collagen-producing cells of normal rat liver. *Proceedings of the National Academy of Sciences, USA* **82**, 8681–8685.

Galambos, J.T. (1972). Natural history of alcoholic hepatitis: III. Histological changes. *Gastroenterology* **63**, 1026–1035.

Gavaler, J.S. (1982). Sex-related differences in ethanol-induced liver disease: Artifactual or real? *Alcoholism: Clinical and Experimental Research* **6**, 186–196.

Gerber, M.A., Krzysztol, K., Miriam, J., Alter, M.J., Sampliner, R.E., Margolis, H.S. and Sentinal Countries Chronic Non-A, Non-B Hepatitis Study Team (1992). Histopathology of community acquired chronic hepatitis C. *Modern Pathology* **5**, 483–486.

Glinsukon, T., Taycharpipranai, S. and Tosulkao, C. (1978). Aflatoxin B$_1$ hepatotoxicity in rats pretreated with ethanol. *Experientia* **34**, 869–870.

Goldberg, S.J., Mendenhall, C.L., Connell, A.M. and Chedid, A. (1977). "Non-alcoholic" chronic hepatitis in the alcoholic. *Gastroenterology* **72**, 598–604.

Goodwin, D.W. (1984). Studies of familial alcoholism: A growth industry. In *Longitudinal Research in Alcoholism* (Edited by Goodwin, D.W., Van Usen, K.T. and Mednick, S.A.), pp. 97–105. Kluwer-Nijhoff Publishing, Boston, MA.

Goodwin, D.W. (1987). Genetic influences in alcoholism. *Advances in Internal Medicine* **32**, 283–298.

Grace, N.D. (1978). Evidence for hepatic toxicity of iron. In *Metals and the Liver: Health and Disease* (Edited by Powell, L.W.), p. 131. Marcel Dekker, New York.

Grant, B.F., DeBakey, S. and Zobeck, T.S. (1991). *Surveillance Report #18: Liver Cirrhosis Mortality in the United States, 1973–1988*. National Institute on Alcohol Abuse and Alcoholism, Alcohol Epidemiologic Data System, Rockville, MD.

Hall, P. de la M. (Ed.) (1985). *Alcoholic Liver Disease: Pathobiology, Epidemiology and Clinical Aspects*. Edward Arnold, London.

Hall, P. de la M. (1987). Alcoholic liver disease. In *Pathology of the Liver* (Edited by MacSween, R.N.M., Anthony, P.P. and Scheuer, P.J.), 2nd edn, pp. 281–309. Churchill Livingstone, Edinburgh.

Hall, P. de la M. (1992). Genetic and acquired factors that influence individual susceptibility to alcohol-associated liver disease. *Journal of Gastroenterology and Hepatology* **7**, 417–426.

Hall, P. de la M., Plummer, J.L., Ilsley, A.H. and Cousins, M.J. (1991). Hepatic fibrosis and cirrhosis after chronic administration of alcohol and "low-dose" carbon tetrachloride vapour in the rat. *Hepatology* **13**, 815–819.

Hall, P., Plummer, J.L., Ilsley, A.H., Ahern, M. and Cmielewski, P. (1994). Influence of excess vitamin A or E on development of cirrhosis in the alcohol/carbon tetrachloride rat model. *Alcoholism: Clinical Experimental Research* **18**, 21A.

Hislop, W.S., Follett, E.A.C., Bouchier, I.A.D. and MacSween, R.N.M. (1981). Serological markers of hepatitis B in patients with alcoholic liver disease: A multi-centre survey. *Journal of Clinical Pathology* **34**, 1017–1019.

Hrubec, Z. and Omenn, G.S. (1981). Evidence of genetic predisposition to alcoholic cirrhosis and psychosis: Twin concordances for alcoholism and its biological end points by zygosity among male veterans. *Alcoholism: Clinical and Experimental Research* **5**, 207–215.

Irving, M., Halliday, J.W. and Powell, L.W. (1988). Association between alcoholism and increased hepatic iron stores. *Alcoholism: Clinical Experimental Research* **12**, 7–13.

Jahn, F., Reuter, A., Danz, M. and Klinger, W. (1993). Age dependent different influence of carbon tetrachloride on biotransformation of xenobiotics, glutathione content, lipid peroxidation and histopathology of rat liver. *Experimental and Toxicology and Pathology* **45**, 101–107.

Jakobovits, A.W., Morgan, M.Y. and Sherlock, S. (1979). Hepatic siderosis in alcoholics. *Digestive Diseases and Science* **24**, 305–310.

Jellinek, E. and Joliffe, N. (1940). Effect of alcohol on the individual: Review of the literature of 1939. *Quarterly Journal of the Studies on Alcoholism* **1**, 110–181.

Johnson, R.D. and Williams, R. (1985). Genetic and environmental factors in individual susceptibility to the development of alcoholic liver disease. *Alcohol and Alcoholism* **20**, 137–160.

Kalvaria, I., Labadarios, D., Shephard, G.S. *et al.* (1986). Biochemical vitamin E deficiency in chronic pancreatitis. *International Journal of Pancreatology* **1**, 119–128.

Kawase, T., Kato, S. and Lieber, C.S. (1989). Lipid peroxidation and antioxidant defence systems in rat liver after chronic ethanol feeding. *Hepatology* **10**, 815–821.

Keegan, A. and Batey, R. (1993). Dietary carbohydrate accelerates ethanol elimination, but does not alter hepatic alcohol dehydrogenase. *Alcoholism: Clinical and Experimental Research* **17**, 431–433.

Kevat, S., Ahern, M. and Hall, P. (1988). Hepatotoxicity of methotrexate in rheumatic diseases. *Medical Toxicology* **3**, 197–208.

Koop, D., Morgan, E.T., Tarr, G.E. and Coon, M.J. (1982). Purification and characterization of a unique isoenzyme of cytochrome P-450 from liver microsomes of ethanol-treated rabbits. *Journal of Biological Chemistry* **257**, 8472–8480.

Krasner, N., Cochran, K.M., Russell, R.I., Carmichael, H.A. and Thompson, G.G. (1976). Alcohol and absorption from the small intestine. 1. Impairment of absorption from the small intestine in alcoholics. *Gut* **17**, 245–248.

Krasner, N., Davis, M., Portmann, B. and Williams, R. (1977). Changing pattern of alcoholic liver disease in Great Britain: Relation to sex and signs of autoimmunity. *British Medical Journal* **1**, 1497–1500.

Kreek, M.J. (1984). Opioid interaction with alcohol. *Advances in Alcohol and Substance Abuse* **3**, 35–46.

Lane, B.P. and Lieber, C.S. (1966). Ultrastructural alterations in human hepatocytes following ingestion of ethanol with adequate diets. *American Journal of Pathology* **49**, 593–603.

Lelbach, W.K. (1975). Cirrhosis in the alcoholic and its relation to the volume of alcohol abuse. *Annals of the New York Academy of Science* **252**, 85–105.

Lelbach, W.K. (1985). The epidemiology of alcoholic liver disease in Continental Europe. In *Alcoholic Liver Disease* (Edited by Hall, P.), pp. 130–166. Edward Arnold, London.

Lefkowitch, J.H., Schiff, E.R., Davis, G.L., Perrillo, P., Lindsay, K., Bodenheimer, Jr., H.C., Balart, L.A., Ortego, T.J., Payne, J., Dienstag, J.L., Gibas, A., Jacobson, I.M., Tamburro, C.H., Carey, W., O'Brien, C., Sampliner, R., Van Thiel, D.H., Feit, D., Albrecht, J., Meschievitz, C., Sanghvi, B., Vaughan, R.D. and the Hepatitis Interventional Therapy Group (1993). Pathological diagnosis of chronic hepatitis C: A multicenter comparative study of chronic hepatitis C. *Gastroenterology* **104**, 595–603.

Leo, M.A. and Lieber, C.S. (1983). Hepatic fibrosis after long-term administration of ethanol and moderate vitamin A supplementation in the rat. *Hepatology* **3**, 1–11.

Leo M.A., Aria, M., Sato, M. and Lieber, C.S. (1982). Hepatotoxicity of moderate vitamin A supplemtation in the rat. *Gastroenterology* **82**, 194–205.

Li, T.-K. and Bosron, W.F. (1987). Distribution and properties of human alcohol dehydrogenase isoenzymes. In *Alcohol and the Cell* (Edited by Rubin, E.), pp. 1–10. Annals of New York Academy of Science.

Lieber, C.S. (1988). Metabolic effects and its interaction with other drugs, hepatotoxic agents, vitamins and carcinogens: A 1988 update. *Seminars in Liver Disease* **8**, 47–68.

Lieber, C.S., DeCarli, L.M. and Rubin, E. (1975). Sequential production of fatty liver, hepatitis and cirrhosis in sub-human primates fed ethanol with adequate diets. *Proceedings of the National Academy of Sciences, USA* **72**, 437–441.

Lischner, M.W., Alexander, J.F. and Galambos, J.T. (1971). Natural history of alcoholic hepatitis: 1. The acute disease. *American Journal of Digestive Diseases* **16**, 481–494.

Loft, S., Olesen, K.-L. and Dossing, M. (1987). Increased susceptibility to liver disease in relation to alcohol consumption in women. *Scandinavian Journal of Gastroenterology* **10**, 1251–1256.

Mackinnon, M., Plummer, J., Ilsley, I., Clayton, C., Ahern, M., Cmielewski, P. and Hall, P. (1993). An animal model of hepatic iron and alcohol interaction with resultant hepatic fibrosis and cirrhosis. *Journal of Gastroenterology and Hepatology* **88**, A13.

MacSween, R.N.M. and Anthony, R.S. (1985). Immune mechanisms in alcoholic liver disease. In *Alcoholic Liver Disease* (Edited by Hall, P.), pp. 193–229. Edward Arnold, London.

Mak, K.M. and Lieber, C.S. (1988). Lipocytes and transitional cells in alcoholic liver disease: A morphometric study. *Hepatology* **8**, 1027–1033.

Marbet, U.A., Stadler, G.A., Thiel, G. and Bianchi, L. (1988). The influence of HLA antigens on progression of alcoholic liver disease. *Hepatogastroenterology* **35**, 65–68.

Marshall, A.W., Kingstone, D., Boss, M. and Morgan, M.Y. (1983). Ethanol elimination in males and females: Relationship to menstrual cycle and body composition. *Hepatology* **3**, 701–706.

Matsuoka, M., Pham, N.-T. and Tsukamoto, H. (1989). Differential effects of interleukin-1 alpha, tumour necrosis factor alpha, and transforming growth factor beta 1 on cell proliferation and collagen formation by cultured fat-storing cells. *Liver* **9**, 71–78.

Mendenhall, C.L., Anderson, S., Weesner, R.E., Goldberg, S.J. and Crolic, K.A. (1984). Protein calorie malnutrition associated with alcoholic hepatitis. *American Journal of Medicine* **76**, 211–212.

Mendenhall, C.L., Seeff, L., Diehl, A.M., Ghosn, S.J., French, S.W., Gartside, P.S., Rouster, S.D., Buskell-Bales, Z., Grossman, C.J., Roselle, G.A., Weesner, R.E., Garcia-Pont, P., Goldberg, S.J., Kiernan, T.W., Tamburro, C.H., Zetterman, R., Chedid, A., Chen, T., Rabin, L. and the Veterans Administration Cooperative Study Group (No. 119) (1991). Antibodies to hepatitis B virus and hepatitis C virus in alcoholic hepatitis and cirrhosis: Their prevalence and clinical relevance. *Hepatology* **14**, 581–589.

Mezey, E. (1980). Alcoholic liver disease: Roles of alcohol and nutrition. *American Journal of Clinical Nutrition* **33**, 2706–2718.

Mills, P.R., Pennington, T.H., Kay, P., MacSween, R.N.M. and Watkinson, G. (1979). Hepatitis Bs antibody in alcoholic cirrhosis. *Journal of Clinical Pathology* **32**, 778–782.

Mills, P.R., Follet, A.E.C., Urquhart, G.E.D., Clements, G., Watkinson, G. and MacSween, R.N.M. (1981). Evidence for previous hepatitis B virus infection in alcoholic cirrhosis. *British Medical Journal* **282**, 437–438.

Monteiro, E., Alves, M.P., Santos, M.L., Quintas, I., Baptista, A., Galvao-Teles, A. and Gavaler, J.S. (1988). Histocompatibility antigens: Markers of susceptibility to and protection from alcoholic liver disease in a Portuguese population. *Hepatology* **8**, 455–458.

Morgan, M. (1982). Alcohol and nutrition. In *Alcohol and Disease* (Edited by Sherlock, S.), pp. 21–29. Churchill Livingstone, London.

Morgan, M.Y. (1985). Epidemiology of alcoholic liver disease in the United Kingdom. In *Alcoholic Liver Disease* (Edited by Hall, P.), pp. 193–229. Edward Arnold, London.

Morgan, M. and Sherlock, S. (1977). Sex related differences among 100 patients with alcoholic liver disease. *British Medical Journal* **1**, 939–941.

Morgan, M.Y., Ross, M.G.R., Ng, C.M., Adams, D.M., Thomas, H.C. and Sherlock, S. (1980). HLA-B8, immunoglobulins and antibody responses in alcohol-related liver disease. *Journal of Clinical Pathology* **33**, 488–492.

Moshage, H., Casini, A. and Lieber, C.S. (1990). Acetaldehyde selectively stimulates collagen production in cultured rat liver fat-storing cells but not in hepatocytes. *Hepatology* **12**, 511–518.

Nalpas, B., Berthelot, P., Thiers, V., Duhamel, G., Courouce, A.M., Tiollais, P. and Brechot, G. (1985). Hepatitis B virus multiplication in the absence of usual serological markers: A study of 146 chronic alcoholics. *Journal of Hepatology* **1**, 89–97.

Nanji, A.A. and French, S.W. (1989). Dietary linoleic acid is required for development of experimentally induced alcoholic liver injury. *Life Sciences* **44**, 223–227.

Nanji, A.A., Mendenhall, C.L. and French, S.W. (1989). Beef fat prevents alcoholic liver disease in the rat. *Alcoholism: Clinical and Experimental Research* **13**, 15–19.

National Health and Medical Research Council of Australia (1987). Is there a safe level of daily consumption of alcohol for men and women? *Recommendation Regarding Responsible Drinking*, 2nd edn. Australian Government Publishing Service, Canberra.

Nei, J., Matsuda, Y. and Takada, A. (1983). Chronic hepatitis induced by alcohol. *Digestive Diseases and Sciences* **28**, 207–215.

Noble, E.P. (1993). The genetic transmission of alcoholism: Implications for prevention. *Drug and Alcohol Review* **12**, 283–290.

Nonomura, A., Hayashi, M., Takayanagi, N., Watanabe, K. and Ohta, G. (1986). Correlation of morphological subtypes of liver cirrhosis with excess alcohol intake, HBV infection, age at death, and hepatocellular carcinoma. *Acta Pathologica Japonica* **36**, 631–640.

Norton, R., Batey, R., Dwyer, T. and McMahon, S. (1987). Alcohol consumption and the risk of alcohol related cirrhosis in women. *British Medical Journal* **295**, 80–82.

Novick, D.M., Enlow, R.W., Gelb, A.M., Stenger, R.J., Fotino, M., Winter, J.W., Yarcovitz, S.R., Schoenberg, M.D. and Kreck, M.J. (1985). Hepatic cirrhosis in young adults. Association with adolescent onset of alcohol and parenteral heroin abuse. *Gut* **26**, 8–13.

O'Keefe, Q.E., Fye, K.F. and Sack, K.D. (1991). Methotrexate and histologic hepatic abnormalities: A meta-analysis. *American Journal of Medicine* **90**, 711–716.

Ohnishi, K. and Okuda, K. (1985). Epidemiology of alcoholic liver disease in Japan. In *Alcoholic Liver Disease* (Edited by Hall, P.), pp. 167–183. Edward Arnold, London.

Ohnishi, K., Iida, S., Iwama, W., Goto, N., Nomura, F., Takashi, M., Mishima, A., Kono, K., Kimura, K., Musha, H., Kototo, K. and Okuda, K. (1982). The effect of chronic habitual alcohol intake on the development of liver cirrhosis and hepatocellular carcinoma: Relation to hepatitis B surface antigen. *Cancer* **49**, 672–677.

Pares, A., Caballeria, J., Bruguera, M., Torres, M. and Rodes, J. (1986). Histological course of alcoholic hepatitis. Influence of abstinence, sex and extent of hepatic damage. *Journal of Hepatology* **2**, 33–42.

Pares, A., Barrera, J.M., Caballeria, J., Ercilla, G., Bruguera, M., Caballeria, L., Castillo, R. and Rodes, J. (1990). Hepatitis C virus antibodies in chronic alcoholic patients: Association with severity of liver injury. *Hepatology* **12**, 1295–1299.

Patek, A.J. (1979). Alcohol, malnutrition and alcoholic cirrhosis. *American Journal of Clinical Nutrition* **32**, 1304–1312.

Pequignot, G., Tuyns, A.J. and Berta, J.L. (1978). Ascitic cirrhosis in relation to alcohol consumption. *International Journal of Epidemiology* **7**, 113–120.

Pickens, R.W., Svikis, D.C., McGue, M., Lykken, D.T., Heston, L.L. and Clayton, P.J. (1991). Heterogeneity in the inheritance of alcoholism. *Archives of General Psychiatry* **48**, 19–28.

Popper, H. and Lieber, C.S. (1980). Histogenesis of alcoholic fibrosis and cirrhosis in the baboon. *American Journal of Pathology* **98**, 695–716.

Poupon, R.E., Heintzmann, F., Valette, I., Gervaise, G., Edouard, A., Monplaisir, N. and Dugoujon, J.M. (1991). HLA Gm systems and susceptibility to alcoholic cirrhosis: A study of mixed-race subjects. *Alcohol and Alcoholism* **26**, 417–424.

Poupon, R.E., Nalpas, B., Coutelle, C., Fleury, B., Couzigou, P. and Higueret, D. (1992). Polymorphism of alcohol dehydrogenase, alcohol and aldehyde dehydrogenase activities: Implication in alcoholic cirrhosis in white patients. *Hepatology* **15**, 1017–1022.

Rankin, J.S., Halliday, M.L., Corey, P.N.J., Coates, R.A. and De Lint, J.E. (1985). Epidemiology of alcoholic liver disease in Australia. In *Alcoholic Liver Disease* (Edited by Hall, P.), pp. 115–129. Edward Arnold, London.

Ricciardi, B.R., Saunders, J.B., Williams, R. and Hopkinson, D.A. (1983). Hepatic ADH and ALDH isoenzymes in different racial groups and in chronic alcoholism. *Pharmacology, Biochemistry and Behaviour* **18**, 61–65.

Rubin, E. and Lieber, C.S. (1967). Early fine structural changes in human liver induced by alcohol. *Gastroenterology* **52**, 1–13.

Rubin, E. and Lieber, C.S. (1968). Alcohol-induced hepatic injury in nonalcoholic volunteers. *New England Journal of Medicine* **278**, 869–876.

Rubin, E. and Lieber, C.S. (1974). Fatty liver, alcoholic hepatitis and cirrhosis produced by alcohol in primate. *New England Journal of Medicine* **298**, 128–135.

Saunders, B. and Phillips, M. (1993). Is "alcoholism" genetically transmitted? And are there any implications for prevention? *Drug and Alcohol Review* **12**, 291–298.

Saunders, J.B., Davis, M. and Williams, R. (1981). Do women develop alcoholic liver disease more readily than men. *British Medical Journal* **282**, 1140–1143.

Saunders, J.B., Wodak, A.D., Haines, A., Powell-Jackson, P.R., Portmann, B., Davis, M. and Williams, R. (1982). Accelerated development of alcoholic cirrhosis in patients with HLA-B8. *Lancet* **i**, 1381–1384.

Saunders, J.B., Wodak, A.D., Morgan-Capner, P., White, Y.S., Portmann, B., Davis, M. and Williams, R. (1983). Importance of markers of hepatitis B virus in alcoholic liver disease. *British Medical Journal* **286**, 1851–1854.

Saunders, J.B., Wodak, A.D. and Williams, R. (1984). What determines susceptibility to liver damage from alcohol? Discussion paper. *Journal of the Royal Society of Medicine* **77**, 204–216.

Savolainen, E.-R., Leo, M.A., Timpl, R. and Lieber, C.S. (1984). Acetaldehyde and lactate stimulate collagen synthesis in cultured baboon liver myofibroblasts. *Gastroenterology* **87**, 777–787.

Schenker, S. and Halff, G.A. (1993). Nutritional therapy in alcoholic liver disease. *Seminars in Liver Disease* **13**, 196–209.

Scheuer, P.J., Asbrafzadeh, P., Sherlock, S., Brown, D. and Dusheiko, G.M. (1992). The pathology of hepatitis C. *Hepatology* **15**, 567–571.

Schuckit, M.A. (1985). Genetics and the risk of alcoholism. *Journal of the American Medical Association* **254**, 2614–2617.

Sherlock, S. (1984). Nutrition and the alcoholic. *Lancet* **i**, 436–439.

Shibuya, A. and Yoshida, A. (1988). Genotypes of alcohol-metabolizing enzymes in Japanese with alcoholic liver diseases: A strong association of the usual Caucasian-type aldehyde dehydrogenase gene ($ALDH^1_2$) with the disease. *American Journal of Human Genetics* **43**, 744–748.

Sorensen, T.I.A. (1989). Alcohol and liver injury: Dose-related or permissive effect? *Liver* **9**, 189–197.

Sorensen, T.I.A., Orholm, M., Bensten, K.D., Hoybye, G., Eghoje, K. and Christoffersen, P. (1984). Prospective evaluation of alcohol abuse and alcoholic liver injury in men as predictors of development of cirrhosis. *Lancet* **ii**, 241–244.

Strubelt, O. (1980). Interactions between ethanol and other hepatotoxic agents. *Biochemical Pharmacology* **29**, 1445–1449.

Strubelt, O., Obermeir, R. and Siegers C.-P. (1978). The influence of ethanol pretreatment on the effects of nine hepatotoxic agents. *Acta Pharmacologica Toxicologica (Copenhagen)* **43**, 211–218.

Sugimoto, M., Hatori, T., Ito, T., Furube, M. and Abei, T. (1985). Characteristic features of liver disease in Japanese alcoholics. *American Journal of Gastroenterology* **80**, 993–997.

Takagi, T., Ishii, H., Takahashi, H., Kato, S., Okuno, F., Ebichara, Y., Yamauchi, H., Nagata, Y., Tashino, M. and Tsuchiya, M. (1983). Potentiation of halothane hepatotoxicity by chronic ethanol administration in rat: An animal model of halothane hepatitis. *Pharmacology, Biochemistry and Behaviour* **18**, 461–465.

Takahashi, H., Wong, K., Jui, L. and French, S.W. (1991). Effect of dietary fat on Ito cell activation by chronic ethanol intake: A long term serial morphometric study on alcohol-fed and control rats. *Alcoholism: Clinical and Experimental Research* **15**, 1060–1066.

Takahashi, H., Johansson, I., French, S.W. and Ingelman-Sundberg, M. (1992). Effects of dietary fat composition on activities of the microsomal ethanol oxidizing system and ethanol-inducible cytochrome P450 (CYP 2E1) in the liver of rats chronically fed ethanol. *Pharmacology and Toxicology* **70**, 347–351.

Takase, S., Takada, N., Enomoto, N., Ysuhara, M. and Takada, A. (1991). Different types of chronic hepatitis in alcoholic patients: Does chronic hepatitis induced by alcohol exist? *Hepatology* **13**, 876–881.

Tanner, A.R., Bantock, I., Hinks, L., Lloyd, B., Turner, N.R. and Wright, R. (1986). Depressed selenium and vitamin E levels in an alcoholic population: Possible relationship to hepatic injury through increased lipid peroxidation. *Digestive Diseases and Sciences* **31**, 1307–1312.

Thacker, S.B., Veech, R.L., Vernon, A.A. and Rustein, D.D. (1984). Genetic and biochemical factors relevant to alcoholism. *Alcoholism (NY)* **8**, 375–383.

Thuluvath, P.J., Wojno, K.J., Milligan, D., Yardley, J.H. and Mezey, E. (1993). Effects of *Helicobacter pylori* (HP) infection and gastritis on gastric alcohol dehydrogenase (ADH) activity. *Hepatology* **18**, 151A.

Tribble, D.L., Aw, T.Y. and Jones, D.P. (1987). The pathophysiological significance of lipid peroxidation in oxidative cell injury. *Hepatology* **7**, 377–386.

Tsukamoto, H., French, S.W., Benson, N., Delgado, G., Rao, G.A., Larkin, E.C. and Largman, C. (1985a). Severe and progressive steatosis and focal necrosis in rat liver induced by continuous intragastric infusion of ethanol and low fat diet. *Hepatology* **5**, 224–232.

Tsukamoto, H., French, S.W. and Largman, C. (1985b). Correlation of cyclical blood alcohol levels with progression of alcoholic liver injury. *Biochemical Archives* **1**, 215–220.

Tsukamoto, H., French, S.W., Reidelberg, R.D. and Largman, C. (1985c). Cyclic pattern of blood alcohol levels during continuous intragastric ethanol infusion in rats. *Alcoholism: Clinical and Experimental Research* **9**, 31–37.

Tsukamoto, H., Gaal, K. and French, S.W. (1990). Insights into the pathogenesis of alcoholic liver necrosis and fibrosis: Status report. *Hepatology* **12**, 599–608.

Tsutsumi, M., Takada, A., Wang, J.-S. and Takase, S. (1993). Genetic polymorphisms of cytochrome P4502E1 related to the development of alcoholic liver disease. *Hepatology* **18**, 124A.

Tuyns, A.J. and Pequignot, G. (1984). Greater risk of ascitic cirrhosis in females in relation to alcohol consumption. *International Journal of Epidemiology* **13**, 53–57.

Umeno, M., McBride, O.W., Yang, C.S., Gelboin, H.V. and Gonzalez, F.J. (1988). Human ethanol-inducible P450IIEI: Complete gene sequence, promoter characterization, chromosome mapping and cDNA-directed expression. *Biochemistry* **27**, 9006–9013.

Van Waes, L. and Lieber, C.S. (1977). Early perivenular sclerosis in alcoholic fatty liver: An index of progressive liver injury. *Gastroenterology* **73**, 646–650.

Villa, E., Rubbiani, L., Barchi, T., Ferretti, I., Grisendi, A., De Palma, M., Bellentari, S. and Manenti, F. (1982). Susceptibility of chronic symptomless HbsAg carriers to ethanol-induced hepatic damage. *Lancet* **ii**, 1243–1244.

Watkins, P.B. (1990). Role of cytochromes in drug metabolism and hepatotoxicity. *Seminars in Liver Disease* **10**, 235–250.

Wilkinson, P., Santamaria, J.N. and Rankin, J.G. (1969). Epidemiology of alcoholic cirrhosis. *Australian Annals of Medicine* **18**, 222–225.

Wilkinson, P., Kornaczewski, A., Rankin, J.G. and Santamaria, J.N. (1971). Physical disease in alcoholism. Initial survey of 1000 patients. *Medical Journal of Australia* **1**, 1217–1223.

Wodak, A.D., Saunders, J.B., Ewusi-Mensah, I., Davis, M. and Williams, R. (1983). Severity of alcohol dependence in patients with alcoholic liver disease. *British Medical Journal* **287**, 1420–1421.

Worner, T.M. and Lieber, C.S. (1985). Perivenular fibrosis as precursor lesion of cirrhosis. *Journal of the American Medical Association* **253**, 627–630.

Yates, W.R., Petty, F. and Brown, K. (1987). Risk factors for alcohol hepatoxicity among male alcoholics. *Drug and Alcohol Dependence* **20**, 155–162.

Zerbe, O. and Gressner, A.M. (1988). Proliferation of fat-storing cells is stimulated by secretions of Kupffer cells from normal and injured liver. *Experimental and Molecular Pathology* **49**, 87–101.

Zettermann, R.K. (1991). Autoimmune manifestations of alcoholic liver disease. In *Autoimmune Liver Disease* (Edited by Krawitt, E.L. and Wiesner, R.H.), pp. 247–260. Raven Press, New York.

Zimmerman, H.J. (1986). Effects of alcohol on other hepatotoxins. *Alcoholism (NY)* **10**, 3–15.

19 New insights into pathogenesis provided by use of specific therapeutic agents

F.J. Lou Carmichael, Hector Orrego and Laurence M. Blendis

Introduction

This chapter addresses the rationale for using the antithyroid drug propylthiouracil in the treatment of alcoholic liver disease. This form of treatment is based on the hypothesis that liver cell necrosis found following alcohol abuse, results from an ethanol-induced increase in liver oxygen consumption that is not compensated for by an increase in oxygen supply. Propylthiouracil has the effect of suppressing the increase in liver oxygen consumption. In both short-term and in long-term clinical trials, propylthiouracil has been used to treat alcoholic liver disease. The problem in analysing the effect of this drug in short-term clinical trials is discussed. The long-term clinical trial resulted in a 62 percent increase in the chances of survival for patients with alcoholic liver disease.

The chapter also discusses the pathogenesis of portal hypertension in alcoholic liver disease. Some of the forms of treatment are described in terms of those directed at reducing portal blood flow and those reducing the intrahepatic resistance to portal blood flow. The treatment of acute alcoholic hepatitis with corticosteroids is briefly discussed. Two recent meta-analyses of the literature have shown an improvement in the rate of survival with this form of therapy in patients with alcoholic hepatitis.

Basis for treatment of alcoholic liver disease with propylthiouracil

Clinical trials with propylthiouracil

Two types of clinical trials have been conducted using propylthiouracil for the treatment of alcoholic liver disease. There have been four short-term clinical trials using propylthiouracil for periods of 3–6 weeks (Orrego *et al.* 1979a; Serrano-Cancino *et al.* 1981; Halle *et al.* 1982; Pierrugues *et al.* 1989). Mortality was not influenced by the drug in these short-term clinical trials, and only one of them showed a significant clinical effect of propylthiouracil (Orrego *et al.* 1979a). All of these trials have serious flaws in design, the most important of which is the difficulty of eliminating a type II error. For a disease with a mortality of 20 percent a year, a drug that decreases mortality by 50 percent would require more than 400 patients to eliminate the possibility of a type II error. All of these clinical trials were well short of this number with a range of 29–133 patients. The only study to show positive results in the propylthiouracil-treated patients had the largest number of patients (Orrego *et al.* 1979a).

In order to decrease this inherent problem with short-term clinical trials, some authors have used samples of patients with extremely high rates of mortality (Serrano-Cancino 1981). This strategy means involving hospitalized patients with very serious complications such as encephalopathy, gastrointestinal bleeding, spontaneous bacterial peritonitis, hepatorenal syndrome, etc. It is possible, therefore, that therapies that could be effective in the treatment of the underlying alcoholic liver disease might not be beneficial in the presence of severe complications that have a pathogenesis and prognosis independent of the underlying alcoholic liver disease. On the other hand, treatments effective for some of the complications, such as lactulose in the case of encephalopathy, might reduce mortality without affecting the basic liver disease. The same could apply to the treatment of severe alcoholic liver disease with corticosteroids that have been reported to be especially effective in patients with encephalopathy (Reynolds *et al.* 1989; Imperiale and McCullough 1990). Therefore, short-term clinical trials are not adequate to assess the efficiency of treatment in patients with chronic conditions such as alcoholic liver disease.

There has been only one long-term clinical propylthiouracil trial conducted to date (Orrego *et al.* 1987). This study, with a maximum follow-up of 2 years, followed 310 compliant patients who received propylthiouracil ($n = 157$) or placebo ($n = 153$). The design of the study included a number of special features, including:

1. The "drop-out" patients were followed for an additional 2 years after leaving the trial.
2. Compliance was assessed daily in every patient by adding riboflavine to both propylthiouracil and placebo capsules and patients mailing daily urine samples in which the fluorescence to riboflavine was determined.
3. Both the presence and concentration of ethanol was determined in the daily urine samples.
4. The data were completely analysed without knowledge of the type of treatment the two groups of patients received. This procedure permitted a maximum of objectivity in making the unavoidable decisions with respect to exclusion of particular patients without knowledge of drug treatment.

The dose of propylthiouracil used in this trial was 300 mg/day and, as mentioned above, both drug and placebo capsules contained 50 mg riboflavine. The propylthiouracil and placebo groups were well matched demographically and with respect to severity of disease. Eighty percent of patients had liver biopsies showing similar histological severity in both groups, 60 percent having alcoholic hepatitis. The frequency of urines containing ethanol and the concentrations were also similar in the propylthiouracil and placebo groups. All of these features were also the same when the propylthiouracil drop-outs were compared with the placebo drop-outs. Moreover, the 2 year follow-up of the drop-outs showed similar mortality in the two groups, a fact that could be interpreted as demonstrating no further protection by propylthiouracil once the drug is discontinued.

As expected, the study ended with patients having different times of follow-up due to drop-outs and mortality. This required the use of statistics that did not need similar length of follow-up, such as Life Table methods (*SPSSX User Guide* 1983) and Proportional Hazard Regression Analysis (Cox Analysis) (Hopkins 1983). The statistical analysis showed that in the total sample, the propylthiouracil group had a cumulative mortality rate half that of the placebo group (0.13 *vs* 0.25; $P < 0.05$). In a subgroup of severely ill patients, 56 patients receiving propylthiouracil and 41 receiving placebo, the cumulative mortality rate was also halved (0.25 *vs* 0.55; $P < 0.03$). Probably the most accurate method of analysis in this type of clinical trial is the Proportional Hazard Stepwise Analysis. With this method, the total sample is matched for severity of disease and for ethanol consumption, resulting in an extremely close similarity between the drug and placebo groups. The cumulative mortality in the propylthiouracil-treated patients was 0.38 (95 per cent confidence interval 0.20–0.83; $P < 0.02$) that of the placebo group (Fig. 19.1). In other words, propylthiouracil reduced the risk of mortality by 62 percent in the complete group. No clinically important side-effects of propylthiouracil were observed at the dose used when compared with the placebo control group.

Ninety-five percent of the patients continued to drink either occasionally or continually and the amount of ethanol consumed had a significant effect on the response to propylthiouracil. When the total patient sample was divided into those in the lower half of urine alcohol concentration (<8 mM), versus those in the upper half (>8 mM), protection by propylthiouracil was observed in those with urine alcohol concentrations below 8 mM. Of course, in the group with high ethanol concentrations, there is the possibility that because of intoxication, the patients might not have been taking the complete dose of propylthiouracil.

Pathogenic basis for treatment with propylthiouracil

The underlying reason for using propylthiouracil in alcoholic liver disease was the finding that normal

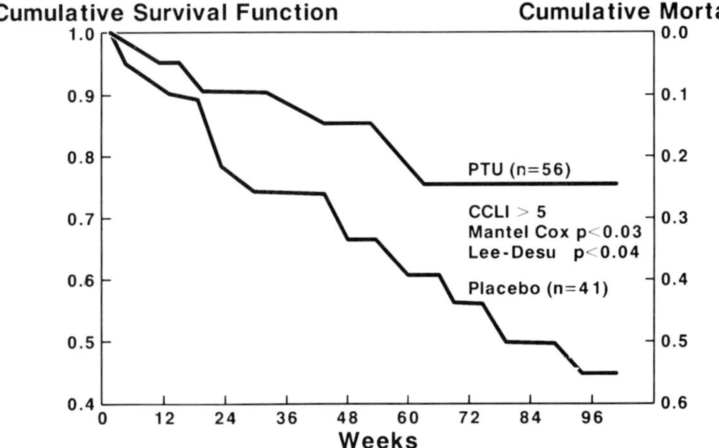

Fig. 19.1   Cumulative mortality rate in patients with CCLI < 5 and in patients with CCLI >5. Reproduced with permission from Orrego *et al.* (1987). *New England Journal of Medicine* **317**, 1421–1427.

thyroid function was necessary for the alcohol-induced increase in liver oxygen consumption, essentially an idea based on the hypoxic theory of alcohol-induced hepatocyte necrosis.

Hypoxic theory of alcohol-induced hepatocyte necrosis

In the liver acinus, the microvascular unit of the liver, blood flows from the portal vein in zone 1 (periportal) to the terminal hepatic vein in zone 3 (perivenular), through the sinusoids (Rappaport 1973) for a distance of 16–20 hepatocytes (Gumucio and Miller 1981; Zajicek *et al.* 1985), delivering oxygen, metabolites and exogenous substances (see also Chapter 14). Since zone 3 is the last zone to be perfused, it is in a state of hypoxia relative to zone 1 (Kessler *et al.* 1973; Quistorff *et al.* 1978; Jungerman and Katz 1982; Matsumara and Thurman 1983). Oxygen tensions in the portal vein have been determined to be 65 mmHg, while those in the hepatic vein are 30 mmHg (Nauck *et al.* 1981). This latter oxygen value represents a mixture of blood from many types of sinusoids, which, in the vicinity of the terminal hepatic vein, can be as low as 2 mmHg (Kessler 1968; Sato *et al.* 1987). Blood flow in some sinusoids is extremely rapid, the so-called "fast sinusoids", while in others it is sluggish (Sato *et al.* 1987; Sherman *et al.* 1990). It is in these latter sinusoids that the more extreme degrees of hypoxia have been obtained. Because of this marked heterogeneity in delivery of blood and therefore of oxygen

to the sinusoids, it is probably a mistake to assume that the oxygen consumption, when measured as the difference in oxygen content between the portal vein and hepatic vein, is truly representative of that occurring in individual sinusoids.

The fact that zone 3 of the liver acinus is in a relative state of hypoxia when compared with zone 1 (Kessler *et al.* 1973; Quistorff *et al.* 1978; Thurman *et al.* 1976; Jungerman and Katz 1982; Sato *et al.* 1983) makes zone 3 more vulnerable to hypoxic injury in conditions where oxygen consumption by the liver is increased without a corresponding increment in the delivery of oxygen (Schaffner 1970; Lemasters *et al.* 1983). For example, this can occur during high fever (Gore and Isaacson 1948), heat overload (heatstroke) (Bowers *et al.* 1978) and in severe hyperthyroidism (McIver and Winter 1943). In these three conditions, necrosis in zone 3 of the liver acinus has been described. Also, the degree of hypoxia in zone 3 can be increased when oxygen delivery to the liver is reduced, for example in conditions of severe anaemia (Song 1957), heart failure (Myers and Hickman 1948), shock (Lefkowitch and Mendez 1986) and anaesthesia (Gelman 1976), where zone 3 necrosis has also been shown to occur. Alcohol must be included as a potential cause of hypoxic liver damage because it is known to increase markedly the rate of oxygen consumption by the liver (Kessler *et al.* 1954; Videla and Israel 1970; Shaw *et al.* 1977; Villeneuve *et al.* 1981; Yuki *et al.* 1982; Ji *et al.* 1983; Bredfeldt *et al.* 1985; Orrego *et al.* 1985; Tsukamoto and Xi 1989), resulting in an increased hypoxia in zone 3 of the acinus

(Quistorff *et al.* 1978; Ji *et al.* 1982; Sato *et al.* 1987). This effect of ethanol has been repeatedly demonstrated in several species, including the rat (Bredfeldt *et al.* 1985) and dog (Villeneuve *et al.* 1981), and during withdrawal in humans (Kessler 1954; Hadengue *et al.* 1988). The same has been shown following the acute, but apparently not the chronic, administration of ethanol in baboons (Jauhonen *et al.* 1982). Furthermore, the alcohol-induced increase in liver oxygen consumption in alcoholic patients remains elevated for 1–2 weeks following the withdrawal of alcohol (Kessler 1954; Hadengue *et al.* 1988).

It has been postulated that when the ethanol-induced increase in oxygen consumption is not accompanied by an increase in oxygen delivery to the liver, the resulting degree of zone 3 hypoxia would be sufficient to produce hepatocyte necrosis in this area. This idea is the basis for the *hypoxic theory* of alcoholic liver necrosis, which states that hepatocyte necrosis ensues only when the increase in liver oxygen consumption induced by ethanol is accompanied by a decrease in oxygen delivery to the organ (Israel and Orrego 1984, 1987).

The hypoxic theory can account for three of the most important characteristics of alcoholic liver necrosis, namely that (1) necrosis occurs in zone 3 (Schaffner and Popper 1970), (2) the hepatocyte necrosis is focal rather than confluent (Green *et al.* 1963) and (3) necrosis does not occur in a majority of human alcoholics (Klatskin 1961) or in most experimental animal models (Lieber and DeCarli 1976; Popper and Lieber 1980; French *et al.* 1983).

The hypoxic theory would predict more necrosis in the areas of the liver acinus which are normally exposed to lower oxygen tensions – in other words, in zone 3. Also, it would predict that, in zone 3, the hepatocytes adjacent to the sinusoids with the lowest oxygen tension would be selectively affected, explaining the focal nature of the damage. Furthermore, the occurrence of necrosis would require the simultaneous presence of two independent factors – the ethanol-induced increase in oxygen consumption, plus a *precipitating* factor limiting oxygen delivery to the liver. Thus, necrosis would be restricted to those alcoholic individuals in whom this combination occurs (Israel and Orrego 1984, 1987).

Among the factors that could precipitate hypoxic hepatocyte necrosis in alcoholics, one should consider the presence of anaemia (Hillman 1975), respiratory diseases (Smith and Palmer 1976), excessive smoking (Rankin and Wilkinson 1971; DiFranza and Guerrera 1990) and sleep apnoea

(Vitiello *et al.* 1987; Taasan *et al.* 1981), all of which have been reported to be more frequent in alcoholics than in the general population. In the case of the animal models, the experimental conditions are frequently designed with the aim of having alcohol as the only variable, thus eliminating any precipitating factors and the likelihood of hepatocyte necrosis.

The postulate of the hypoxic theory – i.e. necrosis results from a combination of the ethanol-induced increase in liver oxygen consumption and failure in a compensatory increase in oxygen delivery – has been tested in experimental models where the chronic administration of ethanol was accompanied by reductions in oxygen delivery to the liver. These experiments have combined ethanol administration with anaemia (Israel *et al.* 1975; Speisky *et al.* 1985), hepatic artery ligation (Kalant *et al.* 1975), reduced inspired oxygen concentration (Israel *et al.* 1975; French *et al.* 1984; Perrisoud *et al.* 1985; Younes *et al.* 1989) and inhalation of carbon monoxide with the formation of carboxyhaemoglobin at blood concentrations similar to those found in heavy smokers (Nanji *et al.* 1989). In all of these situations, ethanol resulted in zone 3 liver necrosis in the rat, a species in which hepatocyte necrosis is not normally observed even following many months of oral alcohol consumption (Lieber and DeCarli 1976; see also Chapter 17).

Tsukomoto and Xi (1989) developed a model where ethanol was administered by continuous intragastric feeding of a liquid diet containing a high proportion of fat. The increase in fat metabolism introduced an added demand for liver oxygen that, when combined with the alcohol-induced increase, resulted in a striking increment in liver oxygen consumption. Although this treatment was accompanied by a 60 percent increase in portal blood flow, this augmented delivery of oxygen to the liver was not sufficient to compensate for the large demand, resulting in a 40 percent decrease in hepatic vein oxygen content. As predicted by the hypoxic theory, in this model, necrosis in zone 3 of the liver acinus was observed.

There is indirect evidence from *in vitro* experiments using perfused livers, that suggests that ethanol at high concentrations (>50 mM) can induce intrahepatic vasoconstriction (Oshita *et al.* 1992). If these data are confirmed *in vivo*, it would raise the possibility that high doses of ethanol would both decrease liver blood flow and increase oxygen consumption by the liver, a combination that should increase the likelihood of producing hepatocyte necrosis.

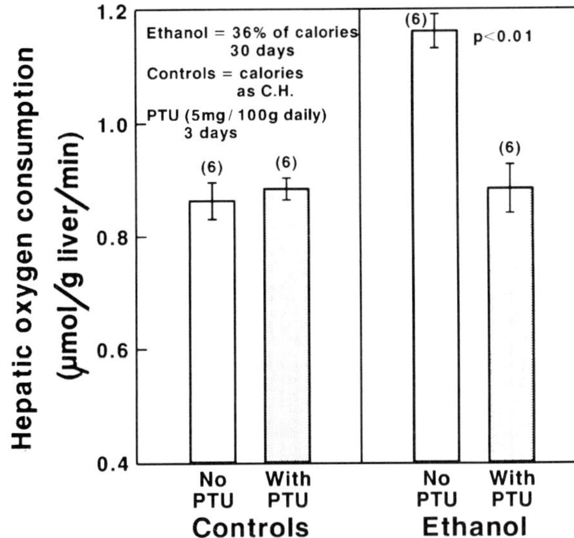

Fig. 19.2 Effect of propylthiouracil on the ethanol-induced increase in liver oxygen consumption.

It should be emphasized that the hypoxic mechanism for zone 3 necrosis is not restricted to hypoxia induced by ethanol. It has been shown to occur following the administration of ureogenic amino acids or thyroid hormones that also increase liver oxygen consumption and result in zone 3 necrosis in conditions of reduced oxygen tension (McIver and Winter 1943; Orrego *et al.* 1978).

From the hypoxic theory it is expected that hepatocyte necrosis should be prevented by (1) suppression of the alcohol-induced increase in oxygen consumption, (2) increasing the delivery of oxygen to the liver, or (3) a combination of these two effects. This led to the use of the antithyroid drug, propylthiouracil, that has been shown to suppress the ethanol-induced increase in oxygen consumption (Israel *et al.* 1975; Britton *et al.* 1979; Yuki *et al.* 1982), and to increase oxygen delivery to the liver (Kawasaki *et al.* 1989; Matsunaga *et al.* 1991).

As mentioned above, the alcohol-induced increase in oxygen consumption has been shown to require normal thyroid function. Thyroid hormones appear to play a *permissive* role without which alcohol administration does not result in enhanced oxygen demands by the liver (Israel *et al.* 1975; Israel and Orrego 1984, 1987). It has been shown experimentally that thyroidectomy and propylthiouracil, suppress the alcohol-induced increase in oxygen consumption (Bernstein *et al.* 1975; Israel *et al.* 1975) (see Fig. 19.2). Furthermore, propylthiouracil but not methimazole, through an effect

that appears to be independent of thyroid function, also increases portal blood flow and thus increases the delivery of oxygen to the liver (Kawasaki *et al.* 1989; Matsunaga *et al.* 1991). Confirming the prediction of the hypoxic theory, propylthiouracil markedly decreases the zone 3 hepatocyte necrosis observed in rats treated chronically with alcohol and submitted to hypoxia (Israel *et al.* 1975; Britton *et al.* 1979) (Fig. 19.3). As would be predicted from the above, propylthiouracil also prevented the zone 3 necrosis that follows the administration of ureogenic amino acids to rats submitted to hypoxia (Orrego *et al.* 1978). This finding is of potential therapeutic importance because it extends the protective effects of propylthiouracil to substances other than alcohol that increase liver oxygen consumption (Fig. 19.4).

The above discussion has been restricted to extrahepatic precipitating factors affecting liver oxygen supply and demand. It is clear, however, that in chronic liver disease, a series of intrahepatic factors could become extremely important in precipitating hepatocyte necrosis. Alcoholic liver disease is characterized by structural abnormalities that seriously interfere with the supply of oxygen to hepatocytes (Orrego and Carmichael 1992). In this situation, the "precipitating factors" have become "in-built" within the liver, i.e. they have become intrahepatic. Among the lesions that interfere with oxygen delivery are:

1. Abnormalities in the sinusoidal endothelium and the space of Disse, such as collagen deposition, sometimes forming a basement membrane under the endothelium of the sinusoids (Schaffner and Popper 1963; Orrego *et al.* 1979b; Horn *et al.* 1985), a decrease in the number of fenestra (Mak and Lieber 1984; Horn *et al.* 1986; see Chapter 15), and a decrease in hepatocyte microvilli which would reduce the surface area for the exchange of nutrients and oxygen (Phillips and Steiner 1966).
2. Enlargement of the hepatocytes compressing the sinusoids (Israel *et al.* 1982a).
3. The obstruction of sinusoids by inflammatory cells. The presence of hypoxia and/or hepatocyte necrosis results in a release of several cytokines and humoral factors that alter leucocyte membranes making them sticky (Perez *et al.* 1984; Schlayer *et al.* 1988; Felver *et al.* 1990; Kubes *et al.* 1990). These cells then adhere to the endothelium, plugging the sinusoids and obstructing blood flow (see also Chapters 14 and 15).
4. The presence of porto-systemic shunts. Although

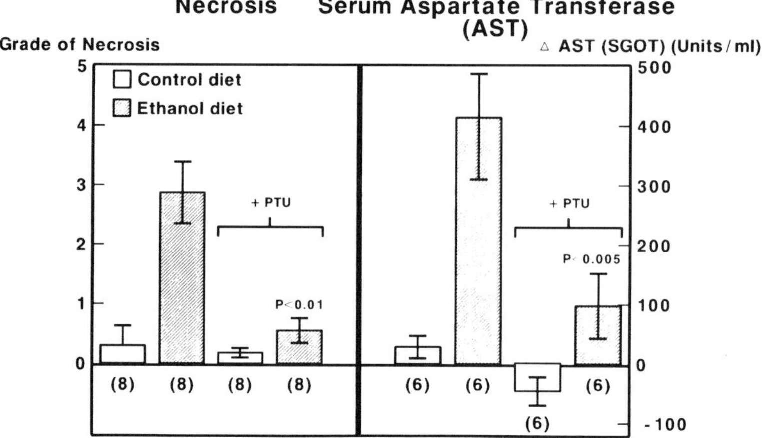

Fig. 19.3 Effects of propylthiouracil on liver damage induced by chronic ethanol and exposure to 5 percent oxygen.

not entirely intrahepatic, these shunts can also contribute to liver hypoxia in alcoholic liver disease. Through these shunts, a substantial proportion of portal blood flow is diverted past the liver into the systemic circulation. This would interfere with the compensatory increase in oxygen delivery following an increase in oxygen demand induced by ethanol or other causes.

The combination of ethanol and "intrahepatic precipitating factors" would eliminate the requirement for an "extrahepatic precipitating factor" and therefore would increase the risk of alcohol-induced liver necrosis even at low levels of oxygen consumption (Fig. 19.5).

Due to the above factors, the liver has been shown to be in a state of chronic hypoxia in alcoholic liver disease (Hayashi *et al.* 1985). This could facilitate the production of necrosis when the demand for oxygen by the liver increases following ethanol intake or from other non-alcoholic causes. The most obvious causes of non-alcohol-related increases in liver oxygen consumption are the daily dietary intake of fat, carbohydrate and protein (Siregar and Chou 1982; Brandt *et al.* 1955; see also Chapter 17). For example, Tsukomoto and Xi (1989) found that a marked potentiation of liver damage occurred when ethanol intake was combined with a high fat diet. This combination led to an increase in liver oxygen consumption that exceeded the compensatory capacity of the ethanol-induced increase in liver blood flow, resulting in the development of zone 3 necrosis. As predicted by the hypoxic theory, this increase in oxygen consumption by the liver may be

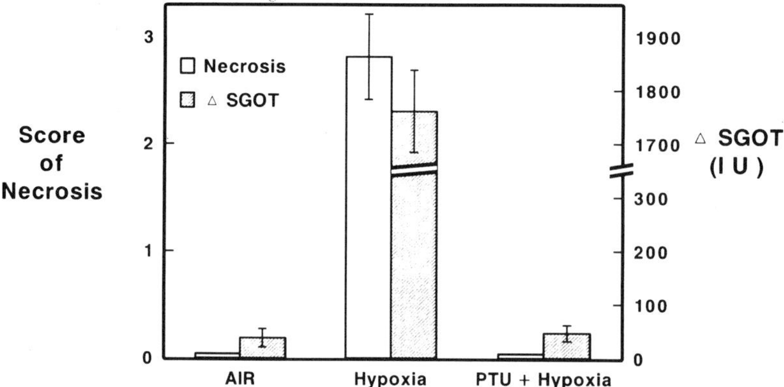

Fig. 19.4 Effect of propylthiouracil on hepatocellular necrosis in rats receiving a high protein diet and hypoxia.

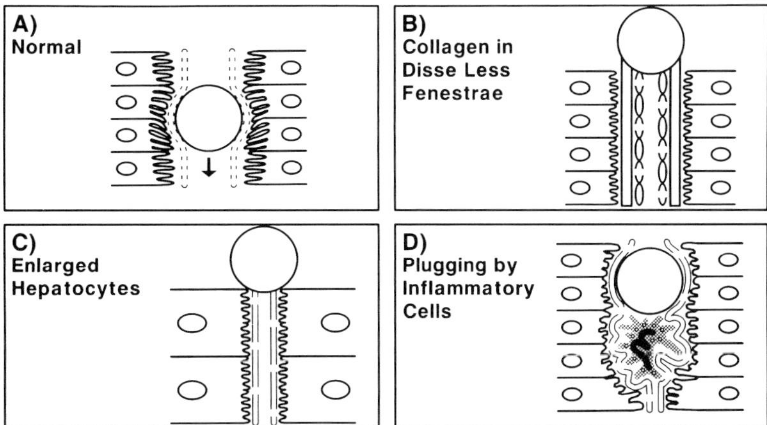

Fig. 19.5   Factors that contribute to hypoxia in alcoholic liver disease.

particularly important with diets containing proteins. Proteins due to ureogenesis (Lundsgaard 1942) have the so-called "specific dynamic action" that results in an added increase in oxygen consumption compared with that of lipid or carbohydrate on a caloric basis. Following the administration of fat, protein and carbohydrate, there is an increase in liver blood flow that increases oxygen delivery to hepatocytes in the normal liver. In alcoholic liver disease with intrahepatic structural abnormalities, however, this increase in blood flow may not reach the hepatocytes and zone 3 hypoxia results.

Functional factors acting on splanchnic haemodynamics and oxygen balance may also play a role in hepatocyte necrosis. For example, the increase in catecholamines that has been observed in the presence of chronic liver disease (Henriksen *et al.* 1984) could result in hypoxic damage to hepatocytes, because while they increase oxygen consumption by the liver (Ji *et al.* 1984) they also decrease liver blood flow (Cousineau *et al.* 1985).

In summary, the hypoxic theory postulates that hepatocyte necrosis will follow any situation in which a combination of an increase in requirement for oxygen by the liver and a decrease in supply to the liver occur. It also postulates that treatments that suppress this increase in liver oxygen consumption, irrespective of the origin (ethanol, protein or catecholamines), should also protect against this type of damage. This is indeed the case following thyroidectomy and the administration of antithyroid drugs. If the beneficial effect of propylthiouracil is specifically restricted to the prevention of necrosis resulting from alcohol, one would not expect protection by propylthiouracil in patients who either

abstain or decrease their drinking to a minimum. However, from the experience of our long-term clinical trial with propylthiouracil, it is clear that this drug also has beneficial effects in these two latter categories of patients (Orrego *et al.* 1987). This would, therefore, indicate that the action of propylthiouracil is not limited to alcohol-induced liver hypoxia and that the risk of hypoxic liver damage following administration of food, the known increase in catecholamines, and other possible causes in patients with alcoholic liver disease could also be reduced following propylthiouracil treatment.

A point that needs clarification is the reason why in most animal models and indeed in the majority of human alcoholics there is no evidence of hypoxic liver necrosis. This is probably the result of a compensatory mechanism that increases oxygen delivery to the liver via the portal vein (McKaigney *et al.* 1985). This increase in portal tributary blood flow has been shown to be mediated by the release of acetate from the liver during ethanol metabolism and the production of adenosine in the splanchnic vasculature as a result of the oxidation of acetate (Carmichael *et al.* 1988; Orrego *et al.* 1988). An increase in liver blood flow has been shown to occur following the intra-arterial and oral administration of both ethanol and acetate and the intra-arterial administration of adenosine (Orrego and Carmichael 1992). In each case, the increase in portal blood flow was completely suppressed by the administration of the adenosine receptor blocker, 8-phenyltheophylline.

It is unlikely that hepatocyte necrosis is due to a single cause. It is more likely that a series of concatenated events result in cell death. This applies, for example, to the possible role of lipid peroxidation and to the release of cytokines in alcoholic liver disease. The evidence for lipid peroxidation playing an initiating role in the production of alcohol-induced hepatocyte necrosis remains controversial, since ethanol has been shown to have a potential role as a free radical scavenger (Klein *et al.* 1983) and has been claimed to increase the resistance of liver membranes to lipid peroxidation (Zidenberg-Cher *et al.* 1991). Also, while the occurrence of alcohol-induced hepatocyte necrosis is not necessarily accompanied by a significant increase in lipid peroxidation (Speisky *et al.* 1985; Inomata *et al.* 1987; Kamimura *et al.* 1992), lipid peroxidation has been observed following the administration of ethanol in the absence of hepatocyte necrosis (Shaw *et al.* 1981; Videla and Valenzuela 1982; Kato *et al.* 1990). Moreover, others have not confirmed the increase in lipid peroxidation following acute exposure (Hashimoto and Recknagel 1968; Reid and Slater 1977; Sullivan *et al.* 1980). Recently, a new view has been presented. It would appear that with liver injury in the presence of fibrosis (Kamimura *et al.* 1992), ethanol administration is associated with increased lipid peroxidation (Yamada *et al.* 1988; Tsukomoto *et al.* 1990). These results support the idea that while lipid peroxidation does not initiate alcohol-induced hepatocyte necrosis, it does play a role in maintaining and increasing liver damage once substantial necrosis and fibrosis have taken place (Castillo *et al.* 1992). It is not the purpose of this review to discuss the exact source or mechanism of production of oxygen free radicals following alcohol consumption (see Chapter 2). However, it has also been claimed that when alcohol is suddenly withdrawn from alcoholic patients with induced cytochrome P4502E1, hepatocytes are more likely to produce lipid peroxides (Castillo *et al.* 1992).

It has been postulated that alcoholic liver disease represents a continuous recruitment of new mechanisms that produce hepatocyte necrosis and result in a vicious cycle of increasing liver damage (Orrego and Carmichael 1992). Thus the possibility of lipid peroxidation playing a role in alcoholic liver disease in the production of hepatocyte necrosis is not contrary to the importance of hypoxia in the generation of liver damage. Hypoxia, when followed by reoxidation (Younes *et al.* 1989; Nagano *et al.* 1990) or when combined with ethanol, results in the production of oxygen radicals (Younes and Strubelt 1987; Kato *et al.* 1990).

Hypoxia and lipid peroxidation could also be associated with the inflammatory responses of the liver to ethanol. Hypoxia has been shown to stimulate the production of oxygen radicals by endothelial and Kupffer cells (Keppler *et al.* 1988). The same appears to be true for migrating neutrophils. As a matter of fact, the production of these radicals by phagocytic cells is one of the mechanisms involved in their microbicidal activity (Baboir 1978).

Stimulation of endothelial and Kupffer cells also results in the release of interleukins (Keppler *et al.* 1988). While normal hepatocytes are resistant to interleukin-induced damage, these cytokines become cytotoxic to hepatocytes under conditions of hypoxia (Trudell *et al.* 1984). Also, endothelial and Kupffer cells release transforming growth factor that is fibrogenic, tumour necrosis factor and platelet activating factor that make neutrophils sticky (Matsuoka *et al.* 1989) and cause them to adhere to the endothelium, obstructing blood flow through the sinusoids (Schlayer *et al.* 1988; Rieder *et al.* 1990; Felver *et al.* 1990; see Chapter 14). This mechanism, as explained above, would result in an added vicious cycle of increasing hypoxia and thus of more release and sensitivity to these cytokines. It is of interest that a correlation exists between blood levels of some of these cytokines and the severity of liver disease (Felver *et al.* 1990). Ethanol itself has been shown to release a chemotactic lipid that induces leucocyte infiltration and thus increases free radicals and leukotrienes in the liver (Matsuda *et al.* 1987). Moreover, it has been found that ethanol inhibits the degradation of leukotrienes which extends their half-life within the liver (Keppler *et al.* 1988; see also Chapter 5).

In summary, lipid peroxidation can result from: (1) hypoxic stimulation of Kupffer and endothelial cells, (2) inflammatory reactions induced by ethanol on hepatocytes, and/or (3) the release of cytokines that attract inflammatory cells.

Clearly, therefore, hypoxia and lipid peroxidation, rather than being mutually exclusive mechanisms, can be conceived as a sequential cascade of effects that lead to hepatocyte necrosis. Interestingly, propylthiouracil can act at a number of different levels of this cascade. As explained above, propylthiouracil can suppress hypoxia in the liver following ethanol administration, an effect that will not only preserve the integrity of the hepatocytes, but will also suppress the release of cytokines and free radicals from Kupffer and endothelial cells. Moreover, propylthiouracil has been shown to reduce the formation of oxygen radicals by human neutrophils, thus acting as an anti-inflammatory agent (Imumura *et al.* 1986). Propylthiouracil can also act after the formation of lipid peroxides as a scavenger of free radicals and decrease hydrogen peroxide generation (Baboir 1978). This effect of propylthiouracil could result from its close structural similarity to thiourea, a well-established hydroxyl radical scavenger (Dorfman and Adams 1973). Propylthiouracil has also been shown to reduce the free radical response and bactericidal action of human neutrophils against bacteria (Repine *et al.* 1984). It has also been claimed to be a substrate for the glutathione-*S*-transferase, acting as a substitute for glutathione (Yamada and Kaplowitz 1980), although this finding remains controversial (Habig *et al.* 1984). Propylthiouracil has been shown to inhibit the depletion of hepatic glutathione induced by azothioprine and to decrease hepatic covalent binding of acetaminophen metabolized in the liver *in vitro* and *in vivo* (Linscheer *et al.* 1980; Raheja *et al.* 1982). These effects of propylthiouracil might be the explanation as to why this drug protects against liver damage induced by non-alcoholic causes such as acetaminophen, carbon tetrachloride (Orrego *et al.* 1976), dichloroethylene (Szabo *et al.* 1977), organomercurials (Szabo *et al.* 1974) and galactosamine (Cooper *et al.* 1984).

Alcohol, liver disease and portal hypertension

The approach to the pathophysiology of the treatment of portal hypertension will be different from that followed with propylthiouracil. There is no single treatment of portal hypertension. On the contrary, treatment has been directed at normalizing the different mechanisms that are thought to be involved in the pathogenesis of the increase in portal pressure. Thus in order to make the presentation of the topic clearer, the discussion of the treatment will be preceded by a brief comment on the pathogenesis of portal hypertension.

From the haemodynamic point of view, the most important abnormality in liver disease is the occurrence of portal hypertension. Portal hypertension is one of the main determinants of death in patients with alcoholic liver disease. Portal hypertension plays an important role in the pathogenesis of some of the most serious complications of alcoholic liver disease, including oesophageal variceal bleeding, ascites, spontaneous bacterial peritonitis and the hepatorenal syndrome. A good correlation exists between the degree of portal hypertension and mortality in alcoholic liver disease (Blake and Orrego 1990). In our experience, the 1 year mortality was 0 percent in 40 patients with portal pressure of less than 10 mmHg, while it was 10 percent in 52 patients with portal pressures between 10 and 20 mmHg, and 30 percent in 56 patients with portal pressures above 20 mmHg.

Pathogenesis of portal hypertension

Portal pressure is the result of an interaction between the hepatic resistance to portal blood flow and the rate of blood flow. Thus, portal pressure can increase following (1) an increase in resistance to portal blood flow, (2) an increase in the rate of portal blood flow or (3) a combination of these factors.

The increase in hepatic resistance to portal blood flow can result from a combination of mechanical and functional abnormalities that decrease the calibre of the intrahepatic vasculature. Thus, portal pressure will result from an interplay of factors acting on portal blood flow and/or resistance at the level of the liver. In any one patient, the importance of these multiple factors in attaining a given degree of portal hypertension may vary greatly.

Increase in hepatic resistance to portal blood flow
Mechanical factors that can increase hepatic resistance to blood flow
Only a few decades ago, the increase in liver resistance observed in alcoholic liver disease (Kelty *et al.* 1950) was attributed to the distortion of the liver vasculature by the formation of fibrous septae (Safran and Schaffner 1967) and/or by compression of the post-sinusoidal veins by the parenchymal nodules that characterize cirrhosis (Blendis *et al.* 1982). This concept did not explain the fact that portal hypertension can occur in the absence of cirrhosis and also that cirrhosis can coexist with normal portal pressures. For example, we have observed that 34 percent of the patients with alcoholic liver disease and portal hypertension do not have cirrhosis on liver biopsy (Blendis *et al.* 1982). Also, this mechanism cannot explain the common observation that portal hypertension decreases soon after withdrawal from alcohol, while the nodularity remains unchanged (Reynolds *et al.* 1960; Leevy *et al.* 1958). Thus, other factors appear to play a more important role in the development and maintenance of portal hypertension.

Four possible determinants of an increased resistance to portal blood flow are (1) necrosis and inflammation, (2) enlargement of hepatocytes, (3) increase in collagen in the space of Disse and (4) terminal hepatic venule fibrosis (see Chapter 3). These abnormalities are frequently seen in alcoholic liver disease and can occur during the early, pre-cirrhotic stages of the disease. All of these result directly or indirectly from prolonged alcohol abuse.

1. *Necrosis.* As explained above, hepatocyte necrosis, the hallmark of alcoholic hepatitis, is accompanied by the accumulation of inflammatory cells within the liver sinusoids that plug the sinusoids and thereby block sinusoidal blood flow (Schlayer *et al.* 1988; Wisse and McCuskey 1986; see Chapter 14), increasing resistance to portal blood flow. It is of interest that four different groups of investigators have shown a good correlation between the severity of alcoholic hepatitis assessed by liver biopsies and the degree of portal hypertension (Orrego *et al.* 1981; Wisse and McCuskey 1986; Poynard *et al.* 1987; Valla *et al.* 1989).

2. *Hepatocyte size.* One of the early effects of ethanol on the liver is an increase in the size of hepatocytes (Israel and Orrego 1987). Hepatomegaly, a common finding in alcoholics, is the result of enlargement of hepatocytes rather than of an increase in cell number (Baraona *et al.* 1975; Israel *et al.* 1982a, b). This increase in liver size is accompanied by a marked decrease in the extracellular and vascular space (Orrego *et al.* 1981; Vidins *et al.* 1985). It has been postulated that, initially, the increase in hepatocyte size distends the infrastructure and the capsule of the liver resulting in an increase in liver size. When the elastic capacity of the liver framework is exceeded, further cell enlargement results in a compression of the vascular and extracelluar compartments. The calibre of the sinusoids is then reduced resulting in more sinusoidal resistance and in an increase in portal pressure (Vidins *et al.* 1985). This effect of enlarged hepatocytes compressing the sinusoids has now been confirmed by different groups of investigators, both in alcoholics and in non-alcoholic experimental models (Vidins *et al.* 1985; Lee *et al.* 1987; Matsuda *et al.* 1987; Shibayama 1988; Valla *et al.* 1989; Van Leeuwen *et al.* 1990). It is of great importance to note that, in our experience, an increase in portal pressure was seen only in animals in which hepatomegaly exceeded a 50 percent increase in liver weight to body weight (Israel *et al.* 1982b; Israel and Orrego 1983). This finding has been confirmed by two other groups of investigators that found no increase in portal pressure in alcohol-fed rats with hepatomegaly of less than 35 percent above the controls (Bredfeldt *et al.* 1981; Mastai *et al.* 1989a).

In humans, we have reported an excellent correlation between hepatocyte size and portal pressures in the range of pressures between 5 and 20 mmHg. In patients with portal pressures above 20 mmHg, there is a plateau in this relationship and the correlation is lost (Blendis *et al.* 1982). This could indicate that in these latter patients, other factors are more important in determining the height of portal pressure. It has also been demonstrated that the sinusoidal space, measured in liver biopsies from patients with alcoholic liver disease and portal hypertension, is significantly reduced (Lee *et al.* 1987). The reduction in sinusoidal area correlates with the degree of portal hypertension. It is important to note that this correlation between hepatocyte size and portal pressure did not exist in patients with non-alcoholic liver disease (Vidins *et al.* 1985).

3. *Space of Disse abnormalities.* As discussed above, alcoholic liver disease is accompanied by serious abnormalities that occur at the level of the sinusoids and the space of Disse (see also Chapters 3, 4, 14, 15 and 17). The combination of these abnormalities can interfere with sinusoidal blood flow resulting in an increase in resistance to blood flow and thus in an increase in portal pressure. The deposition of collagen in the space of Disse would make the walls of the sinusoids more rigid. The calibre of the sinusoids is narrower than the diameter of the erythrocytes (Orrego *et al.* 1981), thus the erythrocytes and leucocytes are squeezed as they flow through the sinusoids; this latter effect would be interfered with when the sinusoids are filled with collagen fibres. Also, this would result in an increased resistance to blood flow through the liver sinusoids and thus to an increase in portal pressure. This has been demonstrated by the finding of a good correlation between the amount of collagen in the space of Disse and the degree of portal hypertension in humans with alcoholic liver disease (Vidins *et al.* 1985; Robert *et al.* 1989) (Fig. 19.6).

4. *Terminal hepatic venule fibrosis.* This term designates a process of fibrosis progressively obstructing the terminal hepatic venules. Terminal hepatic vein sclerosis can occur at an early pre-cirrhotic state of alcoholic liver disease (Miyakawa *et al.* 1985). It has been claimed that this lesion has predictive value in determining progression to cirrhosis in both humans (Van Waes and Lieber 1977; Nakano *et al.* 1982) and baboons (Miyakawa *et al.* 1985). In the baboon, terminal hepatic vein sclerosis correlates with mild elevations of portal pressure in

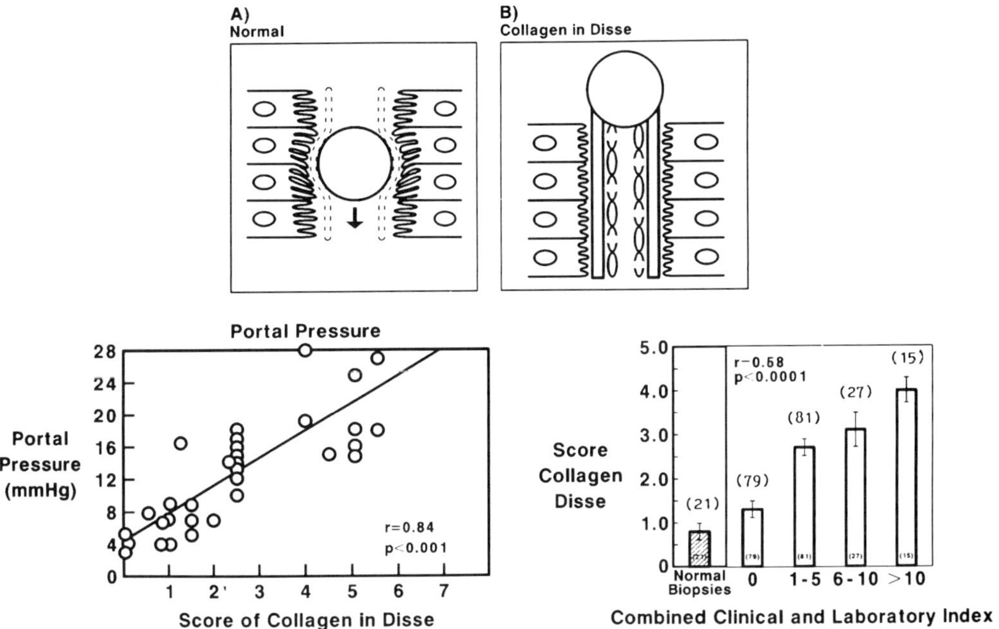

Fig. 19.6 Collagen and liver microcirculation.

the pre-cirrhotic stage, a finding that has not been confirmed in humans with portal hypertension (Orrego *et al.* 1981). Others have found no relationship between terminal hepatic vein sclerosis and the clinical or histological severity of human liver disease (Nasrallah *et al.* 1980; Burt and MacSween 1986). Terminal hepatic vein sclerosis would result in a post-sinusoidal resistance to blood flow; however, there is growing evidence that in alcoholic liver disease the resistance is sinusoidal (Shibayama and Nakata 1985).

Functional factors that can increase hepatic resistance to blood flow
Aside from the mechanical interference with the sinusoidal microcirculation, humeral factors influencing resistance to blood flow include catecholamines (Henriksen *et al.* 1984; Moreau *et al.* 1987), serotonin (Hadengue *et al.* 1987; Cummings *et al.* 1988; Mastai *et al.* 1989b) and methionine enkephalin (Thornton *et al.* 1988). Noradrenaline, when infused intraportally, induces a significant increase in portal pressure (Reilly *et al.* 1981; Lenzen *et al.* 1990), a decrease in the liver vascular space (Cousineau *et al.* 1985) and sinusoidal shunting (Vorobioff *et al.* 1983). Moreover, patients with cirrhosis have significantly elevated circulating levels of noradrenaline (Henriksen *et al.* 1984) and

the administration of phentolamine or clonidine markedly reduces portal pressure in patients with portal hypertension (Mena *et al.* 1963; Moreau *et al.* 1987). A similar association occurs following the administration of the antiserotonin drugs, ketanserin and ritanserin (Hadengue *et al.* 1987; Cummings *et al.* 1988). Plasma methionine enkephalin was found to be increased in patients with oesophageal varices compared with patients without varices (Thornton *et al.* 1988). There is also evidence, although somewhat controversial, showing that calcium channel blocking drugs such as verapamil, can reduce hepatic resistance to portal blood flow and improve the clearance of indocyanine green by the liver (Navasa *et al.* 1988; Vinel *et al.* 1989). The fact that functional factors, amenable to modification by medical interventions, can play an important role in portal hypertension, opens the possibility of a medical treatment of one of the most serious consequences of alcoholic liver disease.

Increase in rate of portal blood flow
Another factor that could play an important role in the production and maintenance of portal hypertension is an increase in the rate of portal blood flow (Blanchet and Lebrec 1982; Vorobioff *et al.* 1983). Since splanchnic blood flow accounts for 20–25 percent of cardiac output, it is difficult to conceive

that the very large elevations in portal pressure seen in alcoholic liver disease could result solely from an increase in portal blood flow. Increases in blood flow, however, can both potentiate the portal pressure effects of an increase in hepatic resistance and also may cancel the possible decompressive effects of the opening of porto-systemic shunts (Vorobioff *et al*. 1983). It has been estimated that in cirrhosis, approximately 60 percent of portal pressure is the result of an increase in liver resistance and that 40 percent can be attributed to an increase in portal blood flow (Benoit *et al*. 1985). The mechanism(s) of this increase in splanchnic blood flow has not been elucidated. Although there is evidence for glucagon playing a significant role, the issue is still controversial (Benoit *et al*. 1986; Sikular and Groszmann 1986; Cerini *et al*. 1989; Silva *et al*. 1990). There is a growing body of literature pointing to an important role of nitric oxide in the hyperdynamic splanchnic circulation that follows the development of portal hypertension (Lee *et al*. 1992; Pizcueta *et al*. 1992; see also Chapter 14). If these observations are confirmed, the possibility of treatment aimed at interfering with the production or release of nitric oxide, might be of importance for the management of portal hypertension in the future.

Corticosteroids for acute alcoholic hepatitis

Two recent meta-analyses have been published incorporating 11 randomized trials assessing the effectiveness of treatment with corticosteroids on mortality in hospitalized patients with acute alcoholic hepatitis (Imperiale and McCullough 1990; Reynolds *et al*. 1989). Both analyses independently found that corticosteroids significantly reduced mortality by 34 percent in a subgroup of the most seriously ill patients that presented with encephalopathy. These findings were recently confirmed by a further study from Paris (Ramond *et al*. 1992). In contrast, in patients with encephalopathy secondary to gastrointestinal bleeding, steroids were found to be detrimental. This is not altogether surprising, since previous studies have shown that the occurrence of bleeding from varices or from peptic ulceration is increased by corticosteroid therapy (Christensen *et al*. 1981). In summary, the meta-analyses and the recent controlled trials, including the Veterans Administration multicentre trial (Carithers *et al*. 1989), confirmed the intitial obser-

vation made 20 years ago that corticosteroids are beneficial to patients with severe acute alcoholic hepatitis, defined as those with spontaneous encephalopathy (Helman *et al*. 1971) or those falling within a discriminatory index (Maddrey *et al*. 1978).

What are the mechanisms that might explain the benefits of steroid therapy in alcoholic hepatitis? Twenty years ago, Leevy and co-workers first suggested that the failure of patients admitted with alcoholic hepatitis to improve in hospital, despite the withdrawal of alcohol, might be due to an immune mechanism (Sorrell and Leevy 1972). Both cellular and humoral factors have been implicated in the pathogenesis of alcoholic liver disease (see Chapter 6):

1. *Cell-mediated immunity*. For example, liver homogenates stimulated the peripheral lymphocytes of such patients, in contrast to patients with steatosis. This phenomenon disappeared when Mallory's hyalin disappeared on liver histology, suggesting that the hyaline might be the cause of *in vitro* lymphocyte transformation (Zetterman *et al*. 1976).

   Although the classical cellular infiltrate in alcoholic hepatitis is with polymorphonuclear leucocytes, there is also a relative increase in intrahepatic T-lymphocytes (French *et al*. 1979), which in turn may secrete a granulocyte and fibroblastic chemotactic factor (Postlewaite *et al*. 1976).
2. *Humoral immunity*. Patients with alcoholic liver disease tend to have polyclonal increases in serum immunoglobulins with disproportionate increases in IgA levels (Feizi 1968) due partly to decreased reticuloendothelial function (Triger and Wright 1973) and polyclonal B cell activation (Berger *et al*. 1979).

Autoantibodies to double-stranded and single-stranded DNA, to smooth muscle actin filaments (Gluud *et al*. 1984) and anti-lymphocyte antibodies have been shown to occur in up to 60 percent of patients with alcoholic liver disease (Laskin *et al*. 1990), similar to the findings in autoimmune disorders such as systemic lupus erythematosis. In contrast, less that 20 percent of control chronic alcoholic patients without liver disease were positive for autoantibodies (Laskin *et al*. 1990). More specifically, antibodies to hepatocyte components other than Mallory's hyaline have been demonstrated in patients with alcoholic liver disease, including liver-specific protein (Meliconi *et al*. 1982) and liver membrane antigen (Anthony *et al.* 1983; Neuberger *et al.* 1984). See Chapter 6 for a detailed discussion.

In patients with alcoholic liver disease who are actively drinking, there are increased levels of acetaldehyde, the first metabolite of alcohol metabolism, both in serum and in the liver (Barry *et al.* 1987; see also Chapter 2). Evidence for lymphocyte sensitization to acetaldehyde and antibody-dependent cytotoxicity against acetaldehyde covalently bound to hepatocyte components (Stevens *et al.* 1981), including that mediated by complement activation, suggest an immune-mediated acetaldehyde hepatotoxicity (Actis *et al.* 1978, Crossley *et al.* 1986). It was hypothesized that acetaldehyde–protein adducts would enable the small acetaldehyde molecule, acting as an hapten, to become antigenic (Sorrell and Tuma 1985; see also Chapter 5). In subsequent experiments, mice chronically fed alcohol exhibited antibodies recognizing proteins labelled *in vitro* with acetaldehyde (Israel *et al.* 1986). These findings have been confirmed in chronic alcoholic patients (Niemela *et al.* 1987). In a study of patients with alcoholic liver disease, antibody titres were significantly higher against protein–acetaldehyde conjugates compared with unmodified protein. The highest titres were found in patients with alcoholic hepatitis, further suggesting an immune pathogenesis for this condition (Niemela *et al.* 1987). The presence of antibodies to other liver components including cytokeratin (Kurki *et al.* 1984) could be due to the presence of acetaldehyde-containing epitopes (Niemela *et al.* 1987).

Recently, Koskinas *et al.* (1992) have linked the two major immune abnormalities in alcoholic liver disease – elevated IgA levels due to increased production by peripheral blood B lymphocytes (Rodriguez *et al.* 1984), and acetaldehyde–liver protein adducts. They demonstrated that IgA antibodies recognize a 200 kDa antigen in 70 percent of patients with alcoholic hepatitis or non-alcoholic liver disease and 20 percent of heavy drinkers without overt liver disease. Thus, another possible cause for the elevated serum IgA levels in alcoholic liver disease may be antigenic stimulation. The above reaction might result in IgA deposition on the sinusoidal membrane of hepatocytes (Van de Wiel *et al.* 1987). This might in turn act as a chemotactic stimulus for neutrophils with the secretion of interleukin-6 and its amplification of immunoglobulin secretion (Deviere *et al.* 1992). The suppression of this chain of events by corticosteroids could

account for its significant therapeutic effect in patients with severe alcoholic hepatitis.

Conclusion

Studies of the various pathogenetic mechanisms of alcoholic liver disease have led to an increased understanding of some of the processes involved in the development of alcoholic liver disease. Furthermore, the efficacy of specific therapeutic agents have, in turn, lent support to these new insights into the pathogenesis. Only with continued research in the pathophysiology of this area will further therapeutic advances be achieved in the future.

References

Actis, G.C., Ponzetto, A., Rizetto, M. and Verme, G. (1978). Cell mediated immunity to acetaldehyde in alcoholic liver disease. *Digestive Diseases and Sciences* **23**, 883–886

Anthony, R.S., Farquharson, M. and MacSween, R.N.M. (1983). Liver membrane antibodies in alcoholic liver disease. *Journal of Clinical Pathology* **36**, 1302–1308.

Baboir, B.M. (1978). Oxygen-dependent microbial killing by phagocytes. *New England Journal of Medicine* **298**, 659–668.

Baraona, E., Leo, M.A., Borowsky, S.A. and Lieber, C.S. (1975). Alcoholic hepatomegaly, accumulation of protein in the liver. *Science* **190**, 794–795.

Barry, R.E., Williams, A.S. and McGivan, J.D. (1987). The detection of aecetaldehyde/liver plasma membrane adduct formed *in vivo* by alcohol feeding. *Liver* **7**, 364–369.

Benoit, J.N., Womack, W.A., Hernandez, L. and Granger, D.N. (1985). Forward and backward flow mechanisms of portal hypertension: Relative contributions in the rat model of portal vein stenosis. *Gastroenterology* **89**, 1092–1096.

Benoit, J., Zimmerman, B., Premen, A.J., Go, V.L.W. and Granger, D.N. (1986). Role of glucagon in splanchnic hyperemia of chronic portal hypertension. *American Journal of Physiology* **25**, G674–G677.

Berger, S.R., Helms, R.A. and Bull, D.M. (1979). Cirrhotic hypergammaglobulinemia, increased rates of immunoglobulin synthesis by circulating lymphoid cells. *Digestive Diseases and Sciences* **24**, 741–746.

Bernstein, J., Videla, L. and Israel, Y. (1975). Hormonal influences on the developement of the hypermetabolic state of the liver produced by chronic administration of ethanol. *Journal of Pharmacology and Experimental Therapeutics* **192**, 583–591.

Blake, J. and Orrego, H. (1990). Monitoring treatment in alcoholic liver disease. *Clinical Chemistry* **3**, 5–13.

Blanchet, L. and Lebrec, D. (1982). Changes in splanchnic blood flow in portal hypertensive rats. *European Journal of Clinical Investigation* **12**, 327–330.

Blendis, L.M., Orrego, H., Crossley, I.R., Blake, J.E., Medline, A. and Israel, Y. (1982). The role of hepatocyte enlargement in hepatic pressure in cirrhotic and non-cirrhotic alcoholic liver disease. *Hepatology* **2**, 539–546.

Bowers, W.D., Hubbard, R.W., Leav, I., Conlon, M., Hamlet, M.P., Magerm, M. and Brandt, P. (1978). Alterations of rat liver subsequent to heat overload. *Archives of Pathology and Laboratory Medicine* **102**, 154–157.

Brandt, J.L., Castleman, L., Ruskin, H.D., Greenwald, J. and Kelly, J.J. (1955). The effect of oral proteins and glucose feeding on splanchnic blood flow and oxygen utilization in normal and cirrhotic subjects. *Journal of Clinical Investigation* **34**, 1017–1025.

Bredtfeldt, J.E., Riley, E.M. and Groszmann, R.J. (1981). Intrahepatic pressure and portal pressure in alcoholic rats. *Hepatology* **1**, 399–402.

Bredfeldt, J.E., Riley, E.M. and Groszmann, R.J. (1985). Compensatory mechanisms in response to an elevated hepatic oxygen consumption in chronically ethanol fed rats. *American Journal of Physiology* **248**, 507–511.

Britton, R.S., Koves, G., Orrego, H., Kalant, H., Phillips, M.J., Khanna, J.M. and Israel, Y. (1979). Suppression by antithyroid drugs of experimental hepatic necrosis after ethanol treatment: Effect on thyroid gland or on peripheral deiodination. *Toxicology and Applied Pharmacology* **51**, 145–155.

Burt, A. and MacSween, R.N.M. (1986). Hepatic vein lesions in alcoholic liver disease: A retrospective biopsy and necropsy study. *Journal of Clinical Pathology* **39**, 63–67.

Carithers, R.L., Herlong, H.G., Diehl, A.M., Shaw, E.W., Combes, B., Fallon, H.J. and Maddrey, W. (1989). Methyleprednisolone therapy in patients with severe alcoholic hepatitis. *Annals of Internal Medicine* **110**, 685–690.

Carmichael, F.J., Saldivia, V., Varghese, G.A., Israel, Y. and Orrego, H. (1988). Ethanol-induced increase in portal blood flow: Role of acetate and A_1 and A_2 adenosine receptors. *American Journal of Physiology* **255**, G417–G423.

Castillo, D., Koop, D.R., Kamimura, S., Triadafilopoulos, G. and Tsukamoto, H. (1992). Role of cytochrome P450 2E1 in ethanol, carbontetrachloride-, and iron-dependent microsomal lipid peroxidation. *Hepatology* **16**, 992–996.

Cerini, R., Koshy, A., Hadengue, A., Lee, S.S., Garnier, P. and Lebrec, D. (1989). Effects of glucagon on systemic and splanchnic circulation in conscious rats with biliary cirrhosis. *Journal of Hepatology* **9**, 69–74.

Christensen, E., Fauerholdt, L., Schlichting, P., Juhl, E., Poulsen, H. and Tygstrup, N. (1981). Aspects of the natural history of gastrointestinal bleeding in cirrhosis and the effect of prednisone. *Gastroenterology* **81**, 944–952.

Cooper, D.S., Cater, E.A., Kieffer, J.D. and Wands, J.R. (1984). Effects of propylthiouracil on D-galactosamine hepatotoxicity in the rat: Evidence for a non-thyroidal effect. *Biochemical Pharmacology* **33**, 3391–3397.

Cousineau, D., Goresky, C.A., Rose, C.P. and Lee, S. (1985). Reflex sympathetic effects on liver vascular space and liver perfusion in dogs. *American Journal of Physiology* **248**, H186–H192.

Crossley, I.R., Neuberger, J., Davis, M., Williams, R. and Eddleston, A.L.W.F. (1986). Ethanol metabolism in the generation of new antigenic determinants on liver cells. *Gut* **27**, 186–189

Cummings, S.A., Kaumann, A.J. and Groszmann, R.J. (1988). Comparison of the hemodynamic responses to ketanserin and prazosin in portal hypertensive rats. *Hepatology* **8**, 1112–1115.

Deviere, J., Content, J., Denys, C., Vandenbussche, P., Le Moine, O., Schandene, J.-P., Vaerman, J.-P. and Dupont, E. (1992). Immunogobulin A and interleukin-6 form a positive secretory feedback loop: A study of normal subjects and alcoholic cirrhotics. *Gastroenterology* **103**, 1296–1301

DiFranza, J.R. and Guerrera, M.P. (1990). Alcoholism and smoking. *Journal of Studies on Alcoholism* **51**, 130–135.

Dorfman, L.M. and Adams, G.E. (1973). Reactions with biological molecules. In *Reacitivity of the Hydroxyl Radical in Aqueous Solution* **46**, 43–56. NSRDS, National Bureau of Standards, Washington, DC.

Feizi, T. (1968). Immunoglobulins in chronic liver disease. *Gut* **9**, 193–198.

Felver, M.E., Mezey, E., McGuire, M., Mitchell, M.C., Herlong, H.F., Veech, G.A. and Veech, R.L. (1990). Plasma tumor necrosis factor alpha predicts decreased long-term survival in severe alcoholic hepatitis. *Alcoholism: Clinical and Experimental Research* **14**, 255–259.

French, S.W., Burbidge, E.J., Tarder, G., Bourke, E., Harkin, C.G. and Denton, T. (1979). Lymphocyte sequestration by the liver in alcoholic hepatitis. *Archives of Pathology and Laboratory Medicine* **103**, 146–152.

French, S.W., Ruebner, B.H., Mezey, E., Tamura, T. and Halsted, C.H. (1983). Effect of chronic ethanol feeding on hepatic mitochondria in the monkey. *Hepatology* **3**, 34–40.

French, S.W., Benson, N.C. and Sun, P.S. (1984). Centrilobular liver necrosis induced by hypoxia in chronic ethanol-fed rats. *Hepatology* **4**, 912–917.

Gelman, S. (1976). Disturbances in hepatic blood flow during anesthesia and surgery. *Archives of Surgery* **111**, 881–883.

Gluud, C., Tage-Jensen, U., Rubinstein, E. and Henriksen, J.H. (1984). Autoantibodies and immunoglobulins in patients with alcoholic cirrhosis *Digestion* **30**, 1–6.

Gore, I. and Isaacson, N.H. (1948). The pathology of

hyperpyrexia: Observations at autopsy in seventeen cases of fever therapy. *American Journal of Pathology* **25**, 1029–1059.

Green, J., Mistilis, S. and Schiff, L. (1963). Acute alcoholic hepatitis: A clinical study of fifty cases. *Archives of Internal Medicine* **112**, 113–124.

Gumucio, J.J. and Miller, D.L. (1981). Functional implications of liver cell heterogeneity. *Gastroenterology* **80**, 393–403.

Habig, W.H., Jakoby, W.B., Guthenberg, C., Mannervik, B. and Van der Jagt, D.L. (1984). 2-propylthiouracil does not replace glutathione or the glutathione transferase. *Journal of Biological Chemistry* **259**, 7409–7410.

Hadengue, A., Lee, S.S., Moreau, R., Braillon, A. and Lebrec, D. (1987). Beneficial hemodynamic effects of ketanserin in patients with cirrhosis: Possible role of serotonergic mechanisms in portal hypertension. *Hepatology* **7**, 644–647.

Hadengue, A., Moreau, R., Lee, S.S., Gaudin, C., Rueff, B. and Lebrec, D. (1988). Liver hypermetabolism during alcohol withdrawal in humans: Role of sympathetic overactivity. *Gastroenterology* **94**, 1047–1052.

Halle, P., Pare, P., Kaptein, E., Kanel, G., Redeker, A.G. and Reynolds, T.B. (1982). Double-blind, controlled trial of propylthiouracil therapy in severe acute alcoholic hepatitis. *Gastroenterology* **82**, 925–931.

Hashimoto, S. and Recknagel, R.O. (1968). No chemical evidence of hepatic lipid peroxidation in acute ethanol toxicity. *Experimental and Molecular Pathology* **8**, 225–242.

Hayashi, N., Kasahara, A., Kurosawa, K., Yoshihara, H., Sasaki, Y., Fusamoto, H., Sato, N. and Kamada, T. (1985). Oxygen supply to the liver in patients with alcoholic liver disease assessed by organ-reflectance spectophotometry. *Gastroenterology* **88**, 881–886.

Helman, R.A., Temko, M.H., Nye, S. and Fallon, H.J. (1971). Alcoholic hepatitis, natural history and evaluation of prednisolone therapy. *Annals of Internal Medicine* **74**, 311–321.

Henriksen, J.H., Ring-Larsen, H. and Christensen, N.J. (1984). Sympathetic nervous system activity in cirrhosis: A survey of plasma catecholamine studies. *Journal of Hepatology* **1**, 55–65.

Hillman, R.S. (1975). Alcohol and hematopoises. *Annals of the New York Academy of Science* **252**, 297–315.

Hopkins, A. (1983). Regression with incomplete survival data. In *BMDP Statistical Software* (Edited by Dixon, W.J.), pp 576–594. University of California Press, Berkeley, CA.

Horn, T., Junge, J. and Christoffersen, P. (1985). Early alcoholic liver injury: Changes of the Disse space in acinar zone 3. *Liver* **5**, 301–310.

Horn, T., Junge, J. and Christoffersen, P. (1986). Early alcoholic liver injury: Activation of lipocytes in acinar zone 3 and correlation to degree of collagen formation in the Disse space. *Journal of Hepatology* **3**, 333–340.

Imperiale, T.F. and McCullough, A.J. (1990). Do corticosteroids reduce mortality from alcoholic hepatitis? A meta-analysis of the randomized trials. *Annals of Internal Medicine* **113**, 299–307.

Imumara, M., Aoki, N., Saito, T., Ohno, Y., Manuyama, Y., Yamaguchi, J. and Yamanoto, T. (1986). Inhibitory effects of antithyroid drugs on oxygen radical formation in human neutrophils. *Acta Endocrinology* **12**, 210–216.

Inomata, T., Ananda, G. and Tsukamoto, H. (1987). Lack of evidence for increased lipid peroxidation in ethanol-induced centrilobular necrosis of rat liver. *Liver* **7**, 233–239.

Israel, Y. and Orrego, H. (1983). On the characteristics of alcohol-induced liver enlargement and its possible hemodynamic consequences. *Pharmacology, Biochemistry and Behaviour* **18**, 433–437.

Israel, Y. and Orrego, H. (1984). Hypermetabolic state and hypoxic liver damage. In *Recent Developments in Alcoholism* (Edited by Galanter, M.), pp. 119–133. Plenum Press, New York.

Israel, Y. and Orrego, H. (1987). Hypermetabolic state, hepatocyte expansion and liver blood flow: An interaction triad in alcoholic liver injury. *Annals of the New York Academy of Science* **492**, 303–323.

Israel, Y., Kalant, H., Orrego, H., Khanna, J.M., Videla, L. and Phillips, M.J. (1975). Experimental alcohol-induced hepatic necrosis: Suppression by propylthiouracil. *Proceedings of the National Academy of Sciences, USA* **72**, 1137–1141.

Israel, Y., Kalant, H., Orrego, H., Khanna, J.M., Phillips, M.J. and Stewart, D.J. (1979). Hypermetabolic state: Oxygen availability and alcohol-induced liver damage. In *Biochemistry and Pharmacology of Ethanol* (Edited by Majchrowicz, E. and Noble, E.P.), pp. 433–444. Plenum Press, New York.

Israel, Y., Orrego, H., Colman, J.C. and Britton, R.S. (1982a). Alcohol-induced hepatomegaly: Pathogenesis and role in the production of portal hypertension. *Federation Proceedings* **41**, 2472–2477.

Israel, Y., Britton, R.S. and Orrego, H. (1982b). Liver cell enlargement induced by chronic alcohol consumption: Studies on its causes and consequences. *Clinical Biochemistry* **15**, 189–192.

Israel, Y., Hurwitz, E., Niemela, O. and Arnon, R. (1986). Monoclonal and polyclonal antibodies against acetaldehyde-containing epitopes in acetaldehyde-protein adducts. *Proceedings of the National Academy of Sciences, USA* **83**, 7923–7927

Jauhonen, P., Baraona, E., Miyakawa, H. and Lieber, C.S. (1982). Mechanism for selective perivenular hepatotoxicity of ethanol. *Alcoholism: Clinical and Experimental Research* **6**, 350–357.

Ji, S., Lemasters, J.J., Christenson, V. and Thurman, R.G. (1982). Periportal and pericentral pyridine nucleotide fluorescence from the surface of the perfused liver: Evaluation of the hypothesis that chronic treatment with ethanol produces pericentral hypoxia. *Pro-*

ceedings of the National Academy of Sciences, USA **79**, 5415–5419.

Ji, S., Lemasters, J.J., Christenson, V. and Thurman, R.G. (1983). Selective increase in pericentral oxygen gradient in perfused rat liver following ethanol treatment. *Pharmacology, Biochemistry and Behaviour* **18**, 439–442.

Ji, S., Beckh, K. and Jungerman, K. (1984). Regulation of oxygen consumption and microcirculation by alfa-sympathetic nerves. *FEBS Letters* **176**, 117–122.

Jungerman, K. and Katz, N. (1982). Functional hepatocellular heterogeneity. *Hepatology* **2**, 385–395.

Kalant, H., Israel, Y., Phillips, M.J., Woo, N., Khanna, J.M. and Orrego, H. (1975). Necrosis produced by hepatic arterial ligation in alcohol-fed rats. *Federation Proceedings* **34**, 719.

Kamimura, S., Gaal, K., Britton, R.S., Bacon, B.R., Triadfilopoulous, G. and Tsukamoto, H. (1992). Increased 4-hydroxynonenal levels in experimental alcoholic liver disease: Association of lipid peroxidation with liver fibrogenesis. *Hepatology* **16**, 448–453.

Kato, S., Kawase, T., Alderman, J., Inatomi, N. and Lieber, C.S. (1990). Role of xanthine oxidase in ethanol-induced lipid peroxidation in rats. *Gastroenterology* **98**, 203–210.

Kawasaki, T., Carmichael, F.J., Giles, G., Saldivia, V., Israel, Y. and Orrego, H. (1989). Effects of propylthiouracil and methimazole on splanchnic hemodynamics in awake and unrestrained rats. *Hepatology* **10**, 273–278.

Kelty, R.H., Baggenstoss, A.H. and Butt, H.R. (1950). The relation of the regenerated hepatic nodule to the vascular bed in cirrhosis. *Mayo Clinic Proceedings* **25**, 17–26.

Keppler, D., Huber, M. and Baumert, T. (1988). Leukotrienes as mediators in diseases of the liver. *Seminars in Liver Disease* **8**, 357–365.

Kessler, B.J., Liebler, J.B., Bronfin, G.J. and Sass, M. (1954). The hepatic blood flow and splanchnic oxygen consumption in alcoholic fatty liver. *Journal of Clinical Investigation* **33**, 1338–1345.

Kessler, M. (1968). Normal and critical O_2 supply of the liver. In *Oxygen Transport in Blood and Tissue* (Edited by Lubbers, D.W., Luft, V.C., Theivs, E. and Witzleb, E.), pp. 242–251. Thieme Verlag, Stuttgart.

Kessler, M., Gornandt, L. and Lang, H. (1973). Correlation between oxygen tension in tissue and hemoglobin dissociation curve in oxygen supply. In *Theoretical and Practical Aspects of Oxygen Supply and Microcirculation of Tissue* (Edited by Kessler, M.), pp. 156–159. University Park Press, Baltimore, MD.

Klatskin, G. (1961). Alcohol and its relation to liver damage. *Gastroenterology* **41**, 443–451.

Klein, S.M., Cohen, G., Leiber, C.S. and Cederbaum, A.I. (1983). Increased microsomal oxidation of hydroxyl radical scavenging agents and ethanol after chronic consumption of ethanol. *Archives of Biochemistry and Biophysics* **223**, 425–432.

Koskinas, J., Kenna, G., Bird, G.L., Alexander, G.J.M. and Williams, R. (1992). Immunoglobulin A antibody to a 200-kilodalton cystosolic acetaldehyde adduct in alcoholic hepatitis. *Gastroenterology* **103**, 1860–1867.

Kubes, P., Ibbotson, G., Russel, J., Wallace, J.L. and Granger, D.N. (1990). Role of platelet-activating factor in ischemia/reperfusion-induced leukocyte adherence. *American Journal of Physiology* **259**, G300–G305.

Kurki, P., Virtanen, I. and Lehto, V.P. (1984). Antibodies to cytokeratin filaments in patients with alcoholic liver disease. *Alcoholism: Clinical and Experimental Research* **8**, 212–215.

Laskin, C.A., Vidins, E., Blendis, L.M. and Soloninka, C.A. (1990). Autoantibodies in alcoholic liver disease. *American Journal of Medicine* **89**, 129–133.

Lee, F.-Y., Albillos, A., Colombato, L.A. and Groszmann, R.J. (1992). The role of nitric oxide in the vascular hyporesponsiveness to methoxamine in portal hypertensive rats. *Hepatology* **16**, 1043–1048.

Lee, S.S., Hadengue, A., Girod, C., Braillon, A. and Lebrec, D. (1987). Reduction of intrahepatic vascular space in the pathogenesis of portal hypertension: *In vitro* and *in vivo* studies in the rat. *Gastroenterology* **93**, 157–161.

Leevy, C.M., Zinke, M., Baber, J. and Chey, W.Y. (1958). Observations on the influence of medical therapy on portal hypertension in hepatic cirrhosis. *Annals of Internal Medicine* **49**, 837–851.

Lefkowitch, J.H. and Mendez, L. (1986). Morphologic features of hepatic injury in cardiac disease and shock. *Journal of Hepatology* **2**, 313–327.

Lemasters, J.J., Ji, S., Stemkowski, C.J. and Thurman, R.G. (1983). Hypoxic hepatocellular injury. *Pharmacology, Biochemistry and Behaviour* **18**, 455–459.

Lenzen, R., Funk, A., Kolb-Bachofen, V. and Strohmeyer, G. (1990). Norepinephrine-induced cholestasis in the isolated perfused rat liver is secondary to its hemodynamic effects. *Hepatology* **12**, 314–321.

Lieber, C.S. and DeCarli, L.M. (1976). Animal models of ethanol dependence and liver injury in rats and baboons. *Federation Proceedings* **35**, 1232–1236.

Linscheer, W.G., Raheja, K.L., Cho, C. and Smith, N.J. (1980). Mechanism of the protective effect of propylthiouracil against acetaminophen toxicity in the rat. *Gastroenterology* **78**, 100–107.

Lundsgaard, E. (1942). The specific dynamic action of amino acids and ammonia salts. *Acta Physiologica Scandinavica* **4**, 330–342.

Maddrey, W.C., Boitnott, J.K., Bedine, M.S., Weber, F.L., Mezey, E. and White, R.I. (1978). Corticoid therapy of alcoholic hepatitis. *Gastroenterology* **75**, 193–199.

Mak, K.M. and Lieber, C.S. (1984). Alterations in endothelial fenestrations in liver sinusoids of baboons fed alcohol: A scanning electron microscope study. *Hepatology* **4**, 386–391.

Mastai, R., Huet, P.M., Brault, A. and Belgiorno, J.

(1989a). The rat liver microcirculation in alcohol-induced hepatomegaly. *Hepatology* **10**, 941–945.

Mastai, R., Rocheleau, B. and Huet, P.M. (1989b). Serotonin blockade in conscious, unrestrained cirrhotic dogs with portal hypertension. *Hepatology* **9**, 265–268.

Matsuda, Y., Sato, H. and Takada, A. (1987). Portal hypertension in alcoholic liver disease related to sinusoidal narrowing by hepatocyte ballooning. In *Microcirculation* (Edited by Tsuchiya, M.), pp. 371–372. Elsevier, Amsterdam.

Matsumara, T. and Thurman, R.G. (1983). Measuring rates of O_2 uptake in periportal and pericentral regions of liver lobule: Stop-flow experiments with perfused liver. *American Journal of Physiology* **244**, G656–G659.

Matsunaga, T., Kawano, S., Okumura, S., Yoshihara, H., Takei, Y., Goto, M., Kukui, H., Oshita, M., Nishimura, Y., Fusamoto, H., Kamada, T. and Sato, N. (1991). Effect of propylthiouracil on sinusoidal hemodynamics and oxygenation: A study by intravital microscopy. *Hepatology* **14**, 160A.

Matsuoka, M., Pham, N.-T. and Tsukamoto, H. (1989). Differential effects of interleukin-1-alpha, tumor necrosis factor-alpha, and transforming growth factor-beta-1 on cell proliferation and collagen formation by cultured fat-storing cells. *Liver* **9**, 71–78.

McKaigney, J.P., Carmichael, F.J., Saldivia, V., Israel, Y. and Orrego, H. (1985). Is glucagon a mediator of ethanol-induced increase in splanchnic blood flow? *Hepatology* **5**, 127A, 978.

McIver, M.A. and Winter, E.A. (1943). Deleterious effects of anoxia on the liver of the hyperthyroid animal. *Archives of Surgery* **46**, 171–185.

Meliconi, R., Perperas, A., Jensen, D., Alberti, A., McFarlane, I.G., Eddleston, A.L.W.F. and Williams, R. (1982). Anti LSP antibodies in acute liver disease. *Gut* **23**, 603–607.

Mena, I., Orrego, H., Barona, E. and Marques, S. (1963). Effects of regitine and reserpine on portal hypertension. *American Journal of Digestive Diseases* **8**, 895–903.

Miyakawa, H., Iida, S., Leo, M.A., Greenstein, J., Zimmon, D.S. and Lieber, C.S. (1985). Pathogenesis of precirrhotic portal hypertension of alcohol-fed baboons. *Gastroenterology* **88**, 143–150.

Moreau, R., Lee, S.S., Hadengue, A., Braillon, A. and Lebrec, D. (1987). Hemodynamic effects of a clonidine-induced decrease in sympathetic tone in patients with cirrhosis. *Hepatology* **7**, 149–154.

Myers, J.D. and Hickman, J.B. (1948). An estimation of the hepatic blood flow and splanchnic oxygen consumption in heart failure. *Journal of Clinical Investigation* **27**, 620–627.

Nagano, K., Gelman, S., Bradley, E.L. and Parks, D. (1990). Hypothermia, hepatic oxygen supply–demand, and ischemia-reperfusion injury in pigs. *American Journal of Physiology* **258**, G910–G918.

Nakano, M., Worner, T.M. and Lieber, C.S. (1982). Perivenular fibrosis in alcoholic liver injury: Ultrastructure and histological progression. *Gastroenterology* **83**, 777–785.

Nanji, A.A., Jui, L.T. and French, S.W. (1989). Effect of chronic carbon monoxide exposure on experimental alcoholic liver injury in rats. *Life Sciences* **45**, 885–890.

Nasrallah, S.M., Nassar, V.H. and Galambos, J.T. (1980). Importance of terminal hepatic venular thickening. *Archives of Pathology and Laboratory Medicine* **104**, 84–86.

Nauck, M., Wolfe, D., Katz, N. and Jungermann, K. (1981). Modulation of the glucagon-dependent reduction of phosphoenolpyruvate carboxy kinase and tyrosine aminotransferase by arterial and venous oxygen concentrations in hepatocyte cultures. *European Journal of Biochemistry* **119**, 657–661.

Navasa, M., Bosh, J., Bru, C., Mastai, R., Zysset, T., Silva, G., Chesta, J. and Rodes, J. (1988). Effects of verapamil on hepatic and systemic hemodynamics and liver function in patients with cirrhosis and portal hypertension. *Hepatology* **8**, 850–854.

Neuberger, J., Crossley, I.R., Saunders, J.R., Davis, M., Portmann, B., Eddleston, A.L.W.F. and Williams, R. (1984). Antibodies to alcohol altered liver cell determinants. *Gut* **25**, 300–304.

Niemela, O., Klajner, F., Orrego, H., Vidins, E., Blendis, L. and Israel, Y. (1987). Antibodies against acetaldehyde-modified protein epitopes in human alcoholics. *Hepatology* **7**, 1210–1214.

Orrego, H. and Carmichael, F.J. (1992). Effects of alcohol on liver haemodynamics in the presence and absence of liver disease. *Journal of Gastroenterology and Hepatology* **7**, 70–89.

Orrego, H., Carmichael, F.J., Phillips, M.J., Kalant, H., Khanna, J.M. and Israel, Y. (1976). Protection by propylthiouracil against carbon tetrachloride-induced liver damage. *Gastroenterology* **71**, 821–826.

Orrego, H., Israel, Y., Carmichael, F.J., Khanna, J.M., Phillips, M.J. and Kalant, H. (1978). Effect of dietary proteins and amino acids on liver damage induced by hypoxia. *Laboratory Investigation* **38**, 633–639.

Orrego, H., Kalant, H., Israel, Y., Blake, J., Medline, R., Rankin, J.G., Armstrong, A. and Kapur, B. (1979a). Effect of short-term therapy with propylthiouracil in patients with alcoholic liver disease. *Gastroenterology* **76**, 105–115.

Orrego, H., Medline, A., Blendis, L.M., Rankin, J.G. and Kreaden, D.A. (1979b). Collagenization of the Disse space in alcoholic liver disease. *Gut* **20**, 673–679.

Orrego, H., Blendis, L.M., Crossley, I.R., Medline, A., MacDonald, A., Ritchie, S. and Israel, Y. (1981). Correlation of intrahepatic pressure with collagen in the Disse space and hepatomegaly in humans and in the rat. *Gastroenterology* **80**, 546–556.

Orrego, H., Blake, J.E., Medline, A. and Israel, Y. (1985). Interrelation of hypermetabolic state, necrosis, anemia, and cell enlargement as determinants of severity in alcoholic liver disease. *Acta Medica Scandinavica* **218**, 81–95.

Orrego, H., Blake, J.E., Blendis, L.M., Compton, K.V. and Israel, Y. (1987). Long-term treatment of alcoholic liver disease with propylthiouracil. *New England Journal of Medicine* **317**, 1421–1427.

Orrego, H., Carmichael, F.J., Saldivia, V., Giles, H.G., Sandrin, S. and Israel, Y. (1988). Ethanol-induced increase in portal blood flow: Role of adenosine. *American Journal of Physiology* **254**, G495–G501.

Oshita, M., Sato, N., Yoshihara, H., Takei, Y., Hijioka, T., Fukui, H., Goto, M., Matsunaga, T., Kashiwagi, T., Kawano, S., Fusamoto, H. and Kamada, T. (1992). Ethanol-induced vasoconstriction causes focal hepatocellular injury in the isolated perfused rat liver. *Hepatology* **16**, 1007–1013.

Perez, H.D., Roll, F.J., Bissel, D.M., Shak, S. and Goldstein, I.M. (1984). Production of chemotactic activity for polymorphic leukocytes by cultured rat hepatocytes exposed to ethanol. *Journal of Clinical Investigation* **74**, 1350–1357.

Perrisoud, D., Maignan, M.F. and Dumont, J.G. (1985). Antinecrotic effect of 3-palmitocyl(+)-catechin against liver damage induced by galactosamine or ethanol in the rat. *Liver* **5**, 55–63.

Phillips, J.M. and Steiner, J.W. (1966). Electron microscopy of cirrhotic modules. *Laboratory Investigation* **15**, 801–817.

Pierrugues, R., Blanc, P., Barneon, G., Bories, P. and Michel, H. (1989). Short-term therapy with propylthiouracil for alcoholic hepatitis. A clinical biochemical and histological randomized trial of 25 patients. *Gastroenterology* **96**, A644.

Pizcueta, M.P., Pique, J.M., Bosch, J., Whittle, B.J.R. and Moncada, S. (1992). Nitric oxide and hyperdynamic circulation in portal hypertension. *British Journal of Pharmacology* **105**, 184–190.

Popper, H. and Lieber, C.S. (1980). Histogenesis of alcoholic fibrosis and cirrhosis in the baboon. *American Journal of Pathology* **98**, 695–710.

Postlewaite, A.E., Snyderman, R. and Kang, A.H. (1976). The chemotactic attraction of human fibroblasts to a lymphocyte derived factor. *Journal of Experimental Medicine* **144**, 1188–1203.

Poynard, T., Degott, C., Munoz, C. and Lebrec, D. (1987). Relationship between degree of portal hypertension and liver histologic lesions in patients with alcoholic cirrhosis. Effect of acute alcoholic hepatitis on portal hypertension. *Digestive Diseases and Sciences* **32**, 337–343.

Quistorff, B., Chance, B. and Takeda, H. (1978). Two- and three-dimensional redox heterogeneity of rat liver: Effects of anoxia and alcohol on the lobular redox pattern. In *Frontiers of Biological Energetics: From Electrons to Tissues* (Edited by Dutton, P.L., Leigh, G.S. and Scarpa, A.), pp. 1487–1497. Academic Press, New York .

Raheja, K.L., Linscheer, W.G., Cho, C. and Mahany, D. (1982). Protective effect of propylthiouracil independent of its hypothyroid effect on acetaminophen toxi-city in the rat. *Journal of Pharmacology and Experimental Therapeutics* **220**, 427–432.

Ramond, M.J., Poynard, T., Rueff, B., Mathurin, P., Theodore, C., Chaput, J.C. and Benhamou, J.-P. (1992). A randomized trial of prednisolone in patients with severe alcoholic hepatitis. *New England Journal of Medicine* **326**, 507–512.

Rankin, J.G. and Wilkinson, P. (1971). Alcohol and tobacco smoking. In *The Health of a Metropolis* (Edited by Krupinski, J. and Stoller, A.), pp. 61–67. Heinemann, Australia.

Rappaport, A.M. (1973). The microcirculatory hepatic unit. *Microvasculature Research* **6**, 212–228.

Reid, A.M.B. and Slater, T.E. (1977). Some effects of ethanol *in vivo* and *in vitro* on lipid peroxidation. *Biochemical Society Transactions* **5**, 1292–1294.

Reilly, F.D., McCuskey, R.S. and Cilento, E.V. (1981). Hepatic microvascular regulatory mechanisms. I. Adrenergic mechanisms. *Microvascular Research* **21**, 103–116.

Repine, J.E., Johansen, K.S. and Berger, E.M. (1984). Hydroxyl radical scavengers produce similar decreases in the chemiluminescence responses and bactericidal activities of neutrophils. *Infection and Immunity* **43**, 435–437.

Reynolds, T.B., Geller, H.M., Kusma, O.I. and Redeker, A.G. (1960). Spontaneous decrease in portal pressure with clinical improvement in cirrhosis. *New England Journal of Medicine* **263**, 734–739.

Reynolds, T.B., Benhamou, J.P., Blake, J., Naccarato, R. and Orrego, H. (1989). Treatment of acute alcoholic hepatitis. *Gastroenterology International* **2**, 208–216.

Rieder, H., Ramadori, G., Allmann, K.-H. and Buschenfelde, K.-H. (1990). Prostanoid release of cultured liver sinusoidal endothelial cells in response to endotoxin and tumor necrosis factor. Comparison with umbilical vein endothelial cells. *Journal of Hepatology* **11**, 359–366.

Robert, P., Champigneulle, B., Kreher, I., Gueant, J.L., Foliguet, B., Dollet, J.M., Bigard, M.A. and Gaucher, P. (1989). Evaluation of fibrosis in the Disse space in non-cirrhotic alcoholic liver disease. *Alcoholism: Clinical and Experimental Research* **13**, 176–180.

Rodriquez, M.A., Montano, J.D. and Williams, R.C. (1984). Immunoglobulin production by peripheral blood mononuclear cells in patients with alcoholic liver cirrhosis. *Clinical and Experimental Immunology* **55**, 369–374.

Safran, A.P. and Schaffner, F. (1967). Chronic passive congestion of the liver in man. Electron microscopic study of cell atrophy and intralobular fibrosis. *American Journal of Pathology* **50**, 447–463.

Sato, N., Kamada, T., Kawano, S., Hayashi, N., Kishida, Y., Meren, H., Yoshihana, H. and Abe, H. (1983). Effect of acute and chronic ethanol consumption on hepatic tissue oxygen tension in rats. *Pharmacology, Biochemistry and Behaviour* **18**, 443–447.

Sato, N., Eguchi, H., Takei, Y., Hijioka, S., Tsuji, T., Matsumura, N. and Hayashi, S. (1987). Microcirculatory aspects of the mechanism of alcoholic liver disease – sinusoidal blood flow and oxygenation at periportal and pericentral regions of hepatic lobules in rats. In *Microcirculation: An Update* (Edited by Tsuchiya, M., Asano, M., Mishima, Y. and Oda, M.), Vol. II, pp. 357–360. Elsevier, Amsterdam.

Schaffner, F. (1970). Oxygen supply and the hepatocyte. *Annals of the New York Academy of Science* **170**, 67–74.

Schaffner, F. and Popper, H. (1963). Capillarization of hepatic sinusoids in man. *Gastroenterology* **44**, 239–244.

Schaffner, F. and Popper, H. (1970). Alcoholic hepatitis in the spectrum of ethanol-induced liver injury. *Scandinavian Journal of Gastroenterology* **5**, 69–78 (suppl. 7).

Schlayer, H.-J., Laaff, H., Peters, T., Woort-Menker, M., Estler, H.C., Karck, U., Schaefer, H.E. and Decker, K. (1988). Involvement of tumor necrosis factor in endotoxin-triggered neutrophil adherence to sinusoidal endothelial cells of mouse liver and its modulation in acute phase. *Journal of Hepatology* **7**, 239–249.

Serrano-Cancino, H., Botero, R., Jeffers, L., Mariani, A., Cowen, G., Ravendhran, N. and Schiff, R. (1981). Treatment of severe alcoholic hepatitis with propylthiouracil. *American Journal of Gastroenterology* **76**, 194A.

Shaw, S., Heller, E.A., Friedman, H.S., Baraona, E. and Lieber, C.S. (1977). Increased hepatic oxygenation following ethanol administration in the baboon. *Proceedings of the Society for Experimental Biology and Medicine* **156**, 509–513.

Shaw, S., Jayatilleke, E., Ross, W.A., Gordon, E.R. and Lieber, C.S. (1981). Ethanol-induced lipid peroxidation: Potentiation by long-term alcohol feeding and attenuation by methionine. *Journal of Laboratory and Clinical Medicine* **98**, 417–424.

Sherman, I.A., Pappas, S.C. and Fisher, M.M. (1990). Hepatic microvascular changes associated with development of liver fibrosis and cirrhosis. *American Journal of Physiology* **258**, H460–H465.

Shibayama, Y. (1988). On the pathogenesis of portal hypertension in cirrhosis of the liver. *Liver* **8**, 95–99.

Shibayama, Y. and Nakata, K. (1985). Localization of increased hepatic vascular resistance in liver cirrhosis. *Hepatology* **5**, 643–648.

Sikuler, E. and Groszmann, R.J. (1986). Hemodynamic studies in long and short term portal hypertensive rats: The relationship to systemic glucagon levels. *Hepatology* **11**, 668–673

Silva , G., Navasa, M., Bosch, J., Chesta, J., Pilar Pizcueta, M., Casamitjara, R., Rivera, F. and Rodes, J. (1990). Hemodynamic effects of glucagon in portal hypertension. *Hepatology* **11**, 668–673.

Siregar, H. and Chou, C.C. (1982). Relative contribution of fat, protein, carbohydrate, and ethanol to intestinal hyperemia. *American Journal of Physiology* **242**, G27–G31.

Smith, F. and Palmer, D.L. (1976). Alcoholism, infection and altered host defences: A review of clinical and experimental observations. *Journal of Chronic Diseases* **29**, 35–49.

Song, Y.S. (1957). Hepatic lesions in sickle-cell anemia. *American Journal of Pathology* **33**, 331–338.

Sorrell, M.F. and Tuma, D. (1985). Hypothesis: Alcoholic liver injury and the covalent binding of acetaldehyde. *Alcoholism: Clinical and Experimental Research* **9**, 306–311.

Sorrell, M.F. and Leevy, C.M. (1972). Lymphocyte transformation and alcoholic liver injury. *Gastroenterology* **63**, 1020–1025.

Speisky, H., Bunout, D., Orrego, H., Giles, H.G., Gunasekara, A. and Israel, Y. (1985). Lack of changes in diene conjugate levels following ethanol induced glutathione depletion or hepatic necrosis. *Research Communications in Chemical Pathology and Pharmacology* **48**, 77–90.

SPSSX User Guide (1983). McGraw-Hill, Chicago, IL.

Stevens, V.J., Fantl, W.J., Newman, C.B., Sims, R.V., Cerami, A. and Peterson, C.M. (1981). Acetaldehyde adducts with hemoglobin. *Journal of Clinical Investigation* **67**, 361–369.

Sullivan, J.G., Jetton, M.M., Hahn, H.J.K. and Burch, R.E. (1980). Enhanced lipid peroxidation in liver microsomes of zinc-deficient rats. *American Journal of Clinical Nutrition* **33**, 51–56.

Szabo, S., Kourounakis, P., Kovacs, K., Tuchweger, B. and Garg, B.D. (1974). Prevention of organomercurial intoxication by thyroid deficiency in the rat. *Toxicology and Applied Pharmacology* **30**, 175–184.

Szabo, S., Haeger, R.J., Moslen, M.T. and Reynolds, E.S. (1977). Modification of 1,1-dichloroethylene hepatotoxicity by hypothyroidism. *Toxicology and Applied Pharmacology* **42**, 367–376.

Taasan, V.C., Block, A.J., Boysen, P.G. and Wynne, J.W. (1981). Alcohol increases sleep apnea and oxygen desaturation in asymptomatic men. *American Journal of Medicine* **71**, 240–245.

Thornton, J.R., Dean, H.G. and Losowsky, M.S. (1988). Do increased catecholamine and plasma methionine encephalin in cirrhosis promote bleeding esophageal varices? *Quarterly Journal of Medicine* **68**, 541–551.

Thurman, R.G., McKenna, W.R. and McCaffrey, T.B. (1976). Pathways responsible for the adaptive increase in ethanol utilization following chronic treatment with ethanol: Inhibition studies with hemoglobin-free perfused liver. *Molecular Pharmacology* **12**, 156–166.

Triger, D.R. and Wright, R. (1973). Hyperglobulinemia in liver disease. *Lancet* **i**, 1494–1496.

Trudell, J.R., Bendix, M. and Bosterling, B. (1984). Hypoxia potentiates killing of hepatocyte monolayers by leukotrienes, hydroperoxyeicosatetraenoic acids, or calcium ionophore A23187. *Biochimica et Biophysica Acta* **803**, 338–341.

Tsukamoto, H. and Xi, X.P. (1989). Incomplete compensation of enhanced hepatic oxygen consumption in rats with alcoholic centrolobular liver necrosis. *Hepatology* **9**, 302–306.

Tsukomoto, H., Gaal, K. and French, S.W. (1990). Insights into the pathogenesis of alcoholic liver necrosis and fibrosis: Status report. *Hepatology* **12**, 599–608.

Valla, D., Flejou, J.F., Lebrec, D., Bernuau, J., Rueff, B., Salzmann, J.-L. and Benhamou, J.-P. (1989). Portal hypertension and ascites in acute hepatitis: Clinical, hemodynamic and histological correlations. *Hepatology* **10**, 482–487.

Van de Wiel, A., Delacroix, D.L., Van Hattum, J., Schuurman, H.J. and Kater, L. (1987). Characteristics of serum IgA and liver IgA deposits in alcoholic liver disease. *Hepatology* **7**, 95–99.

Van Leeuwen, J., Howe, C.S., Scheuer, P.J. and Sherlock, S. (1990). Portal hypertension in chronic hepatitis: Relationship to morphological changes. *Gut* **31**, 339–343.

Van Waes, L. and Lieber, C.S. (1977). Early perivascular sclerosis in alcoholic fatty liver: An index of progressive liver injury. *Gastroenterology* **73**, 646–650.

Videla, L. and Israel, Y. (1970). Factors that modify the metabolism of ethanol in rat liver and adaptive changes produced by its chronic administration. *Biochemical Journal* **118**, 275–281.

Videla, L.A. and Valenzuela, A. (1982). Alcohol ingestion, liver glutathione, and lipid peroxidation: Metabolic interrelations and pathological implications. *Life Science* **31**, 2395–2407.

Vidins, E.I., Britton, R.S., Medline, A., Blendis, L.M., Israel, Y. and Orrego, H. (1985). Sinusoidal caliber in alcoholic and nonalcoholic liver disease: Diagnostic and pathogenic implications. *Hepatology* **5**, 408–414.

Villeneuve, J.P., Pomier, G. and Huet, P.M. (1981). Effect of ethanol on hepatic blood flow in unanesthetized dogs with chronic portal and hepatic vein catheterization. *Canadian Journal of Physiology and Pharmacology* **59**, 598–603.

Vinel, J.P., Caucanas, J.P., Combis, J.M., Cales, P., Voigt, J.J. and Pascal, J.P. (1989). Verapamil has no effect on porto-hepatic pressure gradient, hepatic blood flow and elimination function of the liver in patients with liver cirrhosis. *Journal of Hepatology* **8**, 302–307.

Vitiello, M.V., Prinz, P.N., Personius, J.P., Nuccio, M.A., Ries, R.K. and Koerker, R.M. (1987). History of chronic alcohol abuse is associated with increased nighttime hypoxemia in older men. *Alcoholism: Clinical and Experimental Research* **11**, 368–371.

Vorobioff, J., Bredfeldt, J.E. and Groszmann, R.J. (1983). Hyperdynamic circulation in portal-hypertensive rat model: A primary factor for maintenance of chronic portal hypertension. *American Journal of Physiology* **244**, G52–G57.

Wisse, E. and McCuskey, R.S. (1986). On the interactions of blood cells with the sinusoidal wall as observed by *in vivo* microscopy of rat liver. In *Cells of the Hepatic Sinusoid* (Edited by Kirn, A., Knook, D.L. and Wisse, E.), pp. 477–482. Kupffer Cell Foundation, Rijswijk.

Yamada, S., Fujiwara, K., Masake, N., Ohta, Y., Sato, Y. and Oka, H. (1988). Evidence for potentiation of lipid peroxidation in the rat liver after chronic ethanol feeding. *Scandinavian Journal of Clinical and Laboratory Investigation* **48**, 627–632.

Yamada, T. and Kaplowitz, N. (1980). Propylthiouracil. A substrate for the glutathione-*S*-transferase that competes with glutathione. *Journal of Biological Chemistry* **255**, 3508–3513.

Younes, M. and Strubelt, O. (1987). Enhancement of hypoxic liver damage by ethanol. Involvement of xanthine oxidase and the role of glycolysis. *Biochemical Pharmacology* **36**, 2973–2977.

Younes, M., Wagner, H. and Strubelt, O. (1989). Enhancement of acute ethanol hepatotoxicity under conditions of low oxygen supply and ischemia/reperfusion. *Biochemical Pharmacology* **38l**, 3573–3581.

Yuki, T., Israel, Y. and Thurman, R.G. (1982). The swift increase in alcohol metabolism: Inhibition by propylthiouracil. *Biochemical Pharmacology* **31**, 2403–2407.

Zajicek, G., Oren, R. and Weinreb, M. (1985). The streaming liver. *Liver* **5**, 293–300.

Zetterman, R.K., Luisada-Opper, A. and Leevy, C.M. (1976). Alcoholic hepatitis; cell mediated immunological response to alcoholic hyaline. *Gastroenterology* **70**, 382–384.

Zidenberg-Cher, S., Olin, K.L., Villanueva, J., Tang, A., Phinney, S.D., Halsted, C.H. and Keen, C.L. (1991). Ethanol-induced changes in hepatic free radical defense mechanisms and fatty-acid composition in the miniature pig. *Hepatology* **13**, 1185–1192.

Index